electron microscopy of human blood cells

YASUKAZU TANAKA, M.D.

Clinical Investigator, Veterans Administration;
and Assistant Professor in Residence,
Department of Clinical Pathology and Laboratory Medicine,
University of California, San Francisco;
presently, Senior Investigator,
Department of Pathology and Electron Microscopy,
Metropolitan Institute of Gerontology, Tokyo, Japan

JOSEPH R. GOODMAN, Ph.D.

Research Biochemist, Veterans Administration Hospital;
and Lecturer, Department of Pediatrics,
University of California School of Medicine, San Francisco

electron microscopy of human blood cells

with 230 illustrations

MEDICAL DEPARTMENT
HARPER & ROW, PUBLISHERS
NEW YORK, EVANSTON, SAN FRANCISCO, LONDON

Electron Microscopy of Human Blood Cells

 Printed in the United States of America. For information address Medical Department, Harper & Row, Publishers, Inc., 49 East 33rd Street, New York, N.Y. 10016

First Edition

STANDARD BOOK NUMBER: 06-142523-0
LIBRARY OF CONGRESS CATALOG CARD NUMBER: 76-180703

To Dr. George Brecher,
Professor and Chairman, Department of Clinical Pathology
and Laboratory Medicine, University of California, San Francisco,
for his perpetual interest in blood cell morphology
and his encouragement in the preparation of this book

contents

preface

In an effort to disseminate the latest knowledge on human blood cells to a wider audience, the authors of this volume have drawn together a collection of electron micrographs, along with technics applicable to hematology. These have been presented with a discussion of ultrastructural morphology, cytology, and function of both normal and pathological conditions. Instead of using the standard atlas form, the illustrations and morphological descriptions have been combined with discussions of cytogenesis and function in order to demonstrate more clearly their interrelationships. This was done with the intention of providing material that would be useful in clinical practice and research for hematologists, students of hematology, and those in related disciplines.

Using the electron micrographs that have been collected by us during the past 10 years, we have attempted to use the extensive knowledge gained from light microscopy for developing an understanding of the ultrastructure of human blood cells. Typical pathological cases are often represented by light and electron micrographs from the same patients; only characteristic pictures of proven diagnoses have been used. These micrographs came from specimens at University Hospital, Tokyo Medical and Dental University, Tokyo, Japan; The Clinical Center, National Institutes of Health, Bethesda, Maryland; Veterans Administration Hospitals at Long Beach and San Francisco; and the University of California at San Francisco.

The first of the seven chapters contains basic information on technics applicable to electron microscopy of hematological specimens. Chemicals and compositions of mixtures are cited for their specific merits. The other six chapters deal with established blood and bone marrow cell types, with only these aspects relating directly to cell lines being included in the text. Each of these chapters is divided into five sections; first there is a short historical background and then a section each on morphology, cytogenesis, function, and pathology. The division on morphology presents a brief description of light microscopy and an extensive section on the ultrastructure of each cell type as observed in electron micrographs. Usually this provides the basis for the cytogenetic discussion; these two, in turn, lead to the presentation on function. Some of the pathological entities of human blood cells are only partially represented although the variation of cellular structures is often great. Since it is not possible to present all the deviations from normal conditions, representative cells or structures that appear to relate to the pathology are used in the appropriate place.

The excellent technical assistance of Mmes. D. C. Brindley, J. A. Cushard, and Vibeke Craig is greatly appreciated, as is the manuscript preparation by Nina Wilson. A special acknowledgment goes to Anne M. Schmid for her skilled editorial assistance. We are also very grateful for the careful review and valuable comments by Drs. D. F. Bainton, T. Bradley, G. Brecher, C. Henry, C. F. Piel, M. Sahud, and R. O. Wallerstein.

For the bone marrow specimens used in this book, the authors are indebted to Drs. K. Akazaki, P. P. Carbone, S. D. Douglas, S. Hino, L. D. Petz, F. Stohlman, Jr., and E. J. Van Scott of the clinical staff of the Department of Pediatrics at Moffitt Hospital and the Pathology Department at the Veterans Administration Hospital, both in San Francisco.

Y.T.

San Francisco, California J.R.G

electron microscopy of human blood cells

chapter 1
METHODS

PREPARATION TECHNICS

Many electron microscopic technics described in detail for other tissues (Pease, 1964; Sjöstrand, 1967) can be used in the preparation of hematology specimens. The prime requirements are adequate preservation of cellular details, the structures, and their contents. Ideally, the methods should be as simple as possible, should be reproducible, and should preserve fine subcellular details to the greatest possible degree.

The process of preparing a hematology specimen for routine electron microscopy can be categorized as follows: preparation, fixation, dehydration, embedding, sectioning, and staining. Only some of the typical and more reliable procedures and fixative solutions particularly suited to hematological specimens are listed; more complete information can be found in books specifically designed for electron microscopic technics (Pease, 1964; Sjöstrand, 1967).

Preparation refers to the steps necessary to obtain and process a specimen before exposing it to fixation. This procedure is necessary to assure the quality of the final electron micrographs, particularly when free cells are studied. Very few prefixation procedures are needed for specimens of aspirated bone marrow or biopsy material, whereas peripheral blood or free cell suspensions require a number of preparatory steps in order to concentrate specific cell types.

PERIPHERAL BLOOD

Mature Erythrocytes

The erythrocyte specimen is usually obtained by venipuncture, with the use of either disodium salt of ethylenediaminetetraacetic acid (EDTA) (10% solution) or heparin as anticoagulant (neither anticoagulant has any apparent effect on the morphology of erythrocytes). When venipuncture is difficult, as in a small infant, a few drops of blood obtained by finger- or heel-stick can be put directly into glutaraldehyde fixative and used for erythrocytes only. Erythrocytes are separated by centrifugation (1,000 to 2,500 rpm), and a small portion is fixed by direct addition to the selected fixative; washing the cells with saline or buffer solutions is not required. Erythrocytes infected with parasites—e.g., *Plasmodium*—can be separated by density differences in the albumin flotation method of Ferrebee and Geiman (1946).

Reticulocytes

Reticulocytes can be separated by centrifugation when they are significantly increased in circulating blood. They will concentrate on top of the erythrocyte layer when anticoagulated whole blood is centrifuged at 2,500 rpm for 20 minutes. The purity of the separation should be checked by staining and phase microscopy before fixation. A more complete fractionation of reticulocytes has been reported by Chalfin (1956) by centrifugation at 20,000 g. Kimura *et al.* (1960) centrifuged gum acacia solutions of two different densities (1.068–1.078 and 1.050) to concentrate the reticulocytes in the lighter solution and separated 95% to 100% pure suspensions.

Leukocytes

A good concentration of leukocytes can be obtained by centrifugation of an anticoagulated peripheral blood sample when the leukocyte count is high, as in leukemia, or when a reasonably large specimen (10 ml) is available. In Anderson's (1965) method, glutaraldehyde is used as a fixative and about 10 ml of anticoagulated blood is centrifuged at 2,500 rpm for 20 minutes or 10,000 rpm for 10 minutes. The excess plasma is removed carefully by pipet, then 2% to 5% of the buffered glutaraldehyde solution is layered onto the buffy coat and allowed to fix the cells for 15 minutes. Lower concentrations of glutaraldehyde and buffer appear to give more consistent results (see below, under Fixation). This technic produces good fixation consistency, and the specimens are handled easily. When the leukocyte count is low, narrow tubes (even capillary tubes) can be used to increase the thickness of the buffy coat.

Separation of leukocytes is enhanced by adding such macromolecular substances as dextran, fibrinogen, albumin, nonspecific agglutinin, polyvinylpyrrolidone and phytohemagglutinin to the whole specimen in order to accelerate erythrocyte sedimentation. No significant effects have been reported on the morphology and function of the cells for the short period of exposure to these agents, provided the correct osmolarity is maintained. By this simple method, the solution of choice is mixed with whole blood and left at room temperature for 30 minutes.

A typical procedure includes the *dextran method* (Dausset *et al.,* 1954; Skoog and Beck, 1956) which produces 99% of the erythrocytes or about 85% of the leukocytes and is applicable at 0° C. Similar results are obtained when *fibrinogen* solutions (Minor and Burnett, 1948; Skoog and Beck, 1956) are used at 37° C. The *albumin flotation method* (Vallee *et al.,* 1947; Weiss and Fawcett, 1953) involves the layering of whole blood on top of the solution, then separating the cells by light centrifugation. The separation of lymphocytes from granule-monocytes also can be achieved by passage through a glass column (Rabinowitz, 1964). There has been no critical examination of the effects of these procedures on the ultrastructure of leukocytes; however, these technics are designed to eliminate or minimize the effects of centrifugation on delicate cell structures before fixation.

Less accurate cell separations are obtained by low speed centrifugation (400 to 500 rpm for 5 to 10 minutes) of anticoagulated whole blood. This concentrates most of the erythrocytes on the bottom and leaves the plasma (which contains many leukocytes, platelets, and a few erythrocytes) to be removed. The cells remaining in the plasma are recentrifuged at a higher speed to form a pellet for fixation. The cells also can be fixed in their plasma suspension before the second centrifugation. When this is done, compact pellets are not obtained so easily and subsequent solution changes are made by centrifugations. These steps should be performed in rapid succession to prevent overexposure of the cells to some of the solutions (mainly osmium and some solvents), as the penetration distance becomes the radius of the largest cell; a minute or two is ample time for each solution change after fixation for 10 to 15 minutes.

A very meticulous procedure for the preparation of peripheral blood cells was introduced by Low and Freeman (1958) to avoid the use of anticoagulants and minimize possible artifacts. However, we have found no significant advantage or improvment in morphological detail from the use of this more complicated procedure.

Several methods have been introduced to concentrate the leukocytes when only a small sample is available or when the leukocyte count is very low. Chapman (1962) and Malamed (1963), among others, used capillary tubes to concentrate the leukocytes into a small volume. After fixation, the capillary tubes were broken just below the buffy coat, the layer of cells was dehydrated by centrifugation, and then embedded by routine procedures. To separate pure cell fractions of specific types Marikovsky and Danon (1967) used phthalate esters of 20 different densities, ranging from 1.138 to 1.062, in microhematocrit tubes of 1 by 70 mm, then centrifuged them at 12,000 rpm for 15 minutes. Pure fractions of each blood cell type were obtained and confirmed by electron microscopy, but the quality of fixation in the published prints was not impressive.

Platelets

High concentrations of platelets can be obtained by centrifuging anticoagulated whole blood at 800 rpm for 15 minutes, then removing the supernatant for the formation of a pellet by faster centrifugation.

Free Metastatic Cells

Circulating malignant cells have been separated (Fawcett and Vallee, 1952) by layering anticoagulated suspensions on top of a bovine albumin-saline solution and centrifuging for 5 minutes at 2,000 to 2,500 rpm; this concentrates the lighter metastatic cells at the top of the albumin layer.

BONE MARROW

Bone marrow specimens are usually obtained by needle aspiration; however, in advanced myelofibrosis or malignant proliferations, a Westman-Jensen needle may be used. The needle aspiration produces a suspension of marrow particles in variable amounts of blood, a drop of which can be put directly into a fixative solution. The peripheral blood is separated from marrow particles by gentle agitation. This procedure does not require an anticoagulant, but the aspirate should be examined for marrow particles.

A drop of bone marrow aspirate taken with an anticoagulant is spread on a light microscopy slide and tilted so that the marrow particles are apparent as small refractile spheres. These refractile marrow particles are drawn into a capillary tube (0.9 to 1.1 mm) by putting the capillary on the particle so that capillary action picks up the particles, which are then blown into the fixative solution. The use of an anticoagulant is essential, either in the syringe or in a drop on the slide. When anticoagulants are used, relatively few peripheral erythrocytes are carried along through the subsequent changes and almost no clot fragments are processed mistakenly. Neither heparin nor EDTA appears to have a significant influence on the cellular morphology (we usually use EDTA).

When aspirations are relatively nonproductive and no biopsy is performed, a few particles may be harvested from the syringe and plunger by rinsing them with fixative. Sometimes, a few particles can be collected with a long thin Pasteur pipet from the inside wall of the syringe. Alternatively, the whole specimen can be centrifuged to form a pellet, which can be fixed and processed by the method described for peripheral blood.

Marrow biopsies can be performed when an aspiration is unproductive. The marrow biopsy will produce a specimen which contains some bone spicules that must be separated from the marrow particles. This can be done by spreading the material on a light microscopy slide, diluting the specimen with fixative, and probing the biopsy to free the marrow from the bone spicules. Marrow fragments can be distinguished easily from bone fragments or clots by microscopic examination of fixed particles. Selected particles can then be processed as in bone marrow aspirations.

The bone marrow specimens from infants or from those with aplastic anemia are particularly difficult to prepare for electron microscopy. They usually have a more delicate tissue matrix, are easily fragmented during aspiration, and the particles in the suspension are very small. These small particles can be lost easily in the fluid transfer or embedding steps, are difficult to cut, and usually few cells are found in close continuity.

FIXATION TECHNICS

Fixation is the most critical step in processing any tissue for electron microscopy. The quality of detail in the final micrographs is determined primarily by the condition of the primary fixation. Broken plasma membranes, washed-out figures, coagulated-appearing cytoplasm, and swollen or shrunken cells are artifacts produced at the time of fixation. The two most commonly used fixatives (although a variety of buffers have been combined with them) are osmium tetroxide (osmic acid), which emphasizes membrane structures, and glutaraldehyde, which retains more of the cytoplasmic proteins than the osmium preparations. The best detail of the structures is usually obtained by first fixing with glutaraldehyde then with osmium. Consistency of good cellular detail and time flexibility for starting subsequent steps after the first fixation are the principal advantages of this double-fixation method. Specimens may be left in buffered glutaraldehyde overnight or transferred to buffer solutions after aldehyde fixation if postfixation with osmium is not convenient at that time. Another advantage of glutaraldehyde is its use if cytochemical enzyme localization methods are used before postfixation with osmium. The contrast provided by postfixation with osmium is enhanced by using phosphate buffers that do not interfere with heavy metal localization of an enzyme reaction. These factors make glutaraldehyde fixation the procedure of choice for routine use in clinical hematology.

OSMIUM TETROXIDE (OSMIC ACID)

Final concentration of osmium can range from 0.5% to 2%; most current procedures use 1% in one of the solutions described below.

Veronal-Acetate Solution

Veronal-acetate (Rhodin, 1954) buffered (0.35M) osmium gives a good fixation; however, pH 7.2 to 7.4 is near the end of the effective buffer range of this agent and is not as effective in its buffering capacity as other recommended buffers.

s-Collidine Buffer

The *stock solution* of *s*-collidine as developed by Bennett and Luft (1959) contains:

s-Collidine	
2,4,6-trimethylpyridine	2.65 ml
H_2O, distilled	50.0 ml
HCl 1N	9.0 ml
H_2O, distilled to 2% osmic acid in distilled water	100.0 ml

The *working solution* consists of:

s-collidine buffer	1 part
2% osmic acid	2 parts

The final concentration of osmic acid is 1.33% in 0.67M buffer. This solution has its strongest buffering capacity within the pH range used in electron microscopy. The shelf-life of the 2,4,6-trimethylpyridine is variable, and recently prepared solutions should be used to maintain the quality of the fixation. We store the solutions and 2,4,6-trimethylpyridine in the refrigerator and use equal volumes of *s*-collidine and 2% osmic acid as a working solution.

Phosphate Buffers

Phosphate buffers, prepared according to the method of Millonig (1961) consisted of the following:

2.26% monosodium phosphate	83 ml
2.52% sodium hydroxide	17 ml
H_2O distilled	10 ml
Glucose	0.54 gm
Osmic acid	1.0 gm
or	
$NaH_2PO_4 \cdot H_2O$	2.98 gm
$Na_2HPO_4 \cdot 7H_2O$	30.40 gm
H_2O to	500 ml

This second solution is about 600 mOsm and should be mixed with an equal volume of 2% osmic acid or 2% glutaraldehyde for a final solution of about 300 mOsm.

CHROME OSMIUM

This fixative was first used for electron microscopy by Dalton (1955), and recommended and used extensively by Bessis and Breton-Gorius (1962) for studies of human bone marrow. Prolonged fixation in this solution was found to be less destructive of cell structures, and more background material was retained than by other osmium fixatives. These differences appear to be small compared with the improved detail with glutaraldehyde-osmium procedures.

ALDEHYDE

Formaldehyde and glutaraldehyde are used most frequently.

Formaldehyde

Pease's (1964) method for preparation of the formaldehyde solution follows.
The *buffer solution* contains:

2.26% $NaH_2PO_4 \cdot H_2O$	41.5 ml
2.52% NaOH	8.5 ml

As a *fixative,* the proportions are:

40% formalin in
5.4% glucose solution

The *working solution* consists of:

45 ml buffer solution
and 5 ml fixative,
adjusted to pH 7.3 to 7.6

This has been used successfully on brain tissue (Pease, 1962) and has the advantage of a rapid penetration and good preservation of many enzymatic activities. Many commercial formalin solutions may require purification, since they may contain 10% to 15% methanol and variable amounts of formic acid. This can be avoided by preparing fresh formaldehyde from powdered paraformaldehyde in an alkaline solution at 60° C (Pease, 1964).

Glutaraldehyde

Glutaraldehyde (Sabatini *et al.,* 1963) is used for both bone marrow and peripheral blood cell fixation and eliminates the artifacts which can occur with osmium fixation alone. While the original formula called for relatively high concentrations, we have had better results with final concentrations ranging from 0.5% to 2% glutaraldehyde.

The preparation of *1% glutaraldehyde in phosphate buffer* (Maunsbach, 1966) contains:

$NaH_2PO_4 \cdot H_2O$	2.98 gm
$Na_2HPO_4 \cdot 7H_2O$	30.40 gm
25% glutaraldehyde (or equivalent of other concentrations)	40.0 ml
H_2O distilled to	1,000 ml

The tonicity of this solution is 300 mOsm which is similar to that of serum and can be used for tissue perfusions. However, the osmolarity will change upon standing, depending on the amount of glutaraldehyde degeneration. Commercial glutaraldehyde will develop increasing amounts of glutaric acid during storage, significant concentration of which will affect the quality of fixation. This can be avoided by redistilling the glutaraldehyde or procuring small ampules of solution which are broken open when the solution is needed.

s-Collidine buffer is the same as that described for osmium. It can be used for glutaraldehyde, using equal volumes and 2% glutaraldehyde.

Formaldehyde-glutaraldehyde

Karnovsky's (1965) formula was used to prepare the formaldehyde-glutaraldehyde solution, as follows.

Paraformaldehyde	2 gm
H_2O distilled	17 ml
heated 60° to 70°, stirred to dissolve most of the paraformaldehyde, and cooled	
NaOH 1N	3 drops
Glutaraldehyde, 25%	16 ml
Cacodylate buffer 0.2M	17 ml
$CaCl_2$, 25 mg added within 1 hour of use	

Fixation time is 3 hours for histochemical procedures and 5 to 6 hours for straight morphology. We find this preparation is too concentrated; it has produced good results on hematological specimens only when the final solution is diluted by one-third to one-half with distilled water.

OSMIC ACID AND GLUTARALDEHYDE

The simultaneous use of these fixatives was introduced by Hirsch and Fedorko

(1968) to compensate for the limitation of one fixative by addition of the other. When the preparation is used for peripheral blood, the quality of fixation falls between that produced by either fixative alone. Uranyl acetate solution is used as a whole-tissue stain after fixation steps.

OTHER FIXATIVES

Permanganate fixation was introduced by Luft (1956) and modified by many others. The method emphasizes membranes, but diminishes or destroys many other components of cellular detail.

Methods of *freeze-drying* (Sjöstrand and Baker, 1958; Grunbaum and Wellings, 1960), freeze-substitution (Bullivant, 1965), and current development in technics for frozen sections are particularly useful for enzyme cytochemical reactions.

BUFFER SOLUTIONS

These are used to control the pH of fixatives (buffering capacity) and maintain osmolarity. A number of them hold fixative solutions in the physiological range of pH 7.2 to 7.4. The *s*-collidine buffer has the strongest buffering capacity in this pH range, and the veronal buffer, the weakest. All of them can be adjusted for tonicity or osmolarity, which must be close to that of plasma for use in clinical hematology. This factor is more important in the preparation of blood or bone marrow cells than for solid tissues. Phosphate buffers are perhaps easiest to use; they are more stable and do not react with the aldehydes. The effect of osmolarity is more apparent in aldehyde fixatives than in osmic acid preparations. Maunsbach (1966) suggested phosphate buffers 0.1M to 0.133M for perfusion fixation. We have had good fixation with buffers in this range of concentration with 1% glutaraldehyde in both peripheral blood and bone marrow specimens. Concentrations of slightly less than 0.1M can be used with 2% glutaraldehyde, while higher concentrations produce pronounced shrinkage.

WHOLE TISSUE STAINING

Staining of whole blood specimens with uranyl acetate and phosphotungstic acid after fixation, and before or during dehydration, increases their electron opacity. Kellenberger *et al.* (1958) treated bacteria, and Wallace and Linnane (1964) stained yeast with uranyl acetate before dehydration, to increase the contrast of those structures which contained nucleic acid. Peripheral blood cell specimens were also stained at this stage by Breton-Gorius (1966) to enhance the whole cell image and show better detail of leukocyte granules, particularly the crystalloid structures (15 Å spacing) in human eosinophils. This technic was also used by Hirsch and Fedorko (1968) in their simultaneous fixation method.

FIXATION TIME

Fixation time for both osmium and osmium-dichromate mixtures is usually 1 to 2 hours for bone marrow and 30 minutes to 1 hour for packed peripheral cell specimens. Cells in free suspension are fixed in 10 to 15 minutes. Aldehyde fixation requires the same length of time except that specimens can remain for much longer periods in the fixative without damage to cytoplasmic detail. Specimens fixed in osmium preparations must be processed into dehydration solutions immediately at the end of the specified fixation period, going directly into 50% to 70% alcohol without rinsing in a buffer. Specimens in aldehyde fixatives can be refrigerated for several days, or transferred into isotonic buffers for storage as long as several weeks. When phosphate buffer is used, precipitation of nonphysiologic electron-opaque granules can occur within cells, particularly in tissues stored in buffer for long periods. These dense particles can be eliminated by washing the specimen in another type of buffer or by starting dehydration by rinsing two or three times in alcohol at 50% concentration or lower. The great flexibility of aldehyde fixation and the length of time required to begin dehydration is most useful when the clinical specimen has to be transported and the time exceeds the 2-hour limit for osmium.

Glutaraldehyde fixation at room temperature generally preserves microtubule structures in platelets and leukocytes. However, these structures are lost if the glutaraldehyde fixative is cold (4° C) or if the specimen is fixed in osmium without prior aldehyde treatment (White, 1967).

POSTFIXATION TECHNICS

DEHYDRATION

Dehydration is usually accomplished at room temperature, with increasing concentrations of alcohol starting promptly after fixation in an osmium preparation, and without a rinse in water or buffer. Concentrations of alcohol as low as 35% and as high as 70% have been used successfully for the initial dehydration solution. Inadequate dehydration results in poor penetration of the plastic and therefore, in cutting problems. Once the alcohol is used at any concentration, it is discarded. The volume in each tube is usually from 3 to 8 ml each, and re-use is not worth the risk of contamination. Acetone can be used in the same manner as alcohol for dehydration.

Most plastic embedding mixtures are not miscible with alcohol; therefore, an intermediate solvent, such as propylene oxide or acetone, is usually used. Two short rinses, and a longer period in a mixture of equal volumes of one of these solvents, are sufficient. These dehydration liquids, transition agents, and some of the plastics used in embedding, are also lipid solvents. Therefore, prolonged immersion in any of these solutions, except the final polymerized plastic, enhances the removal of lipids from the specimen and is not recommended.

Dehydration schedules which help to preserve substances which are sensitive to the actions of alcohol, acetone, or propylene oxide solvent have been developed through the use of water-soluble resins (Staubli, 1963; Leduc and Holt, 1965). These procedures are especially desirable on problems which involve lipids, enzyme-cytochemical, or immunocytological processes.

EMBEDDING

The choice of plastic for embedding will affect the appearance of the ultrastructural detail to be seen in the electron micrograph.

Methacrylate

Methacrylate was the first and, for a number of years, the only plastic used in electron microscopy. Prior to its use, thin-sectioning was not practical and, hence, cellular detail was not seen clearly. The major disadvantages are its volatility when hit by the electron beam and its uneven polymerization, which results in a tendency to produce a distortion of structural detail. It is now used for specimens that are difficult to penetrate by the more viscous plastics (methacrylate is nearly as fluid as water) and when adjacent thick sections for specific light microscopic identification are required. Polymerized methacrylate is removed more easily by solvents from thick sections and makes color counterstaining more feasible. Recently Zambernard *et al.* (1969) recommended methacrylate embedding of routine hematological specimens for examination by light microscopy. This has advantages over traditional paraffin embedding since thinner sections can be cut and stained better after the methacrylate is removed. Its ingredients are:

Methyl methacrylate (ethyl)	10% to 20%
Butyl methacrylate	80% to 90%
Activator luperco	2%
or	
Benzol peroxide	2%

The hardness of the polymerized block can be adjusted by the ratio of the two methacrylates; the higher the proportion of methyl or ethyl, the harder the block. Polymerization is stimulated either by heat or by ultraviolet light. It may be used without removing the commercially added inhibitors with sodium hydroxide. Other activators have also been recommended (Shipkey and Dalton, 1959). Partially polymerized mixtures for embedding minimize the ultrastructural distortion produced by uneven polymerization.

Araldite

Araldite was introduced as a possible embedding medium for electron microscopy by Glauert *et al.* (1956) and Glauert and Glauert (1958), and modified by Luft (1961) to the following mixture:

Araldite 502	27 ml
Dodecenyl succinic anhydride (DDSA)	23 ml
Dimethylamino methyl phenol (DMP-30)	1.5% to 2%

This mixture is recommended for high-resolution electron microscopy because it has low background granularity; however, there is a slight increase in opacity because of the very compact character of the plastic and some difficulty in stretching sections on the microtome trough. This mixture, with the added accelerator DMP-30, can be stored in a plastic container in a freezer until needed.

Epon

Epon (Luft, 1961) is used widely. The hardness of the final block can be adjusted by the ratio of two mixtures:

Epon 812	62 ml
DDSA	100 ml
and	
Epon 812	100 ml
Methyl nadic anhydride	89 ml

A 1:1 ratio is used for most tissues of normal consistency, whereas in tougher tissues with a high collagen content the second mixture should be increased to as much as 80% with 1.5% to 2% DMP-30 activator added just before use.

Blocks of this plastic will cut easily, particularly with diamond knives, and thin sections will take heavy metal stains readily. Occasionally, poor polymerization will result in soft blocks that are difficult to cut, usually because of the hydroscopic nature of the chemicals. This can be prevented by using proper storage conditions.

Maraglas

Maraglas, introduced by Freeman and Spurlock (1962) and later improved (Spurlock *et al.,* 1963), consists of:

Maraglas 665	68 ml
Cardolite NC-513	20 ml
Dibutyl phthalate	10 ml
Benzyl dimethylamine	2 ml

This material is not used widely but is

easy to cut and stain, has a low background opacity, and sections can be stretched on the microtome trough.

Vestopal-W

Vestopal-W is produced by the esterification of malic anhydride with glycerol or some other polyhydric alcohol and has been used with specific embedding schedules by Ryter and Kellenberger (1958) and Kurtz (1961). Malic anhydride is not miscible in alcohol; therefore, acetone should be used for dehydration, since it can be replaced by increasing the concentration of the polyester mixture. The material is placed in capsules filled with the pure embedding material and hardened in 12 hours at 60° C. One such mixture is 98.5 ml Vestopal-W, 1.0 ml tertiary butyl benzoate, and 0.5 ml cobalt naphthenate. The advantages of this plastic include fast polymerization, easy cutting and staining, and fine background granularity for high resolution electron microscopy.

Additional embedding media developed recently include a modified epoxy resin (Spurr, 1969) and a water-containing aldehyde-urea resin (Peterson and Pease, 1970).

SECTIONING

The basic principles and technics for the production of thin sections of specimens are detailed by Pease (1964) and Sjöstrand (1967) and are no different for hematological than for other biological specimens. Although dense masses of erythrocytes and cells in free suspension are generally more difficult to cut than solid tissue, the technics remain the same. Experimentation with the speed of the microtome and knife angle usually will solve most problems.

STAINING THICK SECTIONS

Preliminary thick sections are useful in electron microscopy for three major reasons:
(1) to help select the right block and area for thin sectioning, (2) to analyze large areas by light microscopy to avoid possible misinterpretation when smaller thin sections are examined by electron microscopy, and (3) to correlate by light microscopy the cytochemical character of specific cellular constituents with the same structures on adjacent thin sections.

Thick preparations can be mounted on clean microscopic slides without adhesive material and studied by phase microscopy after mounting under a cover slip in a suitable embedding medium. Sections can also be stained with various dyes for examination by light microscopy. Methacrylate-embedded specimens can be stained by many routine methods after removal of the plastic with suitable solvent, or they may be stained directly with the plastic in place. Epon-epoxy resins are more difficult to stain directly, and removal of the plastic is not accomplished easily.

Basic dyes in alkaline solution are perhaps the most popular of those used in routine electron microscopy and stain epon or epoxy sections without removing the embedding medium.

Mallory's Azure II Methylene Blue Staining

Mallory's azure II methylene blue (Richardson *et al.,* 1960) stain solution consists of 1% azure II aqueous solution and 1% methylene blue in 1% borax solution. Sections are stained on a hot plate for a few minutes; the final solution is about pH 11.

Toluidine Blue Staining

Toluidine blue (Trump *et al.,* 1961) staining solution consists of 0.1% toluidine blue in 2.5% sodium carbonate, pH 11. The sections can be stained in a few minutes on a hot plate (about 70° C).

Basic Fuchsin and Alkaline Methylene Blue Staining

Basic fuchsin and alkaline methylene blue (Huber *et al.,* 1968) is a simple polychromatic method for rapid staining and does not require the removal of the embedded plastic. The stain can be used with excellent results in place of hematoxylin-eosin in routine histology.

Solutions:

4% basic fuchsin freshly prepared by dissolving in distilled water at 70° C
2% methylene blue in distilled water
0.1N NaOH

Sections are stained with basic fuchsin for 1 minute on a hot plate and rinsed with distilled water. A mixture of 2 drops of 0.1N NaOH and 1 drop of methylene blue are applied to the completely dried sections and stained for 2 minutes on a hot plate, then rinsed with distilled water and dried.

Giemsa Staining

Giemsa staining is a basic method for clinical hematology for smears and thick plastic sections. The method of Schwalbach *et al.* (1963) may be useful on Vestopal-W and methcrylate blocks; details of solutions and procedures are found in the original publication.

STAINING THIN SECTIONS

The idea that thin sections should be stained with heavy metals to increase contrast for electron microscopy was originally introduced by Watson (1958a, b), and since then, the method has been modified with the use of a variety of metals. Thin sections are stained either for general enhancement of contrast or structure. Lead compounds and uranyl acetate are used to stain for general cell structures and increased contrast.

Lead Staining

Lead is one of the most popular stains used on thin sections and emphasizes the cell membrane and glycogen most effectively. Several modifications are available, but only two of these most widely used are listed:

The *lead citrate* (Reynolds, 1963, modified) staining method has seen many minor modifications. We have found it useful to prepare stock solutions of 5.8 gm lead nitrate ($Pb[NO_3]_2 \cdot 2H_2O$) in 100 ml of H_2O and 3.8 gm sodium citrate in 100 ml of H_2O. Then equal volumes of these solutions are mixed thoroughly and ½ volume of 1N sodium hydroxide is added, the precipitate dissolves, and the solution with pH near 12 is ready for use. If the solution is cloudy, probably a fresh NaOH solution will give a clear solution.

A *simplified lead citrate* (Venable and Coggeshall, 1965) staining solution consists of 0.01 to 0.04 gm lead citrate, dissolved in 10 ml of freshly boiled distilled water, with 0.1 ml sodium hydroxide of 10N added. The solution is ready to use when all the lead citrate is dissolved by vigorous agitation. The staining procedure is similar to that of the Reynold's lead-citrate method.

Lead stain in hematology specimens, particularly tissues fixed with glutaraldehyde, may not demonstrate neutrophilic granules in fine detail. Significant contamination will occur from precipitated lead carbonate formed by carbon dioxide in the air and is a serious problem unless special steps are taken to keep the atmospheric carbon dioxide from the specimen during staining. We pass a slow stream of nitrogen gas from a commercial gas tank over the sections during lead staining.

Uranyl Acetate Staining

Uranyl acetate staining was introduced by Watson (1958a) to enhance general contrast of thin sections. Zobel and Beer (1961) found that a low concentration of uranyl acetate specifically stained structures which contained nucleic acids. This is perhaps one of the most useful stains for the electron microscope, and contamination is usually minimal. The stain increases the contrast of the nuclei and ribosomes, and enhances the neutrophilic granules of myelocytes. Saturated solution of uranyl acetate in distilled water, stored in a brown bottle with a tight stopper, is used. Staining time is 15 minutes to 2 hours in a wet chamber (Petri dish with wet filter paper); stronger staining may be produced by heating. The wet chamber is necessary to prevent the evaporation of water and the precipitation of uranyl acetate from the saturated solution. The stain is also recommended for double-staining with lead compounds. We usually stain with uranyl acetate first, rinse the grids thoroughly with distilled water, then stain with lead.

Phosphotungstic Acid (PTA) Staining

This method was once considered to be effective for general cell structure (Watson, 1958a), particularly for fibrillar structures. The method is simple and usually free of contamination. The stain is now used for collagen and other interstitial fibrils; it is also used widely as a negative stain to emphasize the outline of structures in suspensions.

Specific Methods

There are many technics for the identification of specific material in the cell at the ultrastructural level. Usually, the reaction is made on tissue blocks before embedding and the positive products which form are later identified in thin sections. The most useful methods are *autoradiographic technics* (Caro and van Tubergen, 1962; Salpeter and Bachmann, 1965); *ferritin conjugated antibody technics* for immunocytology (Singer, 1959; Morgan *et al.,* 1961; Rifkind *et al.,* 1962); gold colloid conjugation of antibodies (Faulk and Taylor, 1972); *enzyme cytochemical methods—acid phosphatase* (Holt and Hicks, 1961; Wetzel *et al.,* 1963); *alkaline phosphatase* (Wetzel *et al.,* 1963) and *peroxidase* reactions (Ackerman, 1968; Bainton and Farquhar, 1968). Various cytochemical methods have been introduced for the chemical identity of specific materials found in cells: glycogen (Themann, 1960), iron-containing organelles (Thiery, 1962); mucopolysaccharides (Gasic and Berwick, 1963; Revel, 1964; Hardin *et al.,* 1968); and nucleic acids (Huxley and Zubay, 1961; Watson and Aldridge, 1961; Zobel and Beer, 1961; Albersheim and Killias, 1963; Peters and Giese, 1970; Gautier and Schreyer, 1970). Enzymatic digestion of specific cellular components can be used for the identification of some substances.

SUMMARY

The following is a brief synopsis of the procedures employed in preparation of many of the marrow and peripheral blood specimens used for illustrations in this book. However, these procedures should not be considered as inflexible; variations are used to adjust to the requirements of each situation.

Bone marrow is aspirated with a syringe wet with EDTA or, if no anticoagulant is used in the syringe, a drop of aspirant is spread in an anticoagulant on a microscope slide or dropped directly into the fixative. The marrow particles are fixed in 1% glutaraldehyde in either 0.1M cacodylate or 0.1M phosphate buffer, pH 7.3 for 1.5 or more hours at room temperature. They are postfixed in 1% osmium tetroxide buffered with 0.1M phosphate, 1 to 2 hours, and dehydrated with 50%, 70%, 95%, and 100% (3X) alcohol, then propylene oxide (2X), and 1:1 ratio of propylene oxide and Epon. This is followed by two transfers in 100% Epon, placed in capsules and polymerized by heat.

Peripheral blood is processed as described by Anderson (1965) except 1% glutaraldehyde is used, then processed in the same manner as the marrow particles. Alternately, the peripheral blood is processed as free cells in suspension, as described under Peripheral Blood, Leukocytes.

All specimens are human cells unless otherwise noted. On all specimens we used glutaraldehyde fixative plus postfixation treatment with osmium, and subsequent embedding in Epon, unless stated differently in the legends.

REFERENCES

Ackerman, G. A. Ultrastructure and cytochemistry of the developing neutrophil. *Lab Invest 19*:290, 1968.

Albersheim, P., and Killias, U. The use of bismuth as an electron stain for nucleic acids. *J Cell Biol 17*:93, 1963.

Anderson, D. R. A method of preparing peripheral leucocytes for electron microscopy. *J Ultrastruct Res 13*:263, 1965.

Bainton, D. F., and Farquhar, M. G. Differences in enzyme content of azurophil and specific granules of polymorphonuclear leukocytes. II. Cytochemistry and electron microscopy of bone marrow cells, *J Cell Biol 39*:299, 1968.

Bennett, H. S., and Luft, J. H. S-collidine as a basis for buffering fixatives. *J Biophys Biochem Cytol 6*:13, 1959.

Bessis, M. C., and Breton-Gorius, J. Iron metabolism in the bone marrow as seen by electron microscopy: A critical review. *Blood 19*:635, 1962.

Breton-Gorius, J. Structures périodiques dans les granulations éosinophiles et neutrophiles des leucocytes polynucléaires du sang de l'homme. *Nouv Rev Franc Hémat 6*:195, 1966.

Bullivant, S. Freeze substitution and supporting techniques. *Lab Invest 14*:1178, 1965.

Caro, L. G., and van Tubergen, R. P. High-resolution autoradiography. I. Methods. *J Cell Biol 15*:173, 1962.

Chalfin, D. Differences between young and mature rabbit erythrocytes. *J Cell Comp Physiol 47*:215, 1956.

Chapman, A. L. Preparation of small quantities of blood leukocytes for electron microscopy. *Stain Techn 37*:387, 1962.

Dalton, A. J. A chrome-osmium fixative for electron microscopy. *Anat Rec 121*:281, 1955.

Dausset, J., Nenna, A., and Brecy, H. Leukoagglutinins. V. Leukoagglutinins in chronic idiopathic or symptomatic pancytopenia and in paroxysmal nocturnal hemoglobnuria. *Blood 9*:696, 1954.

Faulk, P. W., and Taylor, M. An immuno-colloid for electron microscopy. *Immunochemistry* 1972.

Fawcett, D. W., and Vallee, B. L. Studies on the separation of cell types in sero-sanguinous fluids, blood and vaginal fluids by flotation on bovine plasma albumin. *J Lab Clin Med 39*:354, 1952.

Ferrebee, J. W., and Geiman, Q. M. Studies on malarial parasites. III. A procedure for preparing concentrates of plasmodium vivax. *J Infect Dis 78*:173, 1946.

Freeman, J. A., and Spurlock, B. O. A new epoxy embedment for electron microscopy. *J Cell Biol 13*:437, 1962.

Gasic, G., and Berwick, L. Hale stain for sialic acid-containing mucins. Adaptation to electron microscopy. *J Cell Biol 19*:223, 1963.

Gautier, A., and Schreyer, M. "Feulgen-like" Electron Stains for Tissue Sections. In *Microscopie Electronique 1970* (Favard, P., ed.). Société Française de Microscopie Electronique, Paris, 1970, vol. 1, p. 559.

Glauert, A. M., Rogers, G. E., and Glauert, R. H. A new embedding medium for electron microscopy. *Nature (London) 178*:803, 1956.

Glauert, A. M., and Glauert, R. H. Araldite as an embedding medium for electron microscopy. *J Biophys Biochem Cytol 4*:191, 1958.

Grunbaum, B. W., and Wellings, S .R. Electron microscopy of cytoplasmic structures in frozen-dried mouse pancreas. *J Ultrastruct Res 4*:73, 1960.

Hardin, J. H., Spicer, S. S., Greene, W. B., and Horn, R. G. Ultrastructural localization of acid mucosubstance in rabbit heterophils and basophils. *J Histochem Cytochem 16*:510, 1968.

Hirsch, J. G., and Fedorko, M. E. Ultrastructure of human leukocytes after simultaneous fixation with glutaraldehyde and osmium tetroxide and "post-fixation" in uranyl acetate. *J Cell Biol 38*:615, 1968.

Holt, S. J., and Hicks, R. M. The localization of acid phosphatase in rat liver cells as revealed by combined cytochemical staining and electron microscopy. *J Biophys Biochem Cytol 11*:47, 1961.

Huber, J. D., Parker, F., and Odland, G. F. A basic fuchsin and alkalinized methylene blue rapid staining for epoxy-embedded tissue. *Stain Techn 43*:83, 1968.

Huxley, H. E., and Zubay, G. Preferential staining of nucleic acid-containing structures for electron microscopy. *J Biophys Biochem Cytol 11*:273, 1961.

Karnovsky, M. J. A formaldehyde-glutaraldehyde fixative of high osmolality for use in electron microscopy. *J Cell Biol 27*:137A, 1965.

Kellenberger, E., Ryter, A., and Sechaud, J. Electron microscope study of DNA containing plasma. II. Vegetative and mature phage DNA as compared with normal bacterial nucleoids in different physiological states. *J Biophys Biochem Cytol 4*:671, 1958.

Kimura, E., Suzuki, T., and Kinoshita, Y. Separation of reticulocytes by means of multi-layer centrifugation. *Nature (London) 188*:1201, 1960.

Kurtz, S. M. A new method for embedding tissues in Vestopal-W. *J. Ultrastruct Res. 5*:468, 1961.

Leduc, E. H., and Holt, S. J. Hydroxypropyl methacrylate: A new water-miscible embedding medium for electron microscopy. *J Cell Biol. 26*:137, 1965.

Low, F. N., and Freeman, J. A. *Electron Microscopic Atlas of Normal and Leukemic Human Blood.* McGraw-Hill, New York, 1958.

Luft, J. H. Permanganate—a new fixative for electron microscopy. *J Biophys Biochem Cytol 2*:799, 1956.

Luft, J. H. Improvements in epoxy resin embedding methods. *J Biophys Biochem Cytol 9*:409, 1961.

Malamed, S. Use of a microcentrifuge for preparation of isolated mitochondria and cell suspensions for electron microscopy. *J Cell Biol 18*: 696, 1963.

Marikovsky, Y., and Danon, D. A micromethod for fixation and embedding of separated blood cell fractions for electron microscopy. *J Ultrastruct Res 18*:176, 1967.

Maunsbach, A. B. The influence of different fixatives and fixation methods on the ultrastructure of rat kidney proximal tubule cells. II. Effects of varying osmolarity, ionic strength, buffer system and fixative concentration of glutaraldehyde solutions. *J Ultrastruct Res 15*:283, 1966.

Millonig, G. Advantages of phosphate buffer for OsO_4 solutions in fixation. *J. Appl Physiol 32*: 1637, 1961.

Minor, A. H., and Burnett, L. A method for obtaining living leukocytes from human peripheral blood by acceleration of erythrocyte sedimentation. *Blood 3*:799, 1948.

Morgan, C., Hsu, K. C., Rifkind, R. A., Knox, A. W., and Rose, H. M. The application of ferritin-conjugated antibody to electron microscopic studies and influenza virus in infected cells. I. The cellular surface. *J Exp Med 114*:825, 1961.

Pease, D. C. Buffered formaldehyde as a killing agent and primary fixative for electron microscopy. *Anat Rec 142*:342, 1962.

Pease, D. C. *Histological Techniques for Electron Microscopy,* 2nd ed. Academic Press, New York, 1964.

Peters, D., and Giese, H. Detection of DNA in Thin Sections. In *Microscopie Electronique 1970* (Favard, P., ed.). Société Française de Microscopie Electronique, Paris, 1970, vol. 1, p. 557.

Peterson, R. G., and Pease, D. C. Features of the Fine Structure of Myelin Embedded in Water Containing Aldehyde Resins. In *Microscopie Electronique 1970* (Favard, P., ed.). Société Française de Microscopie Electronique, Paris, 1970, vol. 1, p. 409.

Rabinowitz, Y. Separation of lymphocytes, polymorphonuclear leukocytes and monocytes on glass columns, including tissue culture observations. *Blood 23*:811, 1964.

Revel, J. P. A stain for the ultrastructural localization of acid mucopolysaccharides. *J Microscopie 3*:535, 1964.

Reynolds, E. S. The use of lead citrate at high pH as an electron-opaque stain in electron microscopy. *J Cell Biol 17*:208, 1963.

Rhodin, J. Correlation of Ultrastructural Organization and Function in Normal and Experimentally Changed Proximal Convoluted Tubule Cells of the Mouse Kidney. Thesis, Karolinska Institutet, Stockholm, 1954.

Richardson, K. C., Jarett, L., and Finke, E. H. Embedding in epoxy resins for ultrathin sectioning in electron microscopy. *Stain Techn 35*:313, 1960.

Rifkind, R. A., Osserman, E. F., Hsu, K. C., and Morgan, C. The intracellular distribution of gamma globulin in a mouse plasma cell tumor (X5563) as revealed by fluorescence and electron microscopy. *J Exp Med 116*:423, 1962.

Ryter, A., and Kellenberger, E. L'inclusion au polyester pour l'ultramicrotomie. *J Ultrastruct Res 2*:200, 1958.

Sabatini, D. D., Bensch, K., and Barrnett, R. J. Cytochemistry and electron microscopy. The preservation of cellular ultrastructure and enzymatic activity by aldehyde fixation. *J Cell Biol 17*:19, 1963.

Salpeter, M. M., and Bachmann, L. Assessment of Technical Steps in Electron Microscope Autoradiography. In *Symposium of the International Society of Cell Biology* (Leblond, C. P., and Warren, K. B., eds.) Academic Press, New York, 1965, vol. 4, p. 23.

Schwalbach, G., Lickfeld, K. G., and Hoffmeister, H. Differentiated staining of osmium tetroxide-fixed, vestopal-W-embedded tissue in thin sections. *Stain Techn 38*:15, 1963.

Shipkey, F. H., and Dalton, A. J. Azodi-iso-butyronitrile (ADIB) as a catalyst for embedding tissues in methacrylate for electron microscopy. *J Appl Physiol 30*:2039, 1959.

Singer, S. J. Preparation of an electron-dense antibody conjugate. *Nature (London) 183*:1523, 1959.

Sjöstrand, F. S., and Baker, R. F. Fixation by freezing-drying for electron microscopy of tissue cells. *J Ultrastruct Res 1*:239, 1958.

Sjöstrand, F. S. *Electron Microscopy of Cells and Tissues. Instrumentation and Techniques.* Academic Press, New York, 1967, vol. 1.

Skoog, W. A., and Beck, W. S. Studies on the fibrinogen, dextran and phytohemagglutinin methods of isolating leukocytes. *Blood 11*:436, 1956.

Spurlock, B. O., Kattine, V. C., and Freeman, J. A. Technical modifications in Maraglas embedding. *J Cell Biol 17*:203, 1963.

Spurr, A. R. A low-viscosity epoxy resin embedding medium for electron microscopy. *J Ultrastruct Res 26*:31, 1969.

Staubli, W. A new embedding technique for electron microscopy, combining a water soluble epoxy resin (Durcupan) with water-insoluble araldite, *J Cell Biol 16*:197, 1963.

Themann, H. Zur elektronenmikroskopischen Darstellung von Glykogen mit Best's carmin. *J Ultrastruct Res 4*:401, 1960.

Thiéry, J. P. Étude des réactions cytochimiques du fer au microscope électronique. *J Microscopie 1*:127, 1962.

Trump, B. F., Smuckler, E. A., and Benditt, E. P. A method for staining epoxy sections for light microscopy. *J Ultrastruct Res 5*:343, 1961.

Vallee, B. L., Hughes, W. L., Jr., and Gibson, J. G. A method for the separation of leukocytes from whole blood by flotation on serum albumin. *Blood 1*:82, 1947.

Venable, J. H., and Coggeshall, R. A simplified lead citrate stain for use in electron microscopy. *J Cell Biol 25*:407, 1965.

Wallace, P. G., and Linnane, A. W. Oxygen-induced synthesis of yeast mitochondria. *Nature (London) 201*:1191, 1964.

Watson, M. L. Staining of tissue sections for electron mocroscopy with heavy metals. *J Biophys Biochem Cytol 4*:475, 1958a.

Watson, M. L. Staining of tissue sections for electron microscopy with heavy metals. II Application of solutions containing lead and barium. *J Biophys Biochem Cytol 4*:727, 1958b.

Watson, M. L., and Aldridge, W. G. Methods for the use of indium as an electron stain for nucleic acids. *J Biophys Biochem Cytol 11*:257, 1961.

Weiss, L. P., and Fawcett, D. W. Cytochemical observations on chicken monocytes, macrophages and giant cells in tissue culture. *J Histochem Cytochem 1*:47, 1953.

Wetzel, B. K., Horn, R. G., and Spicer, S. S. Cytochemical localization of non-specific phosphatase activity in rabbit myeloid elements. *J Histochem Cytochem 11*:812, 1963.

White, J. G. New development in platelet ultrastructural research. *Blood 30*:539, 1967.

Zambernard, J., Block, M., Vatter, R. A., and Trenner, L. An adaptation of methacrylate embedding for routine histopathologic use. *Blood 33*:444, 1969.

Zobel, C. R., and Beer, M. Electron stains. I. Chemical studies on the interaction of DNA with uranyl salts. *J Biophys Biochem Cytol 10*:335, 1961.

chapter 2
ERYTHROCYTES

Cells of the erythrocytic series are highly differentiated elements of the body. During development in the pre- and postnatal blood-forming organs, they synthesize hemoglobin. This enables the mature circulating erythrocyte to transport the oxygen required by all cells of the body.

The interesting story of the red cell discovery is reviewed in a recent monograph by Bessis (1966). Erythrocytes in the blood were first described by Leeuwenhock as small globules, with the use of the first microscope in 1673. Nearly 200 years later (1867) Hoppe-Seyler determined that the role of hemoglobin in erythrocytes was to transport oxygen. The next year Neumann (1868) reported that red corpuscles were formed in the bone marrow from colorless nucleated cells. A comprehensive morphology of blood cells and their possible functions began to develop after Ehrlich (1891) introduced staining technics. Further development of these technics became the basis for modern hematological morphology. Blood group concepts and transfusions were explored from 1900 to 1920, although practical blood transfusion did not develop until World War II, when the system called "blood banking" was established. The basic principles and concepts of this work are now extensively applied in clinical medicine, legal medicine, and general biology.

The general concepts of erythropoiesis and its pathology were developed by 1940, including a major step in the clinical treatment of pernicious anemia based on the work of Minot and Murphy (1926) and Castle and Minot (1936) (summarized by Castle, 1966). The current approaches to the physiology and pathology of various anemias in association with hemoglobinopathies began with the introduction of the concept of "molecular disease" (Pauling *et al.,* 1949) based on a study of sickle cell anemia. The disease was clearly attributed to a genetic abnor-

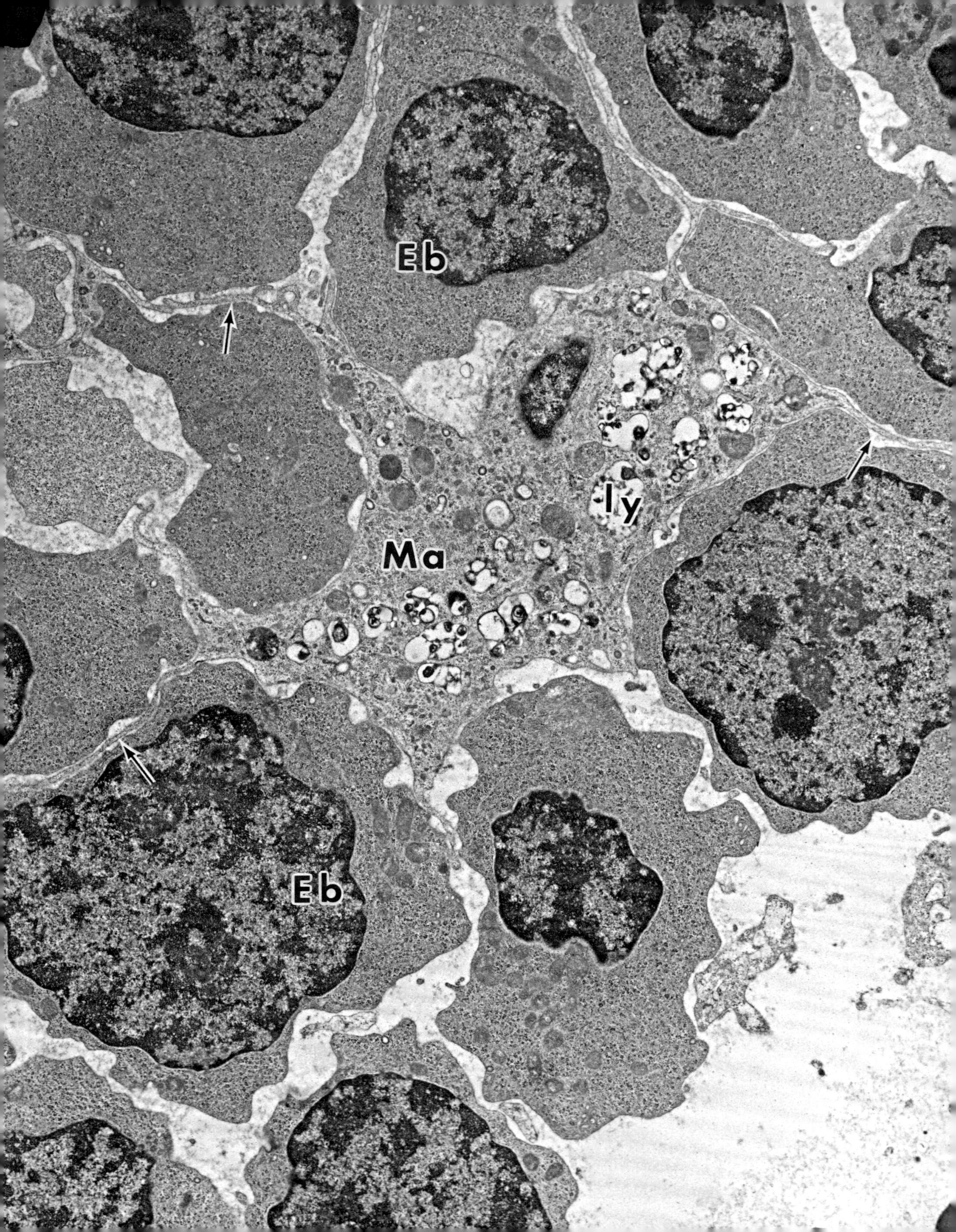

Eb
ly
Ma
Eb

FIGURE 2-2. Erythroblasts at various stages of maturation in Giemsa-stained human bone marrow.
A. A large proerythroblast with several smaller more mature erythroblasts. × *2,000.*
B. Two basophilic erythroblasts and one polychromatic (*arrow*) erythroblast. × *2,000.*
C. Three polychromatic erythroblasts and one orthochromatic (*arrow*) erythroblast. × *2,000.*

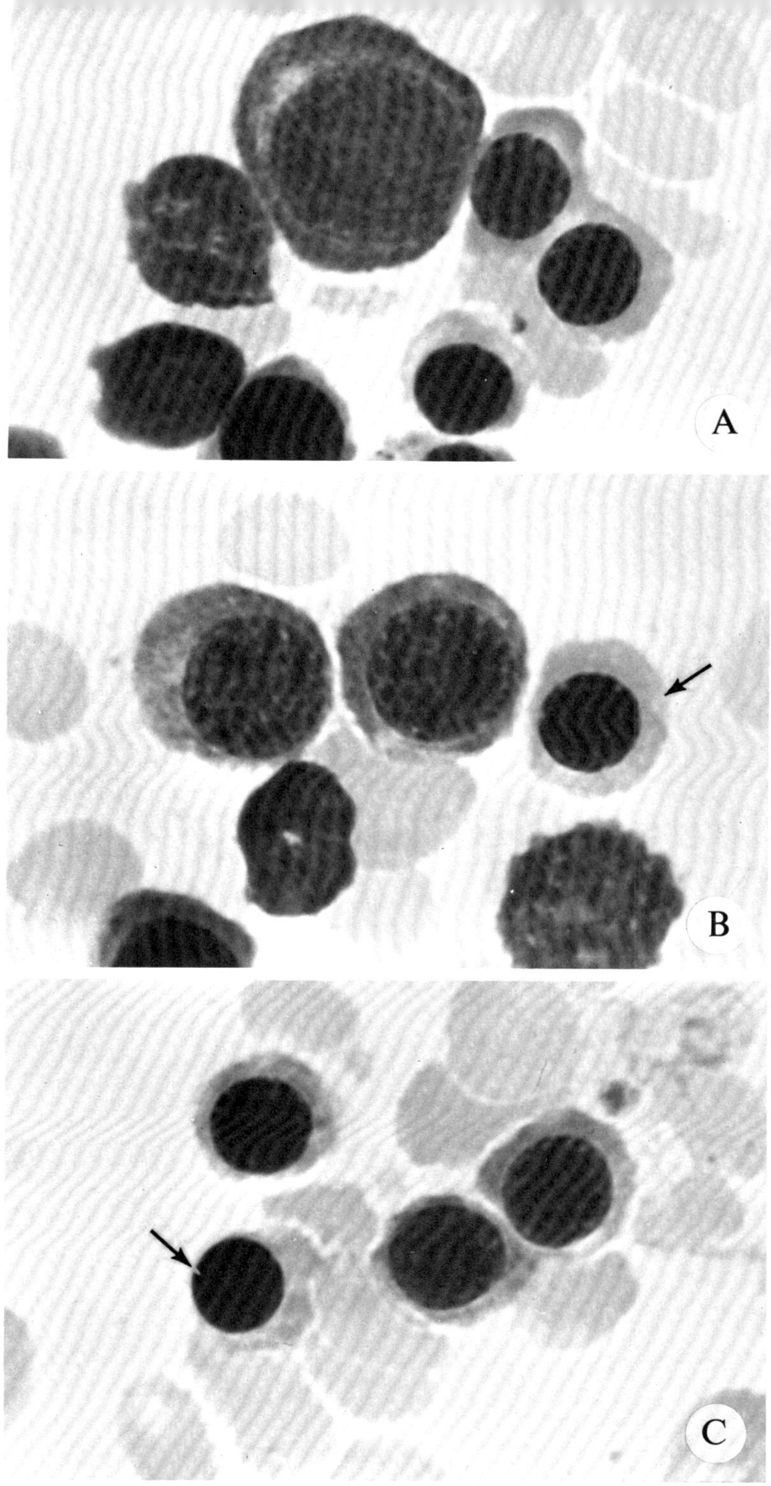

FIGURE 2-1. Erythroblastic island.
Island of erythroblasts (*Eb*) clustered around macrophage (*Ma*), which has a number of thin extensions of cytoplasm (*arrows*) and many lysosomal vacuoles (*ly*). All erythroblast nuclei have moderate condensation of chromatin, and cytoplasm has many polyribosomes and mitochondria. Cytoplasm of each erythroblast has uniform density with some variation from one cell to another. × *6,800.*

mality that controls globin structure in developing erythroblasts.

Circulating red corpuscles were studied as whole-mounted preparations with an electron microscope about 1950, and later in thin sections. Extensive studies on erythroblastic cells have been made by Bessis *et al.* (1957, 1958, 1959a,b, 1961a,b, 1962, 1965).

MORPHOLOGY

In normal adults, erythropoiesis gives a red coloration to bone marrow. The degree of color usually reflects the extent of active erythropoiesis. Erythropoiesis in man and large animals produces clusters of erythrocytic cells in intersinusoidal spaces throughout the marrow, in contrast to granulopoiesis, which produces a diffuse distribution. The cluster of erythrocytic cells, which usually has a central macrophage, is called an "erythroblastic nest" or "island" (Fig. 2-1). In small animals, these islands are near the center of femur marrows, and granulopoiesis is usually distributed around the periphery of the organ (Rohr, 1960). The term "erythroblast" is used to describe nucleated erythroid cells of various degrees of maturation. The recognizable youngest form of this group is the "proerythroblast." Other names have been given to define similar cell types—e.g., erythrogone.

The differences in size of circulating red cells are usually used for the diagnosis of various anemias. It has been speculated that larger erythroblasts (macroblasts or megaloblasts) may give rise to larger erythrocytes called macrocytes. Similarly, proliferation of small erythroblasts, called microblasts, form smaller erythrocytes named microcytes. However, recent cytokinetic studies (Stohlman *et al.,* 1964) suggest that differences in size of circulating erythrocytes may depend on the time for maturation of erythroblasts after stimulation by erythropoietin. Thus, macrocytosis may occur when a step in terminal mitosis is skipped (Stohlman, 1960; Brecher and Stohlman, 1961) and early denucleation occurs in the erythroblast (Seno *et al.,* 1964). This may occur in rapid response to erythropoietin in cases of acute hemolysis or in any excessive stimulation by erythropoietin. Microcytosis, as seen in impaired hemoglobin synthesis in thalassemia, may be due to prolonged maturation of the erythroblasts (Stohlman *et al.,* 1964). Thus, the classic concept, that the difference in size of circulating erythrocytes depends on the size of developing erythroblasts, should be examined for each pathological entity.

Stages of erythroblast maturation are well recognized by light microscopy, and their description at each stage is well established (Fig. 2-2). However, these differentiations are not so apparent by electron microscopy. Erythroblast maturation is a continuous process and electron micrographic criteria do not delineate these stages clearly.

FIGURE 2-3. Ribosomes and hemoglobin in erythroblast cytoplasm.
A. Early erythroblast with many polyribosomes (*arrow, r*) and free ferritin particles (*circles*). × *198,000.*
B. Late erythroblast with fewer polyribosomes (*arrow, r*) and ferritin (*circle*) than in Figure 2-3**A**. × *198,000.*

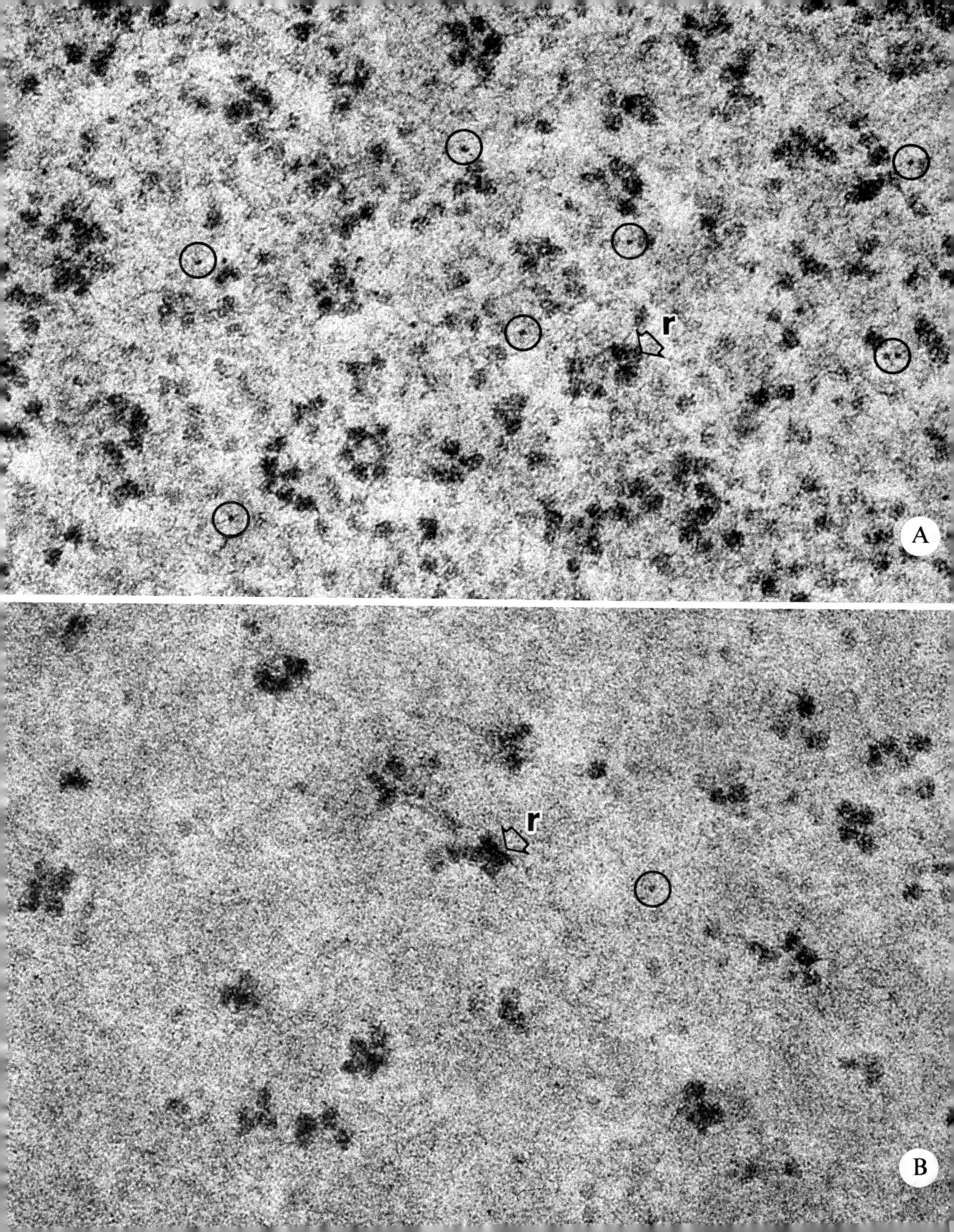
r
A
r
B

ULTRASTRUCTURE OF ERYTHROID CELLS

Erythroblasts, characteristically found in clusters or islands, are commonly disrupted during the preparation of smears (Bessis and Breton-Gorius, 1962), and it is difficult to get a typical example of an island in normal human specimens. Figure 2-1 shows cells from a patient in whom acute erythrocytic regeneration followed chemotherapy for acute lymphocytic leukemia.

Nucleus

In erythroblasts, nuclear chromatin clumping develops early, corresponding to the basophilic stage of light microscopic classification. In nonchromatin areas of the nucleus, there are many electron-dense granules which are considered to contain ribonucleic acid (RNA). Many nuclear pores connect the nucleoplasm and cytoplasm and are particularly apparent between chromatin clumps. The more mature erythroblasts appear to have fewer nuclear pores, suggesting a decrease in nucleocytoplasmic communications during cell maturation. Aldehyde fixatives tend to enhance artificially the space between the two membranes of the nucleus and contribute to the frequent loose nuclear appearance of many erythroblasts.

Cytoplasm

The cytoplasm of erythroblasts contains many polyribosomes in an amorphous matrix (Fig. 2-3*A*) which is presumably hemoglobin. As the cell matures, increasing amounts of this iron-containing protein give the cytoplasm more electron density and the number of polyribosomes diminishes (Rifkind *et al.*, 1964) (Fig. 2-3*B*), particularly in the reticulocyte stage, and even single ribosomes are absent in the mature erythrocyte (Fig. 2-13*B*).

The developing erythroblast has many small pinocytotic vesicles (Fig. 2-4), about 50 mμ in diameter (Policard and Bessis, 1958), which have a single membrane covered on the inner surface by material thought to be mucopolysaccharide or glycoprotein (Fawcett, 1964; Jones, 1965). This layer helps to distinguish between absorptive and nonabsorptive vesicles (Tanaka *et al.*, 1966). The morphological characteristics of these vesicles are similar to the structures in other cells involved in macromolecular absorption (Roth and Porter, 1962). Policard and Bessis (1958) proposed the term "rhopheocytosis" to describe this process. They thought these vesicles were a specific device in erythroblasts, particularly for the transport of ferritin (Bessis and Breton-Gorius, 1959, 1962).

The sequence of development of these pinocytotic vesicles suggests that they start with a tiny dimple on the cell membrane and encave into a very small pocket from the cell surface to form the vesicle. All stages of this process are seen throughout the maturation of erythroblasts and in reticulocytes of many species, including man, rabbit, guinea pig, rat, mouse, chick, duck, and newt. Rarely, similar vesicles are noted in myelocytic or plasma cells of the bone marrow.

FIGURE 2-4. Organelles and vesicles in developing erythroblast.
Portion of erythroblast showing part of nucleus (*N*), the Golgi apparatus (*G*) containing a centriole (*Ce*), several mitochondria (*M*), several small vesicles (*v*) with a fuzzy inner layer, and an early invagination of a pinocytotic vesicle (*pv*). × *90,000.*

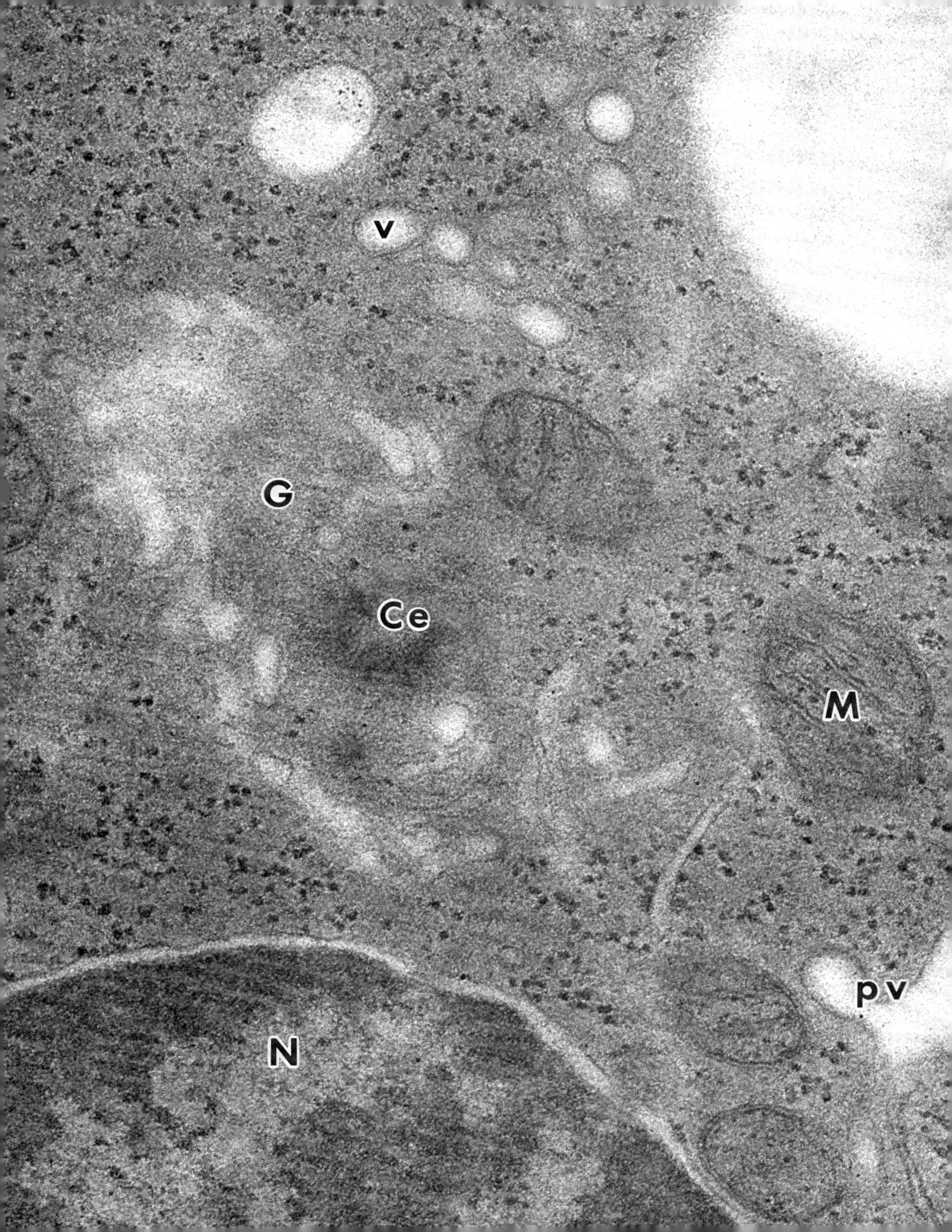
v
G
Ce
M
N
pv

Jones (1964) observed that these diminish as the erythroblasts mature. We have not seen any clear correlation of these factors and have observed many invaginations on the surface of reticulocytes.

The large ovoid mitochondria of erythroblasts (Fig. 2-4) decrease in size and number during the later stages of maturation; some persist in the reticulocyte stage. A striking feature of this organelle is the accumulation of iron compounds between the cristae in some conditions of disturbed hemoglobin synthesis (see under Iron Metabolism, later in this chapter).

The Golgi apparatus in the developing erythroblast is usually observed near the nucleus, and usually consists of several lamellae and vesicles (Fig. 2-4). Frequently, near the middle of the Golgi complex, one or a pair of centrioles is transected. The Golgi apparatus diminishes with cell maturation, and occasionally small vestiges, or even a centriole, are seen in reticulocytes.

Ferritin is found in several places in human erythroblasts, most frequently in vesicles of 0.05 to 0.5μ (Fig. 2-5). Ferritin particles in the larger vesicles appear as a cluster of more than 300 particles in a single cross section or in a loosely scattered form. Some apparent lysosomal vesicles in erythroblasts may also contain ferritin particles and are found in various animal species. They can also be observed as freely dispersed particles in the erythroblast cytoplasm, with the amount tending to decrease with maturation. Only a few particles, if any, are observed in the late reticulocyte stage (Bessis and Breton-Gorius, 1962; Tanaka, 1971). In guinea pig erythroblasts, the number of dispersed ferritin particles remains unchanged in cells of similar maturation, regardless of the amounts of excess iron in the serum (Tanaka, 1971).

Ferritin particles in pinocytotic vesicles of human erythroblasts have been discussed extensively by Bessis and Breton-Gorius (1959a,b; 1962). Ferritin on the surface of pinocytotic depressions is noted rarely (Fawcett, 1964; Ceresa-Castellani and Lanzavecchia, 1966; Berman, 1967; Tanaka, 1970), except in man and guinea pigs, where it is generally restricted to those hypersiderotic conditions in which total iron-binding capacity (TIBC) of transferrin is nearly saturated (Tanaka *et al.,* 1966, 1971b) and rarely in normal iron-loading conditions (Jones, 1965; Tanaka *et al.,* 1966).

The examples in Figure 2-34*A,B* from a siderotic marrow show ferritin in the pinocytotic vesicles of a developing erythroblast. Ferritin particles are clearly discernible on the inner coating of the membrane invagination and in pinocytotic vesicles. Apparently, most of these ferritin particles are subsequently collected in larger vesicles of about 0.1 to 0.3μ in diameter, and most of this ferritin is extruded from the cell (Tanaka, 1970). These ferritin particles may be engulfed from nearby macrophages (Bessis and Breton-Gorius, 1959a, 1962) or synthesized on the cell membrane of erythroblasts (Tanaka *et al.,* 1966, 1971a). The vesicle-bound ferritin particles may represent an excess of iron rather than a primary source of iron for hemoglobin synthesis.

Microtubules, fairly common in erythroblasts when glutaraldehyde is used in

FIGURE 2-5. Small vesicles and ferritin.
Cytoplasm of erythroblast with several small vesicles (*v*) that have fuzzy coat on inner surface, and larger vesicle containing many ferritin particles (*f*). There are a number of polyribosomes (*arrows*). × *180,000.*

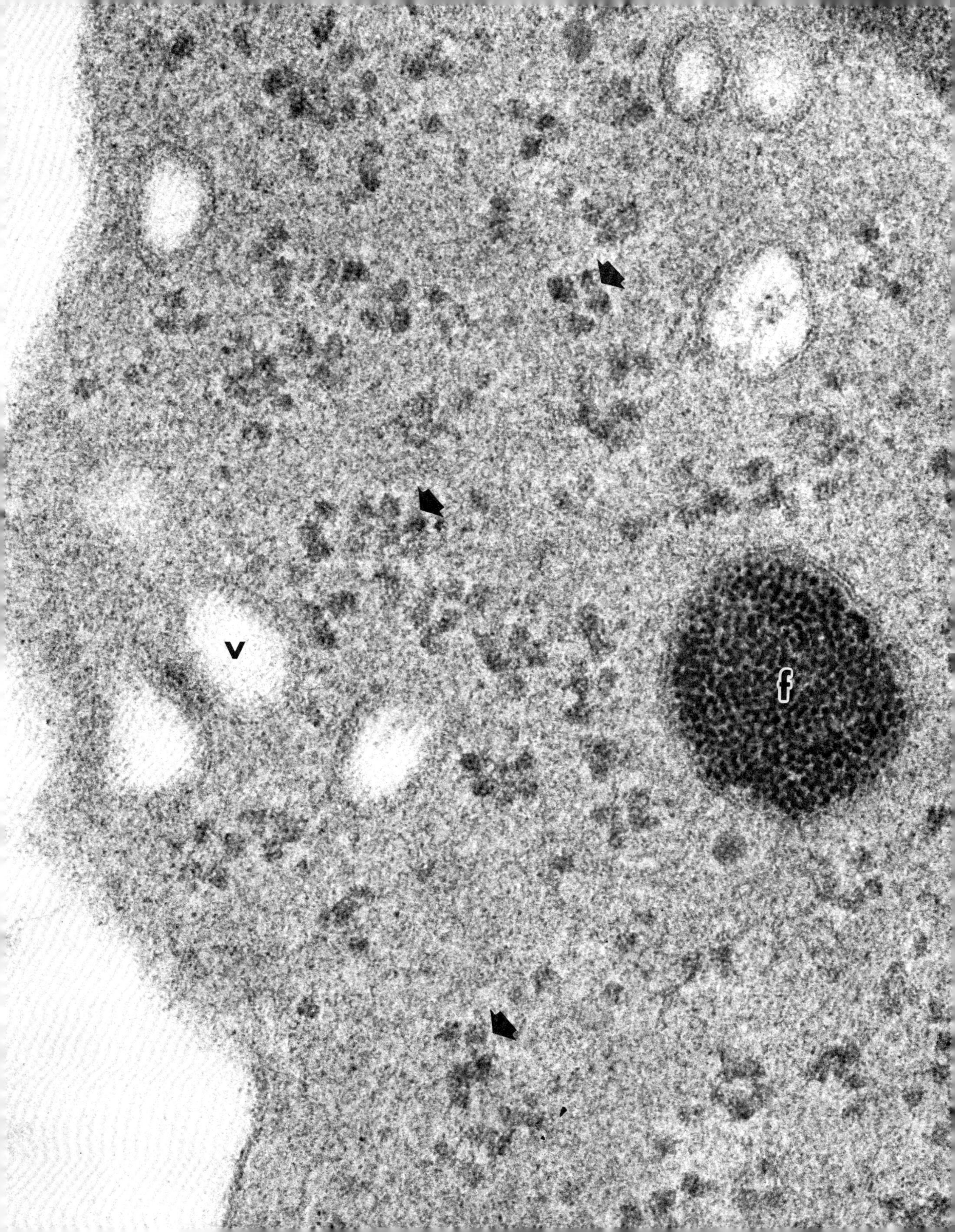
v
f

fixation, may be remnants of spindles from cell division. Less frequently, a cytoplasmic bridge called a "mid-body" (Buck and Tisdale, 1962) connects two erythroblasts (Fig. 2-6). This may be an incomplete cell separation, although the cells seem to have developed an interphase nucleus and have reached relatively late stages of maturation but remain connected. Microtubules are usually visible within this mid-body.

Lamellar or fenestrated membrane structures are infrequent in the early erythroblast (Fig. 2-7*A*) and their significance is unknown. Clusters of *smooth endoplasmic reticulum,* similar to Golgi vesicles but separate from them, have been observed in several erythroblasts in human sideroblastic anemia and guinea pig marrow, but not in normal humans. Their significance is not known. The illustration (Fig. 2-7*B*) is from a guinea pig cell.

Cytoplasmic granules, resembling lysosomal granules of granulocytes, are uncommon in erythroblasts but may be seen in or near the Golgi apparatus in the proerythroblastic stage (Fig. 2-7*C*) (Bessis and Breton-Gorius, 1961b). These single membrane granules are about 0.3μ and contain amorphous material of moderate electron opacity, with an occasional ferritin particle.

MORPHOLOGY OF CELLS AT DIFFERENT STAGES OF MATURITY

Although there are no delineating electron micrographic characteristics within the phases of erythroblastic maturation, a series of continuing changes do take place. The following descriptions are characteristic for cells about median in the proerythroblast stage (Fig. 2-8*A*) and in early (Figs. 2-8*B* and 2-9*A*) and late (Fig. 2-9*B*) erythroblast stages.

Proerythroblasts

Proerythroblasts are the most immature forms identifiable with the light microscope (Fig. 2-2*A*). They are large oval cells about 12 to 19μ, with a central or slightly eccentric large round nucleus. The nucleus is composed of relatively dense strands of chromatin which have a tendency to clump. The chromatin distribution in the nucleus is somewhat coarser than in myeloblastic or megaloblastic cells; thus distinguishing these latter cells from proerythroblasts, the nucleus of which often contains two or three prominent nucleoli. The cytoplasm is strongly basophilic, is sometimes granular in appearance, particularly when the cell is in mitosis, and has a tendency to be more homogeneous and condensed compared with myeloblasts and lymphoblasts.

A small, pale or achroplasmatic area in the cytoplasm appears to correspond to the Golgi apparatus. The cells are occasionally observed in normal human bone marrow (they constitute less than 2 per cent of the total nucleated cells); however, increased numbers are present in abnormal hemopoiesis. By phase microscopy, moderate numbers of mitochondria can be observed around the achroplasmatic zone. The cells have no motility in wet preparation. Electron microscopic features of these cells have been de-

(text continues on page 32)

FIGURE 2-6. Intercellular bridge.
Mid-body or cytoplasmic bridge (*large arrow*) between two erythroblasts. There are many microtubules (*mt*) and a number of ribosomes (*r*). A macrophage (*Ma*) is at right. × *92,000.*

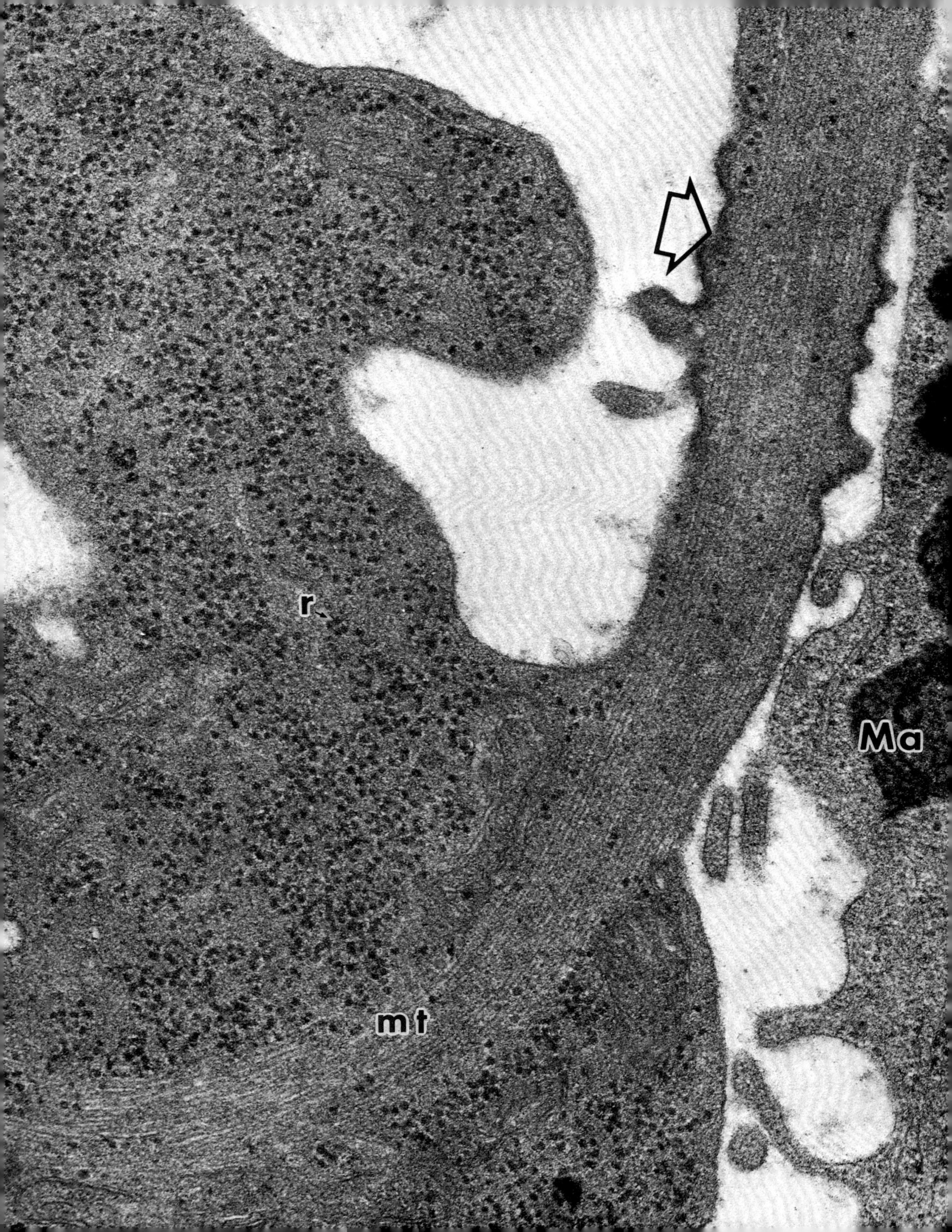
r
Ma
mt

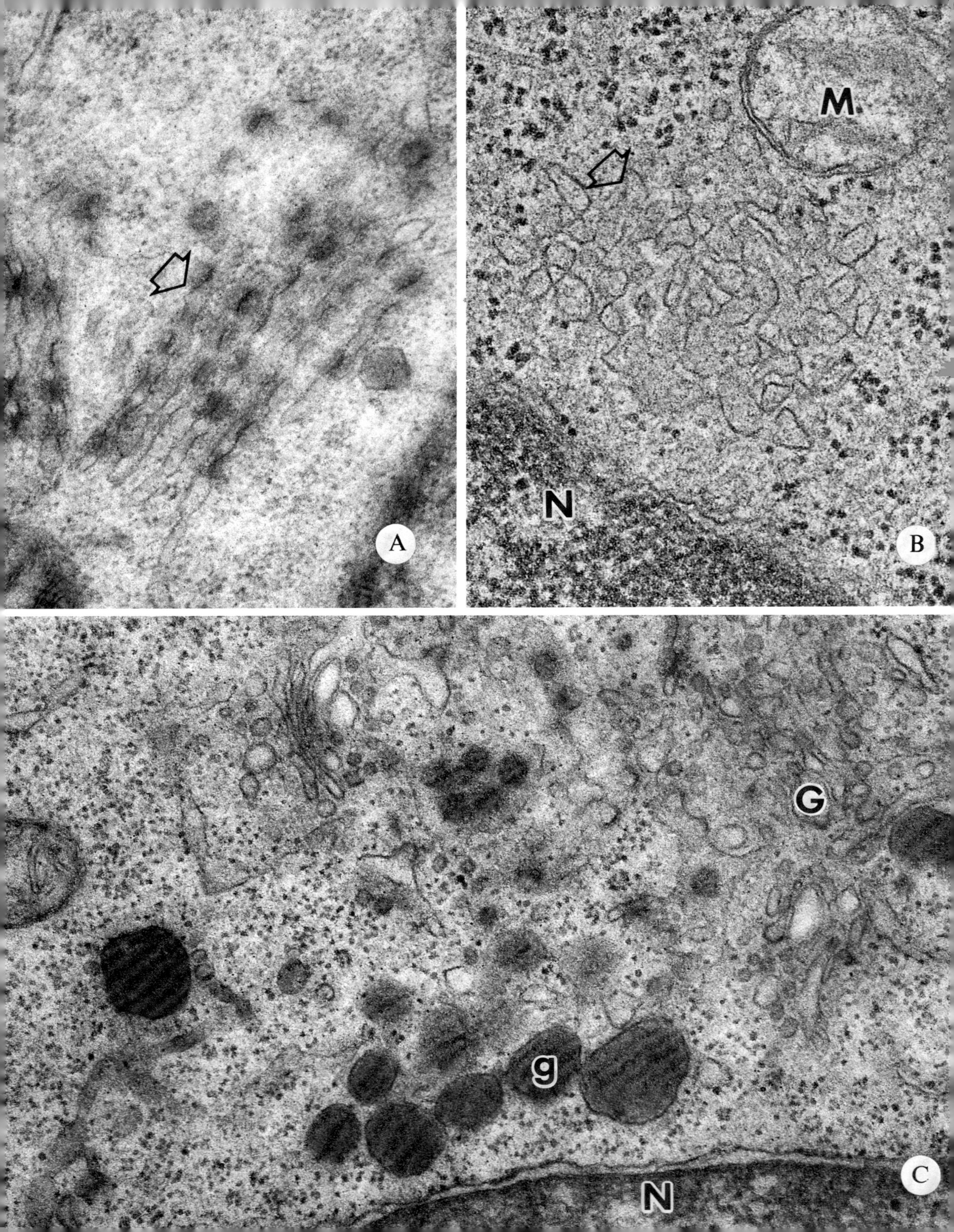
A
M
N
B
G
g
N
C

FIGURE 2-7. Cytoplasmic structures.
A. Cytoplasm with some fenestrated lamellae (*arrow*) and small portion of nucleus. × *58,500.*
B. Cluster of irregular vesicles (*arrow*) between mitochondria (*M*) and nucleus (*N*). × *81,500.*
C. Occasionally a few granules (*g*) are seen near the Golgi (*G*); edge of nucleus (*N*) and mitochondria are also present. × *56,500.*

Figures 2-8 and 2-9 appear on the following pages

FIGURE 2-8. Proerythroblast and early erythroblast.
A. Proerythroblast with scattered chromatin in nucleus (*N*). The pale cytoplasm has numerous polyribosomes and mitochondria (*M*). × *11,500.*
B. Early erythroblasts with condensed chromatin in nucleus (*N*), dense cytoplasm containing many polyribosomes, some mitochondria (*M*), and Golgi complex (*G*). Lymphoblast (*Lb*) is at left. × *11,500.*

FIGURE 2-9. Erythroblasts in metaphase and in late stage.
A. In metaphase. Chromosomes (*Ch*) are spread in fairly dense cytoplasm with no nuclear envelope. Some mitochondria (*M*) are present and pinocytotic vesicles (*pv*) are still being formed. × *12,800.*
B. Late erythroblast nearing stage of enucleation and transformation into a reticulocyte. Chromatin in nucleus (*N*) is condensed, there are few mitochondria (*M*) and polyribosomes, the Golgi complex (*G*) is still present, and several small ferritin-containing vesicles (*v*) are evident. × *20,000.*

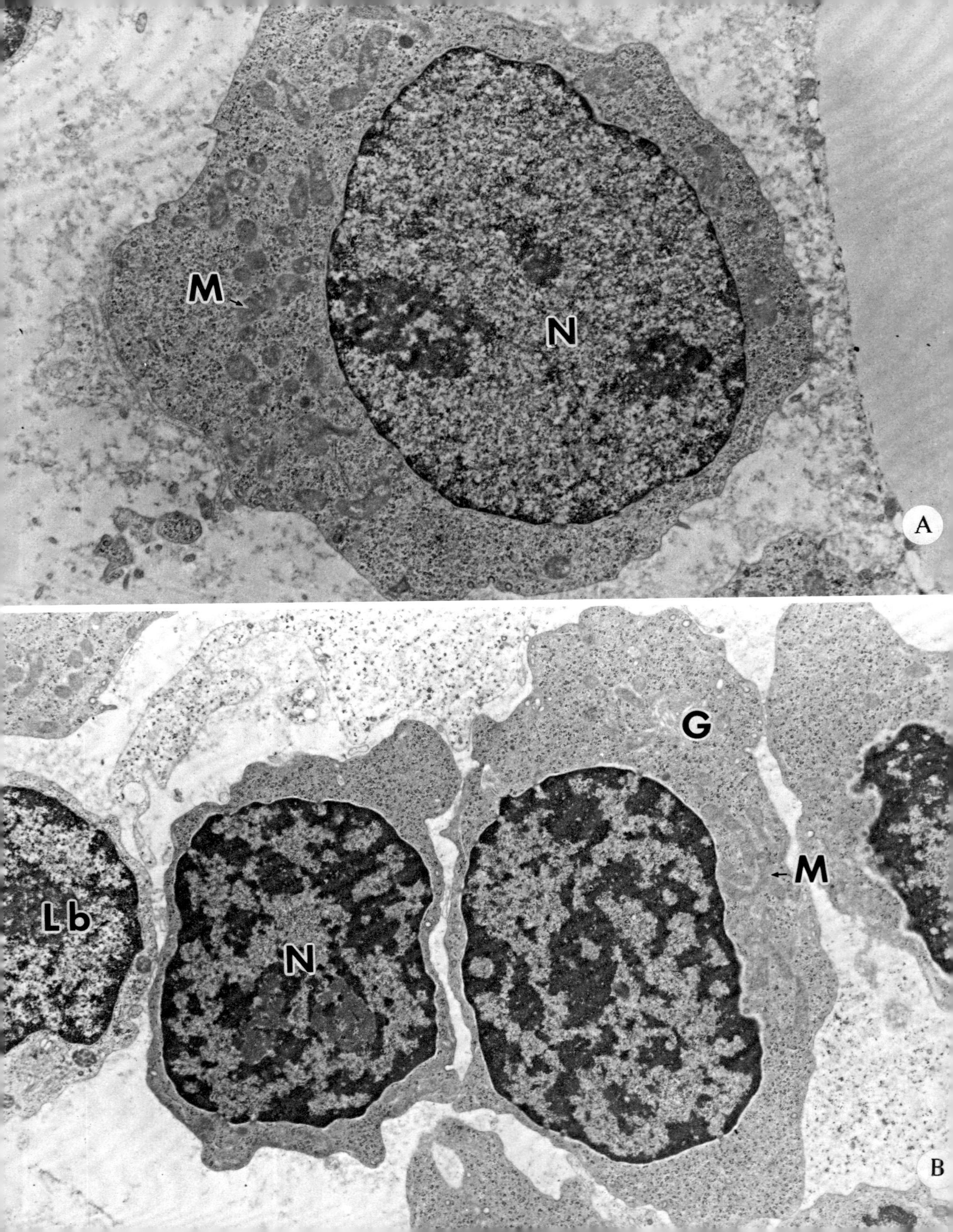
M
N
A
G
Lb
N
M
B

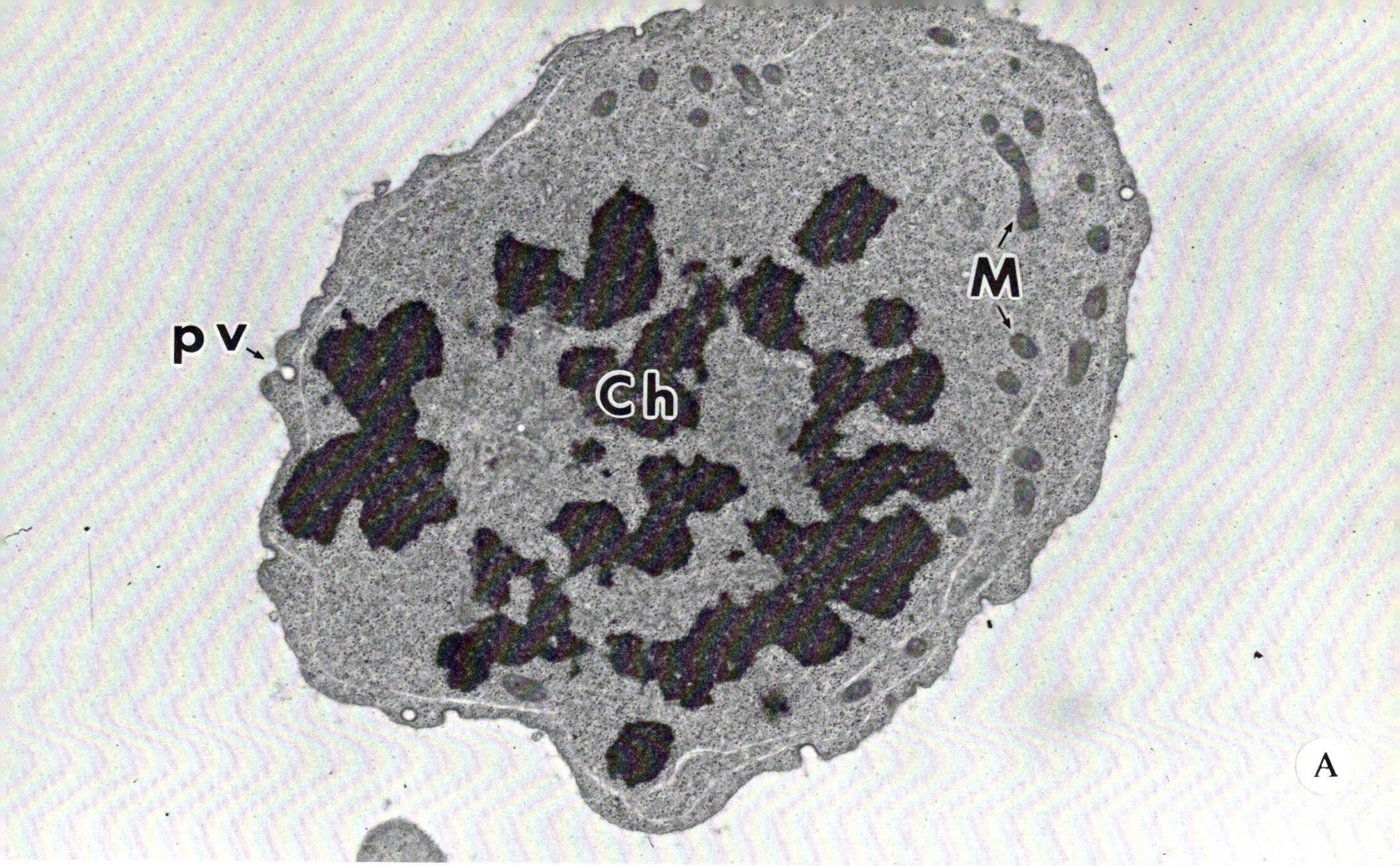
pv
Ch
M
A

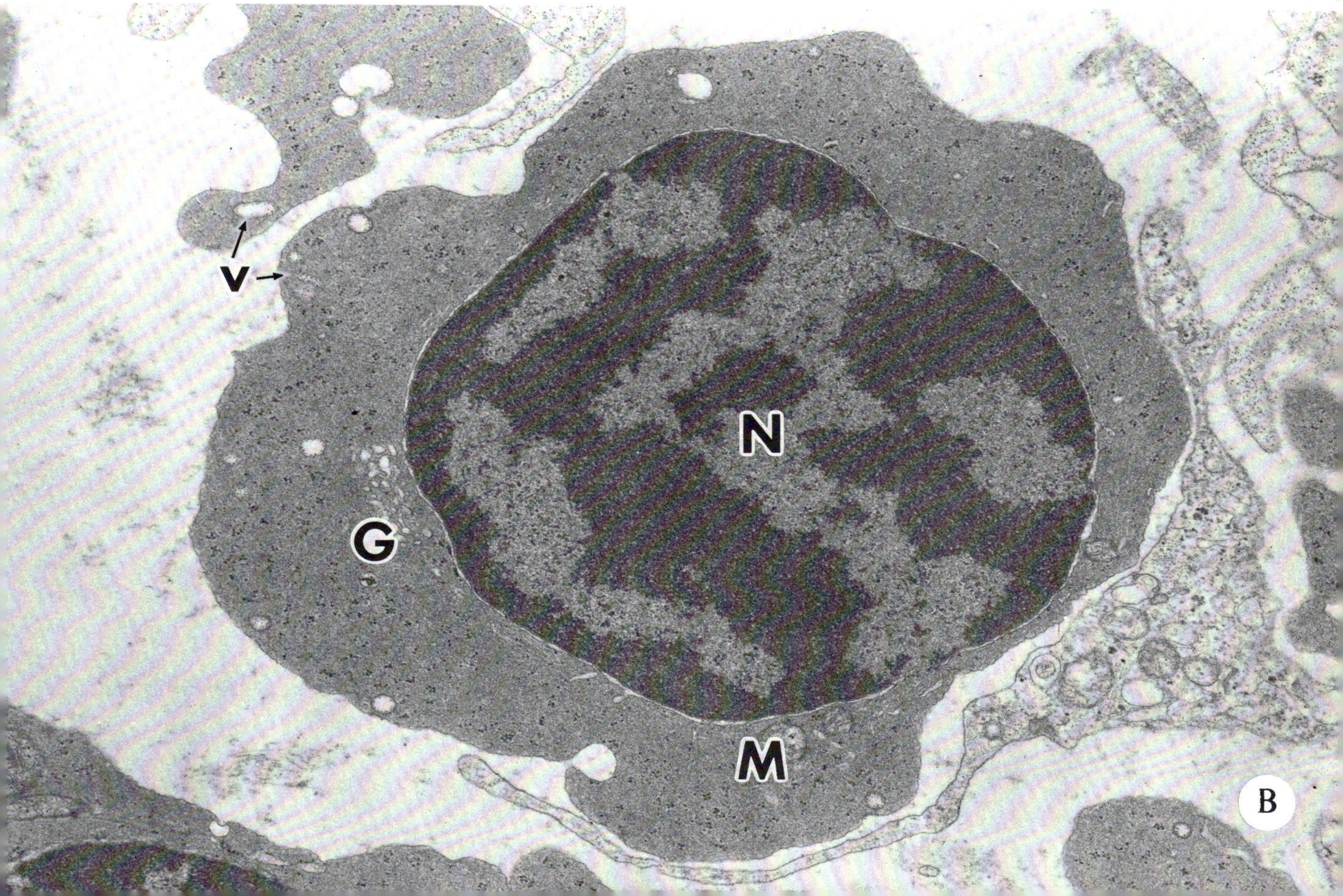
v
N
G
M
B

scribed in both embryonic (Grasso *et al.*, 1962; Zamboni, 1965) and adult erythropoiesis (Bessis and Breton-Gorius, 1961b). The cytoplasm is relatively wider (Fig. 2-7*A*) than that suggested from smears. The cell has a large round nucleus composed of loosely packed chromatin, with distinct nucleoli, which are frequently associated with the nuclear margin. The Golgi apparatus is usually not very large and may have a few granules (about 0.3 to 0.5μ), bound by a single membrane, which contain moderately opaque, amorphous material. Several ovoid mitochondria and abundant polyribosomes in the cytoplasm account for the strong basophilic staining in these cells by light microscopy. Some amorphous material, probably hemoglobin, can be observed between the many polyribosomes. There are also some endoplasmic reticulum in the cytoplasm, rare microtubules and, on occasion, fenestrated lamellae.

Early Erythroblasts

Immature or early erythroblasts (basophilic erythroblasts by light microscopy) have a coarse nuclear chromatin, with some clumping (Fig. 2-2*B*). This distribution may appear as a cartwheel arrangement by light microscopy but is rarely evident by electron microscopy. The nuclear position becomes more eccentric and the nucleoli are less distinct than in the proerythroblast stage. The cells have many polyribosomes dispersed throughout the cytoplasm, with some amorphous material discernible between them. At this stage of maturation cells divide and show more mitotic figures (Fig. 2-9*A*) than at any other stage of erythrocytic development, the Golgi area is present, and mitochondria are well developed.

Later Stages

When the first pinkish gray color appears near the nucleus in stained preparations, the cell is called a *polychromatic erythroblast.* With further differentiation, there is an increase in the amount of hemoglobin, with a corresponding decrease in basophilia, and an increase in chromatin condensation in the nucleus. Irregular lumps of chromatin become more evident and stain very deeply; nucleoli are no longer seen. After each division, the cell becomes smaller and is associated with diminution in size of the nucleus. In this stage of differentiation (when stained supravitally) a maximal number of mitochondria are seen, but their number and size decrease as hemoglobin becomes more plentiful. As maturation proceeds, the basophilia of the cytoplasm is no longer distinctive. When the cytoplasm appears reddish pink, indicating its nearly full complement of hemoglobin, the cell is defined as an *orthochromatic erythroblast.*

In normal marrows, these two cell types are 65 to 80 per cent of total nucleated red cells. However, with the electron microscope it is difficult to make a sharp separation between the orthochromatic and the polychromatic forms. The difference in cytoplasmic staining, as seen by light microscopy, is not substantiated by the differences in cytoplasmic structures by electron microscopy. Ultrastructurally, the most significant difference of the more mature forms is the presence of a large amount of amorphous material (Fig. 2-9*B*) in stroma, presumably synthesized hemoglobin. The distribution of hemoglobin is uniform, particularly after full maturation. The cytoplasm contains a fairly well-developed but not extensive Golgi apparatus and several mitochondria; however, the

Golgi complex decreases as the cells become more mature.

The nucleus of the orthochromatic erythroblast disappears at the final stage of maturation. Two separate mechanisms may be involved in this process: nuclear extrusion (Fig. 2-10*A,B,C*) and nuclear disintegration within the cells. The first mechanism is widely accepted and has been demonstrated by phase microscopy in vitro and by electron microscopy in fixed material (Skutelsky and Danon, 1967). The eliminated nucleus is often observed to be free in extracellular space (Fig. 2-10*C*) and within macrophages (Fig. 2-10*D*). The phagocytosis of eliminated nuclei may take place because there is a decrease in negative electric charge on the surface of a discarded nucleus (Skutelsky and Danon, 1969). The second mechanism proceeds from pyknosis of the nucleus, followed by intracellular karyolysis. In a mature erythroblast, an abnormal nucleus in the shape of budded pieces of nucleoplasm, rosettes, leaves, or double spheres is thought to be evidence of nuclear disintegration. These remnants may be the Howell-Jolly bodies and Cabot's rings seen by light microscopy. Electron micrographic studies, however, do not show remnants of nuclear disintegration in reticulocytes. This problem requires more study, since these unique cells have been seen by light microscopy, though very rarely.

Reticulocytes

After the loss of their nuclei erythroblasts are reticulocytes (Figs. 2-11 and 2-12). Reticulocytes may be slightly larger than a mature erythrocyte. They still contain certain cytoplasmic organelles, such as mitochondria, ribosomes, or even a cluster of vesicles resembling the Golgi apparatus with centrioles (Fig. 2-13*A*). These cytoplasmic structures disapper within a few days in the circulation, and the reticulocytes become matured erythrocytes. The elimination of mitochondria and other remnants of cytoplasmic organelles from the reticulocytes (by the spleen) has been demonstrated by Simpson and Kling (1968). The reticulocytes with their remaining ribosomes, messenger RNA (mRNA) and transfer RNA (tRNA) continue to synthesize hemoglobin, and the residual mitochondria maintain some aerobic metabolism. These structures and their functions are lost as the cell matures into an erythrocyte; however, enzymes synthesized during maturation—including those involved in an aerobic glycolysis—continue throughout the life of the erythrocyte.

The term "reticulocyte" is derived from cytoplasmic characteristics seen with the light microscope when the immature erythrocyte is treated with a supravital stain such as brilliant cresyl blue, Janus green, Nile blue sulfate, new methylene blue, etc. These structures are apparently made of RNA aggregates (Jensen *et al.,* 1965) and may appear as a narrow band traversing the cell, as fine particles evenly distributed throughout the cell, or so densely packed as to give the appearance of a nucleus. They are more prominent in the more immature and less noticeable in nearly mature cells. The reticulum cannot be seen by dark-field illumination or phase microscopy unless the cells are stained. Stained reticulocytes prepared for electron microscopy (Figs. 2-11 and 2-12) show residual mitochondria and amorphous masses, which may be aggregate remnants of ribosomes.

(*text continues on page 38*)

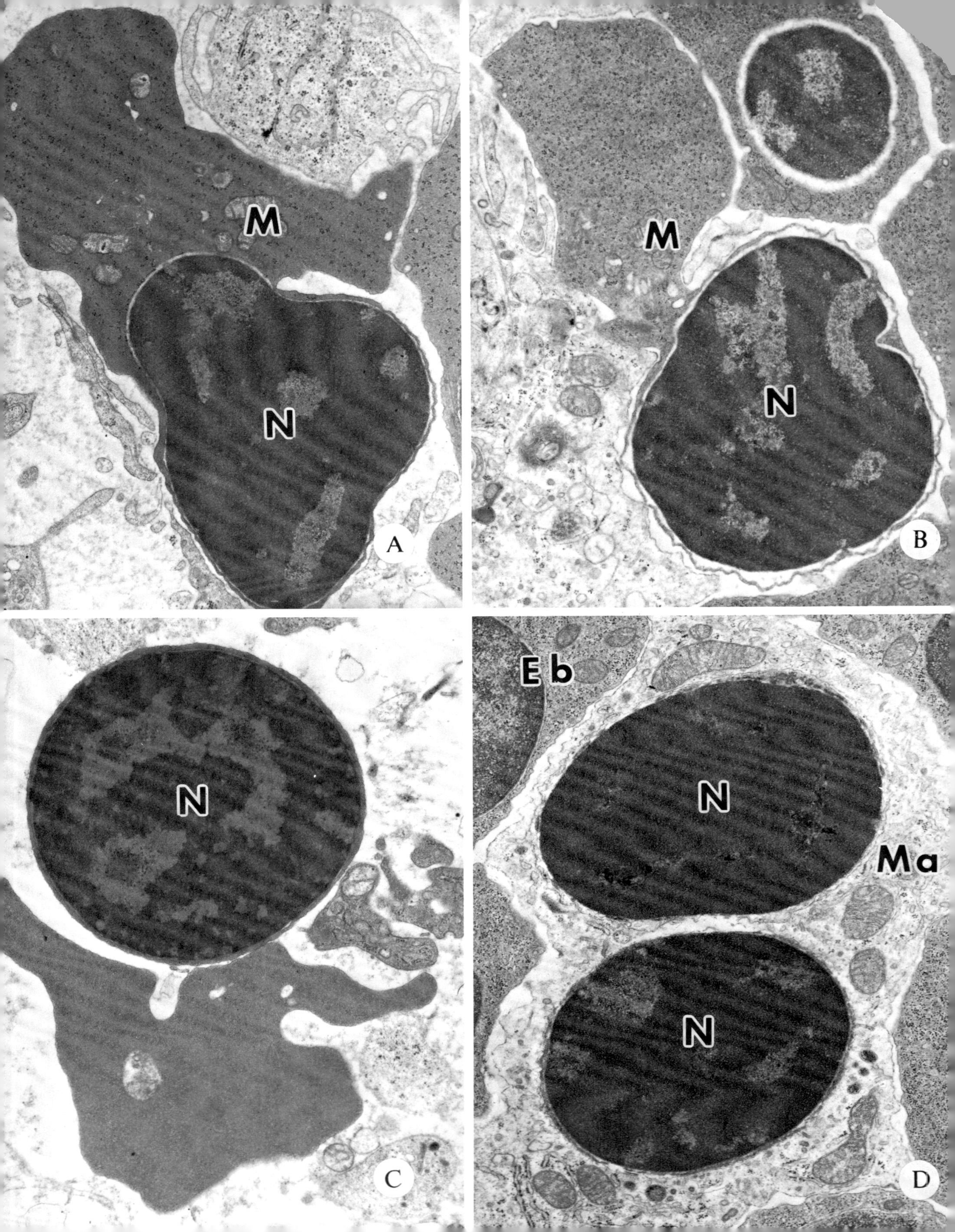
M
N
A
M
N
B
N
C
Eb
N
Ma
N
D

FIGURE 2-10. Process of erythroblast denucleation.
A, B. Guinea pig erythroblasts in last stage of maturation with nuclear margination. Only a very thin sheet of cytoplasm encircles the dense nuclear mass (*N*). Mitochondria (*M*) are concentrated in area adjacent to departing nucleus. **A,** × *13,600;* **B,** × *10,700.*
C. Separation of nucleus (*N*) and remaining reticulocyte in human cell. × *10,700.*
D. Several guinea pig erythroblasts (*Eb*) surround macrophage (*Ma*) which has recently ingested two nuclei (*N*), presumably discharged from erythroblasts when they matured to reticulocytes. × *10,700.*

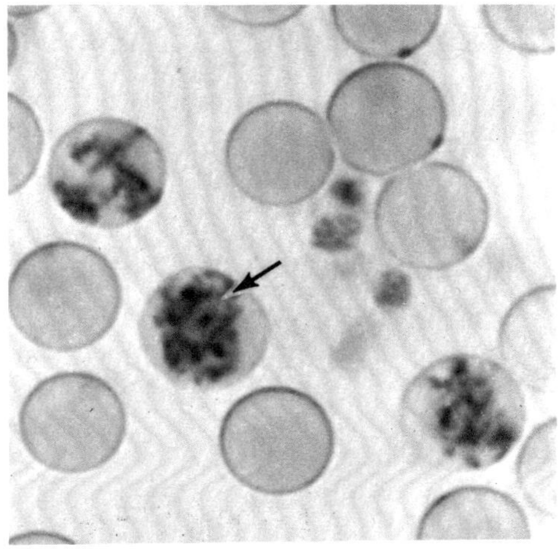

FIGURE 2-11. Reticulocyte.
Reticulocyte (*arrow*) from peripheral blood of guinea pig, stained with brilliant cresyl blue to demonstrate reticulocytes under the light microscope. × *2,000.*

Figures 2-12 and 2-13 appear on the following pages

FIGURE 2-12. Reticulocyte.
Ultrastructure of a reticulocyte from the same specimen as in Figure 2-11. The stained cell contains residue of mitochondria (*M*), a few vesicles, and dense, fine granular material which does not appear to be ribosome per se, but may be residual RNA. × *54,000.*

FIGURE 2-13. Reticulocyte and mature erythrocytes.
A. Reticulocyte (*R*) with numerous polyribosomes, several mitochondria (*M*), and vestiges of Golgi apparatus (arrow). × *18,000.*
B. Mature erythrocytes from peripheral blood, no longer containing ribosomes, mitochondria, or Golgi apparatus. However, occasional small vesicles (*arrow*) and, less frequently, larger vesicles (*v*) are found. × *31,500.*

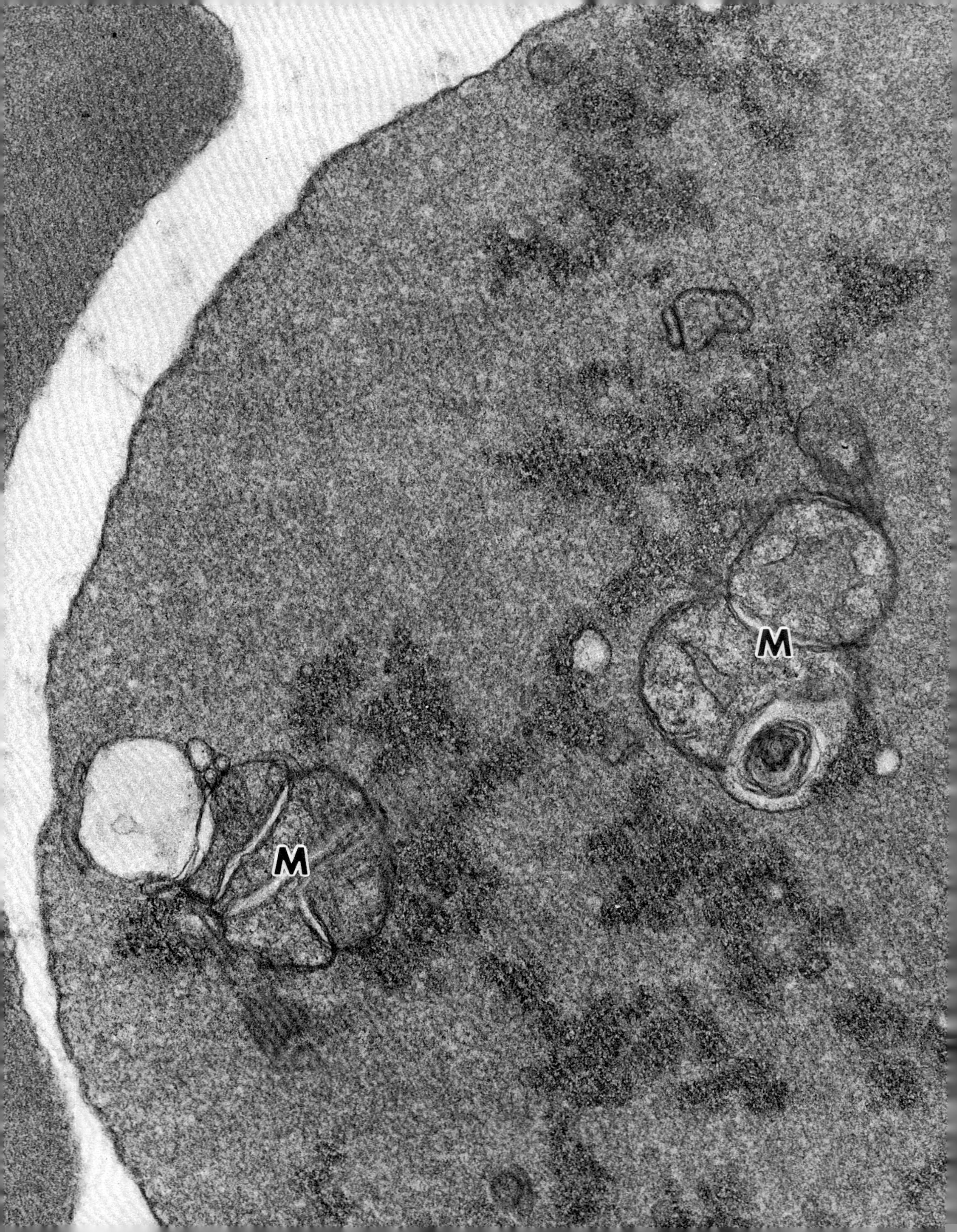
M
M

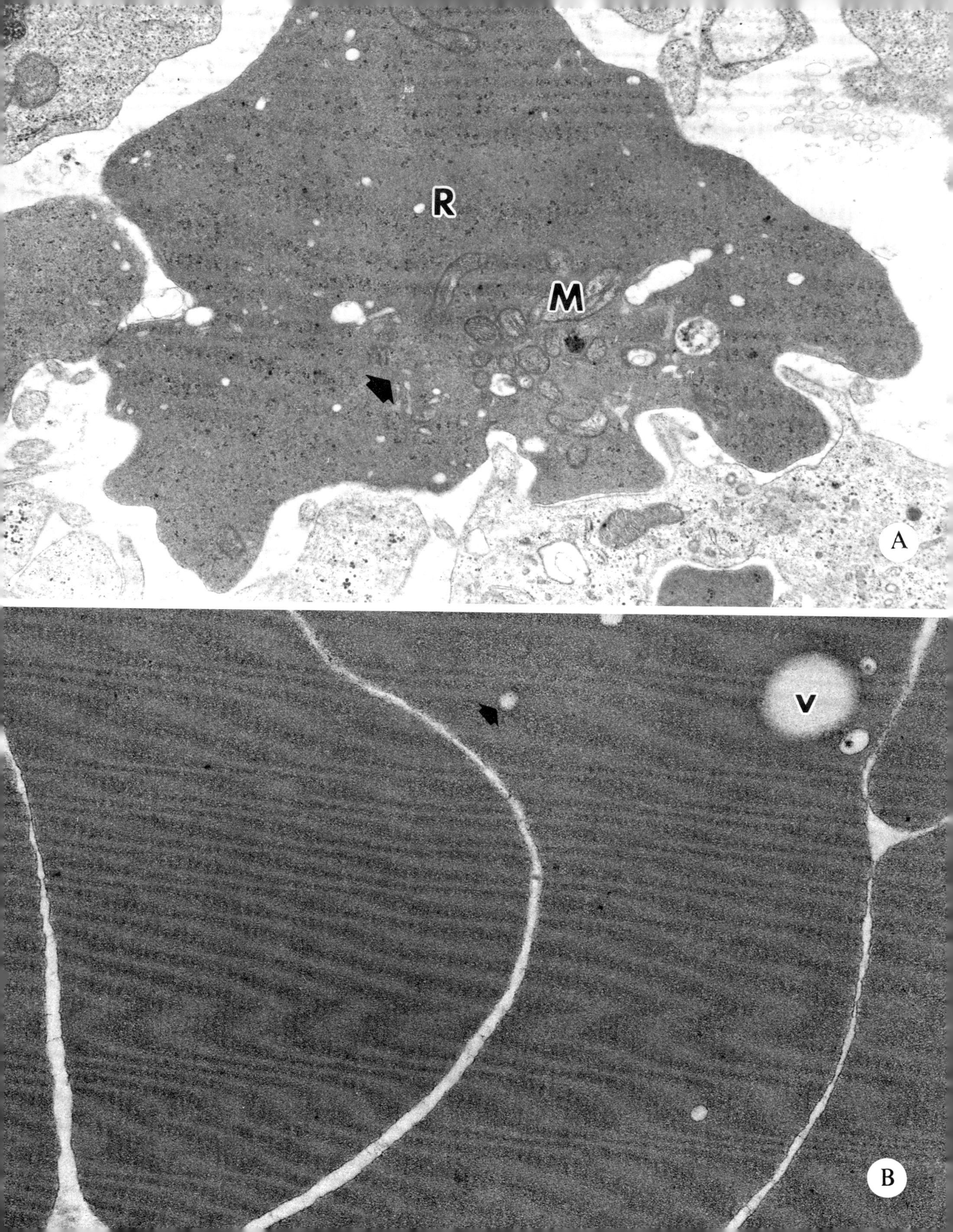
R
M
A
V
B

Erythrocytes

The final stage of maturation in the erythroid series is the circulating erythrocyte (Fig. 2-13*B*), a biconcave disc which is produced when the remnants of cytoplasmic organelles seen in reticulocytes have disappeared. The erythrocytes are extremely flexible and are distorted in response to mechanical forces, but are also elastic and quickly regain their biconcave disc form after removal of the distorting force. This is particularly helpful in easing their flow through small capillaries (Skalak and Brånemark, 1969). The mature erythrocytes without organelles continue to be active metabolically. They utilize glucose via the hexose monophosphate shunt and Embden-Meyerhoff pathway, maintain sodium and potassium gradients, and have a number of enzymatic activities whose functions are not yet clear. A number of genetically determined enzyme deficiencies have been described. These include glucose-6-phosphate dehydrogenase, which has been implicated in some forms of hemolytic anemia, as manifested by erythrocyte hemolysis upon exposure to reducing agents or certain drugs, and pyruvate kinase, which results in erythrocyte distortion and membrane function disorders. As yet, however, no morphological defects have been discerned by electron microscopy.

Aging occurs in mature erythrocytes; all enzymatic activity diminishes in time and the hemoglobin becomes denatured. The average life span of circulating erythrocytes in humans is about 110 days. These aged cells have a change of their surface charge (Marikovsky and Danon, 1969) and become more susceptible to mechanical hemolysis and are also removed from the circulation by macrophages. The fragmentation of aging erythrocytes occurs in normal physiological conditions of circulation, but such fragmentation can also occur in various hematological disorders and can possibly lead to hemolysis (Weed and Reed, 1966). This is possibly more frequent during splenic passage (Koyama *et al., 1964).*

HEINZ BODIES

Inclusions in mature erythrocytes can result when an animal is treated with phenylhydrazine or its derivatives. The production of similar inclusions was first noted by Reiss in 1882 (quoted by Webster, 1949) in erythrocytes of persons poisoned with potassium chloride. The structures were carefully analyzed by Heinz (1890) during his study of the effect of phenylhydrazine on the blood, and his original report described precisely the details of the inclusions, which are now called Heinz bodies. The story of the Heinz bodies has been well reviewed by Webster (1949).

Heinz bodies are round, oval, or serrated granules which are very refractile in wet preparations, vary in size from 1 to 2μ in diameter, and can occur singly or in groups. They are formed by oxidative denaturation of hemoglobin in situ, which leads to several soluble and insoluble sulfhemoglobin-like denaturation products. Heinz bodies are found in the blood of patients suffering from various industrial poisons and in certain hemoglobinopathies. In experimental animals, no Heinz bodies are produced in nucleated red cells or in young reticulocytes—only in mature red cells. The inclusions (Fig. 2-14) can be produced by administration of phenylhydrazine both in vitro and in vivo. By ultrastructural study (Rifkind and Danon, 1965), the collections of small, flocculated, granular, opaque areas of about 0.3μ in diameter appear in the erythrocyte as an initial phase, then become aggregated to form a larger inclusion which can be detected by light microscopy. The initial stage of Heinz body formation occurs near the center of the erythrocyte and migrates to the periphery during confluence. The final inclusions may involve the plasma membrane; however, no hemolysis is observed in vitro. The abnormal inclusions are usually removed by macrophages during the passage through the spleen in vivo (Rifkind, 1965).

Inclusions in thalassemia or Heinz bodies in other hemoglobinopathies are formed by different mechanisms, and may represent an unstable hemoglobin or a qualitative or quantitative abnormality of a peptide chain, which results in a precipitate within the cell. These can be seen in nucleated cells, in contrast to Heinz bodies produced by phenlyhydrazine, which appear only in erythrocytes. Ultrastructurally, no clear distinction is possible between the two different inclusions. However, inclusions in hemoglobinopathies (Figs. 2-25 through 2-27) are usually located in the middle of the erythrocyte, do not involve the cell membrane, and may be associated with many ferritin particles (Figs. 2-26 and 2-27). Iron-laden mitochondria are usually associated with the inclusion in both types.

HEMOLYSIS

The human erythrocyte contains hemoglobin within a membrane which is about 60 to 80 Å thick. No pores or holes can be detected in the intact cell membrane although, when the membrane is studied by shadow-casting technic, the younger cell surface appears more granular (Danon and Marikovsky, 1961). Erythrocytes exposed to various hemolytic agents or immune reactions show holes of various sizes in the membrane (Borsos *et al.*, 1964). These membrane defects can be seen best when the cell fragments are negatively stained by phosphotungstic acid solutions. The holes created by hemolytic agents are larger and show an irregular margin, in contrast to those created by an immune reaction. Hemolysis induced by immune reactions shows many holes in the membrane, fairly uniform in size (about 100 Å). The size of the holes may be affected by the source or number of complement units used, but are not influenced by the source of the type of antibodies (Dourmashkin and Rosse, 1966). By this technic, one unit of antibody complement complex will produce one hole. Hemolysis initiated by the production of a 100-Å hole in the membrane does not induce the escape of hemoglobin since the hole size is not large enough to permit the escape of macromolecules (Dourmashkin and Rosse, 1966). The actual hemolysis may result from the swelling and rupture of the erythrocyte as a result of increased water influx into the damaged cell through the 100-Å holes.

CYTOGENESIS

Erythroid cells are the vehicle for oxygen transport, which is essential for every energy-requiring system of an animal organism. The formation of erythroblasts must start early; they are perhaps the first most differentiated cells to appear in early embryonic life. The site of erythrocyte production, the morphology of developing cells, and the biochemical properties of hemoglobin all change during the course of embryonic development. Since embryonal erythropoiesis and adult erythropoiesis are related, the former will be described briefly.

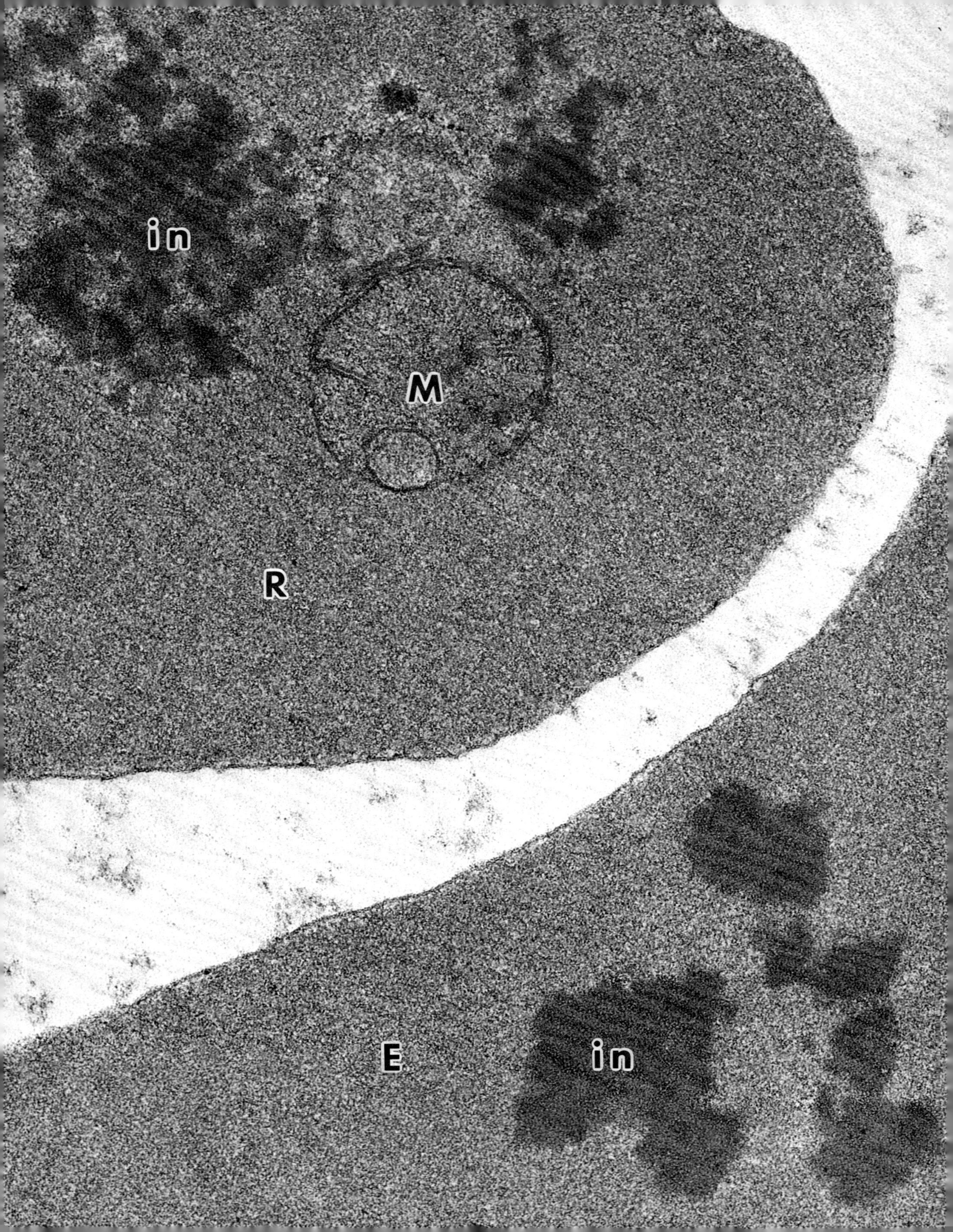
in
M
R
E
in

FIGURE 2-14. Heinz body.
Guinea pig erythrocyte (*E*) and reticulocyte (*R*) with inclusions (*in*) produced by administration of phenylhydrazine. The reticulocyte has residual membranes of a mitochondrion (*M*). × *71,500.*

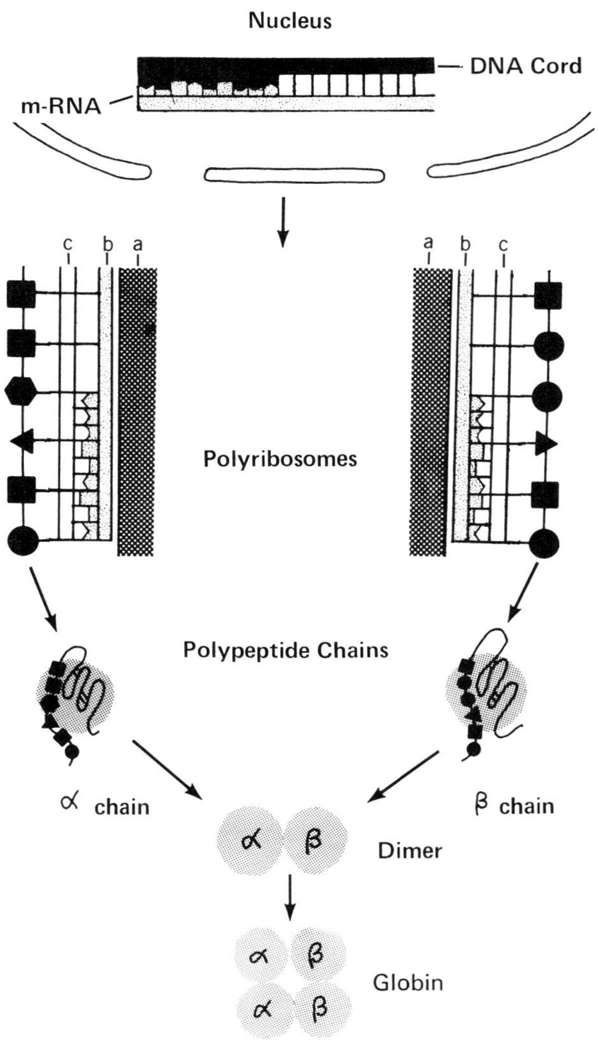

FIGURE 2-15. Globin biosynthesis.
Schematic representation of the biosynthesis of globin. Nuclear DNA (*at top*) codes messenger RNA (mRNA, also *b*) which diffuses to the polyribosomes (*a*) of the cytoplasm. The mRNA (*b*) codes the transfer RNA (*c*) to attach amino acids (opaque figures) in desired sequence to form polypeptide chains.

EMBRYONAL ERYTHROPOIESIS

Yolk Sac Erythropoiesis

Primitive erythropoiesis starts about the third week of embryonic life in blood islands of the human yolk sac (Maximow, 1924; Bloom and Bartelmez, 1940; Knoll and Pingel, 1949). The first primitive blood cells, hemocytoblasts, are produced in mesoderms (Mesenchymal mesoblasts) within an early endothelial tube formed by the transformation of blood islands. By light microscopy, these hemocytoblasts have moderate basophilic cytoplasm and a relatively large nucleus containing spongy chromatin network and several nucleoli. The term "hemocytoblast" has also been used for the blastic cell form of both lymphocytic and myelocytic tissues; however, the two types of cells are functionally different. In supravital preparations, mitochondria are hardly recognized —probably a reflection of their rarity. The exact duration of mesoblastic erythropoiesis is not known, but no blood islands are noted in an embryo of about 5 mm in length, and hemocytoblasts are rarely seen about the seventh to ninth week of embryonic development.

Hemoglobin formation becomes evident in differential primitive blood cells (primitive erythroblasts) that have a fine nuclear chromatin and are larger than adult erythroblasts. These primitive erythroblasts still retain their nucleus even after they lose their mitotic activity. Electron microscopic observations on yolk sac of guinea pigs show that the primitive stem cells, the descendants of primitive blood cells (hemocytoblasts), and primitive erythroblasts form an erythroblastic island around the central macrophages, similar to that described in adult marrows (Sorenson, 1961). However, no erythroblastic islands are observed in chick yolk sac (Breton-Gorius and Stralin, 1967). Ultrastructural characteristics of hemocytoblasts are similar to those reported in hepatic hematopoiesis which will be described in that section.

The cytoplasm of primitive erythroblasts differs little in morphology from that in erythroblasts of adults except for a lower incidence of lipid vacuoles and flattened endoplasmic reticulum in the primitive form (Sorenson, 1961). The primitive blood cell is medium-sized and spherical, and contains abundant ribosomes in the cytoplasm (Jones, 1963). The primitive erythrocytes circulate throughout the embryonic body after yolk sac vessels communicate with intraembryonic circulation. This early erythropoiesis subsides soon after the intrahepatic erythropoiesis occurs in the embryo.

Hepatic Erythropoiesis

The erythropoiesis of the primitive type is succeeded by the second phase, which starts in the third embryonal month—first in the liver, then in bone marrow and spleen. Morphologically, the erythroid elements formed in this stage can hardly be distinguished from those observed in the adult (Ackerman *et al.,* 1961; Grasso *et al.,* 1962; Zamboni, 1965); however, biochemical data have shown that they form fetal hemoglobin (Hb-F), which has a globin of different amino acid composition than that formed by adults. In the liver, the hematopoietic elements arise from the diffuse mesenchymal components concealed between epithelial cells and endothelium, and produce an extravascular hematopoietic nest (Bloom and Fawcett, 1968). There is no convincing evidence for the contribution of endothelial cells to hemocytoblast production in the embryonic liver.

By electron microscopy, the hemocytoblast of human fetal liver has a pale nucleus that contains one or two prominent nucleoli and has evenly distributed chromatin with a finely granulated pattern (Zamboni, 1965). The nuclear margin is often serrated or deeply indented. Mitochondria are present without any recognizable grouping in the cytoplasm. There are a few other cytoplasmic organelles, including a poorly developed Golgi apparatus and some endoplasmic reticulum; however, there are abundant polyribosomes, usually composed of four to six particles arranged in rosettes. The hemocytoblast is thought to differentiate toward both erythrocytic and megakaryocytic lines (Zamboni, 1965).

The erythroblastic nest is composed of immature erythroblasts, which are present in the center of the island and are surrounded by differentiating erythroblasts but lack the central macrophage frequently described in adult erythropoiesis. The erythroblastic differentiation in hepatic hematopoiesis follows the same pattern of cellular development as that observed in adult marrow hematopoiesis (Grasso *et al.,* 1962) as discussed in the previous section.

Bone Marrow Erythropoiesis

Bone marrow appears about the fifth embryonal month, when some of the mesenchyma of primitive bone cartilage is replaced by diffuse proliferation of blood-forming cells. The hematopoietic function of the organ becomes more significant as the embryo grows, and gradually takes over the blood cell generation.

POSTNATAL AND ADULT ERYTHROPOIESIS

In the postnatal stage of normal humans, erythropoiesis is found only in bone marrows; in rodents, such activity is normally seen in the spleen. Recently, differences in morphology and kinetics of transplanted hematopoietic tissues has been demonstrated between fetal, neonatal, and adult erythropoiesis in rodents (Kubanek *et al.,* 1970; Lucarelli *et al.,* 1970). The morphology of the precursor cells is not well documented, but the most immature forms of erythroblasts (proerythroblasts) do not appear to be self-generating (Alpen and Cranmore, 1959). A significant proliferation of mesenchymal cells has been reported in pathological conditions in which impaired erythropoiesis is present and has led to the speculation that mesenchymal cells may be the source of erythroid precursors (Tanaka, 1967). Many investigators in the field of erythroid kinetics regard the mesenchyma of the organ as the primary ancestor of the erythroid compartment and the blastic form, which resembles large lymphocytes, as the possible direct source.

The supply of erythrocytes in humans is regulated so that a fairly constant number circulate. Such control is apparently effective at all stages of cell differentiation—a nearly constant production stream maintains a fairly constant total number in circulation. The mode of proliferation or replacement is equivalent to the cellular regeneration noted in many organs. The total spectrum of erythrocytic cells was designated as "erythron" by Castle and Minot (1936).

By measuring such values as cell cycle of nucleated cells, numbers of each type of erythroid differentiation, mitotic ratio, the amount of hemoglobin synthesized, etc., one can postulate a kinetic model of erythroid proliferation. Recent studies suggest that immature erythroblasts divide four times and that one proerythroblast gives rise to 16 nondividing erythroblast which subsequently mature to red cells (Lajtha and Oliver, 1960).

The total maturation time from one proerythroblast to 16 erythrocytes is estimated to be about 4 to 6 days. Killmann *et al.* (1964) estimate the compartment transit time of human erythroid cells to be 30 hours for proerythroblasts, 12.4 to 63.5 hours for basophilic erythroblasts, 8.8 to 25.0 hours for polychromatic erythroblasts, and 19 hours for orthochromatic erythroblasts. Stohlman *et al.* (1964) speculated that erythroblasts get information to start cell division when the intracellular hemoglobin reaches a certain concentration. In normal erythropoiesis, all divided erythroblasts may eventually mature; however, in some pathological marrows there is no increase in circulating erythrocytes despite the presence of significant erythroid hyperplasia in the bone marrow (Goodman *et al.,* 1968). This impaired production and the loss of defective erythroid cells, which are eventually phagocytosed by marrow macrophages, is called ineffective erythropoiesis. These lysed erythroid cells are considered to be responsible for the formation of the early-labeling fraction of fecal bile pigment (Gray *et al.,* 1950; London *et al.,* 1950).

Marrow erythropoiesis is regulated by various factors, among them erythropoietin (Bonsdorff and Jalavisto, 1948), which is accepted as the major factor in controlling erythroid proliferation. The biochemical nature of the erythropoietin is not known, but it is present in measurable levels in the blood of severely anemic or hypoxic subjects and is excreted in the urine. The biological effect of the substance is to stimulate the stem cell compartment to produce proerythroblasts and accelerate cell maturation at various stages (Stohlman *et al.,* 1964). The primary site of erythropoietin synthesis is not clearly established; however, the kidney plays a significant role in erythropoietin formation. Hypoxia and androsterone are known to produce erythroid hyperplasia, but their activity is considered to be secondary through the increase in erythropoietin production. A direct effect of hemoglobin and heme have been demonstrated on the induction of erythropoiesis (Brown *et al.,* 1963; Sanchez-Medal *et al.,* 1963). The actions of both substances are believed to be independent of erythropoietin.

HEMOGLOBIN

The biochemistry of hemoglobin synthesis has been of interest to geneticists, immunologists, and biochemists as well as hematologists, and its biosynthesis has been studied extensively in reticulocytes of various animals. The main function of the developing erythrocytic cell is to synthesize hemoglobin. Production of hemoglobin begins in the early basophilic erythroblast and continues through the reticulocyte stage. Since 95 per cent of the protein synthesized in circulating reticulocytes is hemoglobin, biochemists have found this cell to be a very useful model for the study of protein synthesis. After bone marrow stimulation, reticulocytes can be obtained from the circulating blood in a fraction that is free of nucleated cells. This results in a preparation in which the major protein production is hemoglobin.

Hemoglobin is a conjugated protein with a molecular weight of 67,000, composed of four heme groups and four polypeptide chains. Each heme has one iron atom. The polypeptide chains in hemoglobin A (the main type of normal adult hemoglobin) are two alpha chains of 141 amino acids and two beta chains of 146 amino acids. Hemoglobin F (the main type in fetal blood) has two alpha and two gamma peptide chains which, like the beta chains, have 146 amino acid units. Another minor component in physiological hemoglobin, called Hb-A2, consists of a pair of alpha and delta chains. The fetal and adult hemoglobin have differences in crystal form, x-ray diffraction, absorption spectra electrophoretic mobility, solubility resistance to alkali, amino acid composition, and immunological specificity. None of these differences are apparent by electron microscopy. Many minor variations in the amino acid sequences of hemoglobin have been found in patients with hemoglobinopathies, some with marked difference in the physical and chemical characteristics of the resulting hemoglobin. These, in turn, can cause gross physiological problems, whereas other changes do not seem to have any significant physiological effect.

The biosynthesis of hemoglobin has three separate biochemical processes: the formation of the globin or polypeptide chains by ribosomes; production of porphyrin—probably in or near mitochondria; and iron incorporation, which also possibly involves the mitochondria. These components are finally assembled to form the hemoglobin molecule.

Globin Production

This is accomplished on polyribosomes dispersed throughout the cytoplasm of erythroblasts, and is typical of the universal process of protein production in many cell systems. RNA of ribosomes (usually in small groups or attached to membranes) produces protein by the combination of amino acids through peptide linkage in predetermined sequences. The amino acids are either absorbed from the extracellular environment or are obtained from intracellular breakdown of polypeptides in the cytoplasm. Reticulocytes and erythroblasts utilize the accumulated amino acids in a pattern that is established from the cell nucleus. This classic process of protein synthesis (Fig. 2-15) starts in the nucleus with the genetically coded information of the chromosomal DNA transferred to a soluble mRNA molecule, by matching nucleotide bases between the two molecules (DNA and RNA). The sequence of three nucleotide bases, called "codon," is specific for an amino acid. In this manner, the proper sequence for amino acid selection is set on the mRNA arrangement of nucleotide bases by the chromosomal DNA and its predetermined nucleotide sequence. The mRNA in the cytoplasm attaches to a ribosome particle, but the nature of this attachment is not clear. Smaller soluble RNA molecules (tRNA), molecular weight about 25,000, combine with an amino-acyl-adenylate-enzyme complex, resulting from a previous reaction of the amino acid and the enzyme. Each tRNA is specific for a particular amino acid and has an anticodon end that corresponds to a specific codon of the mRNA. The spatial arrangement of these three components (the ribosome, mRNA, and the delivering tRNA) have not been defined accurately. However, the arrangement is such that the codon end of the mRNA is matched to its corresponding anticodon of a tRNA, and the series of delivered amino acids are united through their peptide bonds. This process is engineered by the ribosome and requires the presence of an enzyme, Mg^{++}, guanosine triphosphate, and the high energy phosphate system.

The process for this globin synthesis in the erythroblast and reticulocyte starts with the N-terminal amino acid, valine, and continues to add two amino acids per second as the ribosome particle progresses along the mRNA molecule, until growth is complete at the C-terminal.

With the electron microscope, the ribosome (Fig. 2-3) is seen as a particle, or in aggregates up to six, in erythrocytic cells. The clusters of ribosomes or polyribosomes are considered to be on a strand of mRNA. Polyribosomes of reticulocytes have a sedimentation rate of 80S in the ultracentrifuge and are composed of approximately equal amounts of protein and RNA. The mRNA with its coded sequence can be used repeatedly by ribosomes for the production of many hemoglobin molecules. Also, the tRNA, with its anticodon specificity for an amino acid, can repeatedly pick up and deliver its specific amino acid to the ribosome RNA complex for the process of synthesis.

Reticulocytes in vitro form alpha and beta polypeptide chains of globin independently (Fig. 2-15), which then combine to form alpha-beta dimers as an intermediate step in globin synthesis (Tavill *et al.,* 1968). The number of alpha and beta chains synthesized are equal, but a distinctive alpha chain pool has been recognized (Tavill *et al.,* 1968). This has led to the suggestion that newly formed alpha chains are pooled and later released to react with newly formed beta chains on or near their ribosomes. The ratio of alpha or beta chain synthesis is significantly disturbed in thalassemia and leads to a significant excess, usually of the alpha chain.

Porphyrin Production

Heme is synthesized in many types of cells and is incorporated into a number of heme proteins including myoglobins, cytochromes, and catalases. The biochemical pathways of heme synthesis have been established. The sequence of its biosynthesis from amino acids to the final product (coproporphyrin) and the enzymes involved at each step are reasonably well understood (Fig. 2-16). Heme biosynthesis starts with two amino acids: glycine and succinic acid; however, they do not react directly but form complexes which interact. Succinyl coenzyme A is derived from the tricarboxylic acid combination with glycine to form alpha-amino-beta-ketoadipic acid and requires vitamin B_6 (pyridoxine). The product is unstable and loses carbon dioxide to form the delta-amino-levulinic acid (Δ-ALA), a stable heme intermediate which is recovered from urine. The next step involves two molecules of Δ-ALA in the presence of the specific enzyme Δ-ALA-dehydrase. The product is porphobilinogen (PBG), a monopyrrole which subsequently condenses to form a tetrapyrrol and contains all the basic elements of the heme molecule except iron. This intermediate is stable and may also be recovered from urine. The reaction needs four molecules of PBG in the presence of porphobilinogenase to produce uroporphyrinogen III, which can have three isomers. The next direct intermediate is coproporphyrinogen III, which occurs by removal of a carboxyl group from a side chain of uroporphyrinogen III. The product is colorless, does not fluoresce, and cannot bind metals. It is modified by decarboxylation and oxidation to the final product, protoporphyrin IX. Biosynthesis of this material requires, in addition to the above reactions, the presence of hydrogen receptors and either intact mitochondria or enzyme-bearing membranes from them. Iron is inserted into protoporphyrin IX to produce the heme molecule.

Hemoglobin Formation

Heme and globin are synthesized independently in the cytoplasm of developing erythroblasts. The site of globin forma-

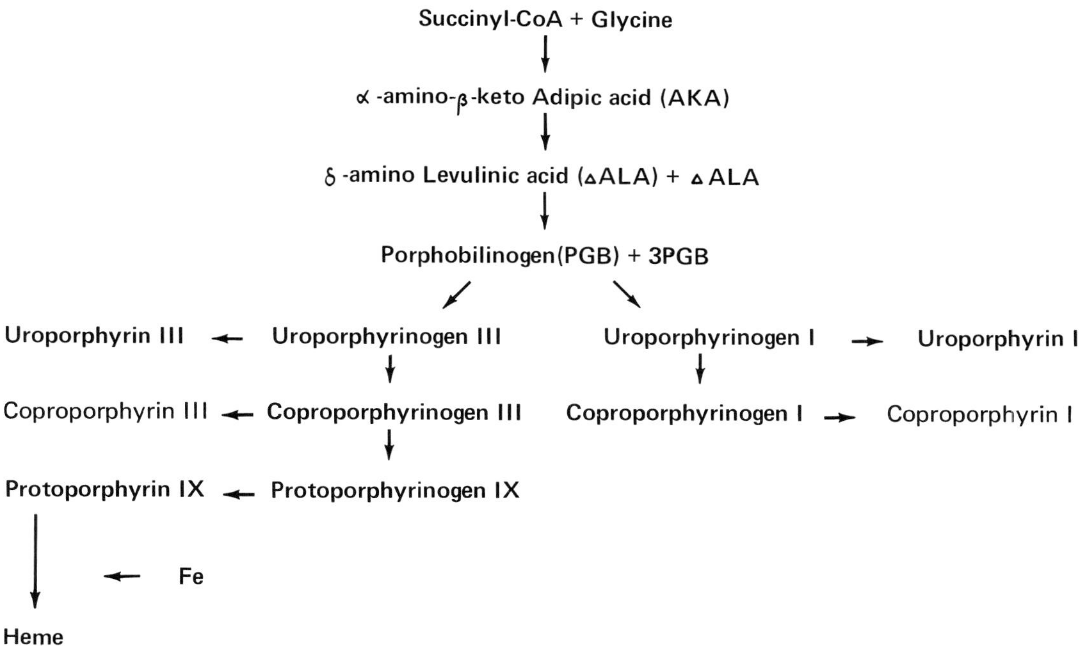

FIGURE 2-16. Biochemical pathways in heme biosynthesis.

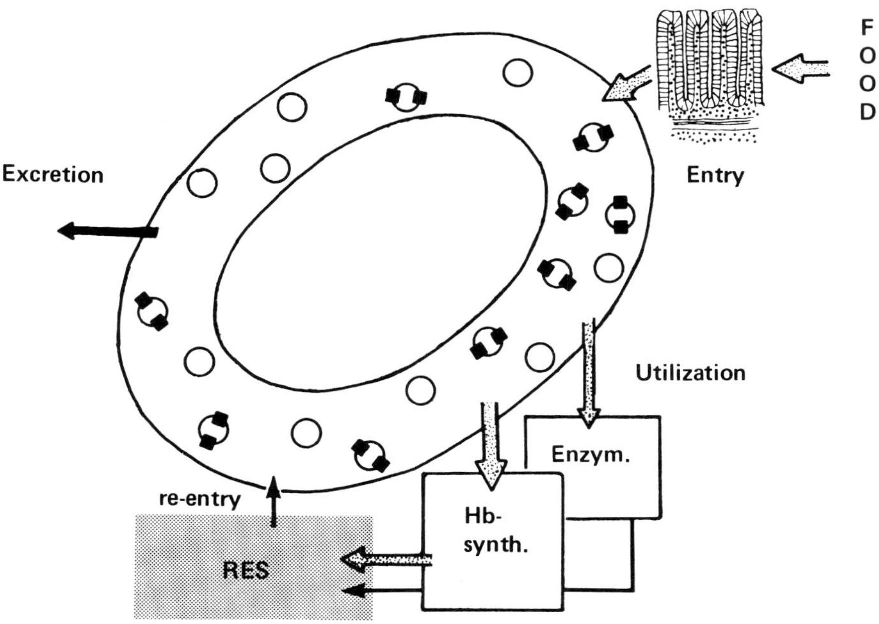

FIGURE 2-17. Schema of iron absorption and turnover.
The transferrin of the circulation is illustrated as open circles with two rectangles representing two iron atoms.

tion is on or near polyribosomes, which are widely distributed in the cytoplasm, while heme is synthesized in or near mitochondria. The conjugation of the heme molecule to each polypeptide chain may occur prior to the formation of the polypeptide polymers or, alternately, heme molecules may attach to the completed globin polymers as the final stage. Globin and heme concentrations affect the rate of synthesis of each other, so that no excess production of either will occur.

In a study of heme and globin synthesis in man, Nathan *et al.* (1961) showed that globin synthesis (estimated by uptake of ^{14}C-glycine) started during an early stage of cell maturation and continued throughout maturation, with a decline in synthetic rate. Heme synthesis, measured by intake of ^{14}C-glycine and ^{59}Fe, showed that the more differentiated erythroblasts formed the largest amounts of heme. By electron microscopy, there is no suggestion from the distribution of increasing electron densities in cells which actively synthesize hemoglobin, to indicate any specific region of the cell area as the probable location of the final step in synthesis. The two portions of the hemoglobin molecule apparently depend on diffusion of one or both of the components for combination, and this takes place throughout the cytoplasm.

IRON METABOLISM

Food iron is absorbed by the mucosa of the upper digestive tract, particularly the duodenum, in a ferrous form (Fig. 2-17). The epithelial cells of these areas have no special affinity for iron, but such luminal factors as pH and redox potential appear to influence iron absorption (Bothwell and Finch, 1962). The transfer of iron through epithelial cells is rapid and is accomplished by an active oxidative process (Mazur *et al.,* 1958; Cheney and Finch, 1960). This iron transfer to the plasma is dependent on a copper-containing enzyme (ceruloplasm) which enables transferrin, a plasma protein, to pick up iron for transport to peripheral tissues (Chase *et al.,* 1952; Lee *et al.,* 1968). The transferrin releases its iron to cells and is not in itself ingested. Once absorbed into the body, iron is firmly retained and only very minor amounts are lost daily through urine and sweating. The absorbed iron is utilized mainly for hemoglobin synthesis while smaller amounts are incorporated into myoglobin and a number of enzymes (mainly cytochromes). The excess iron not immediately used for these processes is stored, mainly in macrophages, as ferritin or hemosiderin. The macrophages also ingest and degradate aging erythrocytes and concentrate the iron for reutilization in new hemoglobin synthesis.

Ferrokinetic studies have shown that nearly all iron utilized in hemoglobin synthesis is supplied from transferrin-bound iron (Lajtha and Suit, 1955; Jandl *et al.,* 1959). The greatest uptake of iron is by the proerythroblast, and the least by the reticulocyte (Lajtha and Suit, 1955), although iron is actively taken up by all stages from proerythroblast to reticulocyte. A small and perhaps insignificant amount may enter as preformed ferritin, a protein molecule rich in iron, in pinocytotic vesicles; however, the contribution of ferritin in vesicles as the iron source for hemoglobin is controversial (Jandl *et al.,* 1959; Bessis and Breton-Gorius, 1962).

Erythroblasts and reticulocytes absorb iron from transferrin, probably at specific sites on the cell surface (Jandl, 1960) (Fig. 2-18). Receptors may be at the points of depression, which are the initial formation point of pinocytotic vesicles; however, this has not yet been established.

The function of these receptors may be totally destroyed in vitro by treatment of proteolytic enzymes or blocked by coating the cell surface with macromolecules or by cyanide; however, lead ions do not affect this iron absorption mechanism (Jandl *et al.,* 1959).

Iron transfer through the plasma membrane probably involves an energy-requiring system (Jandl *et al.,* 1959). Radioactive iron appears in particulate fractions first, then gradually in soluble cytoplasmic cell fractions of ultracentrifuged ruptured reticulocytes (Allen and Jandl, 1960). Greenough *et al.,* (1962) observed that iron diffuses in the cytoplasm and is trapped by a nonheme molecule. The time required for iron transfer and incorporation into hemoglobin molecules is estimated at about 8 minutes. Mazur and Carleton (1963) propose that ferritin in reticulocytes plays an intermediate role for iron in hemoglobin synthesis. This conclusion may not be warranted (Zail *et al.,* 1964; Primosigh and Thomas, 1968). Although ferritin is present in reticulocytes, it is mainly in vesicular structures surrounded by the membrane—i.e., outside the cell—and may not be available for active metabolic processes. Dispersed ferritin may be observed in the cytoplasm of developing erythroblasts and, less frequently, in reticulocytes. Those ferritin molecules could act as holding sites for iron in transit to homoglobin. Mitochondria are considered to be the likely site for iron incorporation into the porphyrin for two reasons: (1) Heme synthetase is mainly in mitochondria, and (2) this organelle accumulates excess iron in some types of impaired hemoglobin synthesis. Recent studies in copper-deficient animals (Goodman and Dallman, 1969) have suggested a possible role for intracellular copper compounds in iron transport and/or mitochondrial utilization of iron.

Transferrin, ferritin, and hemosiderin are proteins which are involved in transport and storage of iron.

Transferrin

Transferrin, a plasma protein with a molecular weight of about 90,000, with an electrophoretic mobility of beta globulin fractions, but a solubility that is closer to albumin, is synthesized in liver cells. It binds two ferric ions in tight chelation by three phenolic groups in combination with bicarbonate ion to form a salmon-red complex. This protein is very stable in psysiological pH ranges, but dissociates at low pH in vitro. The half-life of transferrin in plasma has been estimated at 12 days. The formation of transferrin is genetically controlled at a single locus, although at least 12 different transferrins have been isolated. The concentration of transferrin in plasma responds to various factors, such as erythropoietic activity, erythropoietin, and oxygen tension. Iron is chelated to transferrin in such a way that it is released on the surface of erythroblasts and reticulocytes when the plasma iron saturation is more than 20 per cent. However, above 60 per cent saturation there is an apparent nonspecific or toxic release to other cells, such as erythrocytes and liver cells (Bothwell and Finch, 1962). In humans, iron saturation normally remains between approximately one-third and two-thirds of total iron-binding capacity.

Ferritin

Ferritin, a major form of iron storage in body cells (Fig. 2-19), is a molecule composed of protein called apoferritin, with a molecular weight of about 500,000 and diameter of 100 to 110 Å. The molecule contains up to 23 percent of its weight as

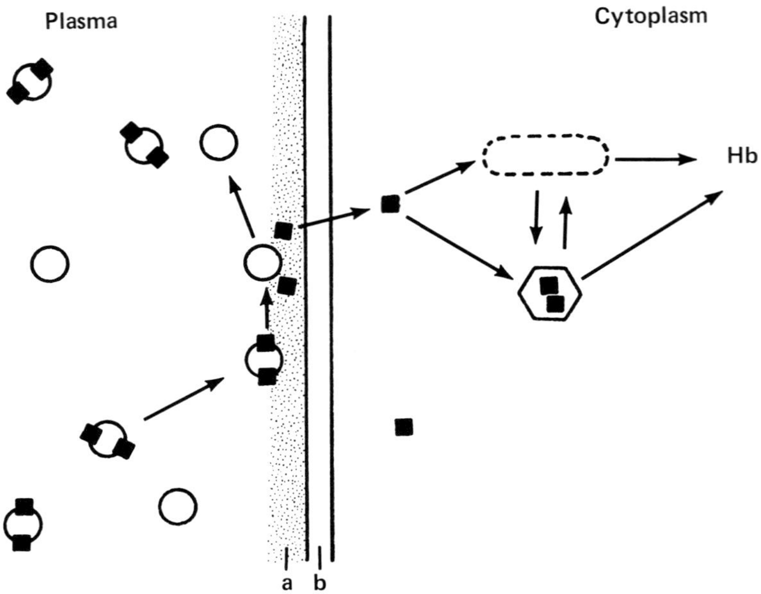

FIGURE 2-18. Iron transport and release on erythroid surface. Iron transport by transferrin and its release, the special coating (*a*) (Jandl, 1960) on the erythroblast or reticulocyte surface (*b*). In the cytoplasm the iron atom may be held as ferritin (*hexagon*) or remain in a soluble form (*oval*). Iron may be utilized from either state for hemoglobin (*Hb*) synthesis.

ferric hydroxyl phosphate ($[FeOOH]_8 \cdot FeOPO_3 H_2$). Iron can be released by various reducing agents, including cystine or hydrosulfate, without denaturation of apoferritin. The iron content in ferritin is probably variable, leading to some variation of the images seen by electron microscopy. Usually the shapes have areas of density suggesting a tetrahedron approximately 55 Å in dimension, though this characteristic has been questioned recently (Haggis, 1965; Haydon, 1969). However, these areas are apparently the dense iron-containing centers of the protein molecule that, by negative staining, is 100 to 110 Å in diameter (Fig. 2-19*B*).

Biosynthesis of apoferritin and ferritin formation occur in a number of organs. In the order of diminishing formation of ferritin, these are spleen, bone marrow, liver, testes, kidney, pancreas, ovaries, and lymph nodes. Apoferritin and ferritin are formed most actively in macrophages, endothelial cells of sinusoids, parenchymal cells of liver, and erythroblasts. Ferritin extracted from reticulocytes and spleen has demonstrated different electrophoretic mobility, a finding that suggests a possible variation in the apoferritin produced in different cells (Gabuzda and Gardner, 1967). Rat liver cells synthesize apoferritin from labeled amino acids and complex it with iron to form ferritin in 4 to 5 minutes (Loftfield and Eigner, 1958). This process is stimulated by the administration of iron to the substrate.

Ultrastructurally, there are two locations of ferritin within cells, either dis-

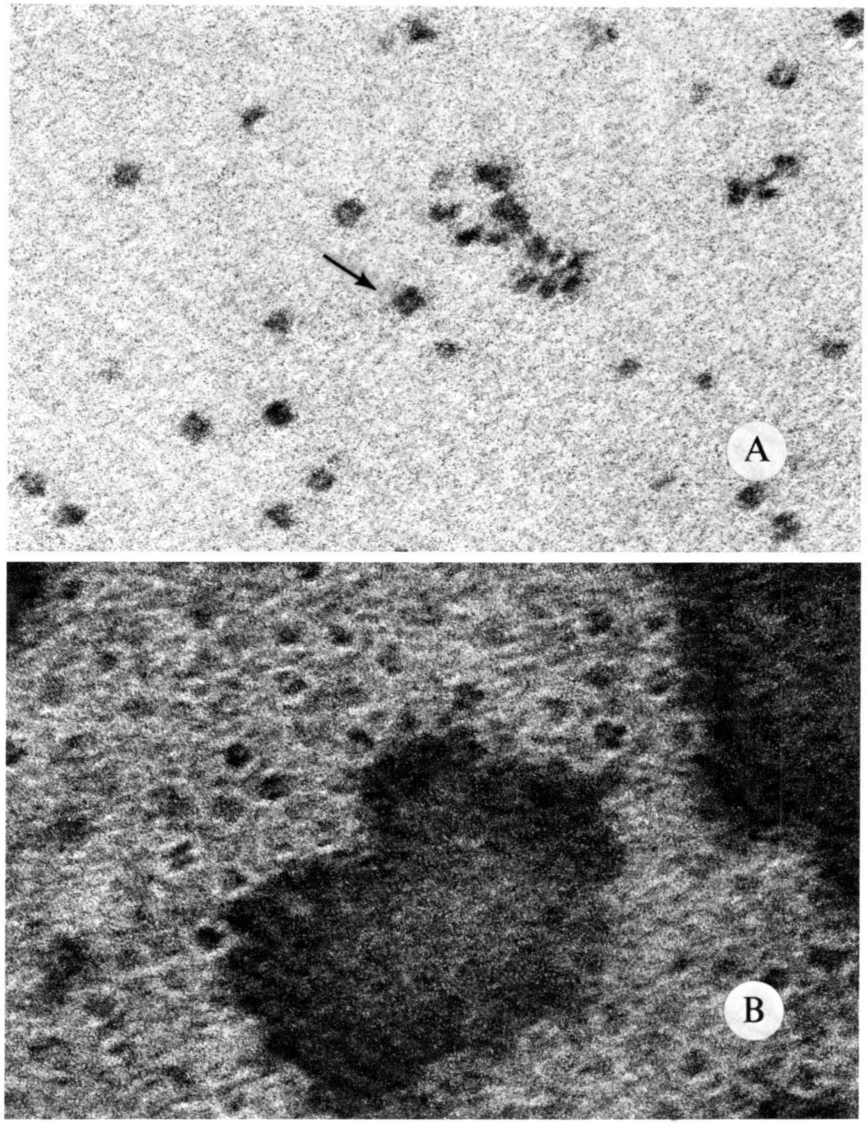

FIGURE 2-19. Isolated ferritin molecules.
A. Electron micrograph showing subunit structures *(arrow)*. × *660,000.*
B. Negatively stained material showing halo of protein around iron-containing, central cores. × *660,000.*

persed freely in the cytoplasm (Fig. 2-20) or contained within single-membrane vesicles (Fig. 2-34*B*). In many tissues the latter form is more common. Macrophages and endothelial cells of liver, spleen, and bone marrow most commonly have ferritin dispersed in their cytoplasm and vesicles. Liver parenchymal cells and erythroblasts may also have both types of ferritin in siderotic conditions; however, no significantly large amounts are noted in normal cells. Ferritin is rarely found in other myelolymphocytic cells even in severe siderotic conditions, except in plasma cells, which accumulate iron when there is siderosis. Ferritin has been demonstrated in vesicles of macrophages in experimental animals with acute siderosis 3 days after iron injections, gradually increasing thereafter. The liver cells of animals which have received large amounts of iron dextran contain dispersed ferritin prior to its appearance in vesicles. After 24 to 48 hours the number of dispersed ferritin molecules becomes stable, in contrast to the gradual increase in ferritin particles in vesicles which also contain ingested iron dextran. Similar correlations in macrophages are not clear since tremendous amounts of dispersed ferritin are present in the cytoplasm after 1 week. Erythroblasts show no increase in dispersed or stromal ferritin, even under severe siderotic conditions. A proposal that apoferritin synthesis in the liver can be inhibited by the administration of actinomycin D, suggests the possibility that the system is operated by nuclear control through mRNA (Drysdale and Munro, 1966; Yoshino *et al.,* 1968).

Hemosiderin

Hemosiderins, a second major form of iron storage, are yellow-to-brown granules noted in the cytoplasm of cells containing iron in ferric form. By electron microscopy, the granules are amorphous masses of irregular density without discernible structure. The iron-containing pigment is derived mainly from hemoglobin of degraded erythrocytes which have been phagocytized. This iron may be stored initially as ferritin, then degraded into hemosiderin, a process that takes 2 to 4 days in macrophages. Iron may be removed completely from hemosiderin in vitro and in vivo. The remaining brown granules are called "hematoidin," the organic complexes of hemosiderins, which are protein- and lipid-containing polysaccharides. It has been speculated that hemosiderins and ferritin are formed independently.

Ultrastructurally, brown granules produced by the injection of large doses of iron appear to consist of ferritin and other forms of iron compounds (Richter, 1959, 1960) compatible with the histochemical characteristics of hemosiderin. Iron-containing substances without definite ferritin form may be produced when the ferritin is treated with proteolytic enzymes (Matioli and Baker, 1963). This suggests that hemosiderin granules found in acute siderosis might be formed by denaturation of ferritin within vesicles which are called "siderosomes" (Richter, 1959; Shoden and Sturgeon, 1963). Iron may also be detected in brown pigments called "lipofuscin," which is nearly indistinguishable from hemosiderin by electron microscopy (Malkoff and Strehler, 1963; Samorajski *et al.,* 1965).

Sideroblasts and Siderocytes

Iron deposits in developing erythroblasts and matured erythrocytes stain blue by the Perl stain on smears. This stain shows iron in the ferric state in hemosiderin and ferritin and does not react with the ferrous iron in hemoglobin. Erythroid cells with these blue-staining granules are called "sideroblasts" if they are nucleated cells and "siderocytes" if they do not have nuclei (Gruneberg, 1941; Kaplan *et al.,* 1954).

Electron microscopically, iron accumulation in developing erythroid cells is classified into two forms: (1) those which cluster or scatter ferritin particles in vesicles of about 0.3 to 0.5μ in diameter, and (2) those which deposit iron in mitochondria (Figs. 2-30 through 2-32). The common types observed in erythroblasts of normal marrows, as well as in some hematological disorders, are accumulations of ferritin in vesicles. The incidence of iron-positive erythrocytes (siderocytes) is very low in circulating blood because iron-containing vesicles tend to be eliminated in passage through the spleen (Crosby, 1957). Hematological disorders in which serum iron is high generally have more ferritin granules in erythroid cells (Kaplan *et al.,* 1954). The second type of iron accumulation was first described by Bessis and Breton-Gorius (1957) in hypochromic hypersiderotic anemia, presently classified as refractory sideroblastic anemia. In this disorder the mitochondria of the erythroblasts accumulate iron between the cristae. When this develops in most mitochondria, with distribution of the stained organelles in a ring around the nucleus (Fig. 2-31), the cells are called "ringed sideroblasts" (Bowman, 1961). These abnormal erythroblasts are most frequently noted in hereditary (Heilmeyer *et al.,* 1962) and acquired sideroblastic anemia (Figs. 2-22 and 2-25) (Bessis and Breton-Gorius, 1957; Sorenson, 1962; Petz *et al.,* 1966). It has been postulated that the defective mitochondrial enzymes involved in heme synthesis are responsible for this phenomenon (Bessis and Jensen, 1965). Iron-laden mitochondria in erythroblasts have been described in other conditions, in patients who had received chloramphenicol treatment (Goodman and Hall, 1966) (Fig. 2-24*A*), and in those with porphyria cutanea tarda (Goodman and Hall, 1966) (Fig. 2-24*C*), mechanical hemolytic anemia (Petz and Goodman, 1966) (Fig. 2-24*B*), severe alcoholism (Grasso and Hines, 1969), and thalassemia (Bessis and Breton-Gorius, 1962). In some conditions, the alteration may be reversible (Goodman and Hall, 1966; Hines, 1969). The phenomenon in these cases may be produced by mitochondrial enzyme defects induced by drug toxicities, correctable when the toxic agent is removed. Human bone marrow rarely shows iron-laden mitochondria in developing erythroblasts of healthy adults, but the presence of such mitochondria is not rare in marrows of certain malignant conditions, such as leukemia or myeloma—with or without treatment. The basis for iron-laden erythroblasts in these conditions is unknown.

Although Bessis and Breton-Gorius (1961) reported that iron-laden mitochondria were common in guinea pig erythroblasts, we have been unable to confirm this observation. Studies of more than 50 guinea pigs, including normal, phenylhydrazine-treated, and iron-loaded by iron dextran injections, produced only one sideroblast. Several cells had a dusty deposition which suggested a fine trace of iron. The incidence could not be interpreted as common. Iron has also been noted in mitochondria of rat liver (Kuff and Dalton, 1957), interstitial cells of bone marrow (Tanaka, 1967), and Sertoli cells of testes following iron injection (Carr *et al.,* 1968). Though iron-laden mitochondria in erythroblasts are regarded as a sign of enzymatic dysfunction, their presence in liver and Sertoli cells is more likely related to the high iron content of the organ.

(*text continues on page 58*)

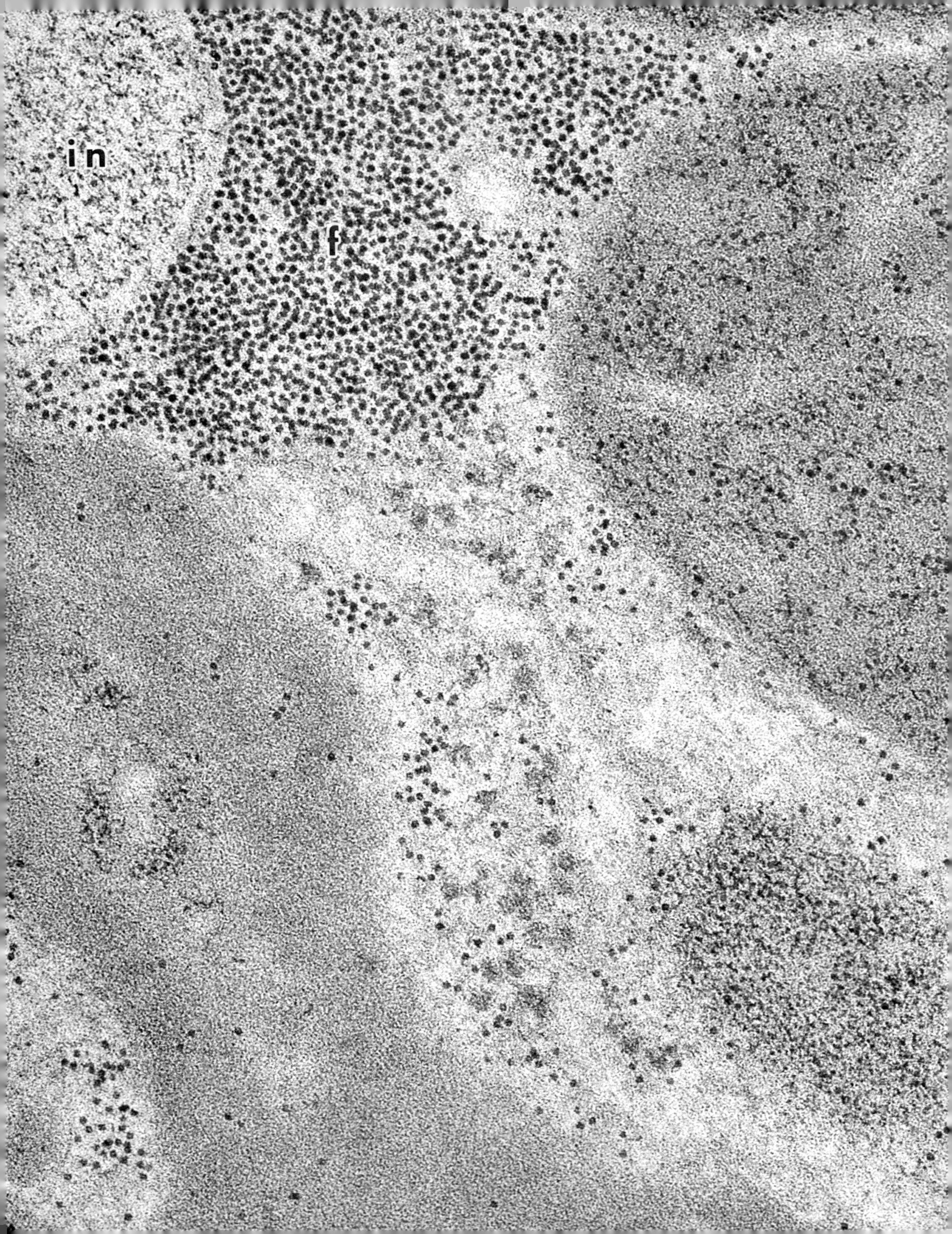
in
f

FIGURE 2-20. Iron-loaded macrophage.
Portion of rat liver macrophage after iron-loading, showing large collection of ferritin (*f*) molecules free in the cytoplasm. Inclusions (*in*) contain some of the injected iron dextran. × *182,000.*

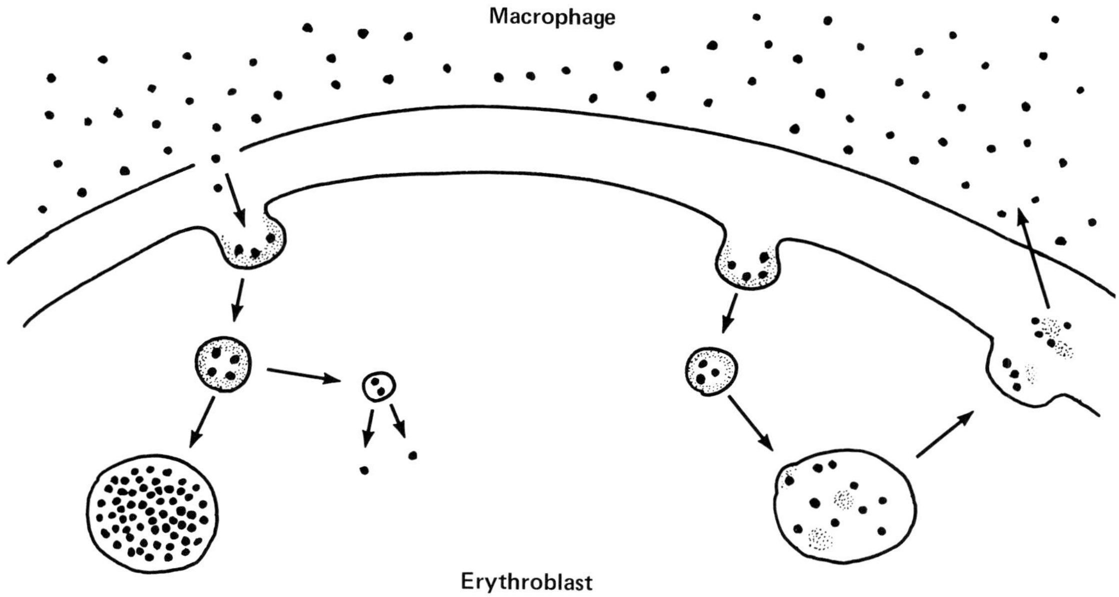

FIGURE 2-21. Ferritin transfer.
Schematic representation of ferritin transfer between a macrophage and an erythroblast. The small dense spots represent ferritin molecules. (*A*) The mechanism proposed by Bessis and Breton-Gorius. (*B*) A probable pathway proposed by Tanaka.

Figures 2-22 and 2-23 appear on the following pages

FIGURE 2-22. Megaloblasts.
Megaloblasts (*Meg*) in different stages of maturation, from patient with vitamin B_{12} deficiency. Mature cell (*upper*) has uniformly granular nucleus (*N*), moderately dense cytoplasm with several mitochondria (*M*), small vesicles, and two larger ferritin-containing vesicles (*arrow*). More immature cell (*bottom*) has pale nucleus (*N*), dense nucleolus (*Nu*), number of mitochondria (*M*), and small vesicles in the cytoplasm. The macrophage (*Ma*) has several small lysosomal vacuoles (*ly*). × *11,300.*

FIGURE 2-23. Degradation of erythroblast.
Macrophage (*Ma*) from same patient as in Figure 2-22 has ingested and started degradation of an erythroblast (*Eb*). The erythroblast has a number of disintegrating mitochondria (*M*). Note many small vesicles (*arrow*) and nucleus (*N*) with scattered masses of chromatin. An eosinophil (*Eo*) is in the vicinity. × *17,600.*

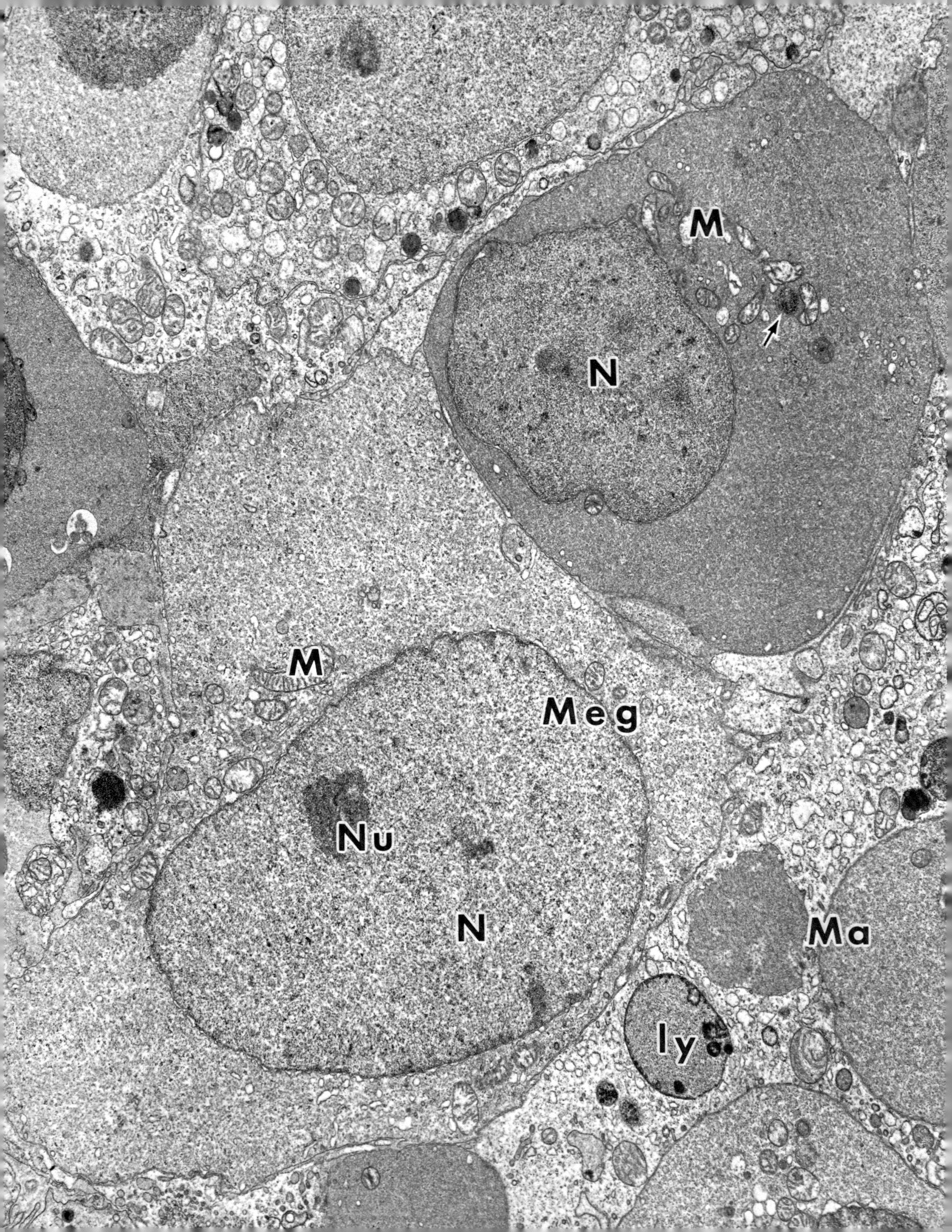
M
N
M
Meg
Nu
N
Ma
ly

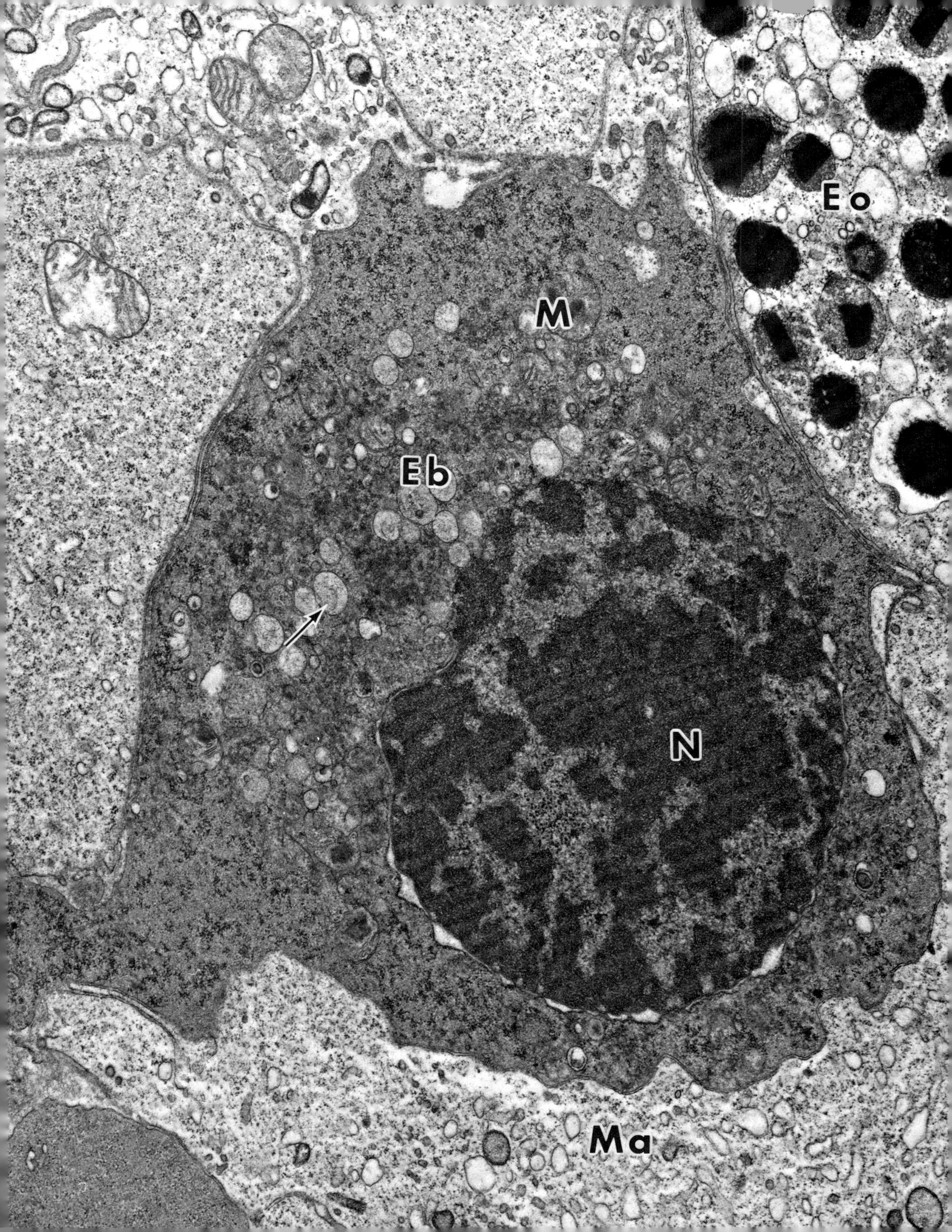
Eo
M
Eb
N
Ma

While the presence of iron-laden mitochondria in developing erythroblasts is well documented (Bessis and Jensen, 1965), it should be stressed that the iron in mitochondria of reticulocytes should be evaluated separately—earlier investigators have not clearly distinguished iron-laden mitochondria in erythroblasts from those in reticulocytes. Iron-laden mitochondria have been noted frequently in reticulocytes in some conditions in which their precursor erythroblasts did not demonstrate this phenomenon (Goodman and Dallman, 1969). Lead poisoning, an example of this phenomenon, may reflect a difference in the lead or iron uptake and metabolism between reticulocytes and erythroblasts.

Erythroblastic Islands

The proliferating erythroblast in both human and animal marrow appears in scattered clusters of cells in the intersinusoidal space. It has been speculated that this island distribution either is due to the immobility of erythroblasts or is important for their maturation. There has been no conclusive evidence that either suggestion is correct.

In electron microscopic studies, Bessis and Breton-Gorius (1959, 1962) examined these erythroblastic islands in hypersiderotic bone marrow and proposed a fundamental role for the macrophages often seen in intimate relationship to erythroblasts. They suggested that the macrophage transfers iron, as ferritin, directly to the erythroblast, and called this process "nursing." They proposed that the bone marrow macrophages ingested damaged or aged erythrocytes and degraded them, concentrating the iron from hemoglobin into ferritin or hemosiderin. The dispersed ferritin was then discharged at the surface and the erythroblast aspirated it through the mechanism of the pinocytotic or rhopheocytotic vesicles (Fig. 2-21). The ferritin contained in small vesicles in the erythroblasts was transported further into the cell, released into the cytoplasm as dispersed ferritin, and utilized as a source of iron in hemoglobin synthesis.

Some modification of this interpretation for the role of ferritin has been suggested. Iron kinetic studies (Pollycove and Mortimer, 1961) show that about 90 per cent of the ^{59}Fe utilized in hemoglobin synthesis is transported by transferrin. Ferritin particles in pinocytotic vesicles are not usually observed in normal human erythropoiesis (Jones, 1965; Tanaka *et al.*, 1966). Although many pinocytotic depressions are seen on the surfaces of erythroblasts of normal marrows, very few have ferritin particles on their surfaces. Ferritin pinocytosis is observed most commonly in pathological states associated with hypersiderosis (Tanaka *et al.*, 1966). In the microgeography of cell juxtaposition, one may find macrophages loaded with ferritin, either in vesicles or free in cells whose cytoplasm may lie beside an erythroblast that has very few or no ferritin-laden pinocytotic depressions along the line of contact. At the same time, erythroblastic ferritin-containing depressions may be present when there is no macrophage cytoplasm apparent. Additionally, there is very little electron microscopic evidence that an excess ferritin uptake results in any increased hemoglobin synthesis. Also, there is no increase in the number of stromal ferritin particles under the conditions which produce a large increase in vesicular bound ferritin.

Other aspects of this problem are apparent when the study of micropinocytosis of ferritin is extended to other species than man. This method of iron access to the erythroblast has been observed only in man and guinea pig (Tanaka, 1970;

Tanaka and Brecher, 1971b). In guinea pig erythroblasts, micropinocytotic ferritin is formed actively in a virtually macrophage-free system in vitro. This appearance of ferritin may be affected significantly by metabolic inhibitors and surface digestion, thus suggesting that ferritin is produced locally by the erythroblast itself (Tanaka and Brecher, 1971a). There is also evidence that ferritin in erythroid cells differs in physicochemical and biochemical properties from ferritin in macrophages (Gabuzda and Pearson, 1969). Further investigation will be required before the mechanisms of intracellular iron movement and metabolism in hemoglobin synthesis are clarified.

PATHOLOGY

NUTRITIONAL DEFICIENCY AND TOXIC ANEMIA

Deficiency of vitamin B_{12} or folic acid results in an anemia characterized by the presence of atypical erythroblasts (megaloblasts) in bone marrow. Clinically, this is typified in pernicious anemia (vitamin B_{12} deficiency), whose etiology was suggested by Minot and Murphy (1926) and has been elaborated by the extensive work of Castle (1966). Other derivations of megaloblastic anemia and their clinical pathological aspects have been summarized by Wintrobe (1967).

Problems relating to the megaloblast and its morphology have been reviewed by Reisner (1958), and ultrastructural aspects of developing megaloblasts in pernicious anemia are available (Ito, 1964). Figures 2-22 and 2-23 are from a patient with typical pernicious anemia whose clinical and hematological signs improved significantly shortly after a single dose of vitamin B_{12}. The nuclei of the megaloblasts in Figure 2-22 do not show the clear chromatin clumping of normal erythroid cells. Electron-opaque spots of various sizes are commonly seen in the nucleus although, occasionally, pronounced differences are observed in the nuclei of the more differentiated erythroid cells. Cytokinetic studies show the presence of cells arrested in development, which are apparently destined to intramedullary death (Wickramasinghe *et al.,* 1969). Some of these defective or dead megaloblasts are phagocytosed by macrophages (Fig. 2-23), a process called "ineffective erythropoiesis" (Goodman *et al.,* 1968). Ultraviolet light microscopy shows a slow rate of RNA disappearance from the cytoplasm and persistence of RNA in the late differentiated forms (Thorell, 1947). By electron microscopy, cytoplasmic ribosomes of megaloblasts appear to be smaller (130 Å or less) than those of corresponding normal erythroblasts (Fig. 2-8). Ferritin deposition in vesicles about 0.3 to 0.5μ is rather common. Upon maturation many of these megaloblasts produce large erythrocytes called macrocytes or megalocytes, which have a low concentration of hemoglobin. Megaloblastic proliferation is converted quickly to normal erythropoiesis after administration of the deficient vitamins. The rapid marrow changes are achieved by the generation of new erythroblasts and improvement of immature erythroid cells which have been least affected by deficient nutrients. (Wickramasinghe *et al.,* 1969).

Insufficient intake of proteins and iron also produces severe anemia with or without marrow aplasia, but such anemia is reversible by administration of the missing nutrient.

A number of toxic agents also produce anemia by inducing suppression of erythroid production which may be sufficiently severe to destroy the capacity of the marrow to replicate. Some effects are reversible when the toxic agent is removed. Lead—at least in respect to its damage to the marrow, if not to other tissues—is in this group. Chloramphenicol, also in this group, causes a mild reversible anemia when used in treatment of certain diseases. These anemias normally do not induce morphologically characteristic changes in cells, except for hypochromia, which is not usually detectable by electron microscopy. However, in some instances iron accumulates within mitochondria.

Pyridoxine deficiency anemia and that created by toxic agents may produce an accumulation of iron within the cristae of the erythroblasts or reticulocytes (Fig. 2-24*A*). The alterations of biochemical mechanisms that results in this deposit are not clear. The significance of iron in mitochondria is discussed above, under Sideroblasts.

HEME SYNTHESIS ABNORMALITY (PORPHYRIA)

Porphyria may be associated with significant hematological abnormalities, in addition to the cardinal sign of skin photosensitivity, including hemolytic anemia and splenomegaly. The basic defect is in the biosynthesis of porphyrin, a precursor of the heme molecule. The disease has been classified into two types: erythropoietic and hepatic, depending upon which organ system is the primary site of the impaired porphyrin synthesis (Watson, 1964).

Abnormalities have been reported in developing erythroid cells in erythropoietic porphyria although most erythroid cells in the marrow appear to be unaffected. These abnormalities include the accumulation of large amounts of porphyrin (Schmid *et al.,* 1955) or hemoglobin (Gross *et al.,* 1965) in the nucleus. Needle-like deposits have been reported in the cytoplasm of both nucleated and non-nucleated erythroid cells (Varadi, 1958), but have not been studied ultrastructurally. Goodman and Hall (1966) reported iron accumulation in mitochondria of developing erythroid cells in porphyria cutanea tarda (Fig. 2-24*C*), a disturbance of hepatic porphyrin synthesis. However, the mitochondria of hepatocytes in these cases had no iron-laden mitochondria.

GLOBIN SYNTHESIS ABNORMALITIES

Sickle Cell Anemia

This genetic abnormality, which transmits erroneous information for hemoglobin synthesis, was originally proposed by Pauling *et al.* (1949) as a specific example of a molecular disease. The abnormal hemoglobin is called Hb-S and the gene is called the Hb-S gene.

The name sickle cell anemia originated from the peculiar transformation of the round mature erythrocytes into a sickle form in vitro, due to crystalloid formation by precipitation of Hb-S in low oxygen tension or by reducing agents. The phenomenon is considered reversible. It is believed to occur in vivo, particularly with low oxygen tension in peripheral vessels or in areas of impaired circulation, leading to its unique clinicopathological manifestations.

Recently, a peculiar configuration of Hb-S in sickled red cells was disclosed by electron microscopy by Murayama (1966), who found microrods of about 170 Å, in whole-mount preparations of sickled cell hemolysates composed of six subunits of about 65 Å in an helical arrangement. He speculated that the rods were twisted filaments of reduced Hb-S molecules. Stetson (1966) observed crystalloid structures, about 150 Å, in cross sections arranged parallel to the axis of sickled red cells in material fixed with glutaraldehyde and embedded in epoxy resins, but not in material fixed with osmic acid—a strong oxidizing reagent. He interpreted the negative-like images of crystalloid as Hb-S. More recently, the observation was extended further by White (1968) who demonstrated bundles of filamentous structures of about 160 to 190 Å in sickled red cells in situ. This structure also was not clearly seen when fixed with osmic acid. Though the crystalloid structures reported by Stetson were electron-lucent images, the positive images of filamentous structures reported by White (1968) could have been similar structures.

Thalassemia

Thalassemia was clearly distinguished by Cooley and Lee (1925) from other hemolytic disorders which showed similar clinical manifestations, so that the name "Cooley's anemia" is used frequently. The thalassemias are a heterogeneous group of inherited red cell disorders. Although the primary genetic defect(s) has not been determined, it is apparent that the abnormality results in impaired synthesis of specific globin polypeptide chains. Thus, in the beta thalassemias, where beta chain synthesis is defective, excess alpha chains may be present in the erythrocytes. These excess alpha chains are unstable and may produce inclusion bodies. In the alpha thalassemias, excess beta chains may be demonstrable by sensitive technics. Accelerated turnover of these excess chains may contribute to the "ineffective erythropoiesis" seen in these disorders.

Beta thalassemia represents the classic form of thalassemia and is fatal at an early age. In heterozygotes, the disease has a mild clinical course but may occur as a genetic complex with other hemoglobinopathies.

Increased amounts of the minor components Hb-F, and occasionally Hb-A2, are found in thalassemia; however, this increase is considered to be a secondary compensatory response to the primary defect in the major hemoglobin component. Bone marrow of thalassemic patients shows significant hyperplasia of erythrocytic cells and an accumulation of iron in interstitial elements. Erythroblasts appear normal, except for the presence of cytoplasmic inclusions. Fessas (1963) studied 24 cases of thalassemia and found inclusions in up to 58 per cent of the total erythroblasts examined. The inclusion in thalassemic erythroblasts can be seen by phase contrast microscopy in living cells as well as in cells supravitally stained by methyl violet. They cannot be detected by the May-Grünwald-Giemsa stain. Specific staining for hemoglobin demonstrates no appreciable difference between inclusions and hemoglobin in the surrounding cytoplasm. Finer inclusions are observed in immature erythroblasts; the larger inclusions in differentiated erythroblasts are believed to be formed by the aggregation of the small particles. The inclusions are thought to be precipitates of excess peptide chains or of denatured hemoglobin. Physical instability of alpha peptide chains under conditions of low ionic strength and oxidation of the heme-iron to the ferric states have been demonstrated. Ultrastructurally, the erythroblasts appear normal except for the inclusion of opaque cytoplasmic material and significant deposition of dispersed ferritin in the cytoplasm (Bessis *et al.,* 1958). Our examination of bone marrows of thalassemic patients confirms descriptions by earlier investigators.

Cells with typical inclusions are shown in Figures 2-25 and 2-26. Inclusions consist of electron-opaque, amorphous, but rod-shaped material in a moderate number of erythroblasts. The precipitates are usually arranged with smaller particles near the middle of the cell and larger aggre-

(*text continues on page 66*)

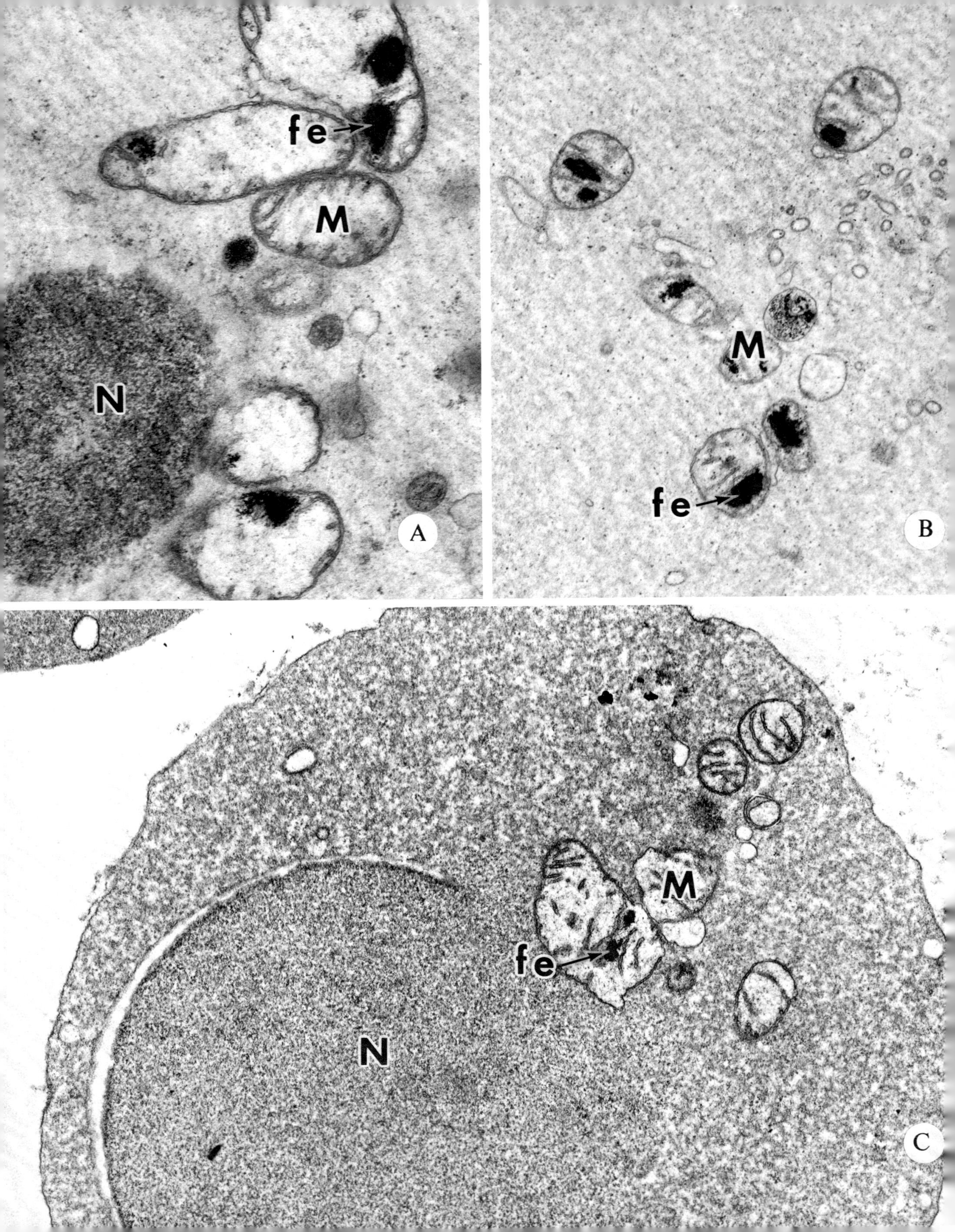
fe
M
N
A
M
fe
B
M
fe
N
C

FIGURE 2-24. Iron accumulations within mitochondria of human erythroblasts in three different anemias.
A. Dense iron deposits (*fe*) from patient who developed anemia when treated with chloroamphenicol. Note distortion of mitochondrial (*M*) structure. Tip of nucleus (*N*) is present. × *31,500.*
B. Iron accumulations (*fe*) in mitochondria (*M*) from patient with hemolytic anemia following a heart valve implant. × *26,500.*
C. Iron accumulation (*fe*) in mitochondria (*M*) of patient with porphyria cutanea tarda. There is an unexplained incomplete nuclear envelope about the nucleus (*N*). Its significance is unknown, and it may not be related to the porphyria. × *24,200.*

Figures 2-25 and 2-26 appear on the following pages

FIGURE 2-25. Erythroblasts from patient with thalassemia showing two types of inclusions (in).
A. Electron-dense spheres, about 0.5μ or less, in two erythroblasts. Part of the nucleus (*N*) is present in one cell. Vesicles (*v*) with ferritin particles (*arrows*) are also present. × *47,500.*
B. Large aggregation of finer precipitates with clustered ferritin (*f*) without limiting membrane. A portion of the nucleus (*N*) has several mitochondria (*M*) near by. × *48,600.*

FIGURE 2-26. Erythroblast cytoplasm from patient with thalassemia.
Inclusions of aggregated dense material are seen and numerous ferritin particles (*arrows*) are freely dispersed in the cytoplasm. × *226,000.*

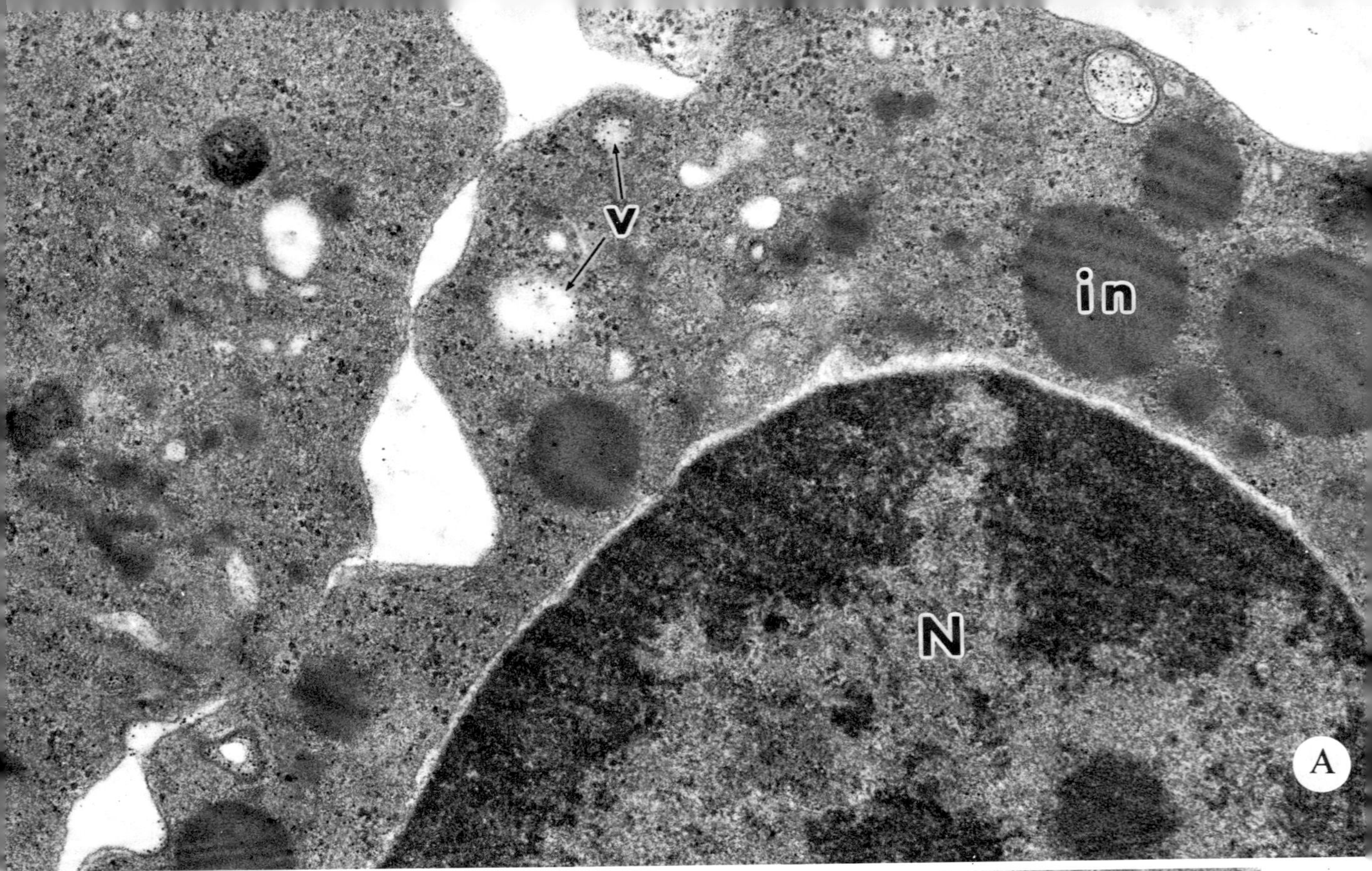
v
in
N
A

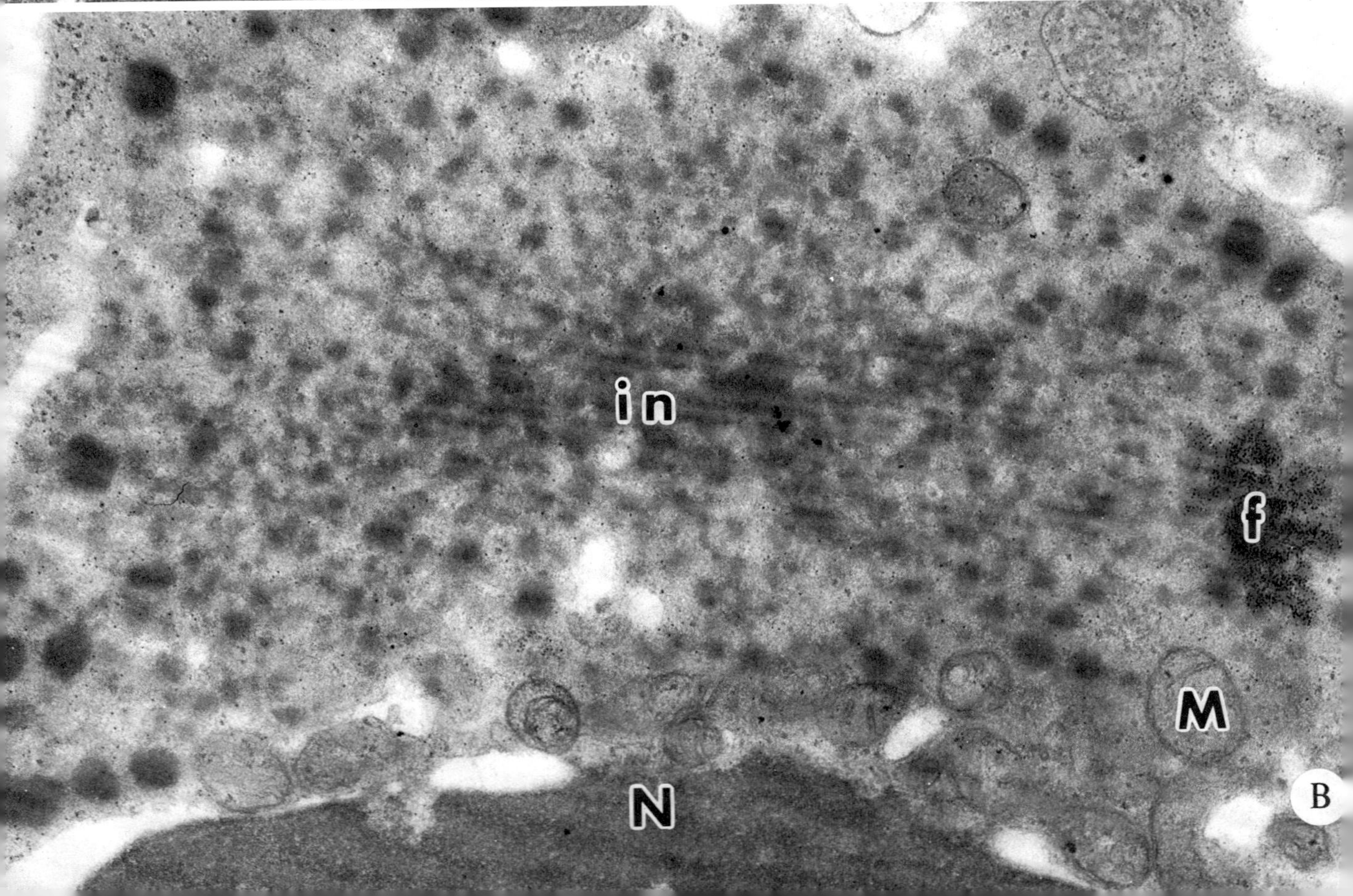
in
f
M
N
B

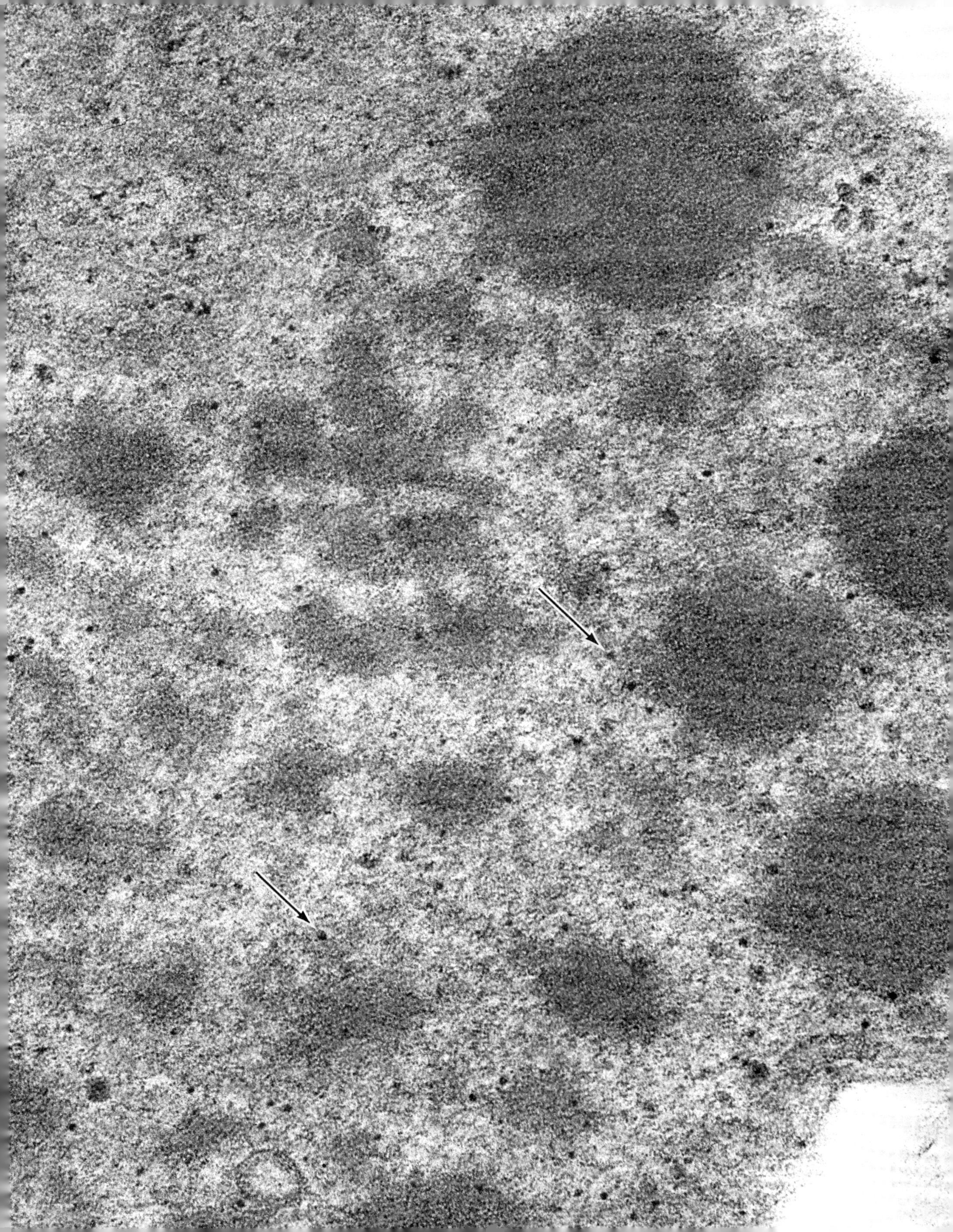

gates in more mature cells nearer the periphery. Small aggregates of electron-opaque, amorphous material are seen in both erythroblasts and erythrocytes. Occasionally, clustered ferritin particles are embedded in these structures (Fig. 2-25*B*) and also in the nonchromatin part of the nucleus. No abnormality is noted in shape and number of polyribosomes except for their relatively small size, and mitochondria are only rarely iron-loaded. Bessis and Breton-Gorius (1959) observed iron-laden mitochondria frequently in erythroblasts of thalassemia; however, this report was later corrected (Bessis and Jensen, 1965) and is now in good agreement with our observation.

The erythrocytes in the peripheral blood of thalassemic patients vary in shape and amount of hemoglobin but only occasionally contain inclusions. The abnormal forms of the erythrocyte are called "teardrops" and target cells. Splenectomized thalassemic patients have fewer teardrop cells but increased erythrocytes with inclusions. This suggests that the teardrop cells are formed during the elimination of inclusions by the spleen (Nathan and Gunn, 1966). Inclusions in mature erythrocytes are believed to be remnants of cytoplasmic inclusions observed in erythroblasts in bone marrows. The hemoglobin content of each thalassemic erythrocyte varies when measured by microspectrophotometry as well as by staining technics (Nathan and Gunn, 1966). Inclusion-bearing cells show strong reaction to Hb-F in specific staining, so that the amount of hemoglobin in each erythroblast may differ quantitatively. Shadow-cast study of erythrocyte ghosts (Hoffman *et al.,* 1956) shows an increased roughness of the surface structure of thalassemic erythrocytes.

Heinz Body Anemia

The presence of the inclusion bodies in matured erythrocytes in hereditary non-specific hemolytic anemia (Lange and Akeroyd, 1958) is similar in morphology to that of Heinz bodies, and this has led frequently to its classification as Heinz body anemia. This group of disorders includes various forms of hemoglobinopathies (Heller, 1966) and an abnormal hemoglobin rather than the enzymatic changes observed in methemoglobinemic patients that produce inclusions in erythrocytes.

Study of the peripheral blood in one of three patients with such inclusions showed no detectable hemoglobin defect (Schmid *et al.,* 1959). The inclusions observed in peripheral blood are morphologically similar to those described in thalassemia, with one large inclusion usually noted in each positive cell. The inclusion is made up of amorphous, electron-opaque, rod-shaped material which aggregates to form a larger inclusion (Fig. 2-27). Frequently, ferritin particles are embedded within these amorphous aggregates, as in the inclusions observed in thalassemia. The erythroid cells with inclusions frequently have mitochondria laden with iron and are included in the aggregates of electron-opaque material. These cells could be reticulocytes; however, no ribosomes are seen. This is quite abnormal when compared with the physiological maturation of reticulocytes in

(*text continues on page 74*)

FIGURE 2-27. Reticulocyte in Heinz body anemia.
Reticulocyte of patient with Heinz body anemia contains aggregate of dense inclusions (*in*), mitochondria (*M*) with iron, and large amounts of ferritin freely dispersed in the cytoplasm. × *97,400.*

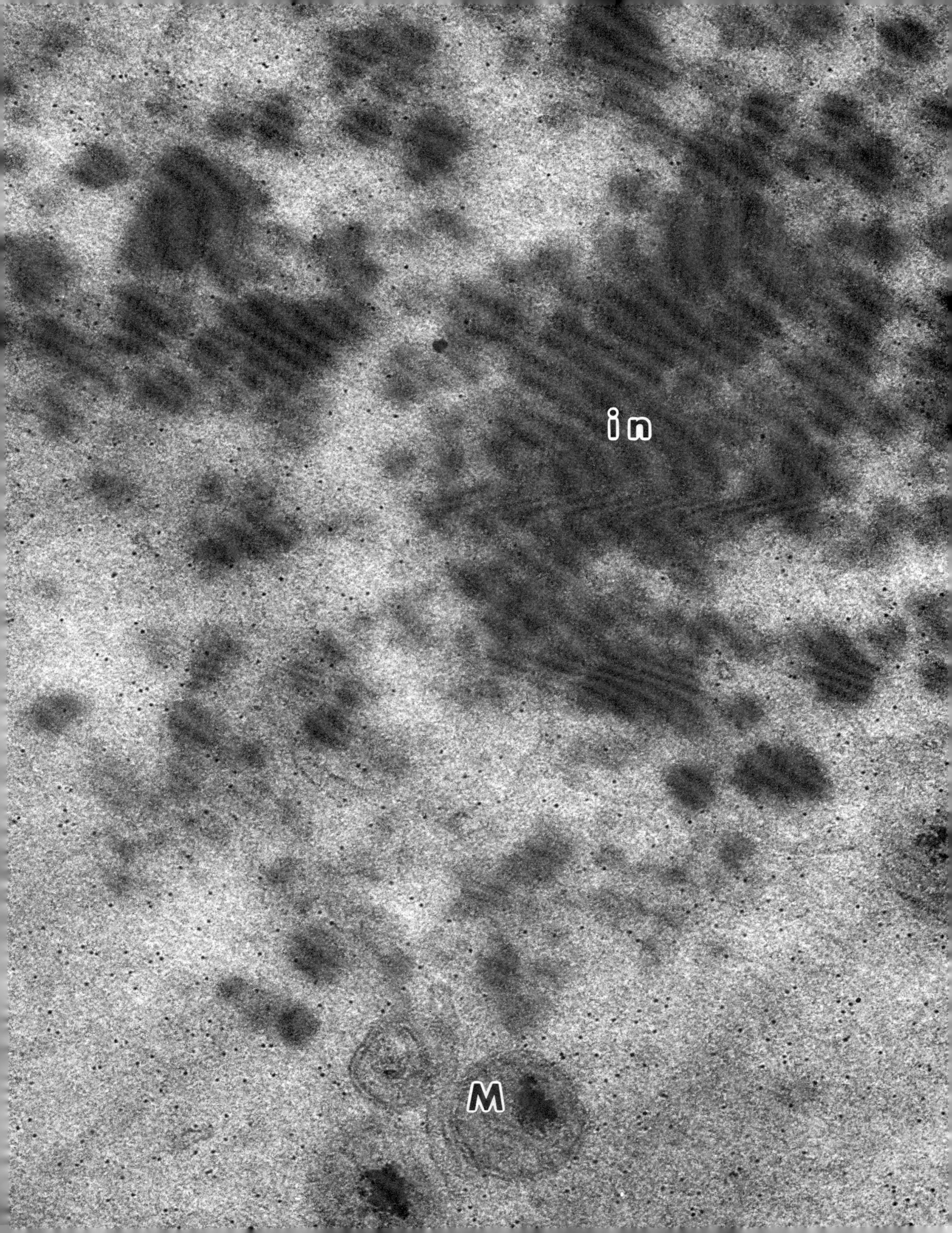
in
M

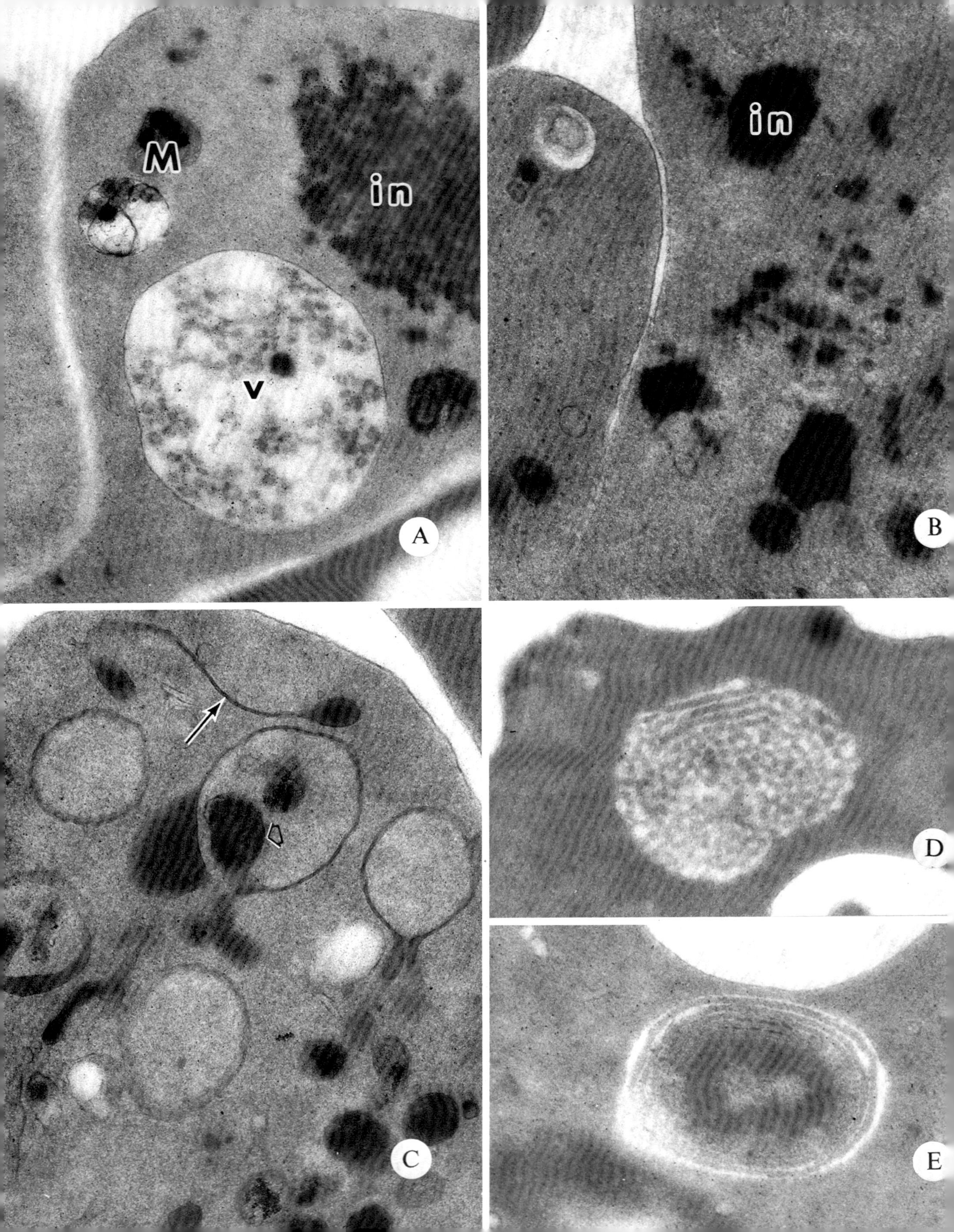
M
in
V
A
in
B
C
D
E

FIGURE 2-28. Erythrocyte inclusions from splenectomized patient with Heinz body anemia.
A. A vacuole (*v*) contains smaller vesicles and some ferritin. There are a residual mitochondrion (*M*) containing some iron and a cluster of dense inclusions (*in*). *× 39,000.*
B. Dense angular inclusions (*in*). *× 39,000.*
C. Unusual double-membrane-bound structures contain electron-dense material within the double membrane (*arrow*) and, in some, within the enclosed lumen (*open arrow*) or vacuolar area. *× 39,000.*
D, E. Inclusions of very small vesicles arrayed in rows (**D**) or in spiral (**E**) configurations. *× 39,000.*

FIGURE 2-29. Bone marrow in sideroblastic anemia.
A. Light micrograph of histological section of bone marrow particle from refractory sideroblastic anemia (H&E stain). Note the immature erythroblasts (*arrows*) with large nuclei and prominent nucleoli. *× 1,000.*
B. Bone marrow smear from same marrow, showing erythrohypoplasia with prominent immature cells. *× 1,000.*

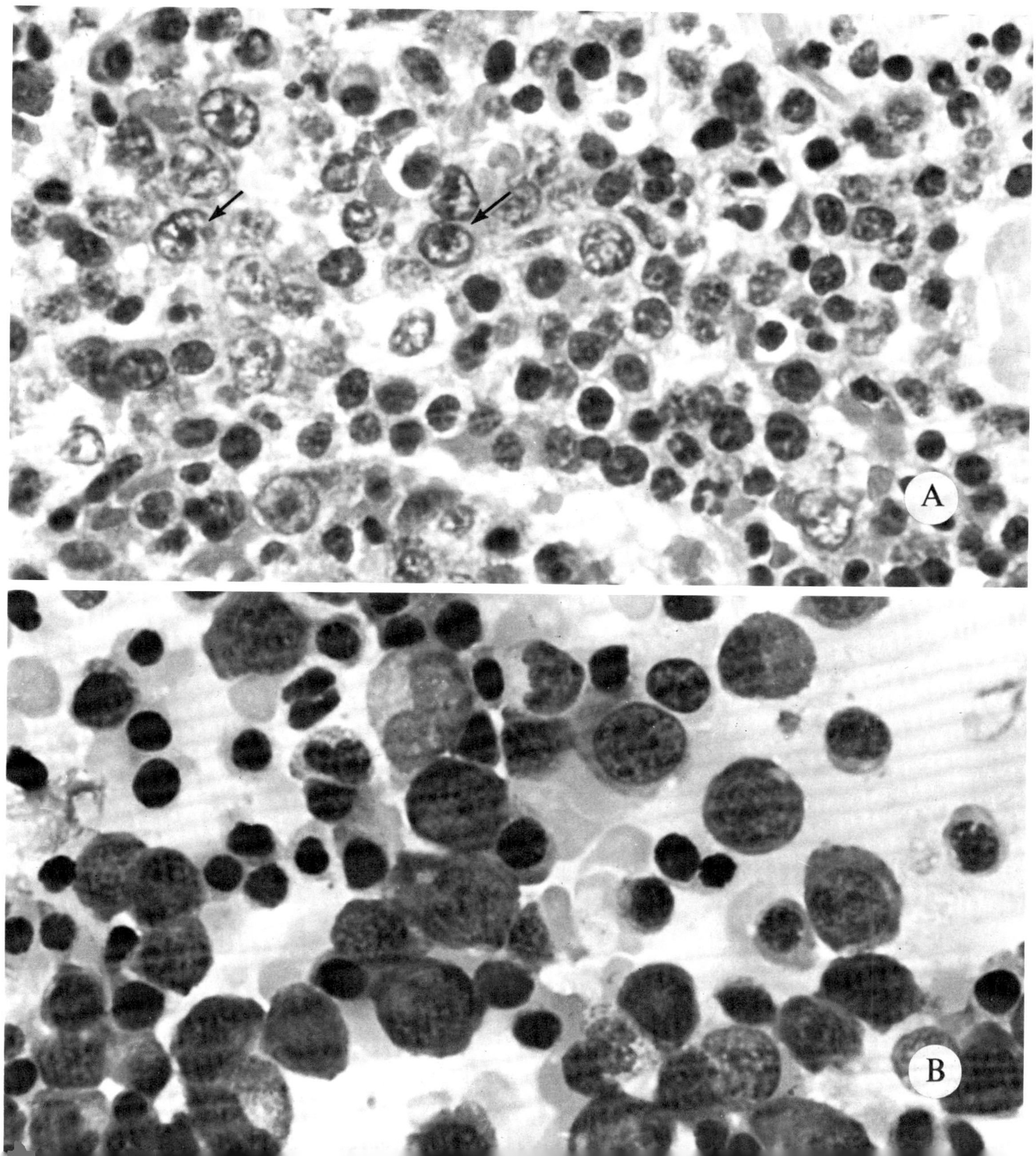

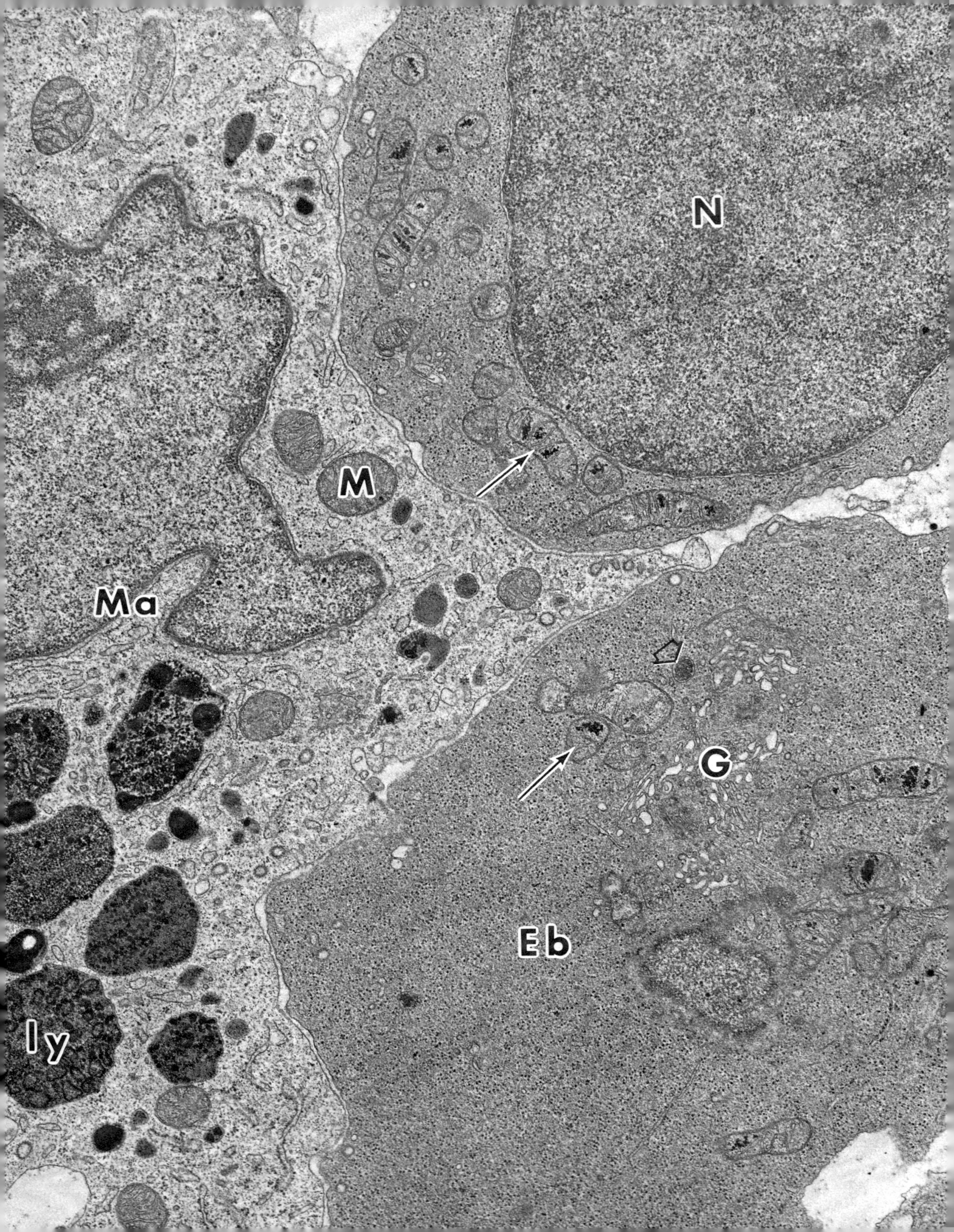
N
M
Ma
G
Eb
ly

FIGURE 2-30. Erythroblastic island.
Erythroblasts (*Eb*) and macrophages (*Ma*) from same marrows as those in Figure 2-29. Mitochondria (*M*) have an accumulation of iron particles between their cristae (*arrows*), the Golgi complex (*G*) is large, and an iron-containing vesicle (*open arrow*) is adjacent. The macrophage has lysosomal vacuoles (*ly*) containing dense material, probably some iron-containing residue from ingested erythrocytic cells. × *18,300.*

Figures 2-31 and 2-32 appear on the following pages ⇨

FIGURE 2-31. Ringed Sideroblast.
Ringed sideroblast from marrow of same patient whose marrow is shown in Figures 2-29 and 2-30. The nucleus (*N*) has ring of iron-containing mitochondria (*M*), some with large dense masses. Numerous vesicles do not appear to contain a significant amount of ferritin. × *25,000.*

FIGURE 2-32. Erythroblasts in sideroblastic anemia.
A. Early erythroblast from same patient as in Figures 2-29 to 2-31, with very large mitochondria (*M*) containing fine granular iron particles that do not appear to be ferritin. Note edge of nucleus (*N*) and some microtubules (*mt*). × *45,000.*
B. Late erythroblast from same patient, with many dense masses of iron in the mitochondria (*M*). Part of the nucleus (*N*) is present. × *60,000.*

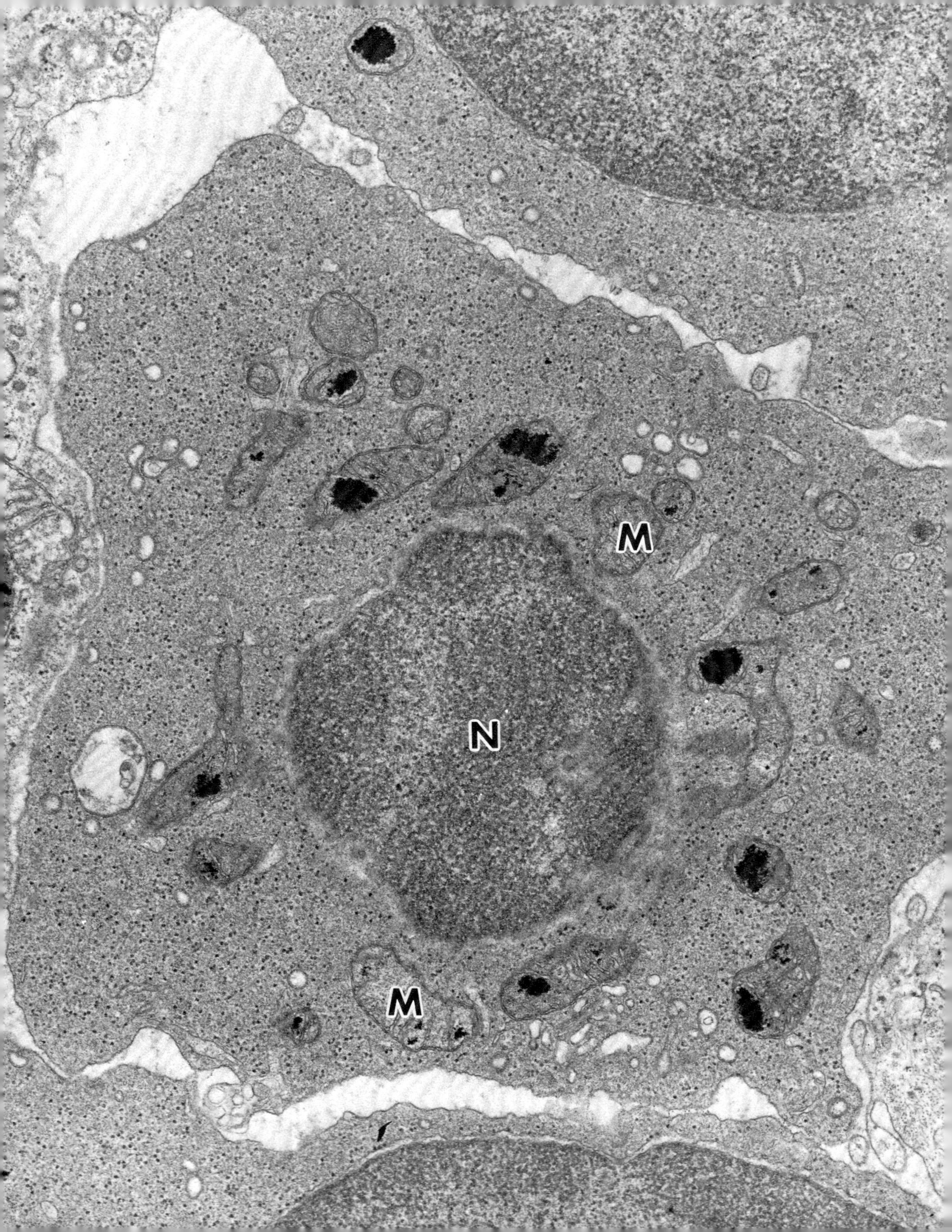
M
N
M

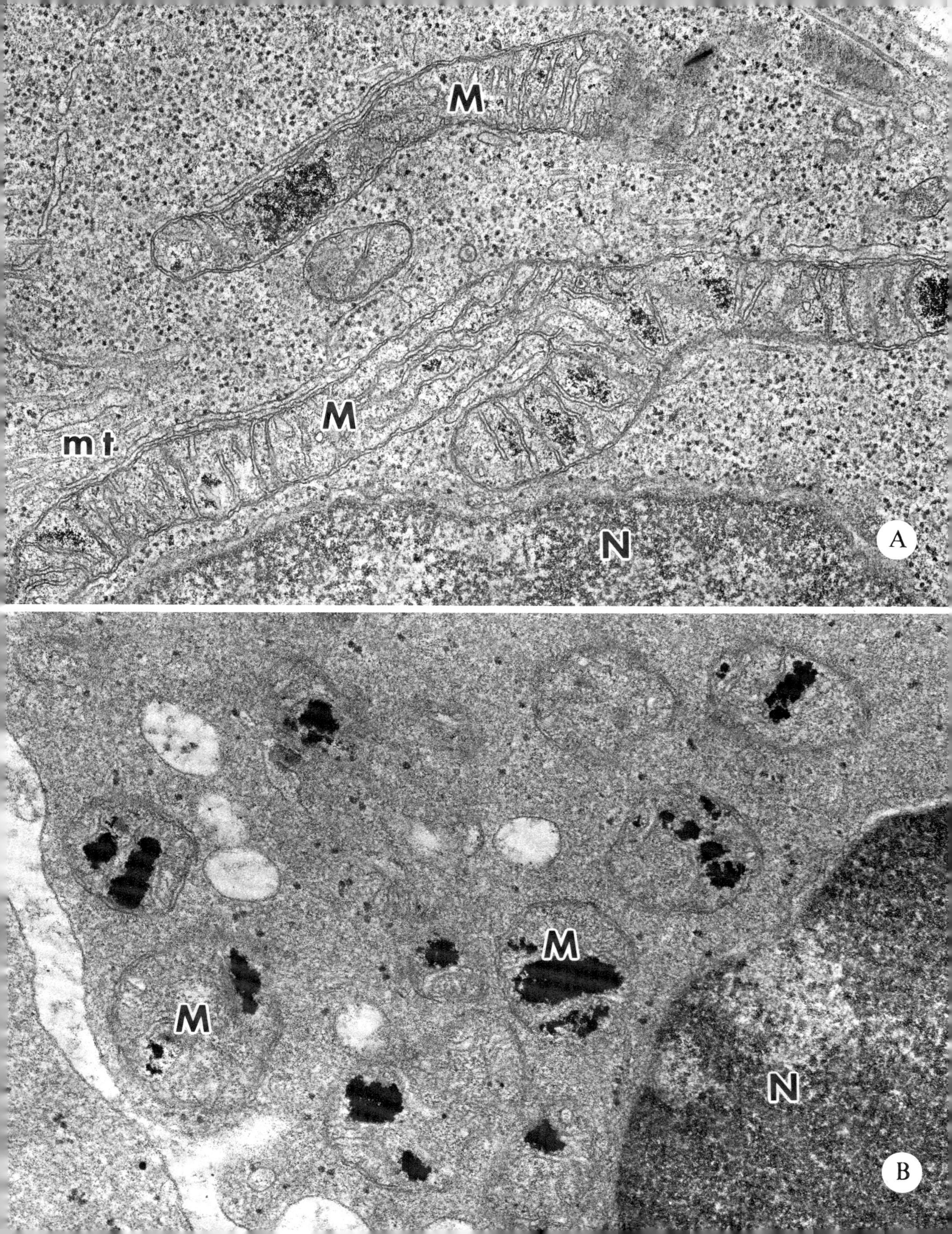
M
M
mt
N
A
M
M
N
B

which mitochondria disappear prior to the complete loss of ribosomes. This suggests either a ribosomal abnormality or a malfunction of the process for the elimination of mitochondria in these reticulocytes. Significant amounts of dispersed ferritin are noted, particularly in erythrocytes with inclusions. Many erythrocytes contain various abnormal structures, some of which are illustrated in Figure 2-28. These abnormal structures may be related to impaired hemoglobin synthesis, and their survival in the cell is due to the absence of the spleen which normally would remove them.

REFRACTORY SIDEROBLASTIC ANEMIA

Sideroblastic anemia is distinguished from other anemias by the presence of ringed sideroblasts (Björkman, 1956; Dacie and Mollin, 1966) and can be either inherited (Heilmeyer *et al.,* 1962) or acquired (Björkman, 1956; Dacie and Mollin, 1966). The inherited disease is rare; it is recognized in early childhood and believed to be due to impaired heme synthesis by an inherited mitochondrial dysfunction which leads to the accumulation of iron in this organelle. Several intermediates of porphyrin synthesis are found in the urine of these patients (Heilmeyer *et al.,* 1962). Most of the reported sideroblastic anemias are of the acquired type and usually occur after middle age. They probably include a variety of disorders and different names have been used by various investigators, which include: normoblastic anemia, refractory sideroblastic anemia, sideroblastic anemia with megaloblastoid change and "myeloproliferative disorders"—particularly the chronic type of Di Guglielmo's syndrome.

The presence of sideroblasts in the acquired type indicates an abnormality of proliferating erythroid precursors. The cause of this is not known, but it is generally classified under the myeloproliferative disorders with a preponderance of erythroid proliferation (Fig. 2-29). The condition frequently leads to myelocytic leukemia, particularly when the megaloblastoid proliferation appears in proliferating erythroid precursors. Dameshek (1965) regarded it as malignant. The significant hematological disorders in this condition are (1) moderate to severe anemia, (2) significant erythroid hyperplasia of bone marrow with a high incidence of ringed sideroblasts, (3) increase in iron absorption and deposition of iron in interstitial elements. There is no remedy available and the outcome is usually fatal.

The contribution of electron microscopy to this disease is perhaps confirmation of the presence of iron-laden mitochondria in the ringed sideroblasts which are characteristic of the lesion. However, it is not known whether the iron-laden mitochondria of erythroblasts represent an essential aspect of this disease. The abnormality may be a manifestation of abnormal erythroid proliferation, an observation first described by Bessis and Breton-Gorius (1959b) and confirmed by many since then (Sorenson, 1962; Petz *et al.,* 1966).

The bone marrow of patients with sideroblastic anemia is usually dominated by proliferating erythroblasts associated with changes in such other elements as megakaryocytes, plasma cells, and interstitial elements, including fixed macrophages. Erythroblastic islands are seen (Fig. 2-30), though a distorted distribution of intermixed young and mature erythroblasts occurs more frequently. A characteristic of the erythroid marrow is the large number of extremely immature forms, which are rather uncommon in physiological marrows. Proerythroblasts are usually noted, together with many intermediate forms between young and mature erythroblasts.

There is no appreciable ultrastructural difference between erythroblasts which proliferate in this condition and in normal marrows except for abnormal mitochondria and a decrease in polyribosomes. Iron-laden mitochondria are common in this disease, but the degree of iron accumulation is variable from one group of proliferating erythroblasts to those nearby. For example, one focus may consist of erythroblasts with significant iron-laden mitochondria in contrast to neighboring cell nests in which no mitochondrial iron is observed in the proliferating erythroblasts. Iron in mitochondria of younger cells is usually dusty in appearance between cristae of the mitochondria (Figs. 2-30 through 2-32). In spite of this, no ferritin particles are clearly identified.

Heavy accumulation of iron is noted in the more mature erythroblasts. The cells with this characteristic usually appear as ringed sideroblasts by Perls' staining of smears. This severe iron accumulation of differentiated erythroblasts deforms and swells the mitochondria and the cristae (Fig. 2-33*A*). In extreme conditions, these damaged mitochondria form inclusions (Fig. 2-33*B*) which may contain other structures, such as tubular endoplasmic reticulum, dispersed ribosomes, and many vesicles that are probably lysosomal in character. No mitochondrial rupture has been noted, which would suggest the release of deposited iron for reutilization in hemoglobin synthesis. Other abnormal cytoplasmic structures are rarely seen in erythroblasts. These include a group of fat droplets (Fig. 2-33*C*) and a cluster of vesicles (Fig. 2-33*D*) that may be a residual of a deformed Golgi apparatus.

Because of the heightened sideremic condition, many other observed morphological characteristics suggest the presence of the excess iron supply and iron deposition in tissues. Erythroblasts have many ferritin particles in their pinocytotic vesicles (Fig. 2-34*A*) and vacuoles (Fig. 2-34*B*), which may represent an attempt to eliminate excess iron. Many ferritin particles are also deposited between adjacent erythroblastic membranes (Fig. 2-34*C*). The phenomenon is closely related to the presence of ferritin in micropinocytotic vesicles of developing erythroid cells (Tanaka and Cushard, 1970). Amorphous material of moderate electron opacity is commonly noted as the background of deposited ferritin particles.

Proliferation of atypical erythroblasts may also be seen. These cells occasionally have an imbalance between nuclear and cytoplasmic maturation. This abnormality may be also observed in the myelocytes. The implications of this are discussed in the next section.

ERYTHREMIC MYELOSIS, ERYTHROLEUKEMIA, DI GUGLIELMO'S SYNDROME

Acute and abnormal proliferation of erythroblasts is frequently called Di Guglielmo's syndrome. The concept of the disease as autonomous and with pure proliferation of erythrocytic cells was first suggested by Di Guglielmo (1928). The condition is considered malignant, as proliferating erythroblasts show various atypical patterns (such as megaloblastoid change and multinucleated and gigantic forms). Originally Di Guglielmo considered the disease to be an entity of erythrocytic abnormality; however, such cases are extremely uncommon (Moeschlin, 1940). Currently, various forms of acute leukoerythroblastic proliferation are included under this concept. The disease often appears first as a mixed proliferation of leukoerythroblasts then terminates

(text continues on page 80)

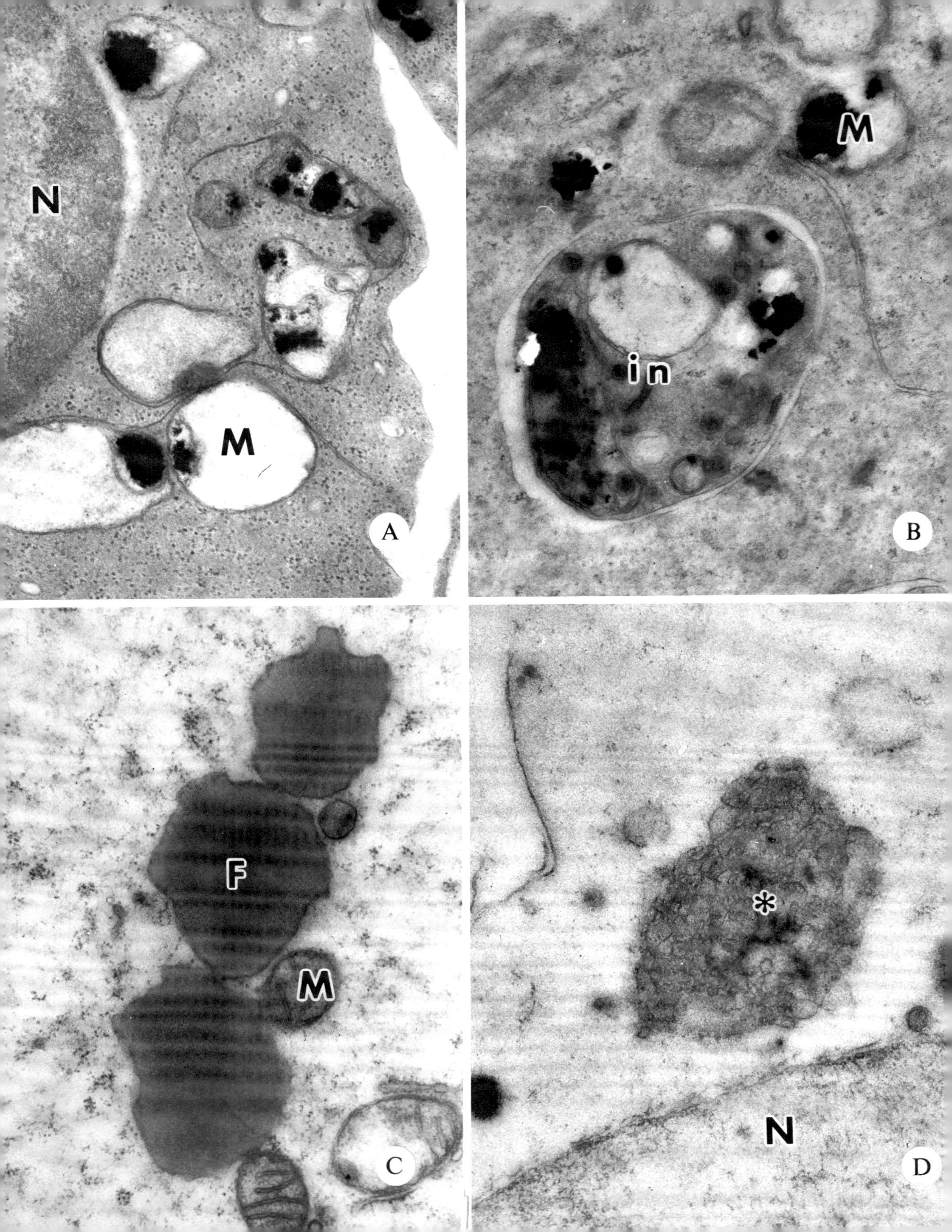
N
M
A
M
in
B
F
M
C
*
N
D

FIGURE 2-33. Erythroblast in sideroblastic anemia.
A. Mitochondrial, (*M*) deformation due to iron deposition in the erythroblast. Portion of nucleus (*N*) shows. × *34,500.*
B. Inclusion (*in*) containing degenerating mitochondria (?) with iron. Another mitochondrion (*M*) also contains iron. × *34,500.*
C. Fat vacuoles (*F*) and three small mitochondria (*M*). × *32,000.*
D. Cluster of small tubules (*asterisk*) near the nucleus (*N*). × *35,600.*

Figures 2-34 and 2-35 appear on the following pages

FIGURE 2-34. Three types of ferritin localization in erythroblasts in sideroblastic anemia.
A. In pinocytotic vesicles (*arrows*). × *89,000.*
B. In a large vesicle (*arrow*), pinocytotic vesicles, and extracellular location. × *75,000.*
C. In extracellular space between adjacent erythroblasts (*arrows*). × *90,000.*

FIGURE 2-35. Large immature cell in erythroleukemia.
The granular nucleus (*N*) has three large dense nucleoli (*Nu*); there are numerous large mitochondria (*M*) and moderate segments of rough endoplasmic reticulum. Identity of the cell is uncertain at this stage of development. × *20,000.*

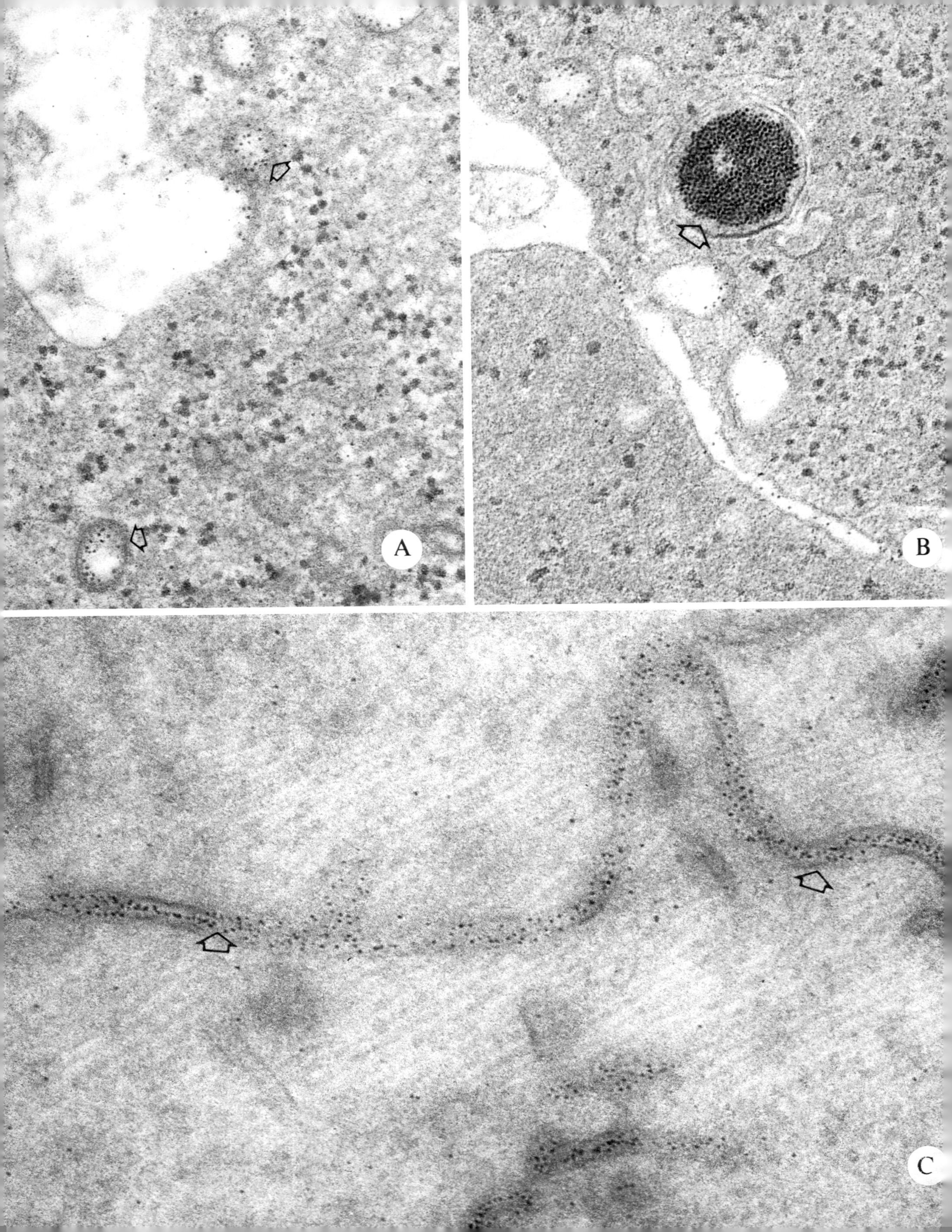
A
B
C

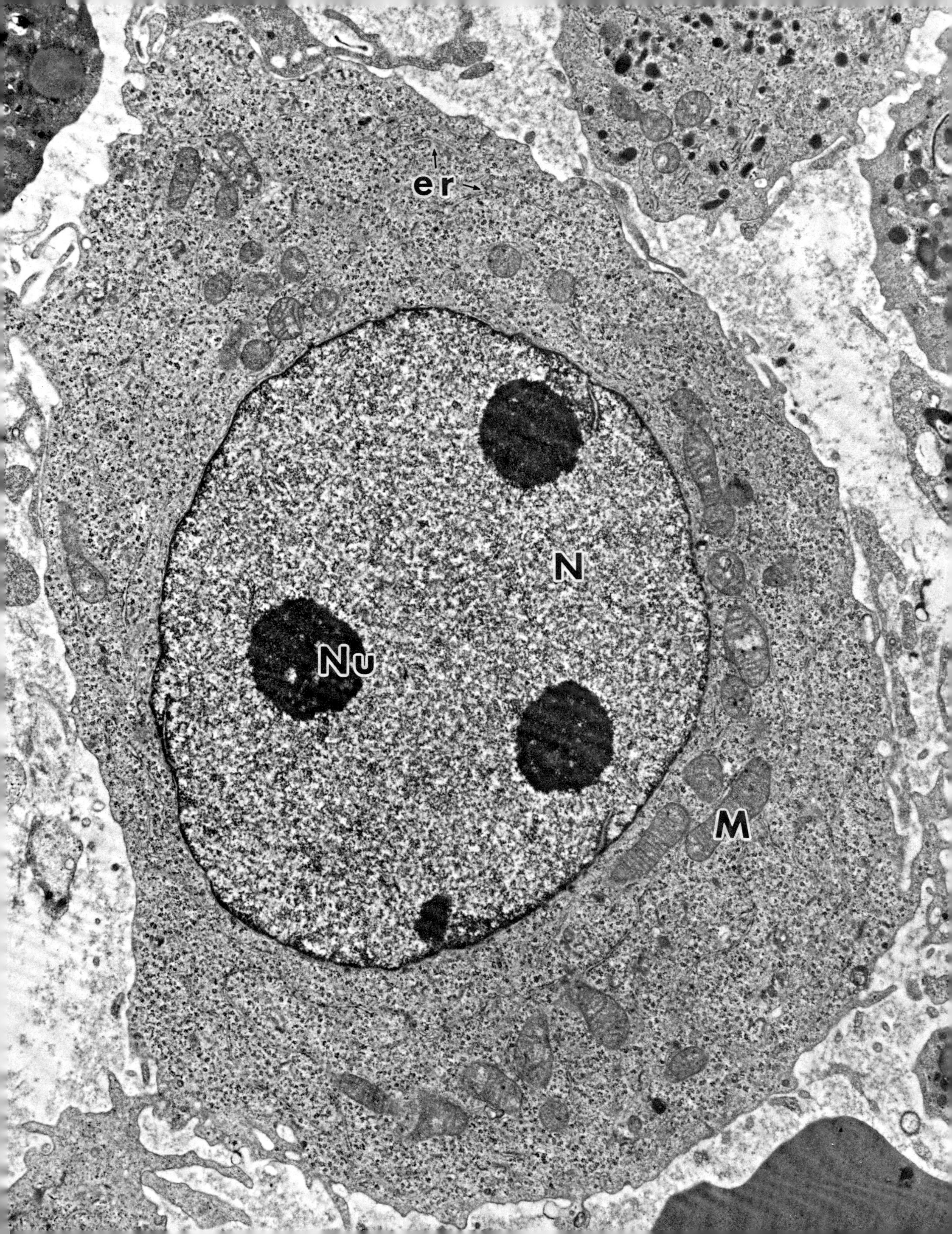
er
N
Nu
M

in acute myelocytic leukemia—i.e., the disease has a polyphasic proliferation. Dameshek and Gunz (1966), distinguished three different hematological stages: erythroblastic erythremic myelosis, mixed erythroblastic and myelocytic proliferation (erythroleukemia), and acute myelocytic leukemia. Any abnormal proliferations which may start with either of the first two of these clinical courses can be included within Di Guglielmo's syndrome. Consequently, certain forms of refractory anemia which are without sideroblasts and which terminate in the leukemic form, can also be included in this concept. However, there is no justification for including all refractory anemias within this concept. The termination of aplastic marrow in typical sideroblastic anemia (Brittin *et al.*, 1968) would not be consistent with this classification.

Since the proliferation is apparently autonomous even if it is not a pure entity, the disease is classed as a malignancy of bone marrow elements. Because of the pleomorphism of the proliferating cells, the malignancy may involve the most immature cellular groups and can develop an abnormal production of several types of blood cells simultaneously. The condition may be analogous to Hodgkin's disease of the lymphocytic line, in which the mother cell of lymphoreticular organs is believed to be involved. As is common in any malignancy, the unique marrow alteration during the course of the disease can be attributed to the following mechanisms:

1. Development of mutation (malignancy) of the stem cell compartment occurs while cell production continues, with final establishment of malignancy in only the myelocytic line; in this sense, abnormal proliferation before establishment of acute myelocytic leukemia may or may not be malignant.
2. Various types of malignant mutants are formed at the beginning, and one group of cells overcomes others during competitive proliferation in the marrow.
3. Both mechanisms are combined.

The second concept is usually more acceptable as the possible mechanism for the establishment of one malignant line of cells. In all representative cases, abnormal proliferation of erythroblasts is recognized throughout the bone marrow and other blood-forming organs. Proliferation of atypical cells tends to form a tiny cluster whose histological features may be considered characteristic of this disease, distinguishing it from myelocytic leukemia. The erythroblasts of these disorders contain large amounts of PAS-positive material, presumably glycogen (Quaglino and Hayhoe, 1960).

Electron microscopic studies make no significant contribution, but only describe various forms of immature elements which are easily identified by light microscopy (Akasaka, 1961). In our unpublished observations, six patients had clinical courses within this category. One patient's bone marrow was consistent with predominant proliferation of erythroblasts, with all types of maturation. The essential alteration was similar to that noted in refractory sideroblastic anemia, except for the absence of iron-laden mitochondria

FIGURE 2-36. Cells in erythroleukemia.
Upper immature cell has more dense cytop'asm, many mitochondria (*M*), much rough endoplasmic reticulum, and a granular nucleus (*N*) containing a large pebbly nucleolus. The other three cells also have granular nuclei (*N*) and one has a large pebbly nucleolus (*Nu*), their cytoplasm has many small granules (*g*), some vacuoles, and mitochondria (*M*). × *11,400.*

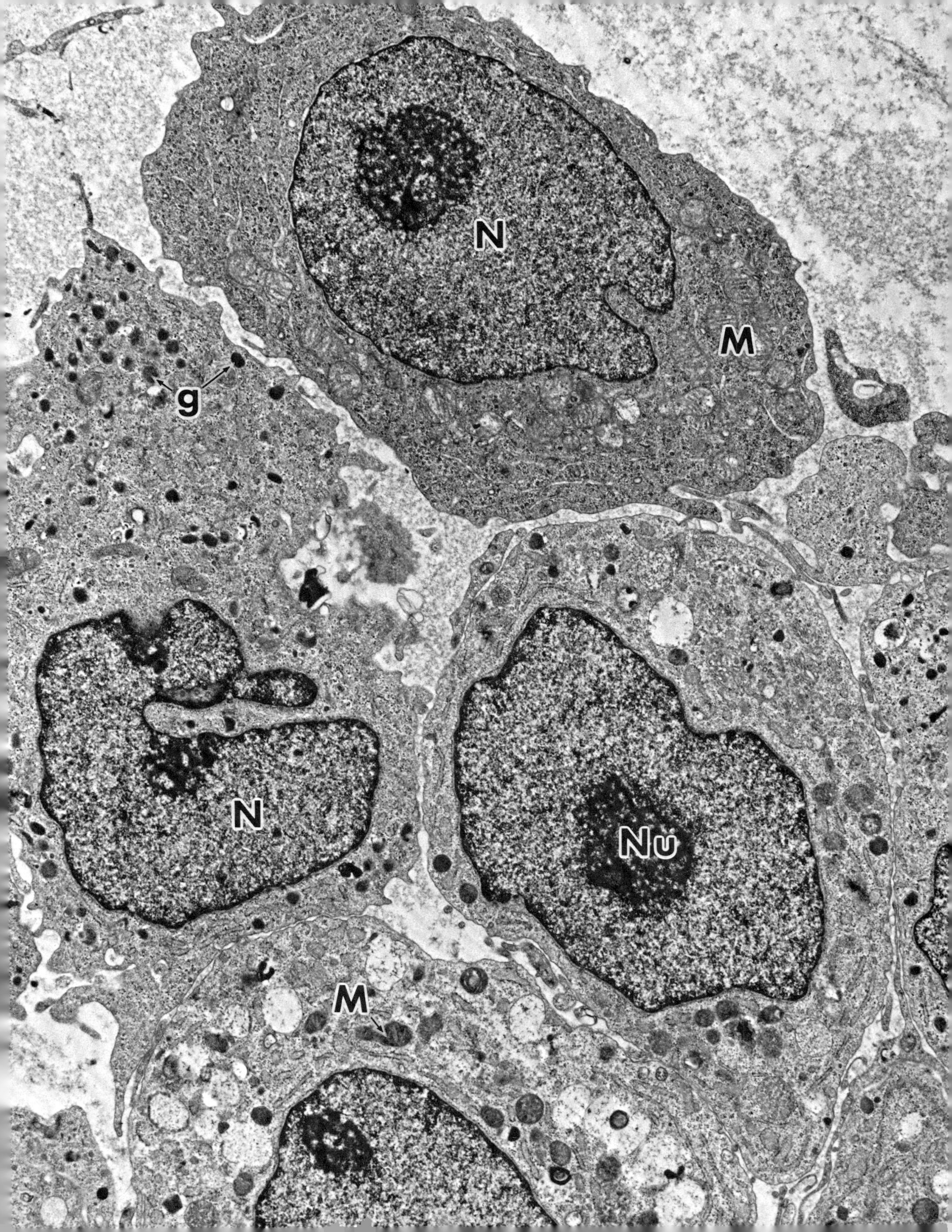
N
M
g
N
Nu
M

in developing erythroblasts. No large number of nucleated erythrocytes appeared in peripheral blood; however, deposition of iron in proliferating macrophages was significantly increased. The patient survived for a long period of time after the onset of the disease, without abnormal proliferation of myelocytes.

Another patient had significant proliferation of erythroblasts in the bone marrow and some nucleated erythrocytes in the peripheral blood. Ultrastructural examination of the bone marrow revealed an absence of iron-laden mitochondria in proliferating erythroblasts; the deposition of iron in the macrophages was not striking. Some areas of the marrow had a proliferation of megaloblastoid cells. Of three marrow specimens examined electron microscopically in a 4-month period, the last two showed proliferation of atypical myelocytic elements; later, an acute myelocytic leukemia developed. Although a significant proliferation of erythrocytic cells was noted before the onset of leukemia, no abnormality of these cells was found by either light or electron microscopy.

Our last four cases were diagnosed as erythroleukemia, or an abnormal erythroid proliferation, which turned into myelocytic leukemia. The marrow showed proliferation of both cell types; however, no significant abnormality was noted in proliferating erythroid cells. Examples from one of these cases are illustrated in Figures 2-35 through 2-37.

FIGURE 2-37. Erythroblasts in erythroleukemia.
A. Binucleated cell of late maturation. Its mitochondria (*arrow*) have masses of iron-containing material between the cristae. The less mature erythroblast (*right*) has several mitochondria, none of which have iron accumulation, and a fairly large Golgi apparatus (*G*). × *10,400.*
B. This group of erythroblasts (*Eb*) around a macrophage (*Ma*) are from same marrow as the cells in Figure 2-37**A**, but have a more normal appearance. × *12,000.*

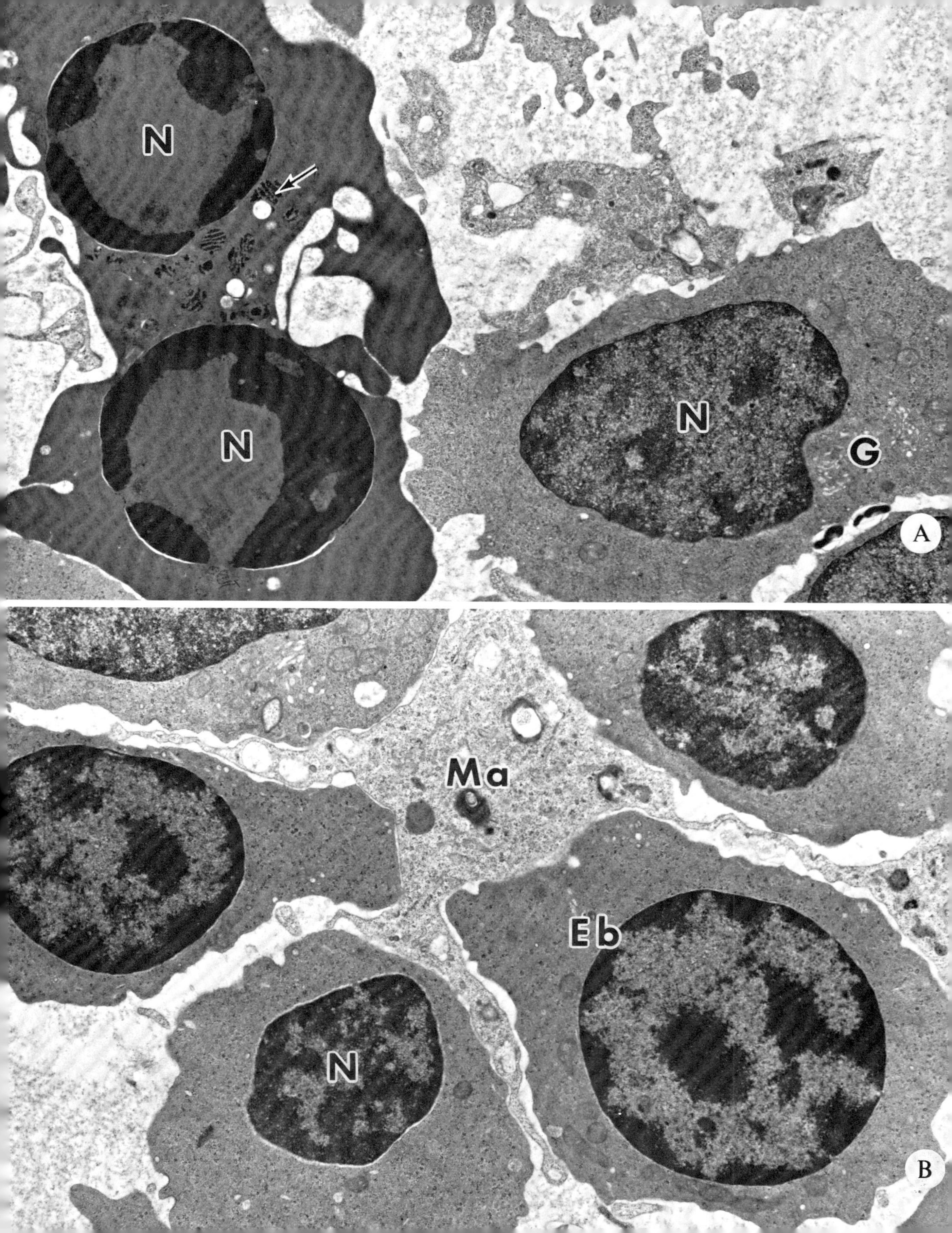
N
N
N
G
A
Ma
Eb
N
B

REFERENCES

Ackerman, G. A., Grasso, J. A., and Knouff, R. A. Erythropoiesis in the mammalian embryonic liver as revealed by electron microscopy. *Lab Invest 10*:787, 1961.

Akasaka, K. An electron microscopic study of blood cells. Ultrastructure of nucleated red cells observed mainly in erythroleukemic cells. *Acta Haemat Jap 24*:519, 1961.

Allen, D. W., and Jandl, J. H. Kinetics of intracellular iron in rabbit reticulocytes. *Blood 15*:71, 1960.

Alpen, E. L., and Cranmore, D. Observations on Regulation of Erythropoiesis and on Cellular Dynamics by Fe^{59} Autoradiography. In *The Kinetics of Cellular Proliferation* (Stohlman, F. Jr., ed.). Grune & Stratton, New York, 1959, p. 290.

Berman, I. The ultrastructure of erythroblastic islands and reticular cells in mouse bone marrow. *J Ultrastruct Res 17*:291, 1967.

Bessis, M., and Breton-Gorius, J. Accumulation de granules ferrugineux dans les mitochondries des érythroblastes. *C R Acad Sc 244:*2846, 1967.

Bessis, M., Alagille, D., and Breton-Gorius, J. Particularitiés des érythroblastes et des érythrocytes dans la maladie de Colley. Étude au microscope électronique. *Rev Hemat 13*:538, 1958.

Bessis, M., and Breton-Gorius, J. Nouvelles observations sur l'ilot érythroblastique et la rhophéocytose de la ferritin. *Rev Hemat 14*:165, 1959a.

Bessis, M. C., and Breton-Gorius, J. Ferritin and ferruginous micelles in normal erythroblasts and hypochromic hypersideremic anemias. *Blood 14*:423, 1959b.

Bessis, M. C., and Breton-Gorius, J. Présence de fer dans les mitochondries des érythroblastes chez la cobaye normal. *Nouv Rev Franc Hemat 1*:356, 1961a.

Bessis, M. C., and Breton-Gorius, J. Ultra-structure du pro-érythroblast. *Nouv Rev Franc Hemat 1*: 529, 1961b.

Bessis, M. C., and Breton-Gorius, J. Iron metabolism in the bone marrow as seen by electron microscopy: a critical review. *Blood 19*:635, 1962.

Bessis, M. C., and Jensen, W. N. Sideroblastic anemia, mitochondria and erythroblastic iron. *Brit J Haemat 11*:49, 1965.

Bessis, M. *Life Cycle of the Erythrocyte.* Sandoz, Basel, 1966.

Björkman, S. E. Chronic refractory anemia with sideroblastic bone marrow. A study of four cases. *Blood 11*:250, 1956.

Bloom, W., and Bartelmez, G. W. Hematopoiesis in young human embryos. *Amer J Anat 67*:21, 1940.

Bloom, W., and Fawcett, D. W. *A Textbook of Histology* (9th ed.). Saunders, Philadelphia, 1968.

Bonsdorff, E., and Jalavisto, E. A humoral mechanism in anoxic erythrocytosis. *Acta Physiol Scand 16*:150, 1948.

Borsos, T., Dourmashkin, R. R., and Humphrey, J. H. Lesions in erythrocyte membranes caused by immune haemolysis. *Nature* (*London*) *202*:251, 1964.

Bothwell, T. H., and Finch, C. A. *Iron Metabolism.* Little, Brown, Boston, 1962.

Bowman, W. D., Jr. Abnormal ("ringed") sideroblasts in various hematologic and non-hematologic disorders. *Blood 18*:662, 1961.

Brecher, G., and Stohlman, F., Jr. Reticulocyte size and erythropoietic stimulation. *Proc Soc Exp Biol Med 107*:887, 1961.

Breton-Gorius, J. and Stralin, H. Formation de cils rudimentaires dans les cellules sanguines, primitives du sac vitellin d'embryons de rat et de poulet. *Nouv Rev Franc Hemat 7*:79, 1967.

Brittin, G. M., Stohlman, F. Jr., and Tanaka, Y. A primary sideroblastic anemia terminating in bone marrow aplasia. *Amer J Clin Path 50*:467, 1968.

Brown, J. R., Altschuler, N., and Cooper, J. A. D. Erythropoietic effect of red cell components and heme-related compounds. *Proc Soc Exp Biol Med 112*:840, 1963.

Buck, R. C., and Tisdale, J. M. The fine structure of the mid-body of the rat erythroblast. *J Biophys Biochem Cytol 13*:109, 1962.

Carr, I., Clegg, E. J., and Meek, G. A. Sertoli cells as phagocytes: an electron microscopic study. *J Anat 102*:501, 1968.

Castle, W. B., and Minot, G. R. *Pathologic Physiology and Clinical Description of the Anemia.* Oxford Univ. Press, New York, 1936.

Castle, W. B. Treatment of pernicious anemia: Historical aspects. *Clin Pharmacol Ther 7*:147, 1966.

Ceresa-Castellani, L., and Lanzavecchia, G. Recherches sur le cyle du fer dans la rate de Triton (Triturus cristatus Laur). *J Microscopie 5*:65, 1966.

Chase, M. S., Gubler, C. J., Cartwright, G. E., and Wintrobe, M. M. Studies on copper metabolism. IV. The influence of copper on the absorption of iron. *J Biol Chem 199*:757, 1952.

Cheney, B., and Finch, C. A. Effect on inosine on iron absorption in rats. *Proc Soc Exp Biol Med 103*:37, 1960.

Cooley, T. B., and Lee, P. Series of cases of splenomegaly in children with anemia and peculiar bone change. *Trans Amer Pediat Soc 37*:29, 1925.

Crosby, W. H. Siderocytes and the spleen. *Blood 12*:165, 1957.

Dacie, J. V., and Mollin, D. L. Siderocytes, sideroblasts and sideroblastic anemia. *Acta Med Scand Suppl 445*:237, 1966.

Dameshek, W. Sideroblastic anemia. Is this a malignancy? *Brit J Haemat 11*:52, 1965.

Dameshek, W., and Gunz, F. *Leukemia.* Grune & Stratton, New York, 1966.

Danon, D., and Marikovsky, Y. Morphologie des membranes des érythrocytes jeunes et âgés. Observations au microscope électronique. *C R Soc Biol 155*:12, 1961.

Di Guglielmo, G. Le eritremie. *Haematologica 9*: 301, 1928.

Dourmashkin, R. R., and Rosse, W. Morphologic changes in the membranes of red blood cells undergoing hemolysis. *Amer J Med 41*:699, 1966.

Drysdale, J. W., and Munro, H. N. Regulation of synthesis and turnover of ferritin in rat liver. *J Biol Chem 241*:3630, 1966.

Ehrlich, P. *Farbenanalytische Untersuchungen zur Histologie und Klinik des Blutes.* Hirschwald, Berlin, 1891.

Fawcett, D. W. Local specialization of the plasmalemma in micropinocytotic vesicles of erythroblasts. *Anat Rec 148*:370, 1964.

Fessas, P. Inclusions of hemoglobin in erythroblasts and erythrocytes of thalassemia. *Blood 21*:21, 1963.

Gabuzda, T. G., and Gardner, F. H. Observations on Fe^{59} labeled bone marrow ferritin. *Blood 29*: 770, 1967.

Gabuzda, T. G., and Pearson, J. Metabolic and molecular heterogeneity of marrow ferritin. *Biochim Biophys Acta 194*:50, 1969.

Goodman, J. R., and Hall, S. G. Accumulation of iron in mitochondria of erythroblasts. *Brit J Haemat 13*:335, 1966.

Goodman, J. R., Wallerstein, R. O., and Hall, S. G. The ultrastructure of bone marrow histiocytes in megaloblastic anemia and the anemia of infection. *Brit J. Haemat 14*:471, 1968.

Goodman, J. R., and Dallman, P. R. Role of copper in iron localization in developing erythrocytes. *Blood 34*:747, 1969.

Grasso, J. A., Swift, H., and Ackerman, G. A. Observations on the development of erythrocytes in mammalian fetal liver. *J Cell Biol 14*:235, 1962.

Grasso, J. A., and Hines, J. D. A comparative electron microscopic study of refractory and alcoholic sideroblastic anemia. *Brit J Haemat 17*: 35, 1969.

Gray, C. H., Neuberger, A., and Sneath, P. H. A. Studies in congenital porphyria. 2. Incorporation of ^{15}N in stercobilin in the normal and in the porphyric. *Biochem J 47*:87, 1950.

Greenough, W. B., III, Peters, T., Jr., and Thomas, E. D. An intracellular protein intermediate for hemoglobin formation. *J Clin Invest 41*:1116, 1962.

Gross, S., Schoenberg, M. D., and Mumaw, V. R. Electron microscopy of the red cells in erythropoietic porphyria. *Blood 25*:49, 1965.

Gruneberg, H. Siderocytes: A new kind of erythrocytes. *Nature (London) 148*:114, 1941.

Haggis, G. H. The iron oxide core of the ferritin molecule. *J. Molec Biol 14*:598, 1965.

Haydon, G. B. Visualization of substructure in ferritin molecules: an artifact. *J Microscopy 89*: 251, 1969.

Heilmeyer, V. L., Merker, H., Molbert, E., and Neidhardt, M. Zur Mikromorphologie der hereditares hypochromen sideroaehretischen Anämie. *Acta Haemat 27*:78, 1962.

Heinz, R. Morphologische Veränderungen der rothen Blutkörperchen durch Gifte. *Virchow Arch Path Anat 122*:112, 1890.

Heller, P. Hemoglobinopathic dysfunction of the red cell. *Amer J. Med 41*:799, 1966.

Hines, J. D. Reversible megaloblastic and sideroblastic marrow abnormalities in alcoholic patients. *Brit J Haemat 16*:87, 1969.

Hoffman, J. F., Wolman, I. J. Hillier, J., and Parpat, A. K. Uutrastructure of erythrocyte membranes in thalassemia major and minor. *Blood 11*:946, 1956.

Ito, K., Ito, N., Sato, S., and Katsunuma, H. Electron microscopic study on the megaloblasts in pernicious anemias. *Acta Haemat Jap 27*:436, 1964.

Jandl, J. H., Inman, J. K., Simmons, R. L., and

Allen, D. W. Transfer of iron from serum iron-binding protein to human reticulocytes. *J Clin Invest 38*:161, 1959.

Jandl, J. H. The agglutination and sequestration of immature red cells. *J Lab Clin Med 55*:663, 1960.

Jensen, W. N., Moreno, G. D., and Bessis, M. C. An electron microscopic description of basophilic stippling in red cells. *Blood 25*:933, 1965.

Jones, O. P. Electron Microscopic Studies of Primitive Erythrocytes. In *Proceedings of the 9th Congress of the European Society of Hematology (Lisbon)*. S. Karger, Basel, New York, 1963, Part II/1, pp. 1–4.

Jones, O. P. Decrease in pinocytosis accompanying maturation of erythroblasts. *Anat Rec 148*: 296, 1964.

Jones, O. P. Selective binding sites for the transfer of ferritin into erythroblasts. I. Preliminary report. *J Nat Cancer Inst 35*:139, 1965.

Kaplan, E., Zuelzer, W. W., and Mouriquand, C. Sideroblasts. A study of stainable non-hemoglobin iron in marrow normoblasts. *Blood 9*:203, 1954.

Killmann, S. A., Cronkite, E. P., Fliedner, T. M., and Bond, V. P. Mitotic indices of human bone marrow cells. III. Duration of some phases of erythrocytic and granulocytic proliferation computed from mitotic indices. *Blood 24*:267, 1964.

Knoll, W., and Pingel, E. Der Gang der Erythropoese beim menschlichen Embryo. *Acta Haemat 2*:369, 1949.

Koyama, S., Aoki, S., and Deguchi, K. Electron microscopic observations of the splenic red pulp with special reference to the pitting function. *Mie M J 14*:143, 1964.

Kubanek, B., Rencricca, N., Porcellini, A., and Stohlman, F., Jr. Growth Patterns of Hemopoiesis Derived from Fetal Liver Transplanted into Heavily Irradiated Mice. In *Hemopoietic Cellular Proliferation* (Stohlman, F., Jr., ed.). Grune & Stratton, New York, 1970, p. 205.

Kuff, E. L., and Dalton, A. J. Identification of molecular ferritin in homogenates and sections of rat liver. *J Ultrastruct Res 1*:62, 1957.

Lajtha, L. G., and Suit, H. D. Uptake of radioactive iron (^{59}Fe) by nucleated red cells *in vitro*. *Brit J Haemat 1*:55, 1955.

Lajtha, L. G., and Oliver, R. A Model of the Erythron. In *Ciba Symposium on Haematopoiesis* (Wolstenholme, G. E. W., and O'Conner, M., eds.). Little, Brown, Boston, 1960, p. 289.

Lange, R. D., and Akeroyd, J. H. Congenital hemolytic anemia with abnormal pigment metabolism and red cell inclusion bodies: a new clinical syndrome. *Blood 13*:950, 1958.

Lee, G. R., Nacht, S., Lukens, J. N., and Cartwright, G. E. Iron metabolism in copper-deficient swine. *J Clin Invest 47*:2058, 1968.

Loftfield, R. B., and Eigner, E. A. The time required for the synthesis of a ferritin molecule in rat liver. *J Biol Chem 231*:925, 1958.

London, I. M., West, R., Shemin, D., and Rittenberg, D. Porphyrin formation and hemoglobin metabolism in congenital porphyria. *J Biol Chem 184*: 365, 1950.

Luccarelli, G., Rizzoli, V., Delsignor, R., Rencricca, N., Porcellini, A., Ferrari, L., Carnevali, C., Howard, D., and Stohlman, F., Jr. Humoral Regulation of Fetal and Neonatal Erythropoiesis. In *Hemopoietic Cellular Proliferation* (Stohlman, F., Jr., ed.). Grune & Stratton, New York, 1970, p. 197.

Malkoff, D. B., and Strehler, B. L. The ultrastructure of isolated and in situ human cardiac age pigment. *J Cell Biol 16*:611, 1963.

Marikovsky, Y., and Danon, D. Electron microscope analysis of young and old red cells stained with colloidal iron for surface charge evaluation. *J Cell Biol 43*:1, 1969.

Matioli, G. T., and Baker, R. F. Denaturation of ferritin and its relationship with hemosiderin. *J Ultrastruct Res 8*:477, 1963.

Maximow, A. A. Relation of blood cells to connective issues and endothelium. *Physiol Rev 4*:533, 1924.

Mazur, A., Green, S., Saha, A., and Carleton, A. Mechanism of release of ferritin iron *in vivo* by xanthine oxidase. *J Clin Invest 37*:1809, 1958.

Mazur, A., and Carleton, A. Relation of ferritin iron to heme synthesis in marrow and reticulocytes. *J Biol Chem 238*:1817, 1963.

Minot, G. R., and Murphy, W. P. Treatment of pernicious anemia by a special diet. *JAMA 87*:470, 1926.

Moeschlin, S. Erythroblastosen, Erythroleukämien und Erythroblastämien. *Folia Haemat 64*:262, 1940.

Murayama, M. Molecular mechanism of red cell "sickling." *Science 153*:145, 1966.

Nathan, D. G., Piomelli, S., and Gardner, F. H. The synthesis of heme and globin in the maturing human erythroid cell. *J Clin Invest 40*:940, 1961.

Nathan, D. G., and Gunn, R. B. Thalassemia: the consequences of unbalanced hemoglobin synthesis. *Amer J Med 41*:815, 1966.

Neumann, E. Ueber die Bedeutung des Knochenmarks für die Blutbildung. *Zbl Med Wiss 6*:689, 1868.

Pauling, L., Itano, H. A., Singer, S. J., and Wells, I. C. Sickle-cell anemia, molecular disease. *Science 110*:543, 1949.

Petz, L. D., Goodman, J. R., Hall, S. G., and Fink, D. J. Refractory normoblastic ("sideroblastic") anemia. Clinical and electron microscopic observations. *Amer J Clin Path 45*:581, 1966.

Petz, L. D., and Goodman, J. R. Ringed sideroblasts and intramitochondrial iron in cases of mechanical hemolytic anemia. *Ann Intern Med 64*: 635, 1966.

Policard, A., and Bessis, M. Sur un mode d'incorporation des macromolécules par la cellule, visible au microscope électronique. *CR Acad Sci 246*: 3194, 1958.

Pollycove, M., and Mortimer, R. The quantitative determination of iron kinetics and hemoglobin synthesis in human subjects. *J Clin Invest 40*: 753, 1961.

Primosigh, J. V., and Thomas, E. D. Studies on the partition of iron in bone marrow cells. *J Clin Invest 47*:1473, 1968.

Quaglino, D., and Hayhoe, F. G. J. Periodic-acid-Schiff positivity in erythroblasts with special reference to Di Guglielmo's disease. *Brit J Haemat 6*:26, 1960.

Reisner, E. H., Jr. The nature and significance of megaloblastic blood formation. *Blood 13*:313, 1958.

Richter, G. W. The cellular transformation of injected colloidal iron complexes into ferritin and hemosiderin in experimental animals: A study with the aid of electron microscopy. *J Exp Med 109*:197, 1959.

Richter, G. W. The nature of storage iron in idiopathic hemochromatosis and in hemosiderosis. Electron, optical, chemical and serologic studies on isolated hemosiderin granules. *J Exp Med 112*:551, 1960.

Riess, L. Ueber Vergiftung mit chlorsaurem Kalium, *Berlin Klin Wschr 19*:785, 1882.

Rifkind, R. A., Danon, D., and Marks, P. A. Alterations in polyribosomes during erythroid cell maturation. *J Cell Biol 22*:599, 1964.

Rifkind, R. A., and Danon, D. Heinz-body anemia, an ultrastructural study. I. Heinz-body formation. *Blood 25*:885, 1965.

Rifkind, R. A. Heinz-body anemia: An ultrastructural study. II. Red cell sequestration and destruction. *Blood 26*:433, 1965.

Rohr, K. *Das menschliche Knochenmark.* Thieme, Stuttgart, 1960.

Roth, T. F., and Porter, K. R. Specialized Sites on the Cell Surface for Protein Uptake. In *Proceedings of the 5th International Congress for Electron Microscopy* (S. S. Breese, ed.). Academic Press, New York, 1962, vol. 2, p. LL4.

Samorajski, T., Ordy, J. M., and Keefe, J. R. The fine structure of lipofuscin age pigment in the nervous system of the aged mice. *J Cell Biol 26*:779, 1965.

Sánchez-Medal, L., Labardini, J., and Loria, A. Hemolysis and erythropoiesis. I. Influence of intraperitoneal administration of whole hemolysates on the recovery of bled dogs, as measured by changes in the total erythrocytic volume. *Blood 21*:586, 1963.

Schmid, R., Schwartz, S., and Sundberg, H. D. Erythropoietic (congenital) porphyria: A rare abnormality of normoblasts. *Blood 10*:416, 1955.

Schmid, R., Brecher, G., and Clemens, T. Familial hemolytic anemia with erythrocytic inclusion bodies and a defect in pigment metabolism. *Blood 14*:991, 1959.

Seno, S., Miyahara, M., Asakura, H., Ochi., O., Matsuoka, K., and Toyama, T. Macrocytosis resulting from early denucleation of erythroid precursors. *Blood 24*:582, 1964.

Shoden, A., and Sturgeon, A. On the formation of haemosiderin and its relation to ferritin. II. A radioisotopic study. *Brit J Haemat 9*:513, 1963.

Simpson, F., and Kling, J. M. The mechanism of mitochondrial extrusion from phenylhydrazine-induced reticulocytes in the circulating blood. *J Cell Biol 36*:103, 1968.

Skalak, R., and Brånemark, P. I. Deformation of red blood cells in capillaries. *Science 164*:717, 1969.

Skutelsky, E., and Danon, D. An electron microscopic study of nuclear elimination from the late erythroblast. *J Cell Biol 33*:625, 1967.

Skutelsky, E., and Danon, D. Reduction in surface charge as an explanation of the recognition by macrophages of nuclei expelled from normoblasts. *J Cell Biol 43*:8, 1969.

Sorenson, G. D. An electron microscopic study of hematopoiesis in the yolk sac. *Lab Invest 10*: 178, 1961.

Sorenson, D. G. Electron microscopic observations of bone marrow from patients with sideroblastic anemia. *Amer J Path 40*:297, 1962.

Stetson, C. A. The state of hemoglobin in sickled erythrocytes. *J Exp Med 123*:341, 1966.

Stohlman, F., Jr. Observations on the changes in

the kinetics of red cell proliferation following irradiation and hypertransfusion. *Blood 16*:1777, 1960.

Stohlman, F., Jr., Lucarelli, G., Howard, D., Morse, B., and Leventhal, B. Regulation of erythropoiesis. XVI. Cytokinetic patterns in disorders of erythropoiesis. *Medicine 43*:651, 1964.

Tanaka, Y., Brecher, G., and Bull, B. Ferritin localization on the erythroblast cell membrane and rhopheocytosis in hypersiderotic human bone marrows. *Blood 28*:758, 1966.

Tanaka, Y. Iron laden mitochondria in reticulum cells of hypersiderotic human bone marrows. *Blood 29*:727, 1967.

Tanaka, Y. Bi-directional transport of ferritin in guinea pig erythroblasts *in vitro. Blood 35*:793, 1970a.

Tanaka, Y. Unpublished data. 1970b.

Tanaka, Y., and Cushard, J. A. Crystalloid array of ferritin particles on the plasma membrane of guinea pig erythroblasts. *J Ultrastruct Res 33*: 436, 1970.

Tanaka, Y. An electron microscopic analysis on stromal ferritin of developing erythroid cells and its significance in impaired hemoglobin synthesis. *Acta Haemat Jap 34:*109,1971.

Tanaka, Y., and Brecher, G. Effect of surface digestion and metabolic inhibitors on appearance of ferritin in guinea pig erythroblasts *in vitro.* Evidences for the production of apoferritin on the erythroblast cell membrane. *Blood. 37*:211, 1971a.

Tanaka, Y., and Brecher, G. Micropinocytotic ferritin in erythroid cells: Species dependency and relation to serum iron levels. *Blood. 38:*431, 1971b.

Tavill, A. S., Grayzel, A. I., London, I. M., Williams, M. K., and Vanderhoff, G. A. The role of heme in the synthesis and assembly of hemoglobin. *J Biol Chem 243*:4987, 1968.

Thorell, B. The relation of nucleic acids to the formation and differentiation of cellular proteins. *Sympos Quant Biol 12*:247, 1947.

Varadi, S. Haematological aspects in a case of erythropoietic porphyria. *Brit J Haemat 4*:270, 1958.

Watson, C. J. Porphyrin Metabolism. In *Disease of Metabolism* (5th ed.) (Duncan, G., ed.). Saunders, Philadelphia, 1964.

Webster, S. H. Heinz body phenomenon in erythrocytes. A review. *Blood 4*:479, 1949.

Weed, R. I., and Reed, C. F. Membrane alterations leading to red cell destruction. *Amer J Med 41*:681, 1966.

White, J. G. The fine structure of sickled hemoglobin *in situ. Blood 31*:561, 1968.

Wickramasinghe, S. N., Chalmers, D. G., and Cooper, E. H. Arrest of cell proliferation and protein synthesis in megaloblasts of pernicious anemia. *Acta Haemat 41*:65, 1969.

Wintrobe, M. M. *Clinical Hematology* (6th ed.). Lea & Febiger, Philadelphia, 1967.

Yoshino, Y., Manis, J., and Schachter, D. Regulation of ferritin synthesis in rat liver. *J Biol Chem 243*:2911, 1968.

Zail, S. S., Charlton, R. W., Torrance, J. D., and Bothwell, T. H. Studies on the formation of ferritin in red cell precursors. *J Clin Invest 43*: 670, 1964.

Zamboni, L. Electron microscopic studies of blood embryogenesis in humans. II. The hemopoietic activity in fetal liver. *J Ultrastruct Res 12*:525, 1965.

chapter 3
GRANULOCYTES

Granulocytes of both peripheral blood and myeloid tissues in man can be classified into three major categories—neutrophils, eosinophils, and basophils—on the basis of the staining character of their cytoplasmic granules. Mast cells—cells that contain larger metachromatic granules and are observed near the vasculature of various organs—are considered to be akin to basophils and, therefore, are included in the granulocyte category and discussed with the basophils. The appearance of granules in circulating leukocytes in other animal species may differ from their appearance in man, probably a reflection of the chemical variations of their granular constituents. Small granules of an azurophilic nature can be observed in all types of granulocytes. However, they cannot be said to characterize granulocytes since they occasionally are seen in other marrow cells, such as plasma cells, lymphocytes, megakaryocytes, and monocytes. Though they appear similar on staining, their chemical constituents may differ in different cell lines. Each major group of leukocytes is described separately.

NEUTROPHILIC GRANULOCYTES

Neutrophilic granulocytes (neutrophils) constitute the major group of circulating granulocytes in the normal human. Because of their highly segmented nuclear appearance, they are also called polymorphonuclear leukocytes.

White corpuscles in the circulating blood were recognized for many years before Ehrlich (1879a, 1891) introduced the tinctorial staining method. The presence of large numbers of white cells in the blood of leukemic patients and in inflammatory pus was established by 1850. The role of bone marrow in production of normal and leukemic white cells was proposed by Neumann (1868, 1870) and later confirmed by many others.

Cells with nonsegmented nuclei in the bone marrow were defined as myelocytes by Ehrlich (1898). Three types of marrow cells were identified by their granules, similar to the three granule types of peripheral blood cells. The term "myeloblasts" was introduced by Naegeli in 1900, to define the most immature compartment of all myeloid elements; however, the same term is now used for definition of immature granulocytes only. Various methods of staining, such as the panoptical staining technic of both May and Grünwald (1902) and Giemsa (1904, 1910), supravital staining (Cowdry, 1915), and the peroxidase reaction (Graham, 1916, 1919) were introduced successively. These technics have contributed significantly to the development of modern hematology and clinical diagnoses of hematological disorders.

Metchnikoff (1884) introduced the concept that phagocytosis by leukocytes is a primary body defense in inflammation. This concept led Aschoff (1924) to propose a theory of a reticuloendothelial system in which circulating leukocytes (monocytes) were considered to be one of the most powerful defenses against invading microorganisms. Granulated leukocytes with their varied and easily identified cell characteristics have been the subject of extensive pathophysiological studies. The classic view of granulocyte function as a defense against infection has been confirmed beyond doubt. Additional information about the range of their proteolytic and hydrolytic enzymes and the chemical content of granules will be discussed.

MORPHOLOGY

The differentiation of neutrophils in the bone marrow can be followed by gradual changes of both nuclear and cytoplasmic characteristics (Fig. 3-1). Five stages are distinguished by light microscopy in marrow: myeloblasts, promyelocytes, myelocytes, metamyelocytes, and juvenile forms of matured granulocyte.

MYELOBLASTS

Myeloblasts (Figs. 3-2 and 3-3) are the most immature form found in the three major types of granulocyte. In smears they are about 10 to 25μ in diameter with a large, centrally located nucleus containing two to four distinctive nucleoli. The chromatin net is fine and reticular. In panoptical staining the cytoplasm is stained blue, occasionally has a reticular foamy appearance but no cytoplasmic granules. Identification of these cells becomes more certain when a few granules are present. In wet preparations, myeloblasts have a snail-like movement (Rich *et al.,* 1939). The cells show a positive reaction for both peroxidase and nonspecific esterase (Leder, 1964) which can be used to distinguish them from lymphoerythrocytic precursors, although the extremely immature myeloblasts may show no peroxidase reaction.

Few electron micrographs are available of non-neoplastic human myeloblasts

FIGURE 3-1. Light micrographs of granulocytes at various stages of maturation.
A. Myeloblast from bone marrow. × *2,000.*
B. Early promyelocyte from bone marrow. × *2,000.*
C. Promyelocyte (*arrow*) and myelocyte from bone marrow. × *2,000.*
D. Three myelocytes from bone marrow. × *2,000.*
E. Myelocyte (*arrow*), metamyelocytes, and juvenile forms from bone marrow. × *2,000.*
F. Mature neutrophil from peripheral blood. × *2,000.*

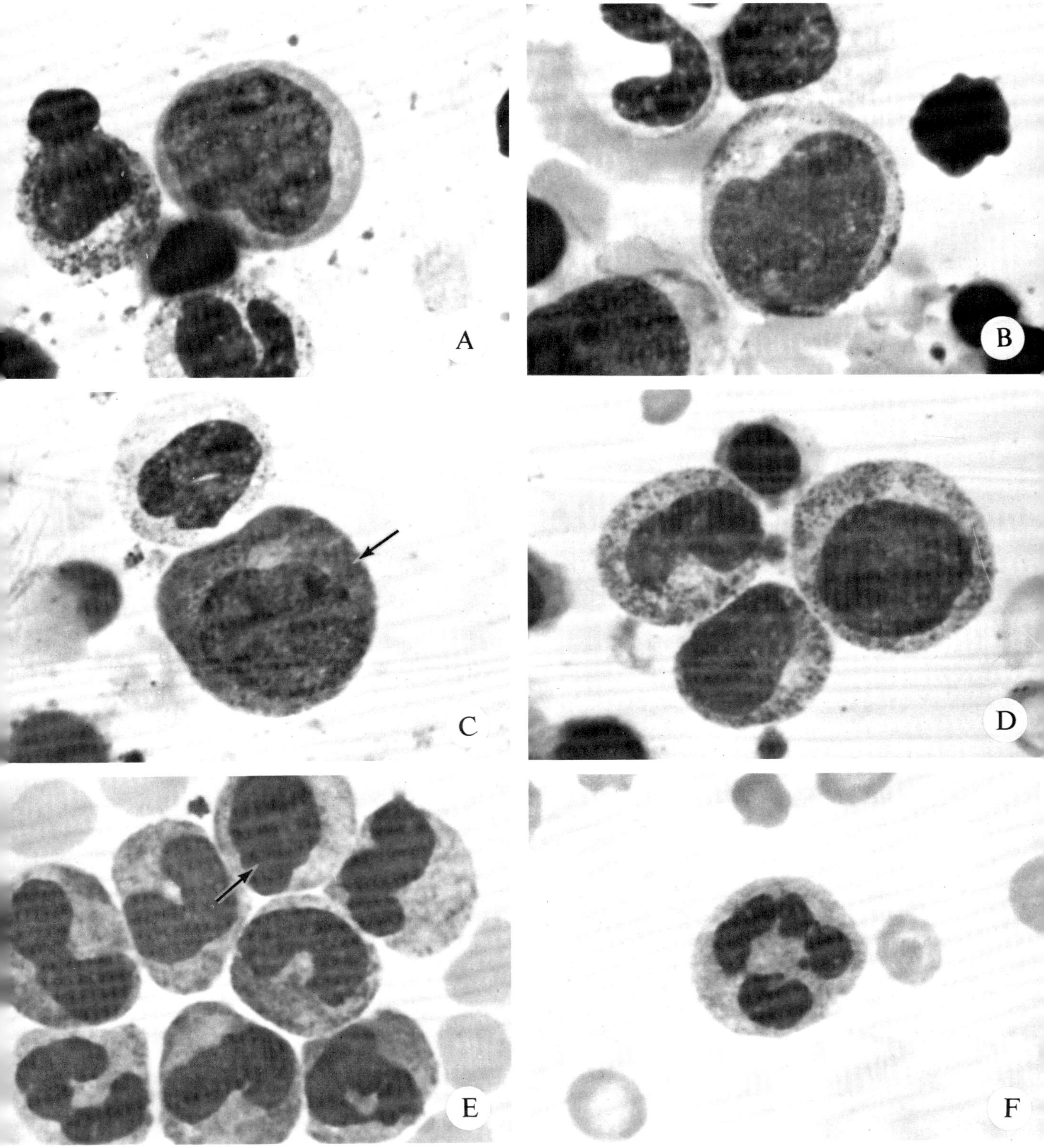
A
B
C
D
E
F

(Bessis and Thiéry, 1961a; Capone *et al.*, 1964). The myeloblast is a large cell with a round to slightly angular nucleus. The nucleolus of the myeloblast is usually located near the nuclear center without apparent attachment to the rim, as is seen frequently in proerythroblasts. The cytoplasm is moderately wide and contains many mitochondria and abundant polyribosomes. In contrast to proerythroblasts, the Golgi apparatus is well developed, and there are usually signs of early granular formation (Fig. 3-4). A large amount of tubular endoplasmic reticulum is also present. The cell membrane has frequent small invaginations. No ferritin particles are found in the vesicles, but small electron-opaque granules of possible azurophilic type are seen commonly in the cytoplasm. These granules may be too small to be detected by light microscopy. Infrequently, intracytoplasmic fibrils (Fig. 3-9*A*) are also noted in myeloblasts and promyelocytes. Their significance is not apparent, although they are more commonly present in more mature cells in leukemia. Myeloblasts form no cell clusters and localize in intersinusoidal spaces (Fig. 3-2).

PROMYELOCYTES

Promyelocytes (Fig. 3-5) are the next least differentiated of the granulocytes. Cell morphology is significantly altered from myeloblasts, and the differences may be observed by both light and electron microscopy. In smears, promyelocytes are cells of about 20 to 25μ in diameter, with bluish cytoplasm filled with abundant purplish-red (azurophilic) granules. Granules may cover the entire nucleus, and make it indistinctive. Two to three nucleoli may be detected. Because of its characteristic appearance, identification of this cell is made easily.

Electron microscopic studies show round-to-ovoid granules scattered throughout the cytoplasm that are heterogeneous in density and degree of granularity. The nucleus is usually round or oval and includes indistinct nucleoli. Many profiles of endoplasmic reticulum, some distended, are seen consistently, a particularly characteristic feature in the promyelocyte. Moderate numbers of ribosomes are also present. The formation of azurophilic granules at the promyelocyte stage is defined as "primary granulogenesis" by Wetzel *et al.* (1967a) (see discussion of granulogenesis in section on neutrophils). Azurophilic granules in human granulocytes contain a sulfate-mucopolysaccharide substance and cationic proteins (Dunn and Spicer, 1969). Cytochemically, vesicles of the Golgi apparatus, the endoplasmic reticulum, and azurophilic granules appear to be strongly positive with the peroxidase reaction (Wetzel *et al.*, 1967b; Ackerman, 1968; Bainton and Farquhar, 1968b; Dunn *et al.*, 1968). Spicer and Hardin (1969) define promyelocytes as the cells which primarily produce azurophil granules, the development of which terminates when the specific granulogenesis begins.

MYELOCYTES

Differentiation of granulocytes continues through promyelocytes to myelocytes (Figs. 3-6 through 3-8) and into metamyelocytes, which subsequently become neutrophils. This sequential maturational staging can be traced easily by light microscopy (Fig. 3-1). It is difficult however, to identify specific stages in single cells at the ultrastructural level, because of the difficulty in visualizing the whole nuclear shape—a key feature of myelocyte classification. In smears, the myelocyte is 16 to 25μ in diameter and contains a

(*text continues on page 100*)

Figures 3-2 through 3-7 appear on the following pages

FIGURE 3-2. Myeloblast.
Myeloblast (*center*) from case of granulocytic hyperplasia. The large ovoid nucleus (*N*) with indistinct nucleolus (*Nu*) is in an eccentric location. Cytoplasm has large mitochondria (*M*), a Golgi complex (*G*), many polyribosomes, and only a few profiles of endoplasmic reticulum. Four myelocytic cells (*My*) show various degrees of maturation. There is also a portion of a macrophage (*Ma, center left*) and an erythroblast (*Eb, top*). × *13,300.*

FIGURE 3-3. Myeloblast.
Myeloblast with more detail than in Figure 3-2. Nucleus (*N*) has a fine dispersion of chromatin, the Golgi apparatus (*G*) is near the slight hof of nucleus, several dense granules (*g*) and mitochondria (*M*). Rest of cytoplasm is dominated by polyribosomes and some endoplasmic reticulum (*er*). × *20,000.*

FIGURE 3-4. Golgi apparatus in myeloblast.
Golgi (*G*) area in this myeloblast suggests its role in early formation of granules (*arrows*). Edge of nucleus (*N*) and centriole (*Ce*) are also present along with many ribosomes. Mitochondria (*M*) are at top. × *104,000.*

FIGURE 3-5. Promyelocyte.
Promyelocyte showing large vesicular nucleus (*N*) and cytoplasm which has developed endoplasmic reticulum (*er*) and numerous round granules (*arrows*) whose content has variable density. Mitochondria (*M*) are intermingled. × *13,700.*

FIGURE 3-6. Early myelocyte.
Early myelocyte showing extensive granular formation around Golgi apparatus (*G*). The nucleus (*N*) is beginning to develop some chromatin concentration along the nuclear membrane. There are numerous large round granules with granular or flocculent content (a) and a second class of small dense granules (*b*); many granules have densities ranging between these two. A few large ovoid mitochondria (*M*) are around the periphery of the Golgi complex. × *28,000.*

FIGURE 3-7. Maturing myelocyte.
Myelocyte which appears a little more mature than the one in Figure 3-6. Nuclear chromatin is more condensed, but the nucleus (*N*) is still rounded. The cytoplasm contains the same types of granules as are seen in Figure 3-6 but the smaller dense type is becoming more dominant. The Golgi complex (*G*) and endoplasmic reticulum are still present but appear to be less prominent. Parts of four other myelocytes (*My*) are on the periphery. × *14,700.*

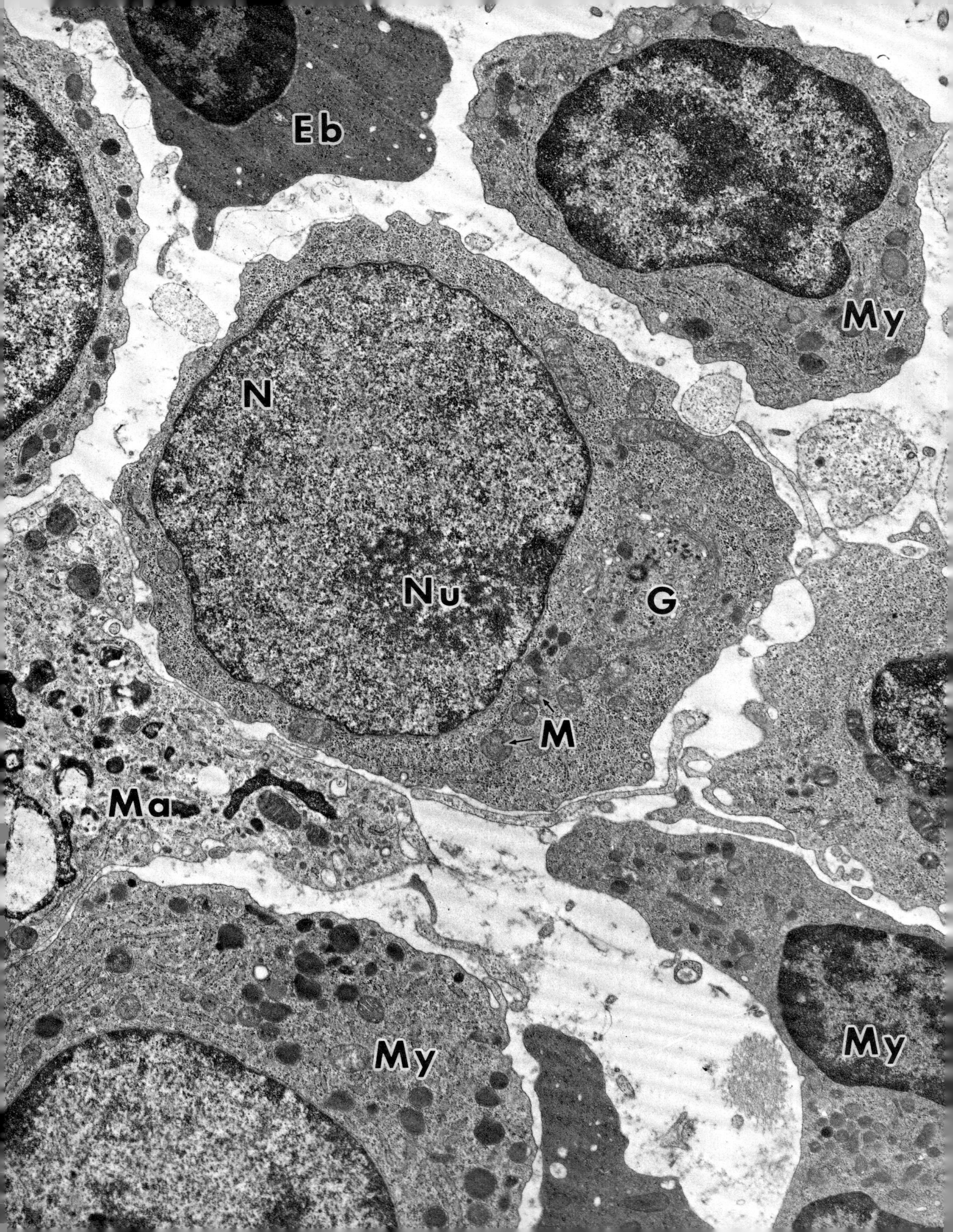

Eb
My
N
Nu
G
M
Ma
My
My

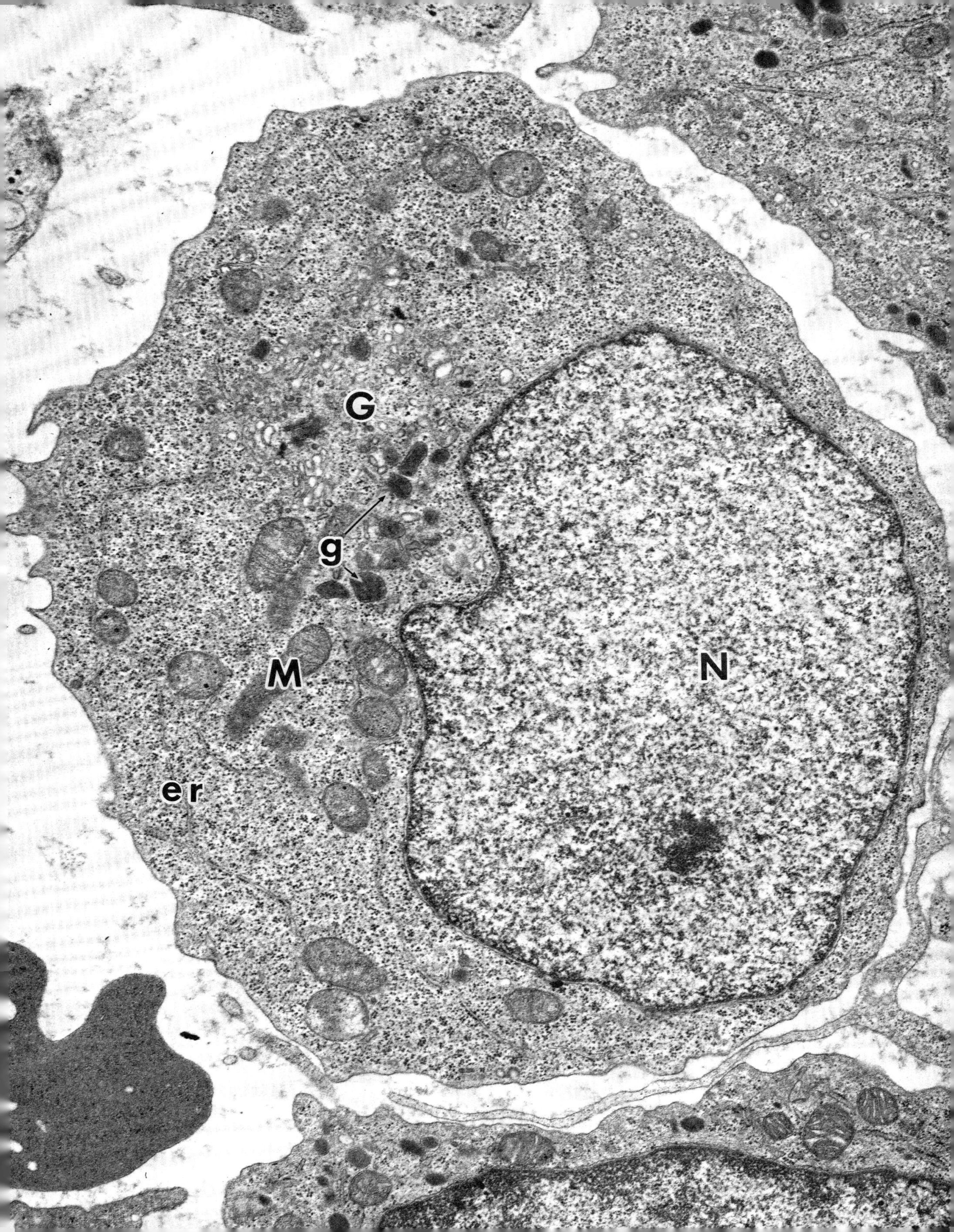
G
g
M
N
er

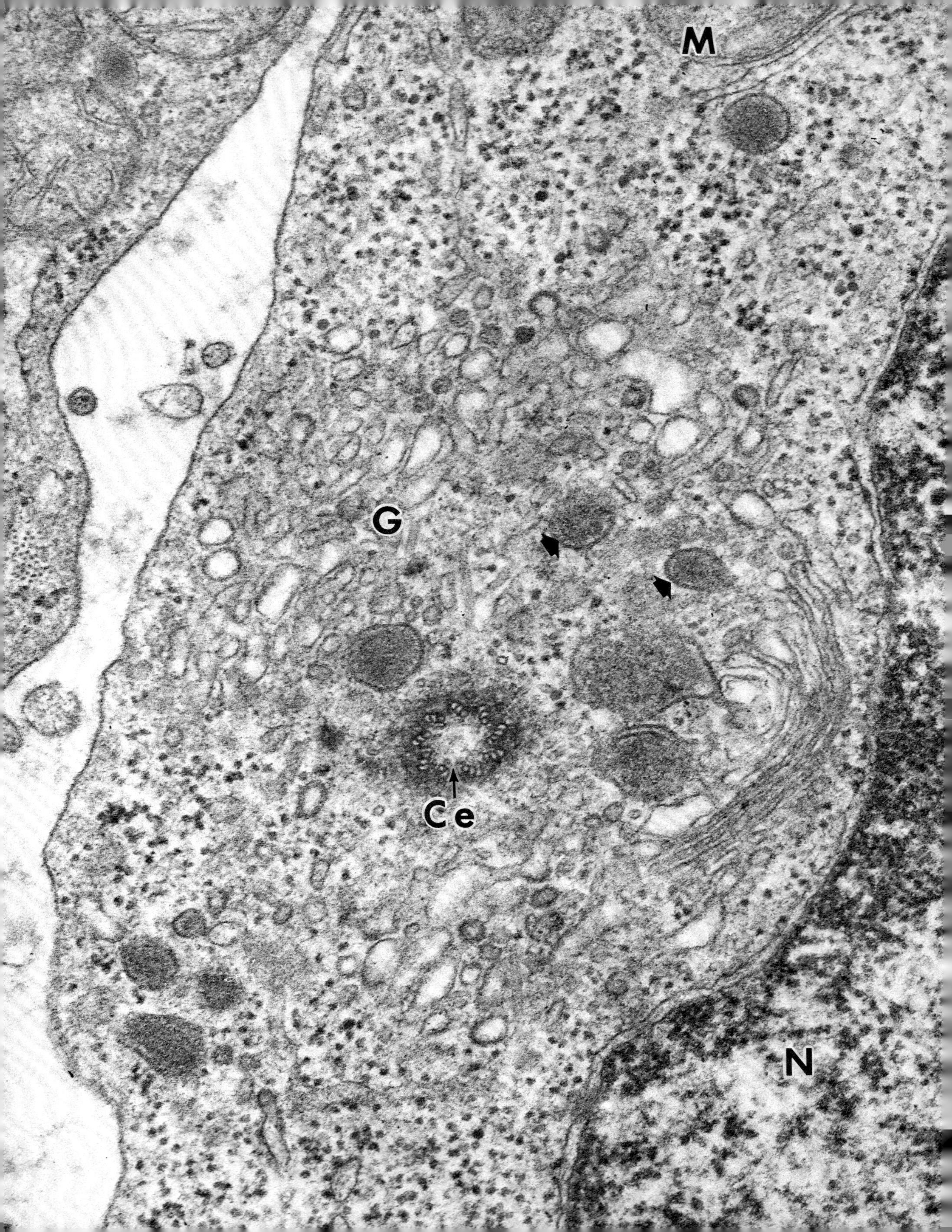
M
G
Ce
N

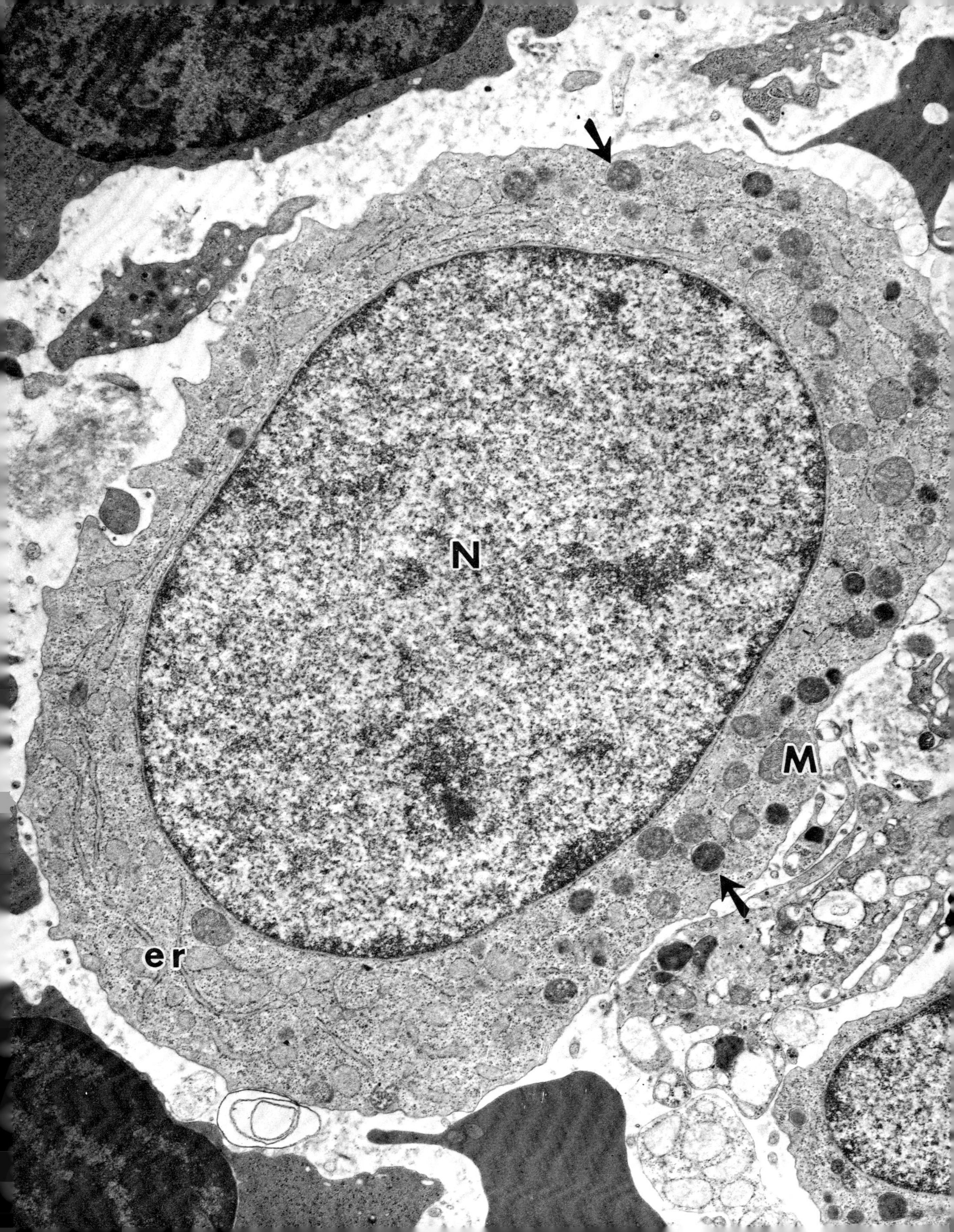

N
M
er

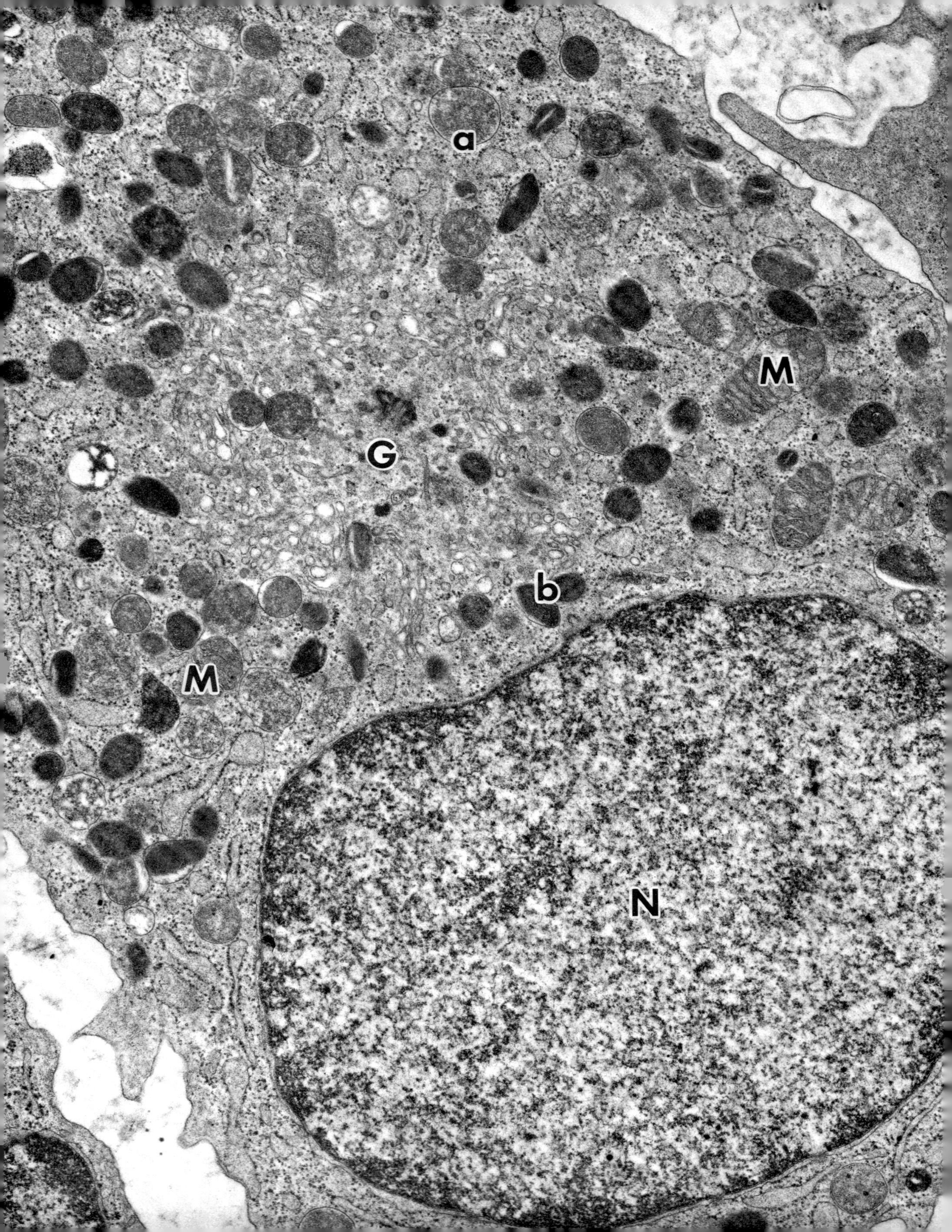
a
M
G
b
M
N

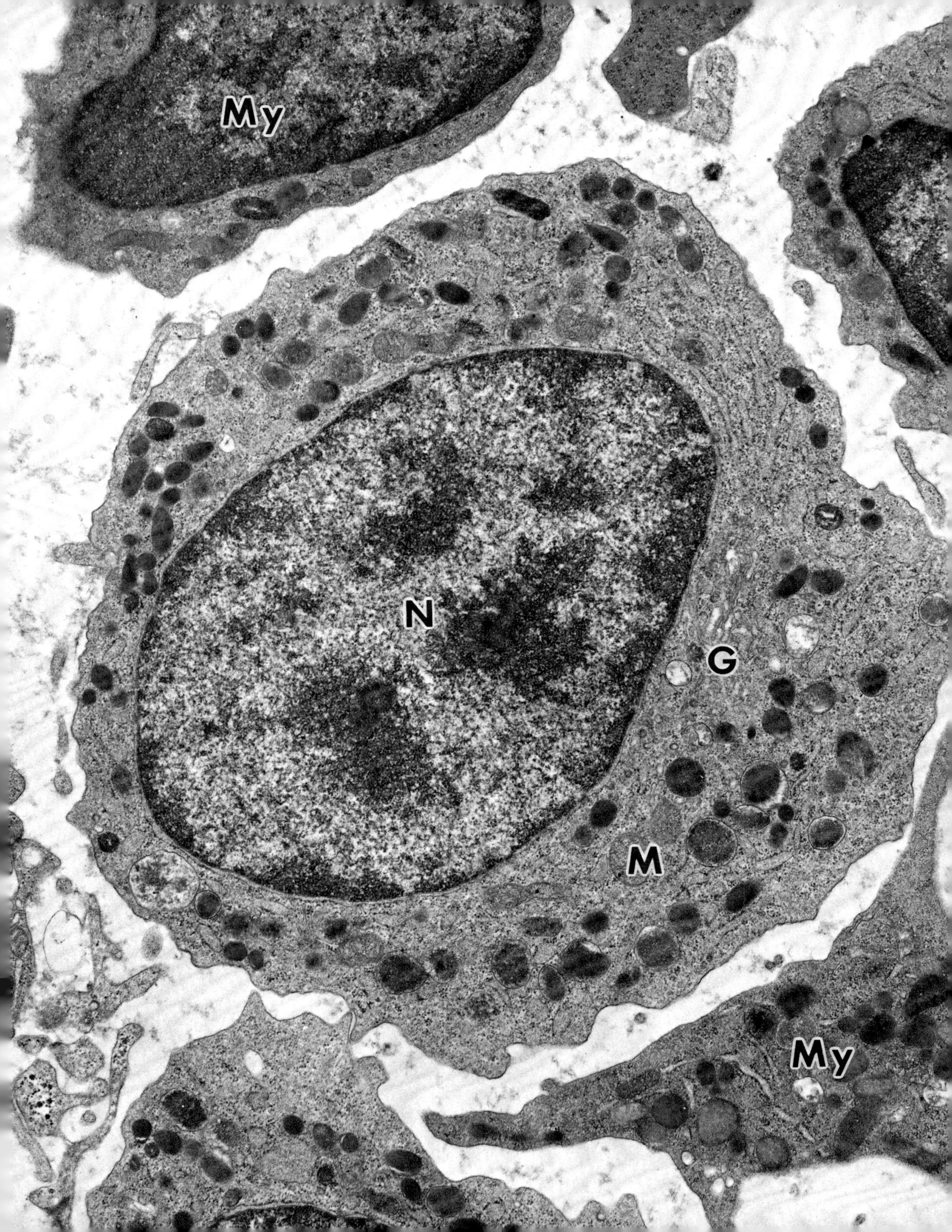
My
N
G
M
My

round nucleus with coarse chromatin distribution and no nucleolus. The cytoplasm appears as light orange in color and contains many finer granules of both azurophilic and neutrophilic type. It has been speculated that azurophilic granules transform into specific granules during myelocyte maturation. However, recent electron-microscopic investigations on rabbit heterophils have shown that azurophilic and specific granules are formed independently in the Golgi apparatus (Bainton and Farquhar, 1966; Wetzel *et al.,* 1967a).

This view is further extended in the granulogenesis of human leukocytes (Dunn *et al.,* 1968). The number of azurophilic granules per rabbit heterophil decreases during the myelocyte differentiation as the rate of production decreases and cellular division reduces the concentration. However, specific granules increase throughout the myelocyte stage as their rate of production increases (Bainton and Farquhar, 1968b). Examples of early myelocytes and more differentiated forms are illustrated in Figures 3-6 through 3-8. The early myelocytes start producing specific granules, a process termed "the secondary granulogenesis" (Wetzel *et al.,* 1967a). Figure 3-6 shows this active formation of granules around the Golgi apparatus of the early myelocyte. The small dense granules and the endoplasmic reticulum of the promyelocytic stage are still present, and the chromatin distribution of the nucleus still maintains its vesicular appearance. As the cells mature, the condensation of nuclear chromatin is more apparent (Figs. 3-7 and 3-8), the cells decrease in size (Figs. 3-7 and 3-8) and many cytoplasmic granules are observed. The endoplasmic reticulum and ribosomal content diminish, and the mitochondria are smaller and fewer in number (Figs. 3-7 and 3-8). Occasionally, there is an aggregaiton of lamellated endoplasmic reticulum resembling that described as the Döhle body (McCall *et al.,* 1969) (Fig. 3-9*B*).

METAMYELOCYTES

When the nucleus becomes horseshoe- or sausage-shaped (Fig. 3-10), the cells are called metamyelocytes. Electron microscopically, the nucleus of the metamyelocyte shows advanced chromatin condensation and no nucleoli. The cytoplasm has many heterogeneous granules (for morphology see section on neutrophils). Remnants of endoplasmic reticulum which are observed in promyelocytes are seen occasionally in late myelocytes, and the mitochondria become fewer, smaller, and more slender in shape. Dispersed glycogen particles and amorphous background material are evident as the differentiation proceeds. A moderate number of small vesicles are distributed throughout the cytoplasm along with scattered ribosomes.

NEUTROPHILS

The immature neutrophils (at the completion of the metamyelocyte stage) are stored in the bone marrow before migration into the circulation. They still show

FIGURE 3-8. Maturing myelocytes.
Two myelocytes, more mature than those in Figures 3-6 and 3-7, have nuclei (*N*) with a significant condensation of chromatin. There are large numbers of granules (*g*) in the cytoplasm which appear to have shifted to types with more homogeneous and less dense matrix. × *28,000.*

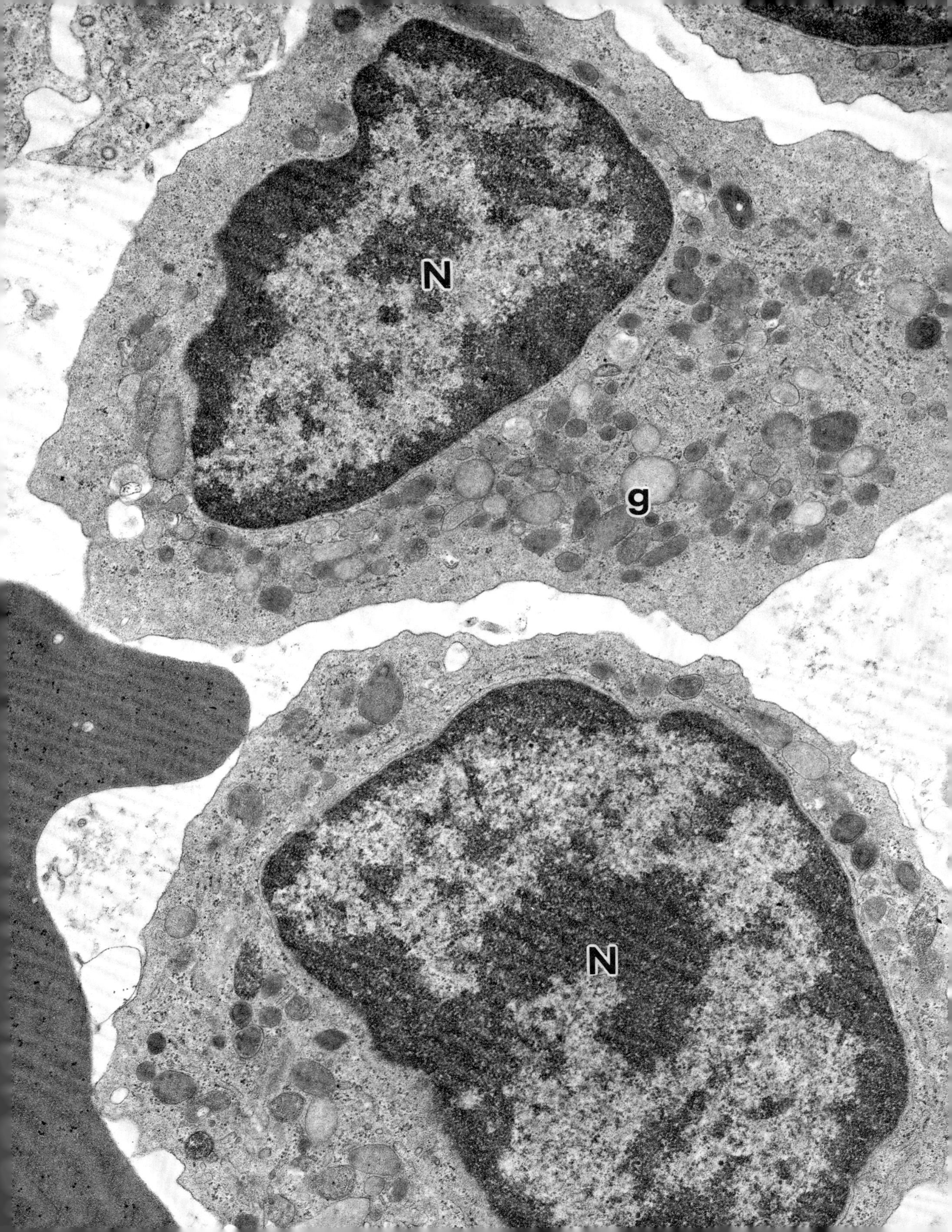
N
g
N

an unlobulated but slender or crescent-shaped nucleus, often called band or juvenile forms. An example of an immature neutrophil in the bone marrow is shown in Figure 3-11.

In smears, matured neutrophils of the peripheral circulation are 10 to 12μ in diameter (Fig. 3-1*F*). The number of nuclear lobes may indicate the relative maturation of the neutrophil. Quantitative alteration in the number of circulating segmented neutrophils can be used as an aid in diagnosis or estimation of prognosis in diseases. The cytoplasm is filled with fine granulations which have an affinity for neutral dyes. Histochemically, mature neutrophils are positive in peroxidase (Graham, 1919; Kaplow, 1965) and alkaline phosphatase (Takeuchi and Utsunomiya, 1952; Kaplow and Burstone, 1964); however, the exact localization of most of these enzymes is controversial. The cytoplasm of neutrophils is diffusely and strongly PAS-positive because of the presence of a large number of glycogen particles which serve as the major energy source for active anaerobic metabolism during phagocytosis. The cells are actively motile and engulf various foreign and degenerating intrinsic substances. This feature will be discussed in the section on function.

Electron micrographs of mature neutrophils have appeared repeatedly in many publications. The nucleus shows significant lobulation and advanced chromatin condensation (Fig. 3-12). The thin bridges connecting adjacent lobes appear as chromatin threads, covered on both sides by nuclear membranes similar to those of the nuclear bleb seen in Figure 3-15. The cytoplasm contains rudimentary Golgi vesicles, and a few thin mitochondria and individual glycogen particles are dispersed among many membrane-bound cytoplasmic granules with their heterogeneous morphology. Ribosomes and endoplasmic reticulum are noted less frequently; moderately electron-opaque, amorphous background material is usually present.

Ultrastructural characteristics of granules in human neutrophils are rather controversial (Breton-Gorius, 1966; Watanabe *et al.,* 1967; McCall *et al.,* 1969). This is due partially to the differences in fixatives, embedding materials, or even staining methods used. However, the major problem is more likely to be the lack of extensive information on the granule morphology correlated with adequate cytochemical localization methods. The water-soluble content of the granules may escape when improper methods are used in fixation, which could create considerable distortion in the final appearance of the granule. It has been established that most granules in human neutrophils are a mixture of azurophilic and specific granules.

The following summary will indicate the state of confusion based on current observations. According to Breton-Gorius (1966), granules in mature neutrophils and myelocytes in man can be classified into two major populations: large electron-lucent, and small electron-dense types. The first, called type A, was considered to be a specific granule with a periodic lamellar array of membranes spaced at about 100 Å. The second or dense type, called type B, was considered to be the azurophilic granule, also with the periodic array of about 100 Å. Watanabe *et al.,* (1967) and McCall *et al.* (1969) fixed human leukocytes with similar methods and came to the conclusion that small granules with lighter appearance were possibly specific granules. These granules were pleomorphic (Watanabe *et al.,* 1967) and negative in peroxidase reaction without any internal periodicity (McCall *et al.,* 1969).

(text continues on page 108)

Figures 3-9 through 3-12 appear on the following pages

FIGURE 3-9. Fibrils and lamellated endoplasmic reticulum in mature cells.
A. Fine fibrils (*fb*) near the nucleus (*N*) of a promyelocyte. The many dense particles are ribosomes, and some endoplasmic reticulum (*er*) is present. × *79,000.*
B. Lamellated endoplasmic reticulum (*er*) in a myelocyte, which resembles the structures found in mature cells interpreted as Döhle bodies. Granules (*g*) are near by. × *75,000.*

FIGURE 3-10. Metamyelocyte.
In the metamyelocyte the nucleus (*N*) is no longer ovoid and has heavy margination of chromatin, with only a few nuclear pores (*arrows*). The cytoplasm has a large number and several types of granules, a number of pale translucent ones, and some with the flocculated content commonly seen in promyelocytes. The Golgi apparatus (*G)* and residual endoplasmic reticulum and mitochondria are still discernible. × *27,000.*

FIGURE 3-11. Early neutrophil.
Juvenile neutrophil in bone marrow with essentially the same cytoplasm as metamyelocyte in Figure 3-10, and a heterogeneous group of granules. However, the nuclei (*N*) has developed a large indentation out of the plane of the cut, or initial lobulation has taken place. The scattered small dense particles are probably glycogen. There is a centriole (*Ce*) and a few mitochondria (*arrows*). × *29,000.*

FIGURE 3-12. Neutrophil.
Typical neutrophil from peripheral blood with granules (*g*) in cytoplasm, and two lobes of nucleus (*N*) transected. Granules are fairly uniform in size and electron-opaque; a few (as at *asterisk*) are quite dense, and one (*arrow*) has an internal crystalloid structure. The cytoplasm has a relatively dense background with scattered glycogen particles. × *27,200.*

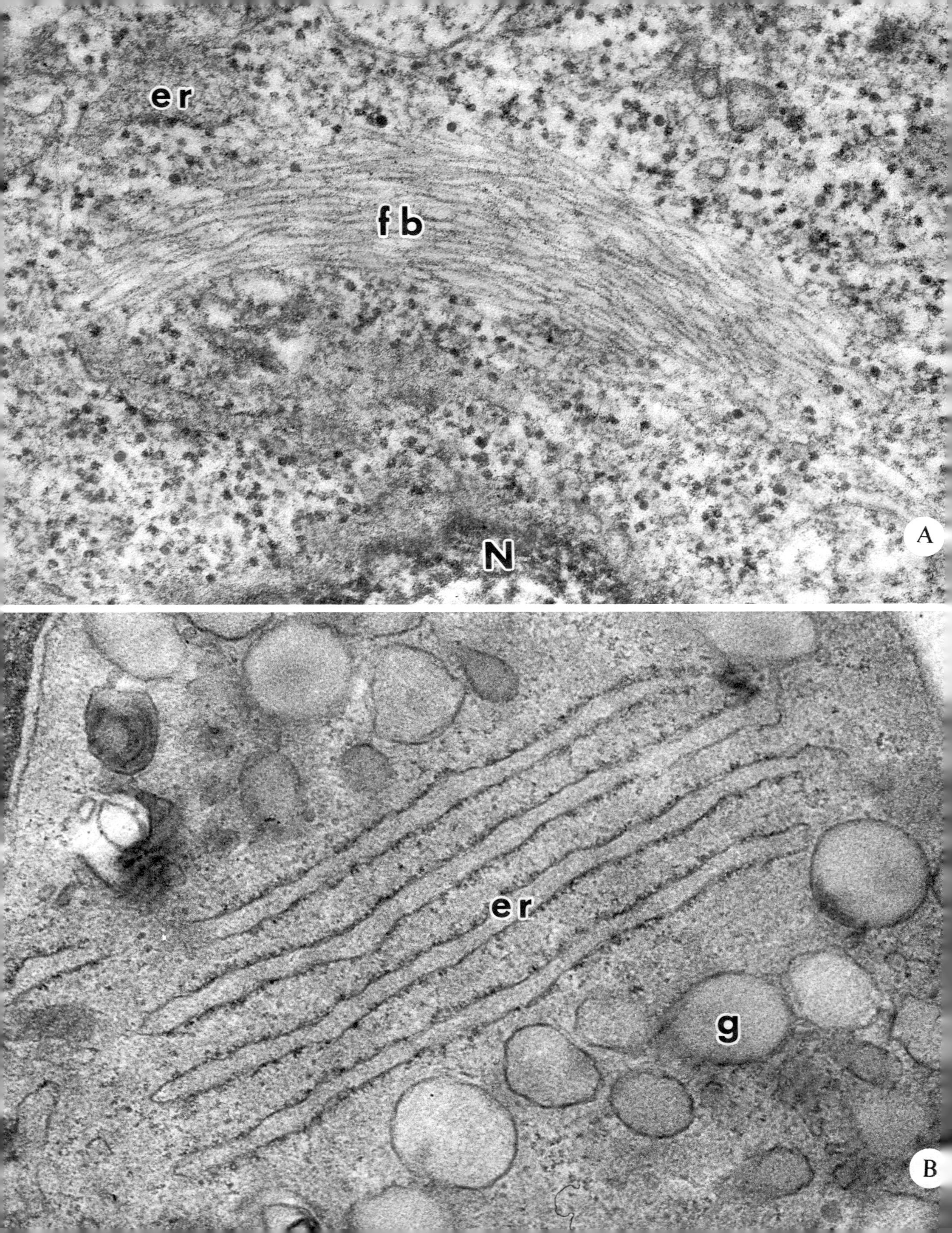
er
fb
N
A
er
g
B

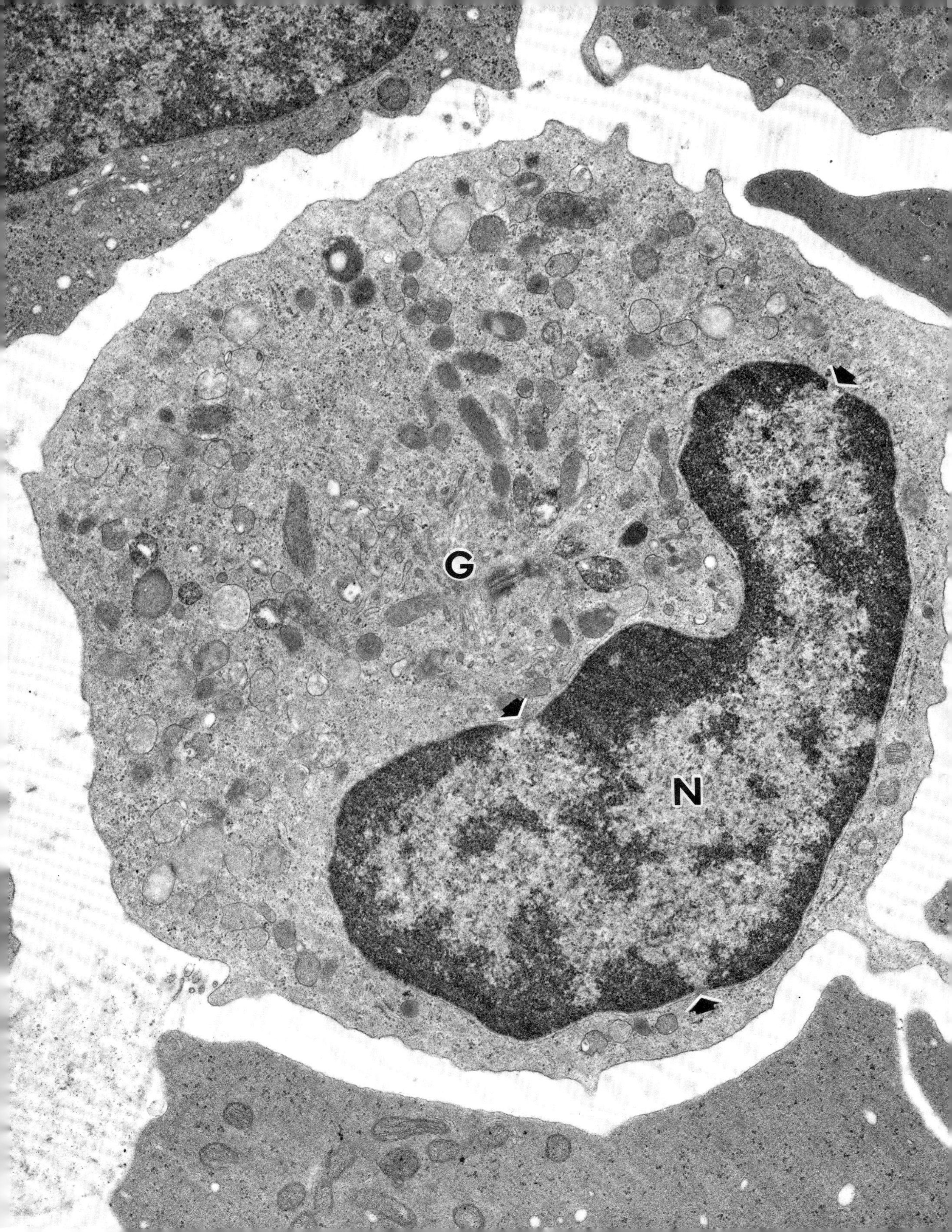
G
N

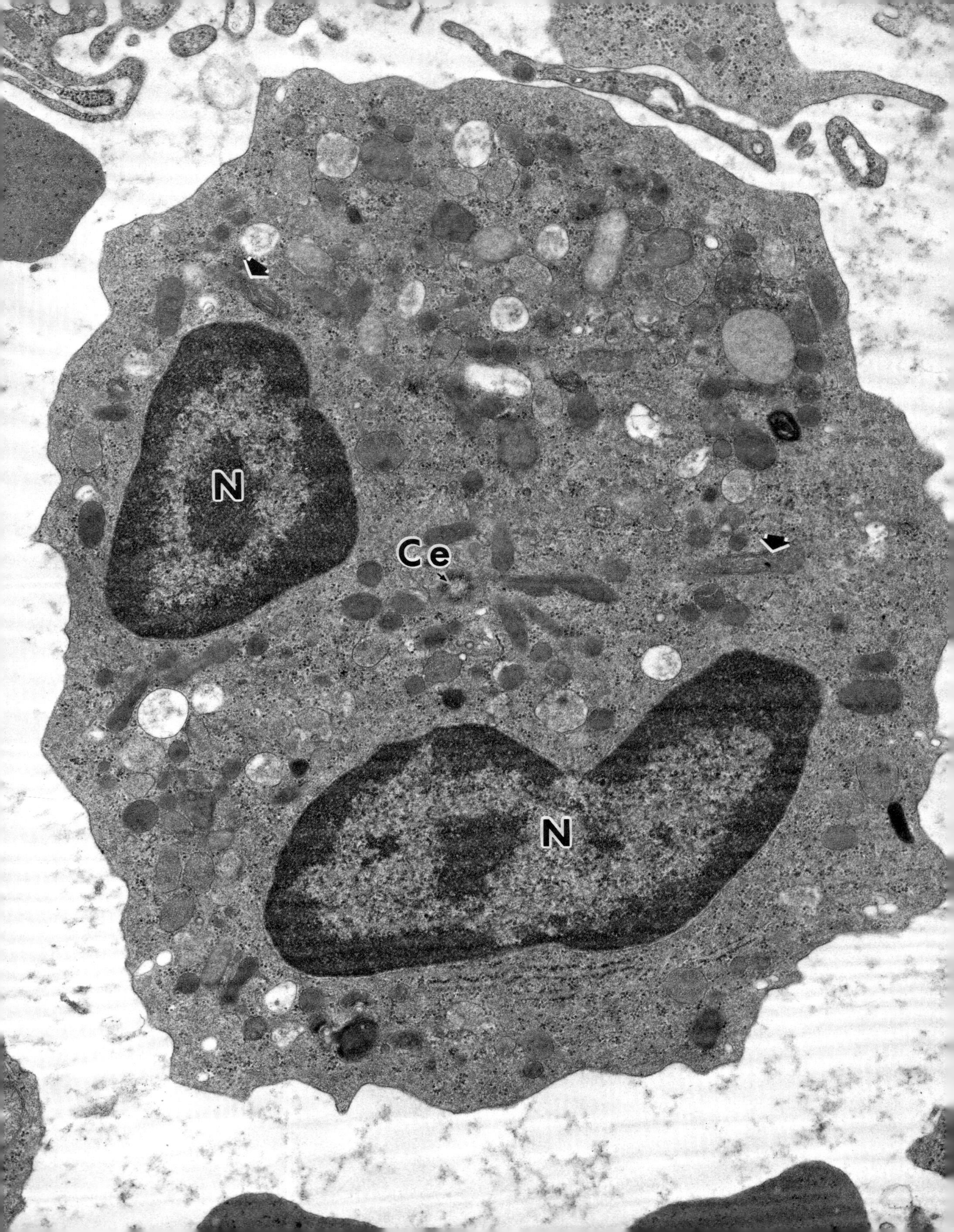
N
Ce
N

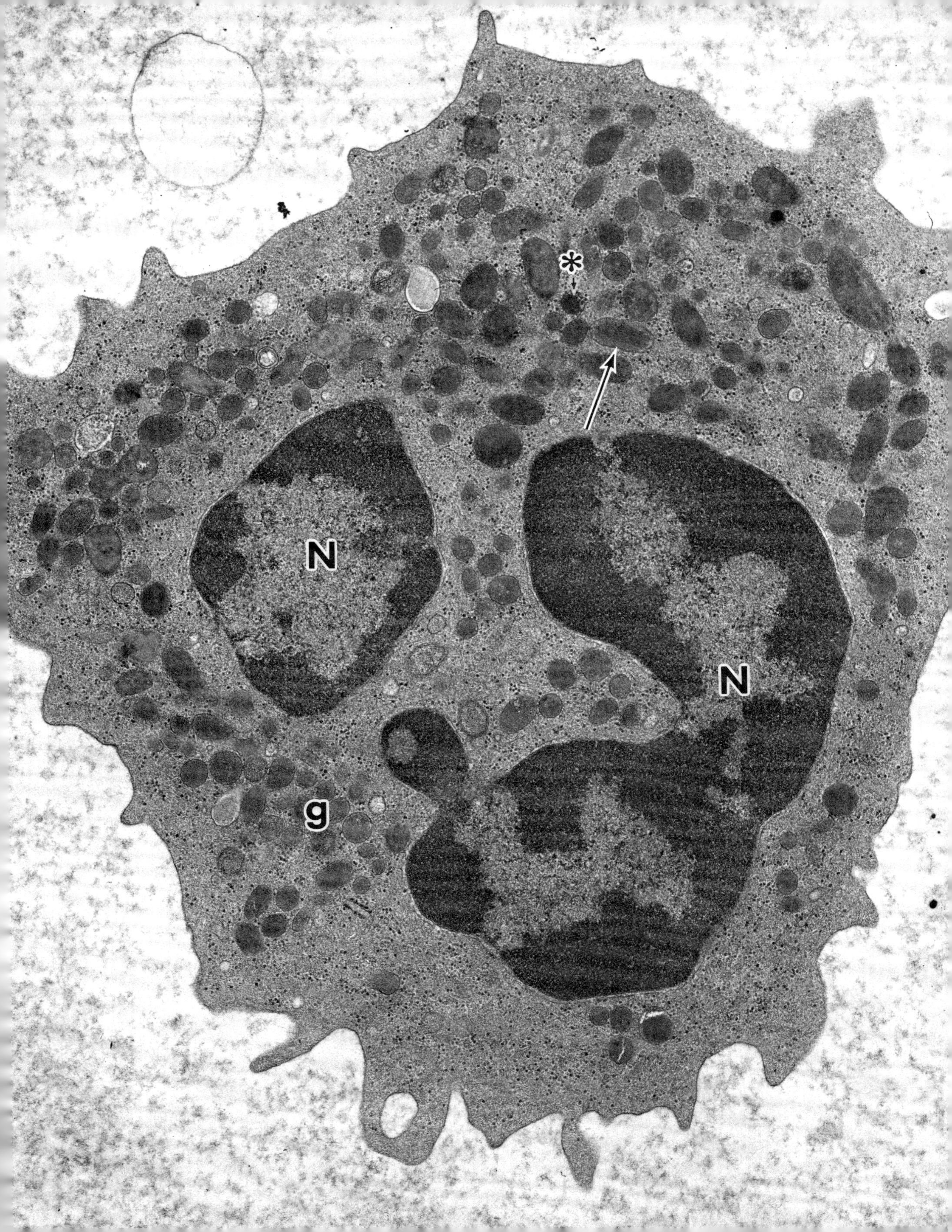

*
N
N
g

They stated that the internal crystalloid array might be seen in the larger dense granules with peroxidase-positive nature, and were the azurophilic granules.

Watanabe *et al.* (1967) distinguished a third type of granule which contained internal bars and appeared electron-lucent. Granules of this morphology are probably the type classified as the specific granule by Breton-Gorius (1966). These granules are heterogeneous in shape, electron-lucent and, at times, have lamellar, rod-form internal structures. The electron-opaque granules, probably the azurophilic type, vary in size and frequently show internal crystalloid array. Any schematic classification or differentiation of granulocytes based primarily on granule morphology does not appear to be warranted at this time.

An example of a mature neutrophil shows at least two types of granules (Fig. 3-13), a large dense type and a lighter, smaller type, similar to those described by Watanabe *et al.* (1967) and McCall *et al.* (1969). One of the dense granules shows a crystalloid pattern (*arrow,* Fig. 3-13). Dense granules with crystalloid or filamentous patterns are also common in the myelocytes, as in Figure 3-14. A comparison of granules in the progression of maturing granulocytes suggests that granules in human neutrophils may alter their morphology considerably during differentiation. The observations may be summarized as follows: (1) Round granules with loosely flocculated content of various electron opacity predominate in the promyelocytic stage (Fig. 3-5). (2) Smaller and more elliptical electron-opaque types are more prevalent in the early myelocytes (Figs. 3-6 and 3-7). (3) Increased electron-lucent types with heterogeneous morphology are more common in the later myelocytes (Figs. 3-8 and 3-10). The biochemical nature and the morphogenesis of human neutrophilic granules in developing myelocytes remains to be clarified.

In contrast to the observations on human neutrophils, there has been good agreement among many investigators on the morphological and histochemical analyses of rabbit heterophils. The granulogenesis of rabbit heterophils may be divided into three major stages: the primary, in both myeloblast and promyelocyte; the secondary, in myelocyte; and the tertiary, in mature heterophils (Wetzel *et al.,* 1967a). Primary granulogenesis is defined as the formation of azurophilic granules. Morphologically, they are round to oval and consist of homogenous electron-dense material (Bainton and Farquhar, 1966; Wetzel *et al.,* 1967a), histochemically, they are PAS-positive (Horn and Spicer, 1964) and contain readily water-soluble sulfated mucopolysaccharides and a strong basic protein. Granules appear to be positive in peroxidase (Bainton and Farquhar, 1968a; Dunn *et al.,* 1968), acid phosphatase (Wetzel *et al.,* 1967b; Bainton and Farquhar, 1968b), arylsulfatase, beta galactosidase, beta glucuronidase, nonspecific esterase, and 5-nucleotidase (Bainton and Farquhar, 1968a).

Tertiary granules in mature leukocytes are acid phosphatase-positive but are un-

FIGURE 3-13. Cytoplasm of neutrophil.
Portion of neutrophil showing greater cytoplasmic detail and parts of nucleus (*N*). There are a number of larger dense granules (*g*), one of which has an internal crystalloid pattern (*arrow*), and smaller lighter ones (*asterisk*). × *63,000.*

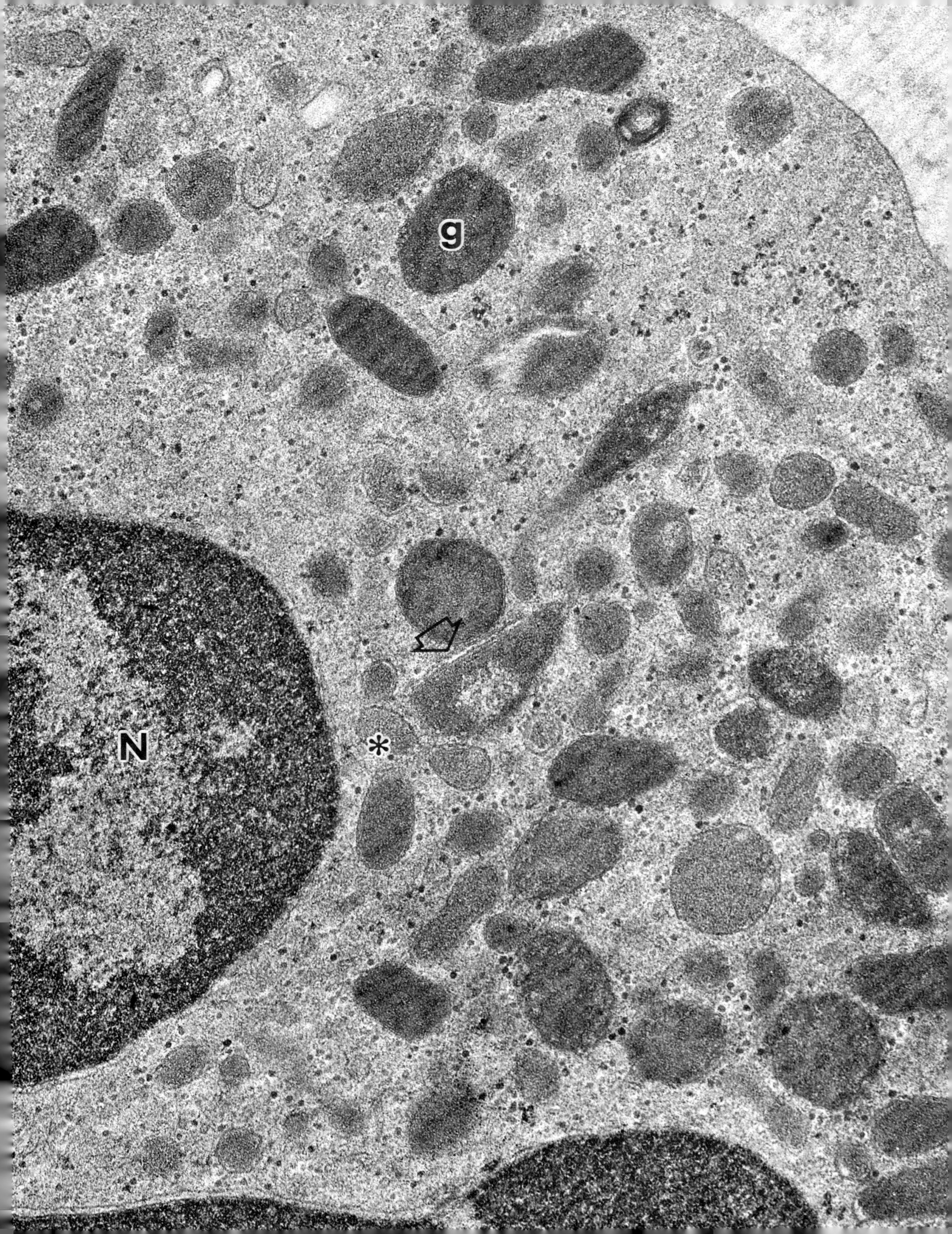
g
N
*

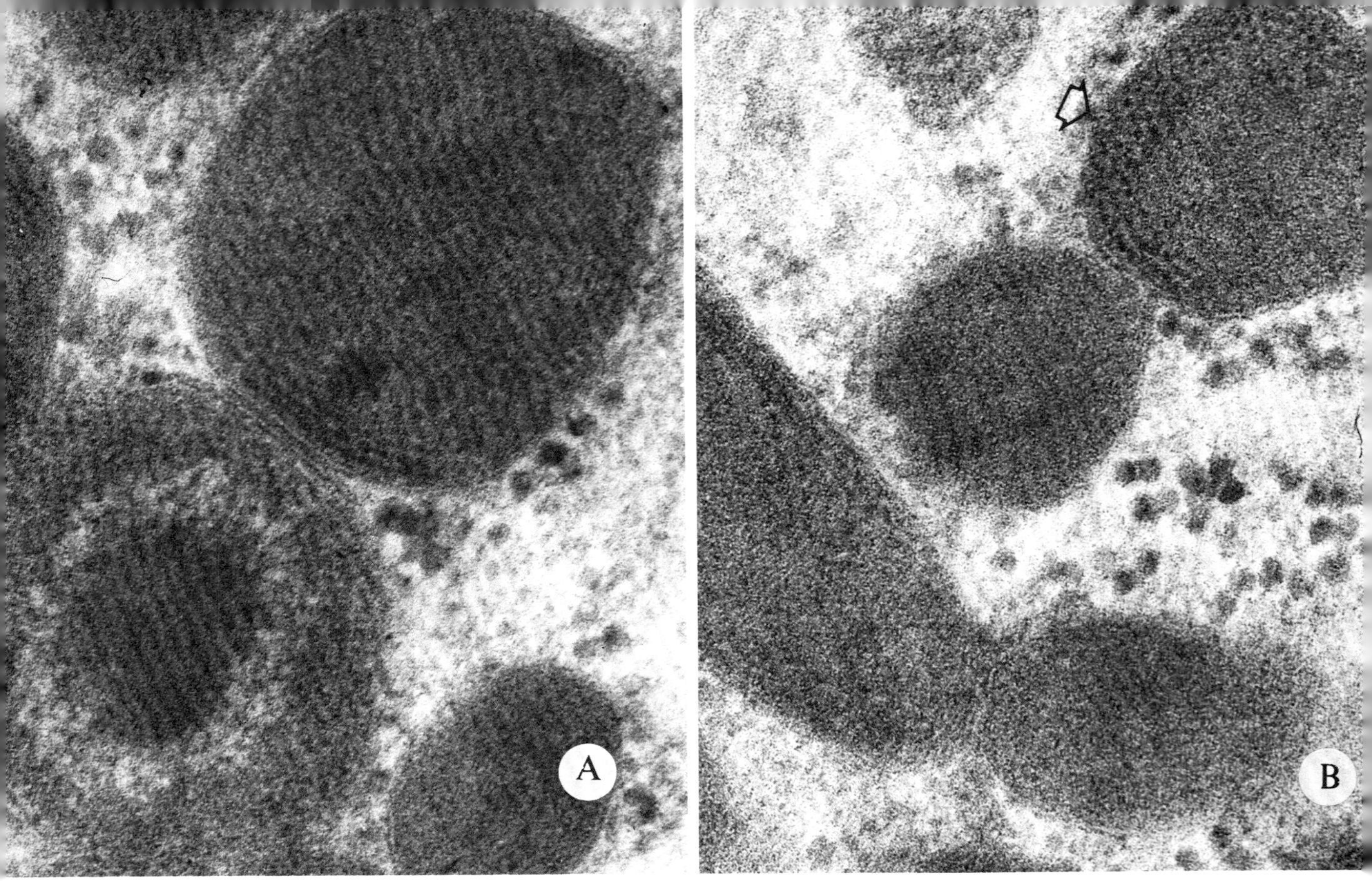

FIGURE 3-14. Patterns in dense granules of myelocytes.
A. Lamellar. × *189,000.*
B. Lamellar structure in granule (*left*) and a periodic array of dots (*arrow*). × *189,000.*

related to azurophilic type granules (Wetzel *et al.,* 1967a). The Golgi apparatus has a key role in formation of all these granules (Bainton and Farquhar, 1966, 1970; Wetzel *et al.,* 1967a). A similar distribution of peroxidase in neutrophil granules has been shown in cat myelocytes (Ackerman, 1968).

Most investigators agree on the presence of the following enzymes in the separated granules of neutrophils from different animal species: acid phosphatase, alkaline phosphatase, nucleotidase, ribonuclease, deoxyribonuclease, beta glucuronidase, cathepsin, lysozymes, and dopa-oxidase (Cohn and Hirsch, 1960; Ohota, 1964; Hirschhorn and Weissman, 1965; Olsson, 1969; Baggiolini *et al.,* 1969, 1970). Some of these enzyme activities have also been found with varying degrees of activity in the mitochondrial fraction. At present, the exact site of a specific enzyme activity in neutrophils awaits further clarification before a specific granule can be designated for a specific enzymatic role. These correlations may become more certain when there is more quantitative information on the effects of fixatives and separation procedures on enzyme activities, and when the problems of cross-contamination between separated cell fractions are solved.

Since Cohn and Hirsch (1960) demonstrated the presence of various enzymes in granules of leukocytes, the lysosomal nature of granules has been proposed (Weissman, 1964), a concept well supported by the functional involvement of granules during phagocytosis. Initially, the lysosomal activity was thought to be in the specific granules of the leukocyte (Weissman, 1964). However, recent investigation on rabbit heterophils has shown that the azurophilic granules contain various enzymes and are compatible with the functional concept of the lysosome (Bainton and Farquhar, 1968b; Baggiolini *et al.,* 1969, 1970). This view may also apply to the role of azurophilic granules in human leukocytes.

SEX CHROMOSOMES AND NUCLEAR APPENDAGES

Somatic diploid cells of humans contain 22 pairs of autosomal chromosomes and one pair of sex chromosomes, X and Y—the female has a pair of X chromosomes, the male an X and Y chromosome. The Y chromosome has a specific binding activity to quinacrine mustard (Caspersson *et al.,* 1970), a phenomenon which suggests a possible chemical differentiation between individual chromosomes. The only morphologically known difference between the two chromosomes is their shape and size. Barr and Bertram (1949) demonstrated a deeply stained spot of 0.7 to 1.2μ in the nucleus near the nuclear membrane in the somatic cells of females and suggested a difference in the nuclear morphology of somatic cells between the two sexes. This structure is known as the "Barr body" and has been used for the determination of genetic sex (Moore *et al.,* 1953). Later, Davidson and Smith (1954) found a nuclear projection resembling a drumstick in neutrophils of females but not in males, which differed from those resembling tennis rackets or small clubs. The rich chromatin in the extra X chromosome of the female may be responsible for the drumsticks. Nuclear appendages have been studied extensively by Kosenow and Scupin (1956), who classified them into four groups: (1) drumstick, (2) sessile nodules, (3) ambiguous projections, and (4) racket form. Nuclear projections of groups 3 and 4 are seen in leukocytes of both D_1 trisomy (Huehns *et al.,* 1964) and irradiated subjects (Duplan *et al.,* 1969). The nuclear appendages in irradiated subjects may be distinguished from genetically determined drumsticks and sessile nodules (Mehes, 1966) and should be considered nonspecific. The nuclear appendages observed in D_1 trisomy and X-irradiated subjects have been studied by electron microscopy (Lutzner and Hecht, 1966; Duplan *et al.,* 1969). The chromatin appendage in D_1 trisomy consists of a projection with a characteristic configuration described as coiled (Lutzner and Hecht, 1966). Many chromatin clefts in the nucleoplasm are also found near the nuclear periphery and are considered responsible for a bulging in the nuclear margin. Irradiated subjects occasionally show nuclear projections which appear to be of the simple type, resembling the nuclear bleb described in leukocytes of malignancy-bearing subjects (Clausen and von Hamm, 1969). An example of this type of nuclear bleb is seen in Figure 3-15. The thin strip of chromatin is bound on both sides by membranes, and the bleb contains cytoplasm, including granules and occasional mitochondria.

TOXIC GRANULES

Many large bluish granules appear in circulating leukocytes in severe bacterial infections. These are called "toxic" granules and are associated with such other toxic phenomena as the "left shift" of the nucleus, Döhle bodies, and vacuolated cytoplasm. Several electron-microscopic studies on this topic have appeared (Zucker-Franklin, 1966; Fedorko, 1967; McCall *et al.,* 1969). These granules are interpreted as phagocytized materials (Zucker-Franklin, 1966) or autophagic inclusions (Fedorko, 1967). Toxic granules appear as electron-dense large granules of either ellipsoid or oval-shape, whose morphology differs little from that of azurophilic granules of normal leukocytes (McCall *et al.,* 1969). Biochemical analysis on enzymes of toxic granulocytes does not show any significant abnormality except for the presence of high alkaline phosphatase activity in the granulated fraction and higher acid phosphatase activity in the supernate of ruptured cells, without an increase in total acid phosphatase activity. The mechanism of toxic granule formation is unknown. Postulated mechanisms include denaturation of preexisting granules (Fedorko, 1967), defective granule synthesis (Fedorko, 1967), an unknown mechanism relating to stimulation or degeneration of the cells (Koszewski *et al.,* 1967; McCall *et al.,* 1969), and cellular immaturity (McCall *et al.,* 1969).

DÖHLE BODY

Patchy blue coloration in the cytoplasm of mature granulocytes is observed in various pathological conditions where maturation of myelocytes is distorted by various infections or exposure to cytotoxic agents. This structure, described by Döhle (1911), is known cytochemically to contain RNA and thought to be a vestige of the basophilic material of early myelocytes. McCall *et al.,* (1969) found that the structure consisted of lamellar aggregates of rough endoplasmic reticulum, similar to that shown in Figure 3-9*B* and observed in the early myelocytes. This is a variant of the conclusion made on the Döhle body observed in the May-Hegglin anomaly.

CYTOGENESIS

Granulocyte kinetics have been analyzed by various technics, including mitotic index (Killmann *et al.,* 1964), cinematography (Boll, 1958), and cell-labeling by radioactive phosphorus (Craddock *et al.,* 1955; Bierman *et al.,* 1961), radioactive thymidine (Cronkite and Fliedner, 1964; Cronkite, 1969) and di-isopropylfluorophosphate (Athens *et al.,* 1959; Cartwright *et al.,* 1964).

The committed blastic form of granulocytes the myeloblasts, may originate from a common ancestor of myelo-erythro-megakaryocyte. The myeloblast differentiates to promyelocytes, which subsequently become myelocytes. The cells in these three stages are considered to be capable of mitosis and are grouped as the "mitotic or proliferating pool." It is not known how many mitoses occur

FIGURE 3-15. Nuclear bleb in myelocyte.
The nuclear bleb, a thin chromatin sheet, is covered by nuclear envelope on both sides. Cytoplasmic granules, both in and out of the bleb, have a double membrane and dense glycogen (*gy*) particles which are randomly scattered throughout. × *79,000.*

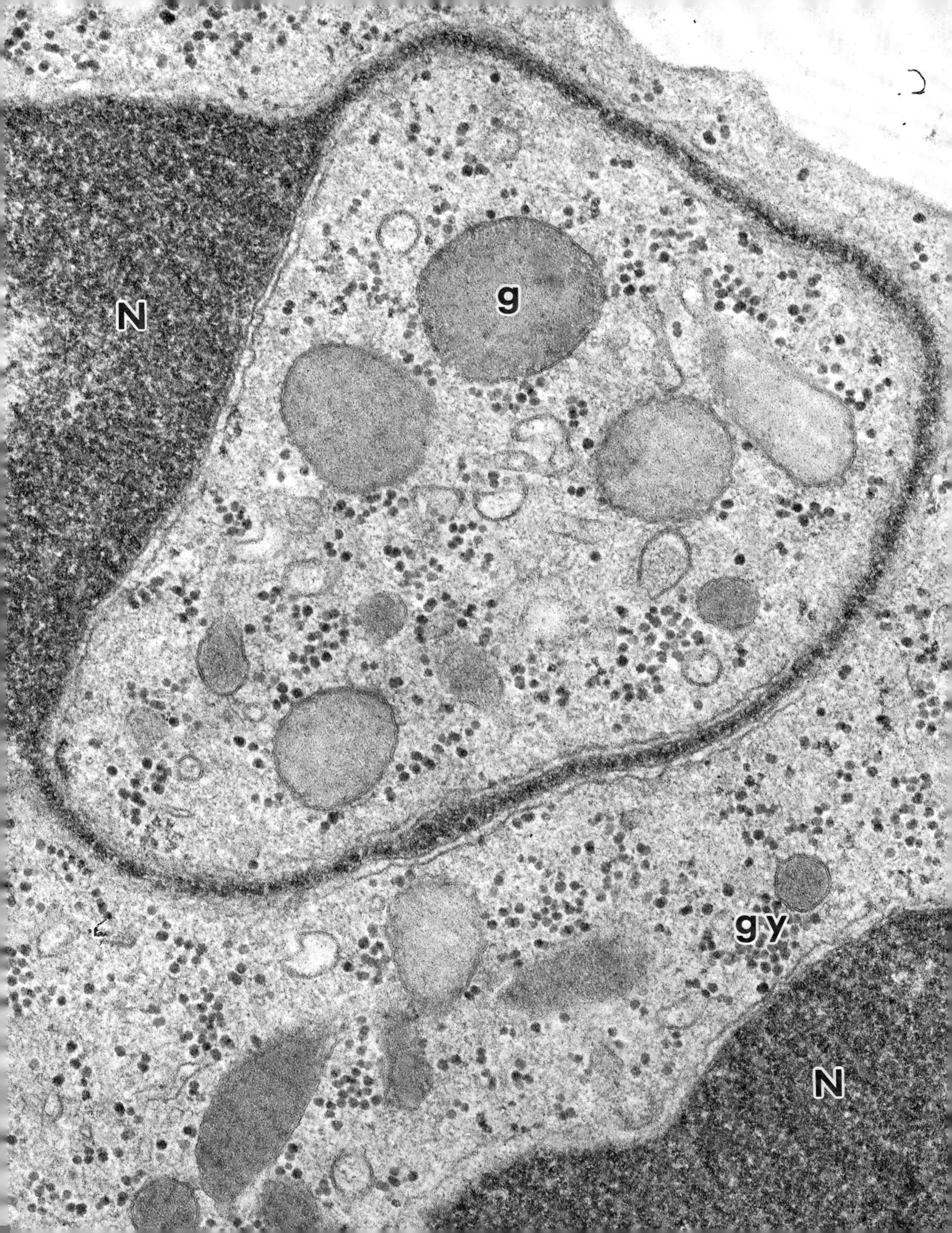
N
g
gy
N

during myelocyte differentiation or how many mature granulocytes are derived from a single myeloblast. Comparing data obtained by an in vivo di-isopropylflouro-phosphate experiment with a theoretical model, Athens (1969) proposed that at least three or four mitoses are involved in the myelocytic state or, alternately, that a self-generating mechanism is present in immature cells at each stage of differentiation (Cartwright *et al.,* 1964). Studies of granulokinetics in humans, based on mitotic indexes (Killmann *et al.,* 1964) estimate that transit times for each stage are 23.3 hours for myeloblasts, 78.3 to 26 hours for promyelocytes, and 126 to 37.4 hours for myelocytes. Total transit time in the proliferating pool is 228 to 87 hours (Cronkite and Fliedner, 1964). Cells in the metamyelocytic stages are considered to be incapable of division and transit time is estimated as 33 hours (Cronkite and Fliedner, 1964). Cells which are incapable of mitosis but which are retained in myeloid tissues are called the "maturation or nonproliferating pool"; in them the total transit time is about 6 days (Cronkite and Fliedner, 1964) or 4.2 days (Cartwright *et al.,* 1964). Cells stored in myeloid tissues may be released by administration of proper stimulants, such as endotoxin (Athens *et al.,* 1959). Exhaustion of this compartment may create peripheral leukopenia, as in severe infection (Athens, 1969). Neutrophilic granulocytes leave the blood in a random or exponential manner, rather than according to age; half-life is estimated as 6 to 8 hours in normal subjects. These migrated leukocytes may be stored in a marginal pool whose cell capacity is about twice that of the circulating pool. Reentry of emigrated leukocytes in normal conditions is believed to be insignificant. The total life span of mature granulocytes is estimated to be 6.5 (Cronkite and Fliedner, 1964) to 11.4 days (Cartwright *et al.,* 1964); the value may differ slightly from one pathological condition to another.

A steady progression in granulocyte maturation keeps a fairly constant peripheral leukocyte count; therefore, abnormal deviation of counts in either direction is a basis for suspicion of disease. Morley (1966) reported a periodic oscillation of several days in granulocyte counts in normal males. A feedback mechanism from blood neutrophils to the production compartment and to the rate of neutrophil release has been suggested for this periodic variation in peripheral neutrophil counts.

FUNCTION

Neutrophils actively phagocytize bacteria, fungi, and other foreign and intrinsic pathological substances, a most primitive body defense mechanism against invaders. Metchnikoff (1884) evaluated the phenomenon accurately and observed that it occurred widely, even in very primitive animal species. The process has been investigated extensively by various methods, including microcinematography and light, phase, and electron microscopy.

Phagocytosis of bacteria begins when microorganisms contact the plasma membrane of granulocytes and bacteria are engulfed in the pseudopods of the phagocytes (Goodman and Moore, 1956) (Fig. 3-16*A*). Phagocytes (granulocytes, histiocytes, monocytes, etc.) recognize and discriminate the objects, possibly by chemotaxis or sometimes by surface electric charge. For example, bacteria and fungi are actively engulfed by leukocytes (Fig. 3-17); however, phagocytosis of viral agents appears to be minimal. After ingestion, cytoplasmic granules which contain various hydrolytic enzymes, fuse to

Figures 3-16 and 3-17 appear on the following pages

FIGURE 3-16. Phagocytosis of bacteria (*E.coli*) by neutrophils.
A. Early phase of phagocytosis. Two pseudopods engulfing bacteria, one showing initial contact (*1*) and the second, closure of pseudopod (*2*) about the bacterium. Some bacteria are free in the extracellular space (*asterisks*) and others are seen within neutrophils (*arrows*) cytoplasm. × *25,400.*
B. Cytoplasmic residuals (*asterisks*) in neutrophil after degradation of phagocytosed bacteria. Mitochondria (*M*) is present. × *37,600.*

FIGURE 3-17. Phagocytosis by neutrophil.
Recently ingested bacteria in neutrophil from same preparation as that in Figure 3-16. They are contained within vesicles into which cytoplasmic granules coalesce (*arrow*) and release their enzymes. Two bacteria (*asterisks*) have already lost their distinct ribosomes, although their outer cell wall is still identifiable. × *43,300.*

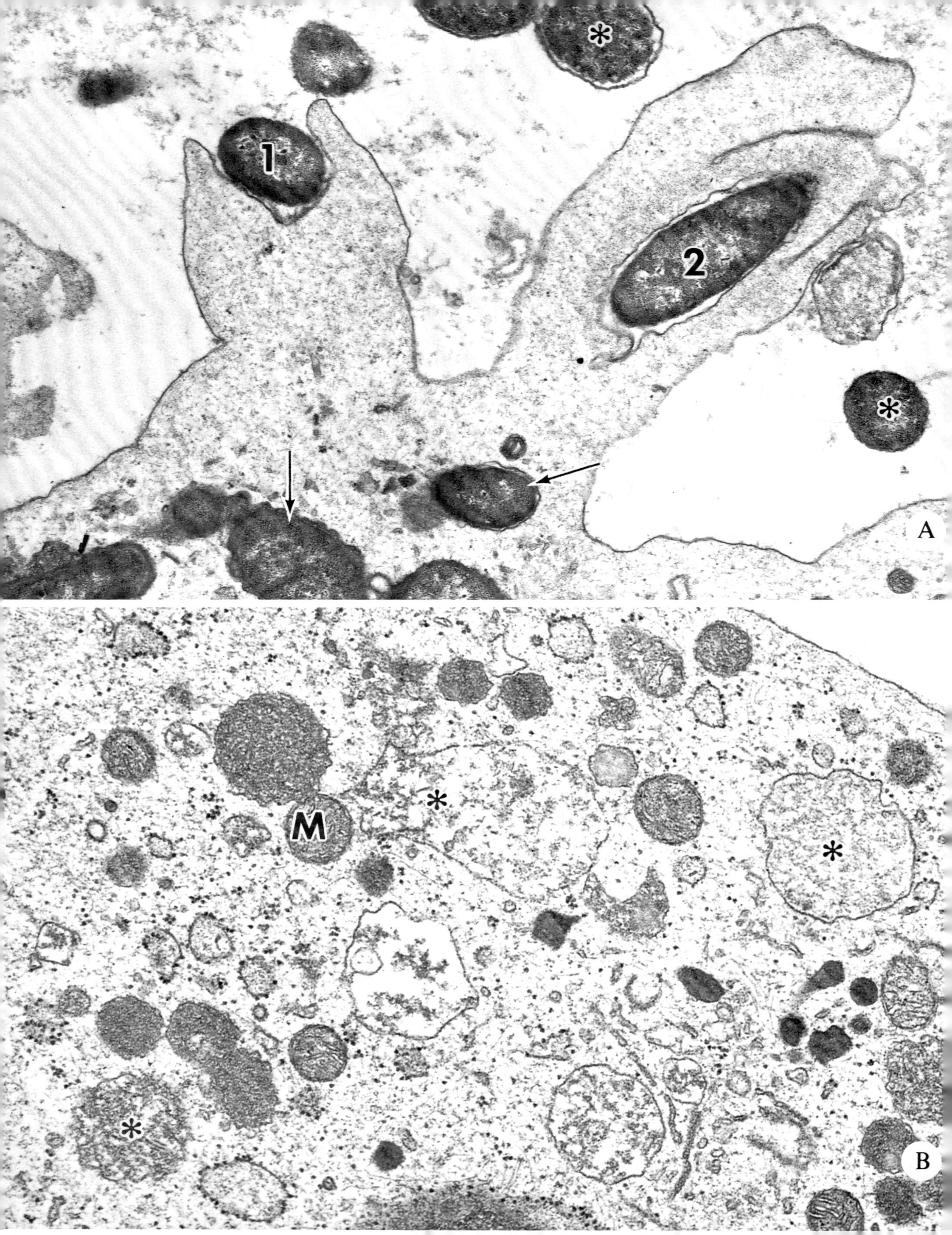
1
2
A
M
B

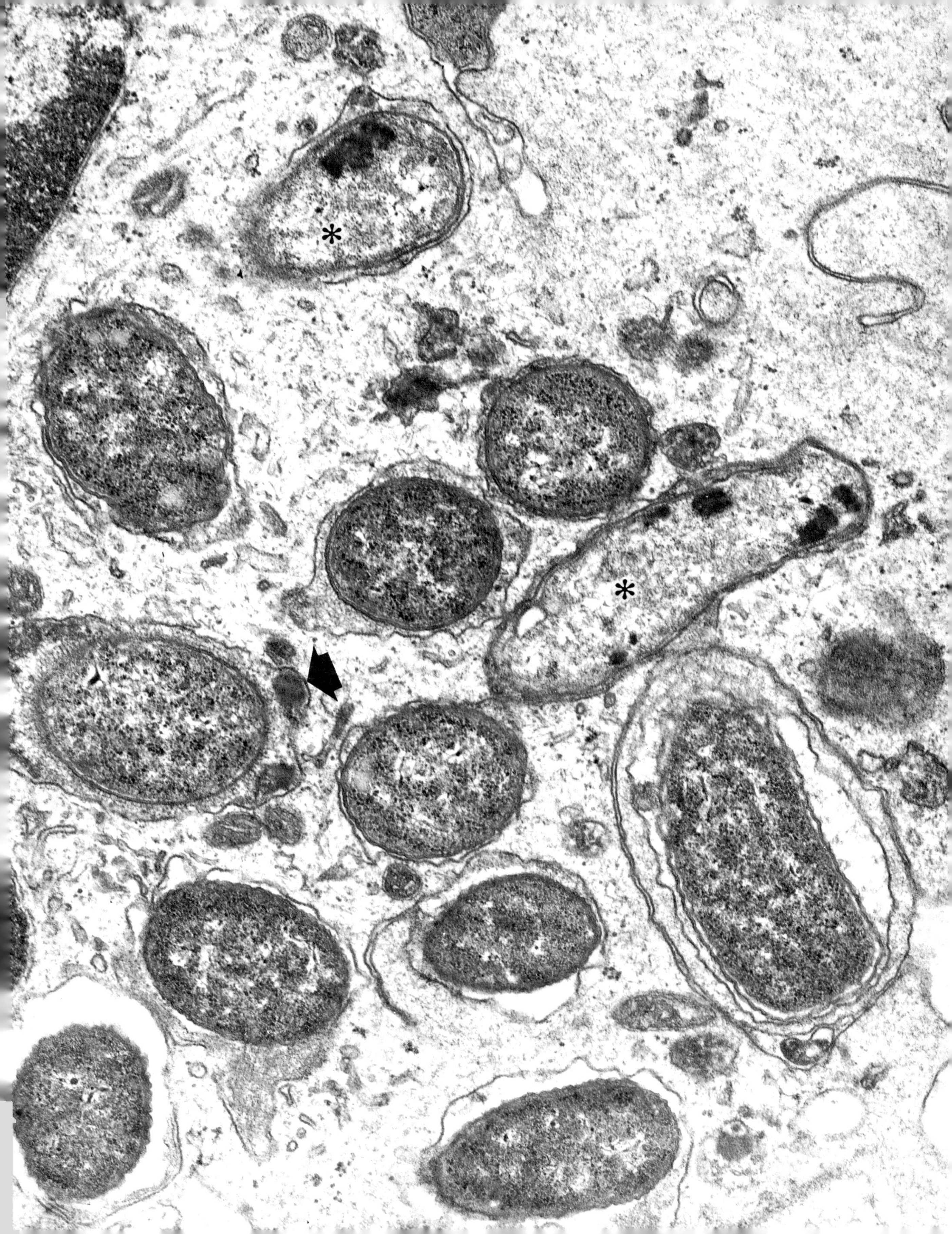

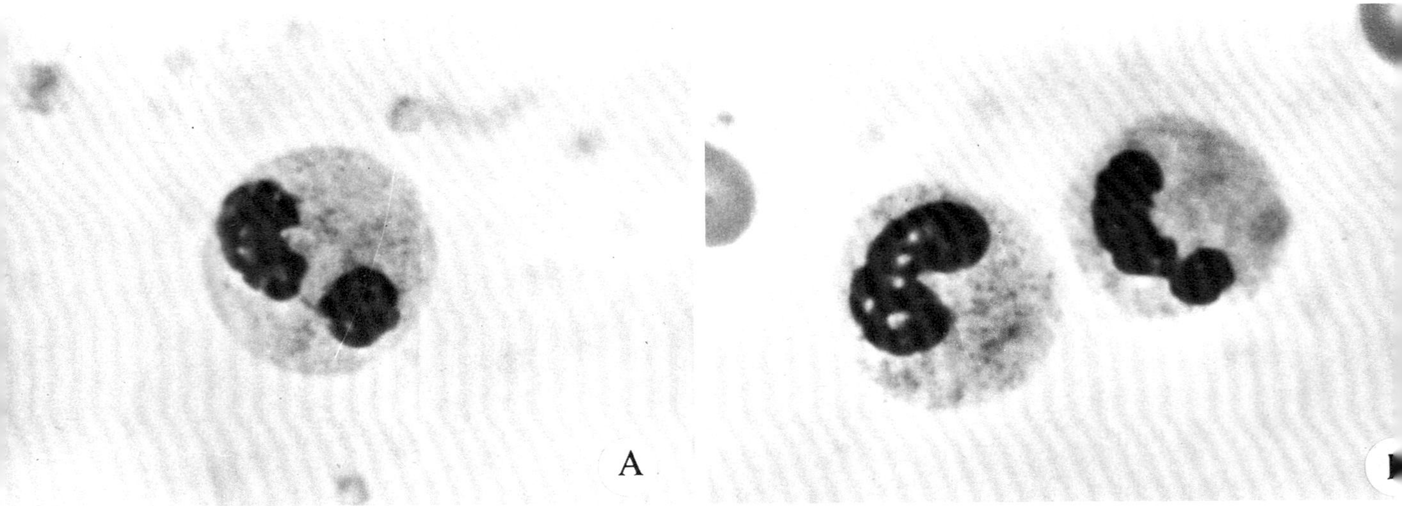

FIGURE 3-18A, B. Pelger-Huët anomaly.
Light micrographs of leukocytes from a Pelger-Huët nuclear anomaly. × *2,000.*

FIGURE 3-19. Pelger-Huët anomaly.
Electron micrograph from same case shown as Figure 3-18. The only apparent abnormality is the shape of the nucleus (*N*) and its dense chromatin. There are numerous granules (*g*) in the cytoplasm. At top is a platelet (*P*). × *46,200.*

nearby vacuoles which contain the engulfed material, the bacteria, etc. (Hirsch, 1962; Lockwood and Allison, 1963; Zucker-Franklin and Hirsch, 1964) (Fig. 3-17). This process occurs within one minute (Zucker-Franklin, 1968). Delivery of a bactericidal substance—phagocytin—from the granules may be initiated by the pH of engulfed material (Cohn and Hirsch, 1960). Some of the basic and cationic proteins of granules may serve as neutralizing agents of anionic components of microorganisms (Spicer and Hardin, 1969). Bacteria are digested by the hydrolytic enzymes of granules (lysosomes) and only amorphous residues remain (Fig. 3-16*B*). During the combat with ingested material, granulocytes utilize most of their granules (Hirsch and Cohn, 1960). The granule-depleted cells do not appear to regenerate granules and are short-lived defenders at the locus of acute inflammation or infection (Spicer and Hardin, 1969).

The role of granulocytes in inflammation, other than that of phagocytosis, has also been explored. Initially, granulocytes release one or more of the following: vasoactive peptide kinin (Melmonk and Cline, 1968), an inflammation-accelerating cationic protein (Janoff and Zweifach, 1964), anticoagulant substances (Saba *et al.,* 1967), and histamine which is released from granulocytes upon stimulation by proper antigens in allergic individuals (Pruzansky and Patterson, 1967). However, the releasing mechanisms of these materials are not clearly understood (see basophil-mast cell section). Neutrophils, when properly stimulated, are also known to form and release a neutral protein

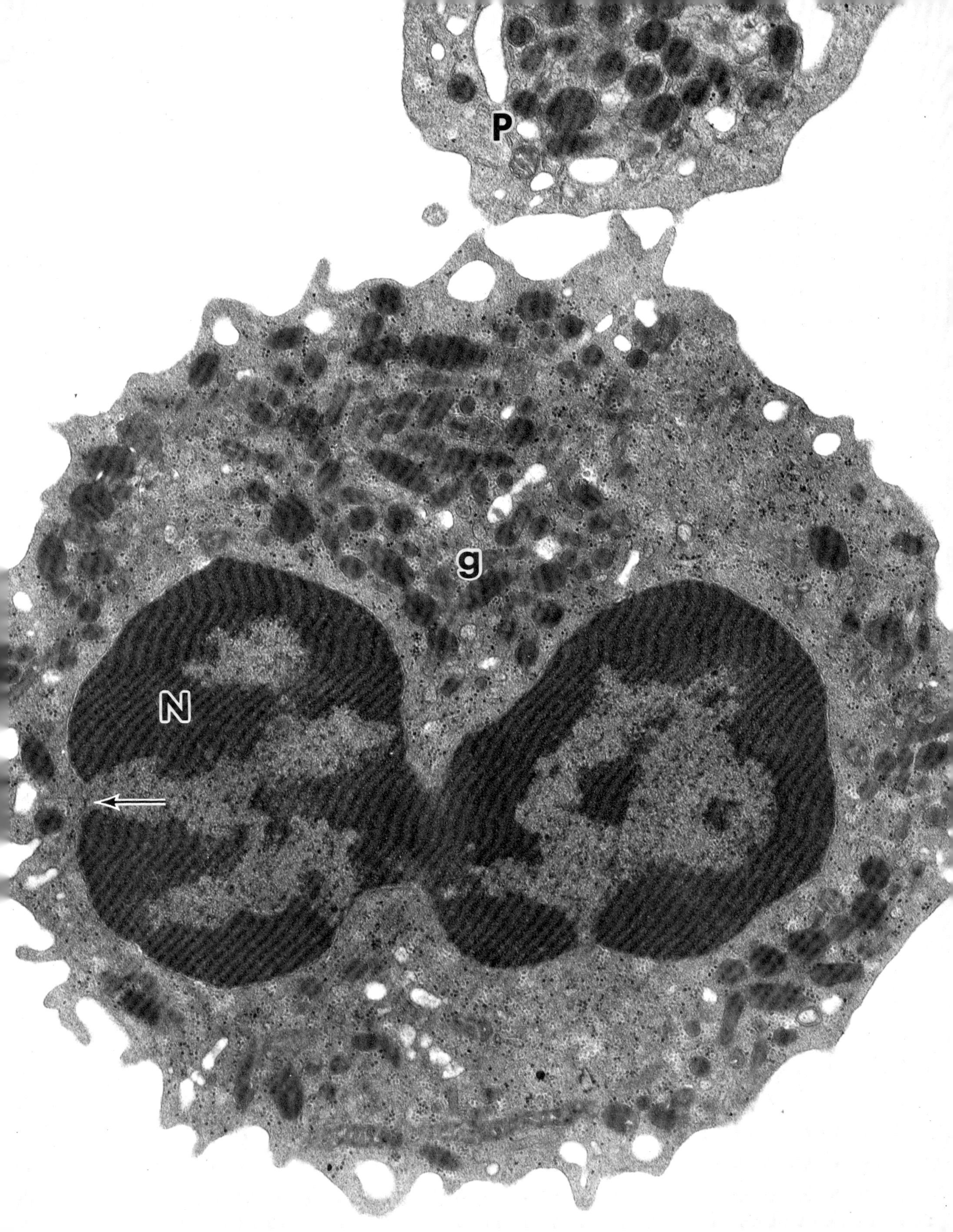
P
g
N

(leukocytic pyrogen) which stimulates the hypothalamic thermoregulatory center to raise body temperature (Bornstein and Woods, 1969).

PATHOLOGY

ANOMALIES IN LEUKOCYTES

Qualitative and quantitative anomalies of circulating leukocytes have been studied by hematologists since Huët in 1932 speculated on an inherited anomaly of nuclear lobulation. A well-documented review was published by Davidson (1968) indicating about 15 different types. Electron microscopic studies have been made on some of these leukocyte anomalies.

Pelger-Huët Nuclear Anomaly

Hyposegmented nuclei of circulating leukocytes were described by Pelger in 1928; Huët (1932) suspected that the disorder was hereditary; it was found to be relatively common, occurring in about 1 per 6,000 population (Davidson, 1968). The nucleus of leukocytes in heterozygous individuals has a characteristic rodlike, dumbbell, or peanut shape, with coarse clumping of the nuclear chromatin (Fig. 3-18). In the homozygote the nucleus is round, with coarse chromatin clumps. The nuclei of monocytes and lymphocytes in the homozygote show similar chromatin condensation. No functional abnormalities have been detected in these leukocytes. The genesis of this nuclear anomaly is not understood. The leukocytes of this disorder have been used as tracers in studies of granulocyte kinetics (Rosse and Gurney, 1959) because of their unique morphology. Figure 3-19 is from a heterozygous form of the Pelger-Huët anomaly. No significant abnormality is found in the cytoplasmic structure.

Similar nuclear anomalies have been observed in man during various disease states, including infections and malignancies (Dorr and Moloney, 1959) and a similar nuclear abnormality was discovered in rabbits (Harm, 1953). The condition is lethal or accompanied by skeletal anomalies in the homozygote. The anomalous leukocytes show round nuclei rather than the bilobulated nuclei of heterozygotes.

May-Hegglin Anomaly

Döhle bodies in leukocytes associated with giant platelets were discovered as a hereditary trait by May in 1909, confirmed by Hegglin in 1945, and by many others since then. Hereditary aspects of the anomaly are now well established (Wassmuth *et al.,* 1963). Cytochemically, Döhle bodies are RNA-containing structures (Wassmuth *et al.,* 1963) that may be related to an impaired maturation of leukocytes; ultrastructural studies show that the Döhle bodies consist of electron-opaque granules of about 200 Å, fibrillar structure of 50 Å, and an associated amorphous substance (Jordan and Larsen, 1965; Lusher *et al.,* 1968). Granules of about 200 Å which appear as clusters in Figures 3, 5, and 6 of the Jordan and Larsen (1965) report are ribosomes rather than glycogen. No abnormalities are reported in other cytoplasmic organelles, including mitochondria and granules (Jordan and Larsen, 1965; Lusher *et al.,* 1968).

The May-Hegglin anomaly is frequently associated with a bleeding tendency. Only slight quantitative and qualitative abnormalities have been reported on the circulating platelets. Ultrastructural investigation reveals no abnormalities in platelet structure except for giant size (Jordan and Larsen, 1965;

Lusher *et al.,* 1968). There is no clear indication that leukocytes of this disorder are functionally impaired except for the one report by Rebuck *et al.* (1963), which showed some defective phagocytosis.

Chediak-Steinbrinck-Higashi Anomaly

This familial panleukocyte abnormality, with giant granules and usually fatal course at an early age, was first reported by Steinbrinck in 1948. Independently, a well-written report of granulocyte morphology was made by Chediak in 1952. Anomalous giant granules in leukocytes, a pigment anomaly of the skin and hair (albinism), photophobia, and neuropathy are frequently associated with this disorder. The impaired function of leukocytes in body defense results in high susceptibility to infections, induction of hepatosplenomegaly, and general lymphadenopathy. Peripheral leukocyte counts vary from hypo- to hypercellular, and children usually die within 10 years. Giant granules in peripheral leukocytes are characteristic of this disorder (Fig. 3-20). They are negative in alkaline phosphatase and positive in peroxidase (Higashi, 1953) and acid phosphatase. The PAS reaction is negative. Similar giant granules are seen in lymphocytes as well as monocytes.

Ultrastructural investigations have been made by several investigators (Bessis *et al.,* 1961; White, 1966a, b; Douglas *et al.,* 1969). Abnormal granules of the leukocytes are similar to coexisting normal-looking granules except for their large size and high incidence of disintegration in internal structure (Fig. 3-21). These granules show a strong acid-phosphatase reaction and are considered to be lysosomes (White, 1966a). It has been suggested that the essential defect of this disorder is either in lipid metabolism or membranes (Windhorst *et al.,* 1966), but there have been no conclusive observations in either category. This disorder has been noted to have a high incidence of acute leukemia and susceptibility to viral infections (White, 1966b).

A leukocyte abnormality has been reported in mink (Leader *et al.,* 1963; Padgett *et al.,* 1964), cattle (Padgett *et al.,* 1964), and beige mice (Lutzner *et al,* 1967), with cytological and pathoanatomical characteristics similar to those reported in human cases.

MYELOCYTIC LEUKEMIA

Malignant proliferation of granulocytes, defined as myelocytic leukemia is fatal. The duration of illness and type of proliferating cell classifies myelocytic leukemia into acute and chronic forms. Because of its high mortality, there has been extensive research and many excellent reviews are available on this condition.

Abnormal increase in white cells was recognized for many years before the classification of blood cells was established. Discovery of leukemia is credited to Velpeau (1827), Bennett (1845), and Virchow (1845) (all cited by Dameshek and Gunz, 1964). The term "leukemia" was introduced by Virchow in 1847 (cited by Dameshek and Gunz, 1964) and many of his original views on the nature of leukemia are still considered valid in contemporary medical science. The introduction of staining methods for blood cells led to extensive studies on this disease, and finally lymphatic leukemia was separated from the granulocytic form. Later, monocytic leukemia was also identified (Reschad and Schilling-Torgau, 1913), and the classification of different types of human leukemia was established. Modern investigations of leukemia have produced exhaustive studies into its etiology, particularly in relation to viral carcinogenesis and methods of early diagnosis and therapy. As yet, there are no definitive conclusions in any of these fields; however, it is expected that leukemia will be included in the category of curable diseases in the future.

Acute Myelocytic Leukemia

Extensive proliferation of abnormal immature granulocytes in bone marrow suppresses the prolifieration of other myeloid elements and there is severe anemia, bleeding tendency, and high susceptibility of infections. The onset of acute leukemia is abrupt, of short duration, and usually terminates within a few months. The presence of malignant cells in peripheral blood can be detected easily by routine smears (Fig. 3-22). The extensive number of immature cells in the bone marrow confirms the diagnosis. Morphologically abnormal cells are highly immature and granule formation is defective or impaired. Extensive coverage of morphology based on light microscopic investigation is available (Dameshek and Gunz, 1964). Morphologically, the cells resemble myeloblasts. They also have been called leukemic myeloblasts or paramyeloblasts (frequently in the European literature). As is common in immature forms, the cells show a large nucleus with prominent nucleoli and a strong basophilic but scanty cytoplasm. About 50 percent of cases of leukemia have some cells that contain needle-shaped cytoplasmic inclusions called Auer bodies (Fig. 3-28), which help to identify the myelocytic nature of the proliferating cells. The very small proliferating cells are sometimes called micromyeloblasts. Proliferating cells in myelocytic leukemia show a strongly positive reaction in the peroxidase test and serve to affirm the cytogenesis of the malignant cells.

Electron microscopic studies on cells of acute myelocytic anemia have appeared repeatedly (Freeman and Samuels, 1958; Low and Freeman, 1958; Marchal *et al.,* 1959; Ackerman *et al., 1960;* Braunsteiner and Pakesch, 1960; Freeman, 1960, 1966; Bessis and Thiéry, 1961b; Akasaka, 1963; Anderson, 1966; Ito, 1966; McDuffie, 1967a; Seman and Seman, 1968; Bessis and Breton-Gorius, 1969; Smetana *et al.,* 1969) and confirm the resemblance between the malignant cells and immature myeloid elements observed by light microscopy. Morphologically, cells in acute myelocytic leukemia vary from myeloblastic to promyelocytic forms (Figs. 3-23 through 3-25); with a large, centrally located nucleus. The nucleus is frequently lobulated or deeply indented (Fig. 3-23); nucleoli are common (Figs. 3-23*A,* 3-24*A,* 3-25*A*) and the nuclear bodies observed are believed to be rudimentary nucleoli. The chromatin in the nucleus is diffusely reticular, but condensation near the nuclear rim or some patchy forms are sometimes seen (Figs. 3-23 through 3-25). Occasionally, nuclear blebs or projections (Fig. 3-26*A*) and lamellated structures are found on the nuclear rim (McDuffie, 1967b). The cytoplasm appears relatively wider than normal and contains various organelles. Polyribosomes, which are responsible for cytoplasmic basophilia, are diffusely distributed (Figs. 3-23 through 3-25). Electron-opaque granules of small sizes, similar to those observed in early promyelocytes, are observed frequently in the cytoplasm of leukemic cells (Fig. 3-26*B*), even in cases in which no granules are detectable by light microscopy. The Golgi apparatus is moderately developed, and there are active signs of granulogenesis and possible formation of some azurophilic granules (Fig. 3-27). Usually, no specific granules are seen. Cells in acute myelocytic leukemia are considered to have impaired differentiation of the secondary granulogenesis (Spicer and Hardin, 1969). In general, there appears to be a lack of coordination between the maturation of the nucleus and the cytoplasmic organelles.

Unlike immature cells of the erythroid series, abnormal myeloid cells show many profiles of endoplasmic reticulum (Figs. 3-23 and 3-25*A*); occasionally, the development of this structure is so extensive that the whole image of leukemic cells resembles that of myeloma cells (Fig. 3-25*A*). The large amounts of endoplasmic reticulum may be an exaggerated expression of similar structures commonly noted in the promyelocyte stage. Application of peroxidase at the ultrastructural level demonstrates the presence of enzymes in the nuclear envelope, endoplasmic reticulum, Golgi area, and formed granules. This positive reaction corresponds to a similar phenomenon reported by light microscopy. Activity of excess myeloperoxidase enzymes formed in malignant cells is considered to be responsible for the coloration of proliferating foci in chloroma. Several abnormal cytoplasmic characteristics have been described.

Auer bodies (Fig. 3-28) studied by electron microscopy (Freeman, 1960, 1966; Kondo *et al.*, 1966; McDuffie, 1967a) show an apparently abortive azurophilic granule which is positive for both acid phosphatase and peroxidase. The inclusions appear singly or in multiples. Occasionally, a tubular or periodic array of about 100 Å may be detected in the structure. Needle-like structures of considerably smaller types may also be seen in leukemic cells, the morphology of which is essentially similar to that of Auer bodies except for their extremely small size.

The presence of *fibrillar structures* (Fig. 3-29) in leukemic leukocytes was

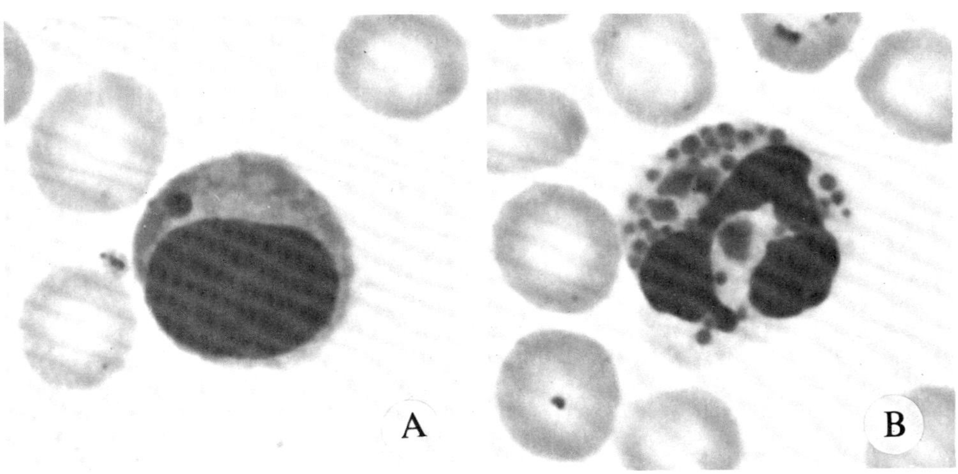

FIGURE 3-20. Chediak-Steinbrinck-Higashi anomaly.
Light micrographs of Chediak-Steinbrinck-Higashi anomaly show giant granules in lymphocyte (**A**) and neutrophil (**B**). × *2,000.*
Courtesy of Dr. S. Hino.

(*text continues on page 130*)

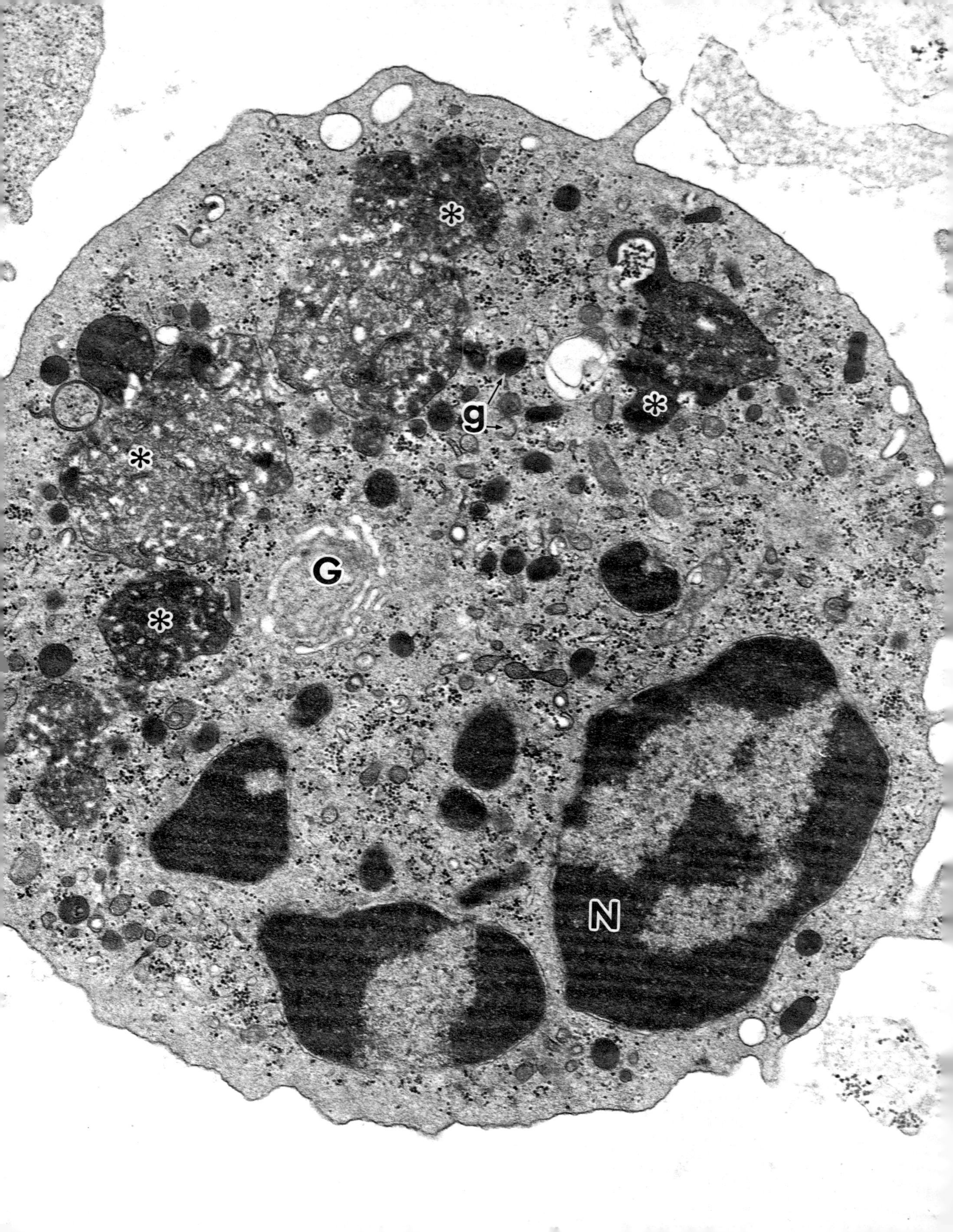

*
g
*
*
G
*
N

FIGURE 3-21. Chediak-Steinbrinck-Higashi anomaly.
Electron micrograph of neutrophil of Chediak-Steinbrinck-Higashi anomaly. The very large granules (*asterisks*) have heterogeneous content, both granular and amorphous in appearance. Normal light and dense granules (*g*), glycogen, and a vesicular Golgi complex (*G*) are present. Nucleus (*N*) is at lower right. × *29,000.*
Specimens provided by Dr. S. Douglas.

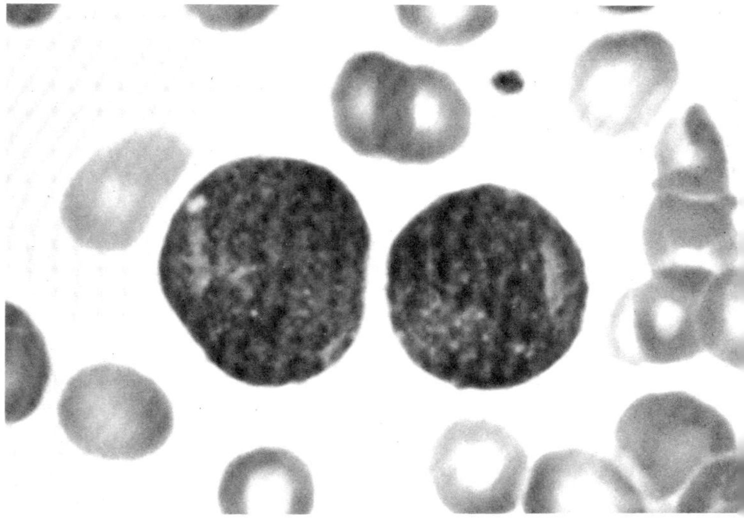

FIGURE 3-22. Malignant cells in acute myelocytic leukemia.
Light micrograph of acute myelocytic leukemic cells from peripheral blood. × *2,000.*

Figures 3-23 through 3-26 appear on the following pages

FIGURE 3-23. Acute myelocytic leukemia.
Proliferating cells from bone marrow in acute myelocytic leukemia (same case as shown in Figure 3-22), with characteristics of myeloblasts seen in Figure 3-3, except for the presence of highly indented nuclei (*N*) and numerous cytoplasmic extensions (*asterisks*). This irregular surface suggests mobility of these leukemic cells. Fat vacuoles (*arrows*) are also present, as are several mitochondria (*M*). × *17,600.*

FIGURE 3-24. Marrow cells in acute myelocytic leukemia.
A. Immature cell from bone marrow of patient with acute myelocytic leukemia has characteristics of a hemocytoblast. It is not certain if this is a malignant immature stem cell proliferating in the marrow or a normal hemocytoblast reacting to leukemic stimulus to produce a benign proliferation. The cytoplasm contains mainly large mitochondria (*M*) and polyribosomes while the nucleus (*N*) has a large nucleolus (*Nu*). × *16,000.*
B. In a second case of acute myelocytic leukemia, an immature cell has developed more endoplasmic reticulum (*er*) and a few granules (*arrows*). Some mitochondria (*M*) are present. Chromatin in nucleus (*N*) is diffuse. × *15,700.*

FIGURE 3-25. Cells in acute myelocytic leukemia.
A. Leukemic cell has extensive rough endoplasmic reticulum (*er*) and cisternae containing amorphous substance. There are a very large Golgi complex (*G*), many free ribosomes and polyribosomes, a few granules (*arrow*), and mitochondria (*M*) in the cytoplasm. The nucleus (*N*) contains a large nucleolus (*Nu*). Well-developed endoplasmic reticulum gives the general appearance of an atypical plasma cell. × *16,700.*
B. In an atypical cell from another patient with leukemia there are abundant small round mitochondria (*M*), generally vesicular cytoplasm, and scattered dense glycogen particles. × *17,300.*

FIGURE 3-26. Acute myelocytic leukemic cells.
A. Nuclear (*N*) bleb (*B*) in leukemic cell has a peculiar internal lamellated structure. × *56,000.*
B. Cytoplasmic detail of cell in Figure 3-25**A**, showing endoplasmic reticulum (*er*). Note granules (*g*), edge of nucleus (*N*), and mitochondria (*M*). × *43,400.*

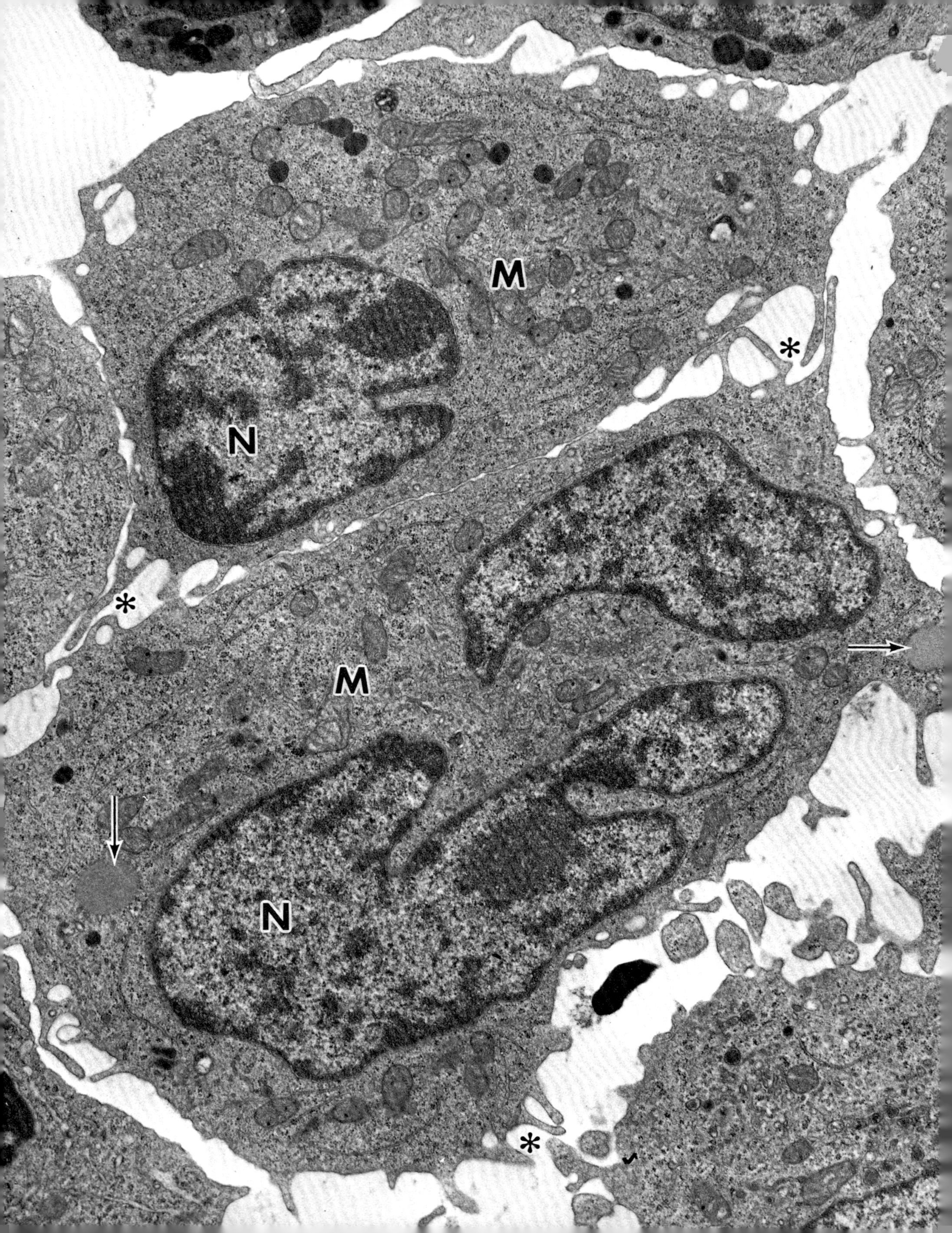
M
N
*
*
M
N
*

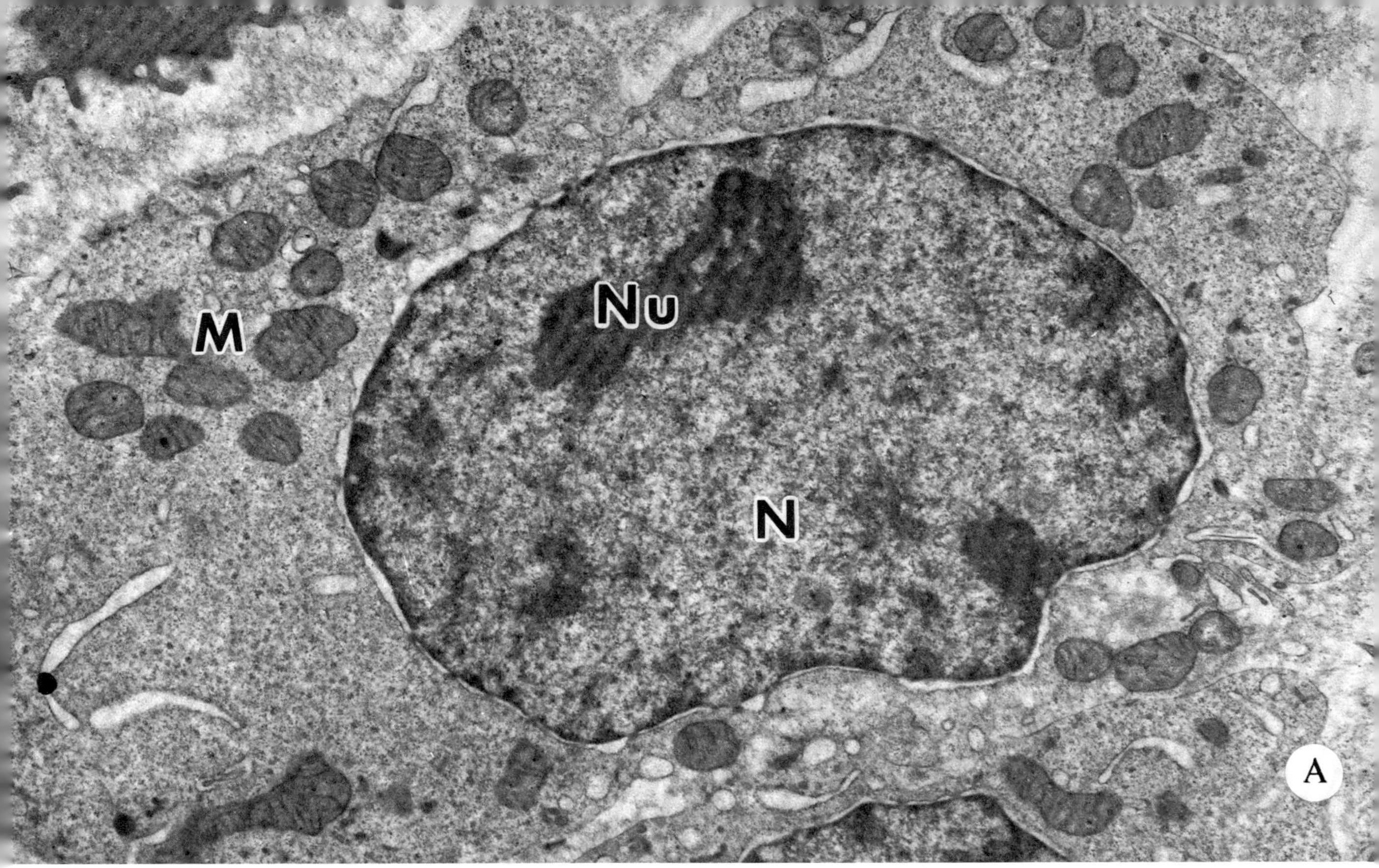
Nu
M
N
A

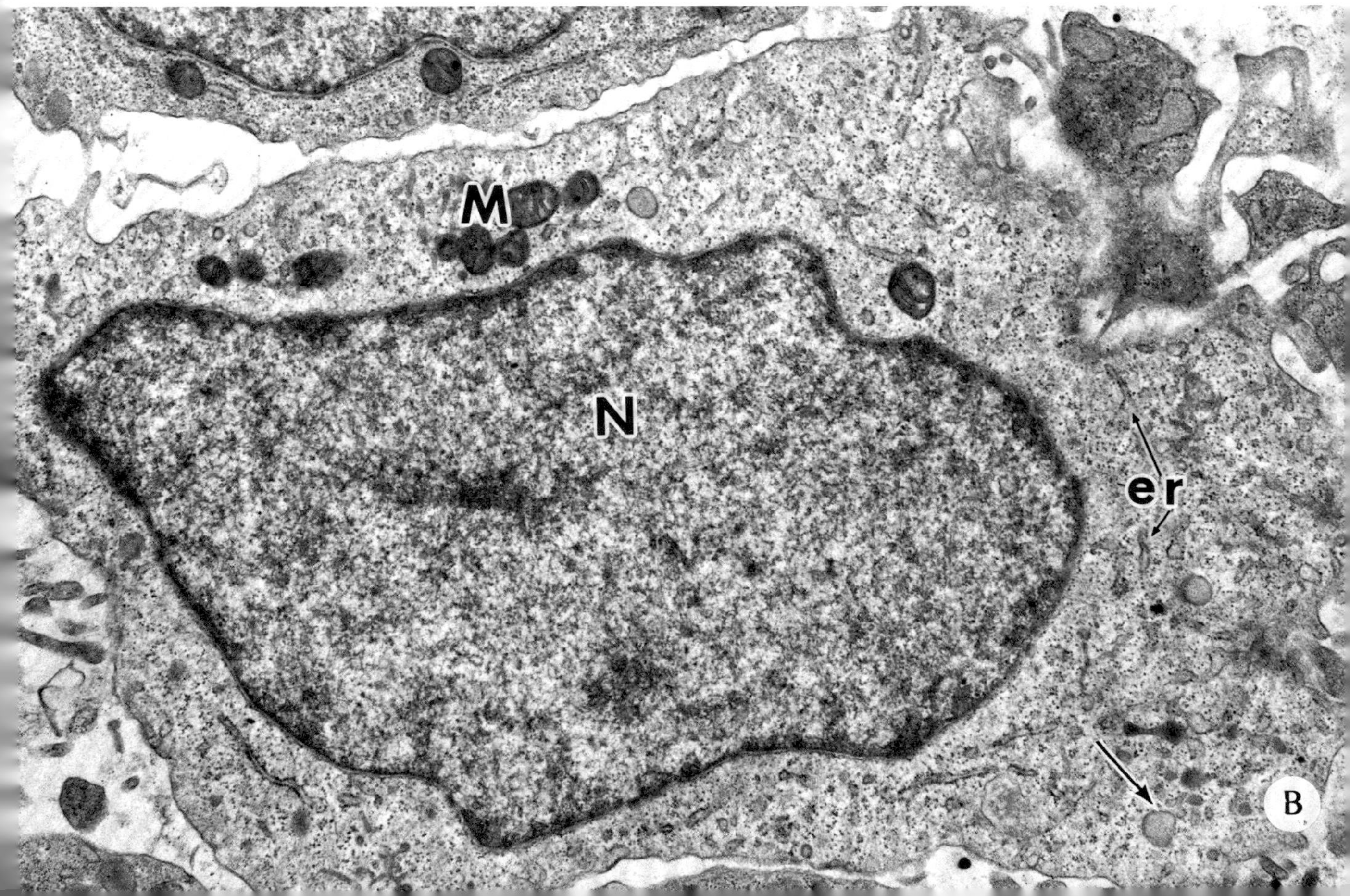
M
N
er
B

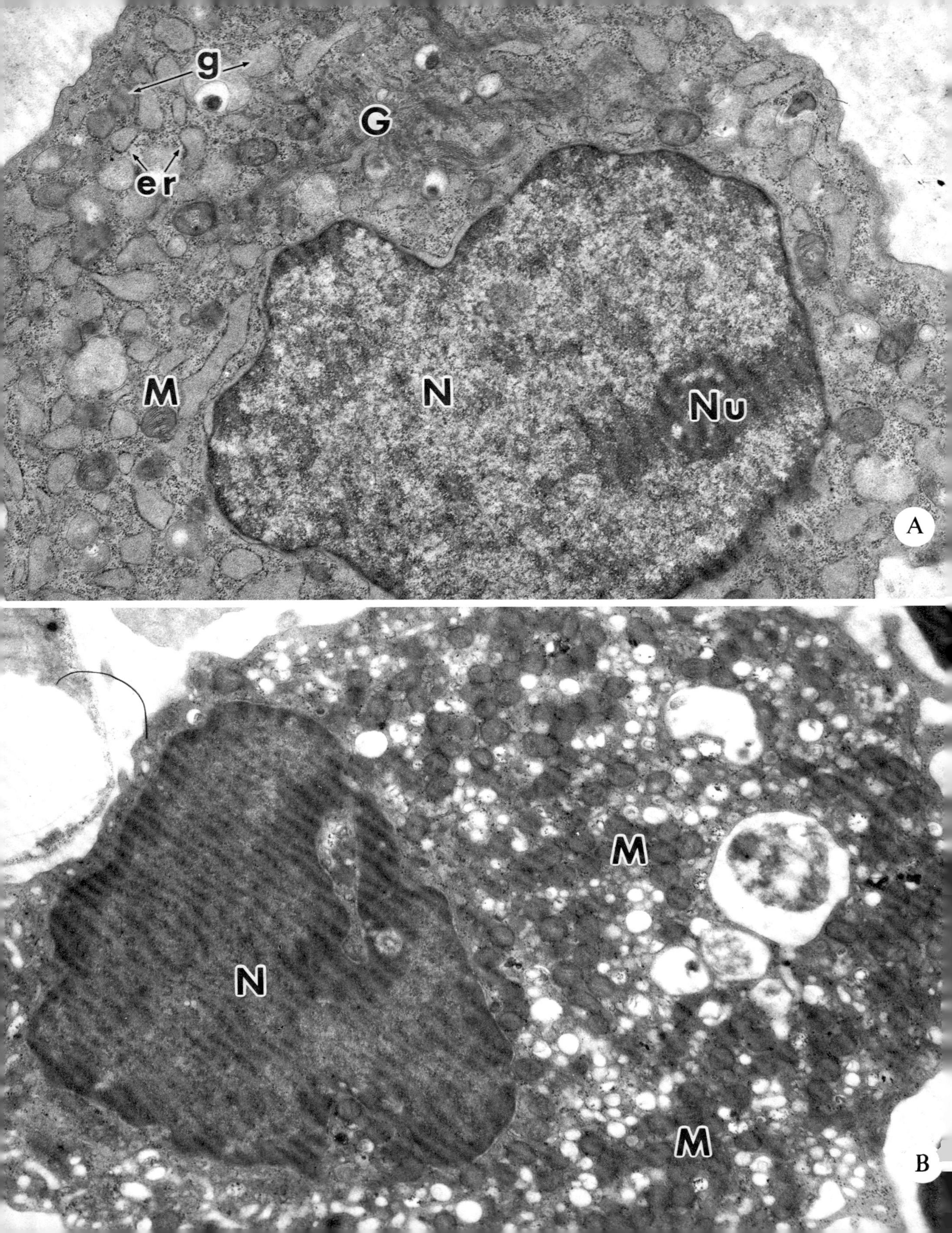
g
G
er
M
N
Nu
A
M
N
M
B

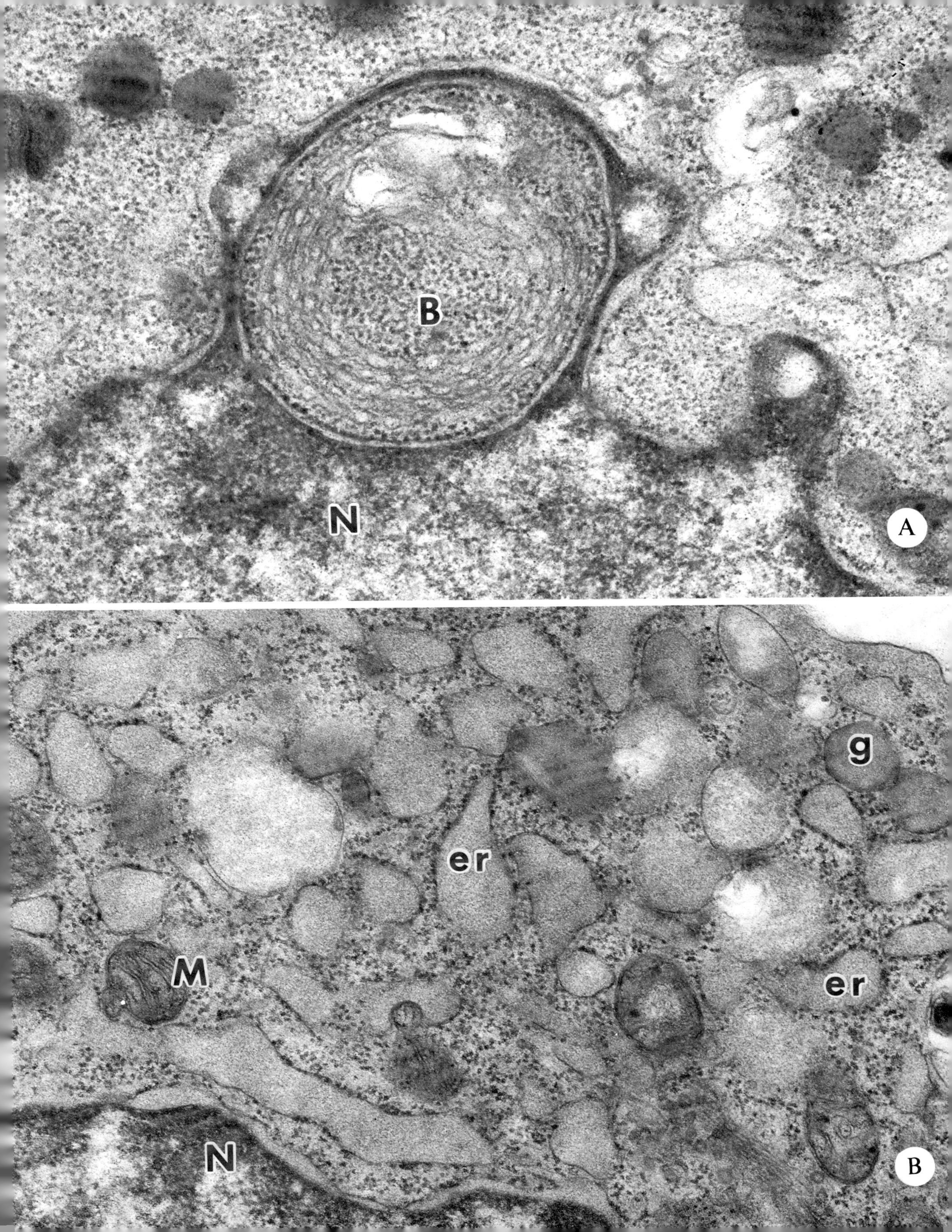
B
N
A
g
er
M
er
N
B

first noted by Bessis and Breton-Gorius in 1955 and described as a crescent zone. Later, Freeman and Samuels (1958) studied the same structure more precisely. The structure can also be detected by phase microscopy and is known to appear frequently in cells of monocytic leukemia, but its significance is not known. Fibrillar structures, both bundles and individual forms, may be seen in the cytoplasm of malignant cells (Anderson, 1966). They are not known to be related to the fibrils described above. Fibrillar bundles are also reported in the nucleus of leukemic granulocytes (Bessis and Breton-Gorius, 1969), the nature of which is also unknown.

Pseudoviral inclusions (Figs. 3-30 and 3-31)—small vesicles of about 30 to 70μ resembling the type C particles described by Bernhard (1960)—are noted in cells of myeloma (Sorenson, 1961) and both myelocytic and lymphocytic leukemia (Tanaka *et al.,* 1967). The structure corresponds to the cytoplasmic inclusions described by Terrasse *et al.* (1958) in leukemic cells. These structures are known to be PAS-positive after saliva digestion, metachromatic, alcian blue-positive, and contain proteins and acid phosphatase (Tanaka *et al.,* 1967). They are negative in RNA and DNA. These cytochemical data are compatible with a lysosomal structure and not viral in nature. Other unusual inclusions (Fig. 3-32) which may or may not be viral have been observed in the cisterna of endoplasmic reticulum in malignant cells of acute promyelocytic leukemia (Ogawa, 1968). This observation was confirmed by Matsuoko *et al.* (1969). The structures appear as honeycomb in one direction of sectioning or, alternatively, as dense lines about 100 Å wide, periodically arranged with about 200 Å spacing. This has been reported only in acute promyelocytic leukemia which accompanies coagulopathies. The structure is limited to the rough endoplasmic reticulum and does not appear to be associated with either the Golgi apparatus or granules. Its significance is not apparent (see discussion on viral particles in Chap. 5).

Chronic Myelocytic Leukemia

Granulocytic malignancy with predominantly mature forms, classified as chronic myelocytic leukemia (Fig. 3-33) has a gradual onset and a better survival time than the acute type. Proliferating cells which appear in peripheral blood are highly differentiated and are difficult to distinguish from physiological cells. The patient may have slight to moderate hepatosplenomegaly due to the peripheral accumulation of the malignant cells. The progress of the disease is dependent on therapy; however nearly 80 per cent of the cases eventually develop an acute myeloblastic crisis which leads to early death. The blastic crisis of chronic myelocytic leukemia could be regarded as the onset of another malignancy. However, persistence of the Philadelphia (Ph) chromosomes after blastic change is against such a conclusion (Kundel *et al.,* 1963). The bone marrow is filled with granulocytes

FIGURE 3-27. Golgi complex of acute myelocytic leukemia cell.
Golgi area (*G*) of acute myelocytic leukemia cell shows elaboration of early granules (*arrows*). More mature types of granules (*g*) are seen near by. The edge of the nucleus (*N*) and mitochondria (*M*) are present. × *53,500.*

(*text continues on page 138*)

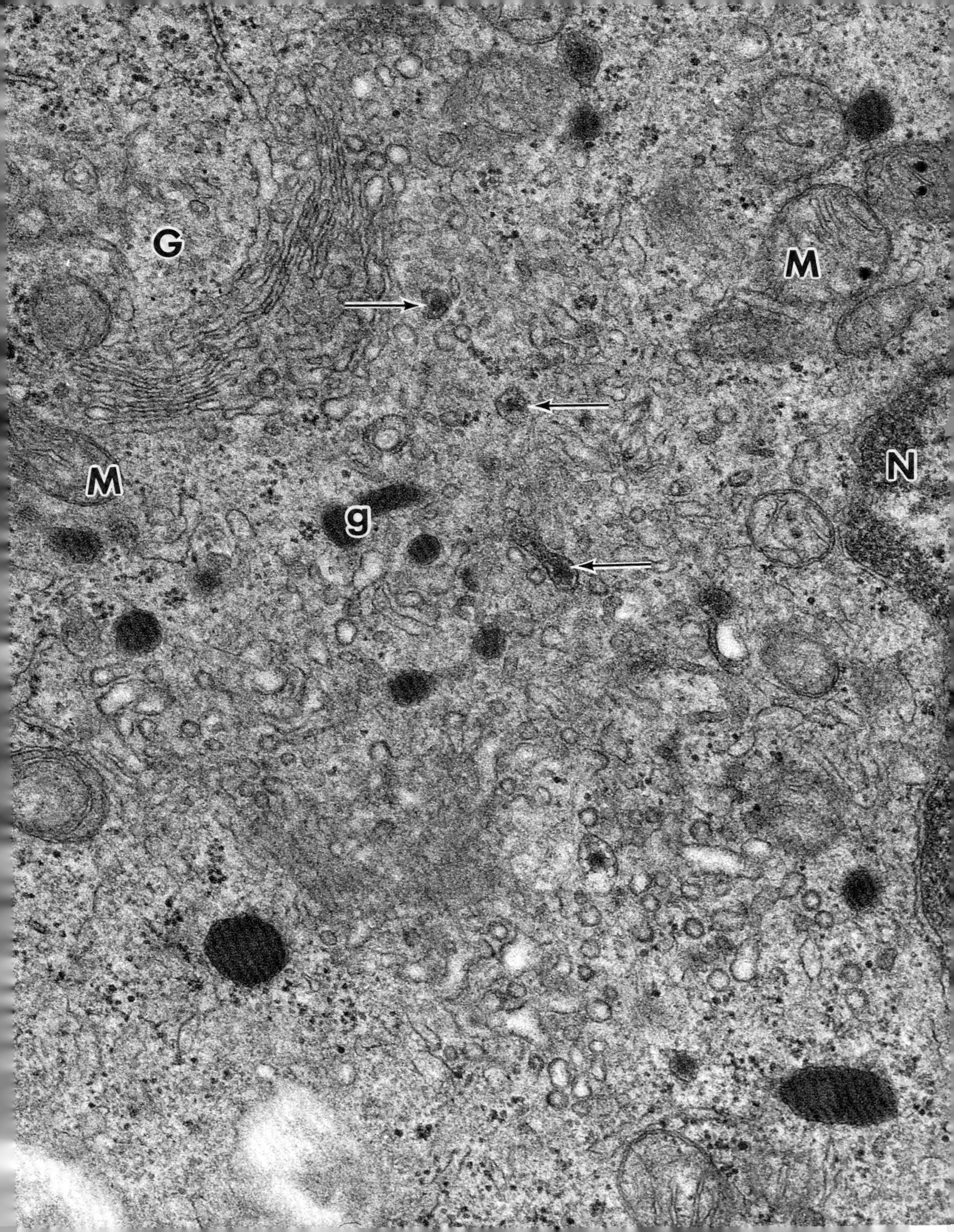
G
M
M
N
g

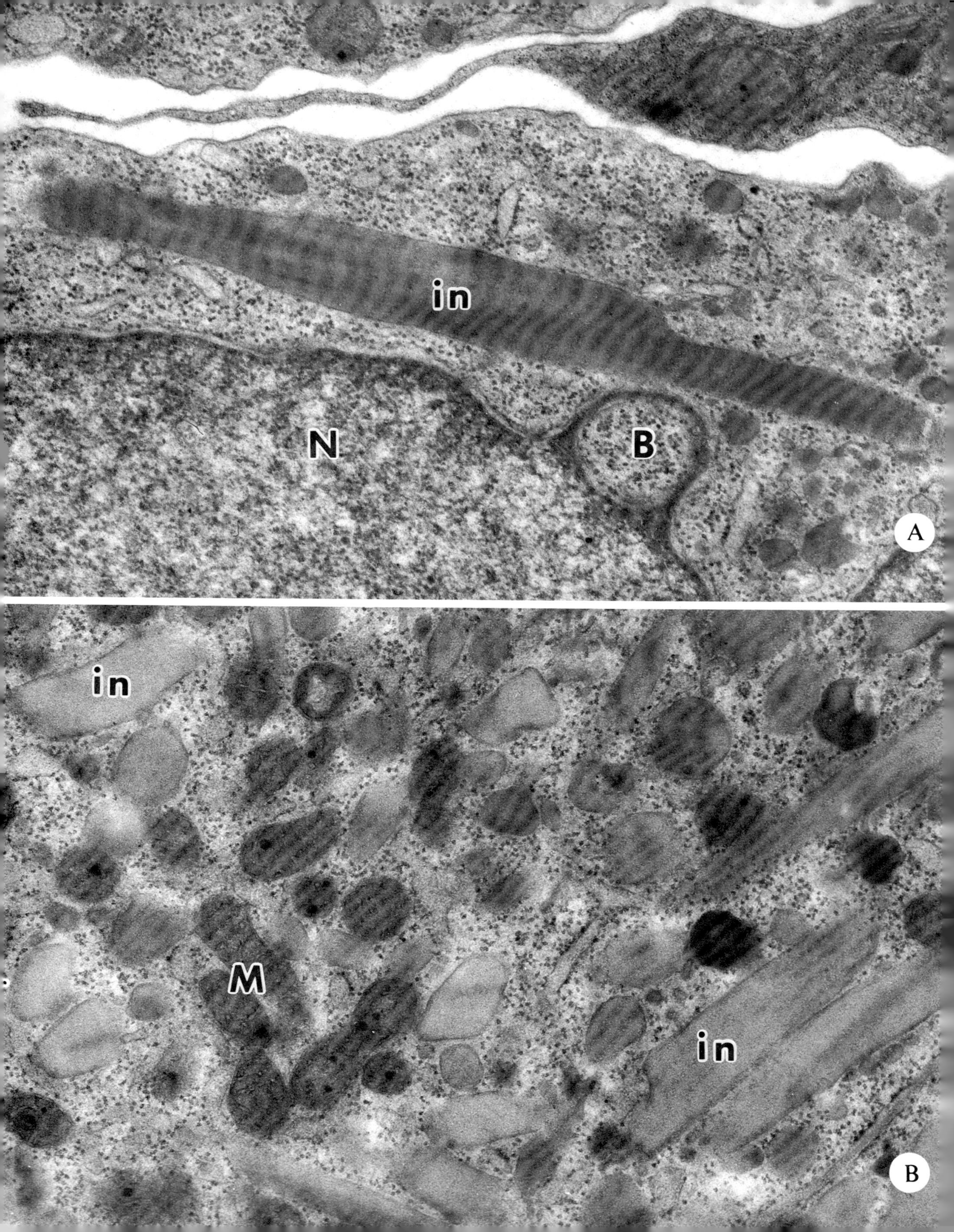
in
N
B
A
in
M
in
B

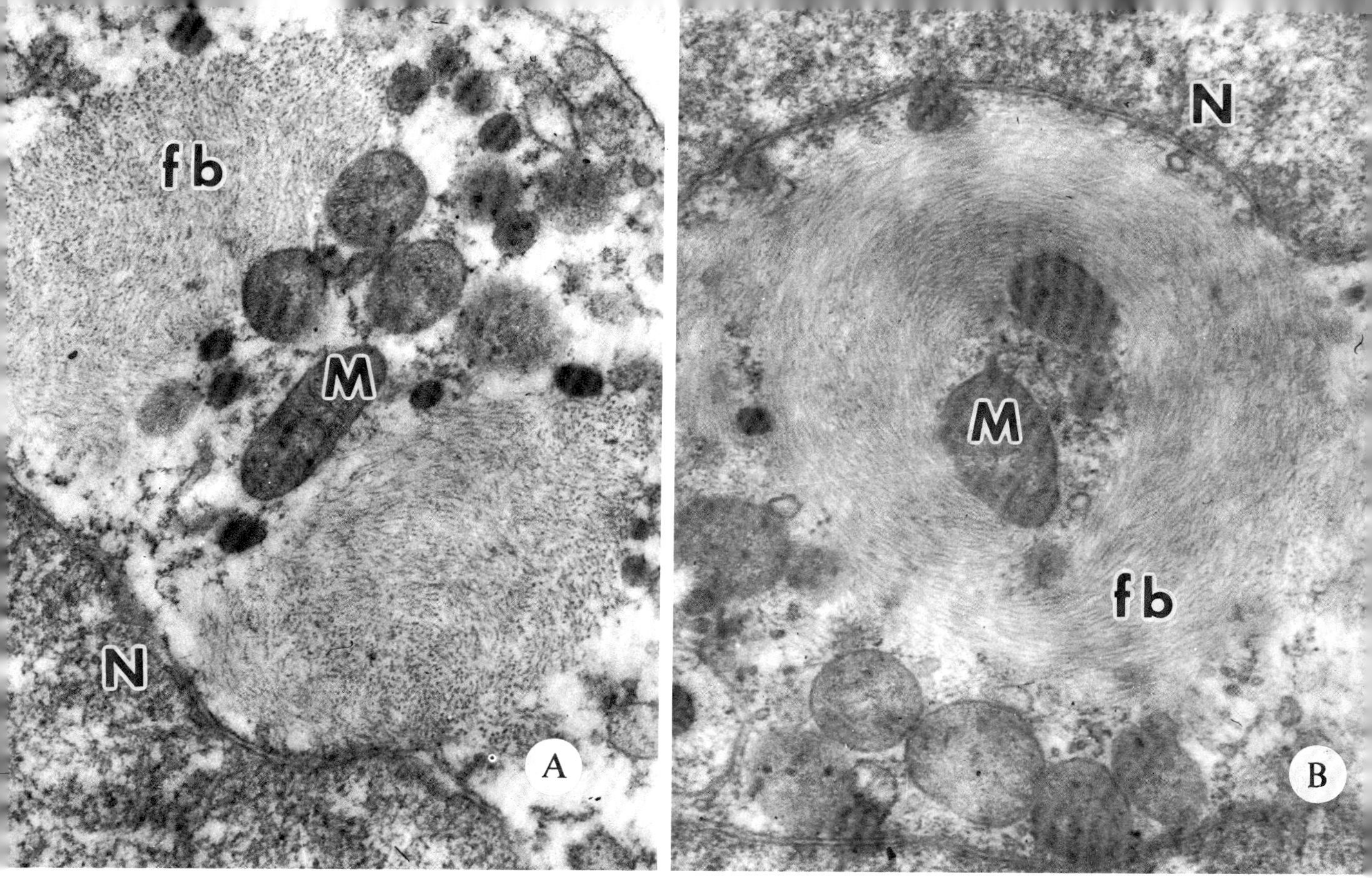

FIGURE 3-29. Free fibrillar material in leukemia cells.
Such material is sometimes found in cytoplasm of myelogenous leukemia cells, frequently near the nucleus (*N*), often doughnut-shaped and sometimes with mitochondria (*M*) in the "hole."

A. Cross-section to plane of fibers (*fb*). × *16,000.*

B. Parallel to plane of fibers (*fb*). × *16,000.*

Reprinted with permission from Kundel, D. W., Tanaka, Y., Tijo, J. H., Whang, J., and Fishbein, W. N. *Nouv Rev Franc Hemat 3:*844, 1963.

FIGURE 3-28. Auer bodies in acute myelocytic leukemia cells.

A. A single needle-shaped inclusion (*in*) with some variation in density. Nucleus (*N*) has a bleb (*B*). × *41,000.*

B. More electron-lucent multiple crystalloid inclusions (*in*). Mitochondria (*M*) are present. × *43,000.*

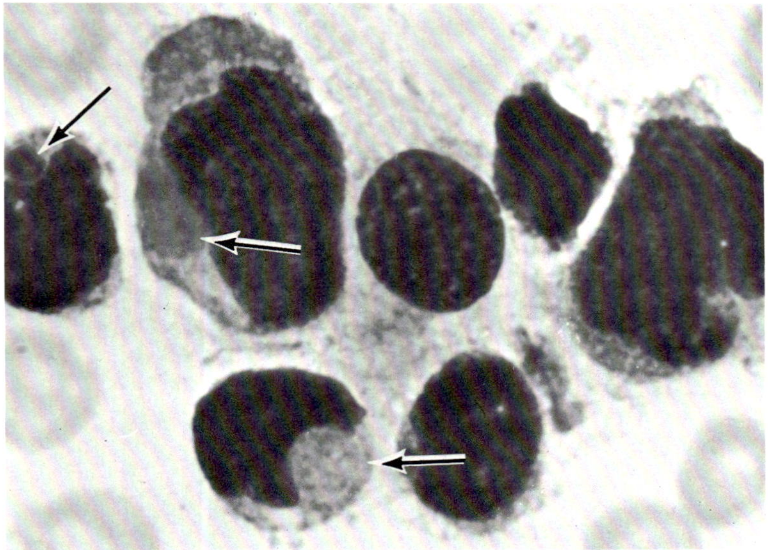

FIGURE 3-30. Inclusions in acute myelocytic leukemia.
Light micrograph of large unusual inclusions (*arrows*) in acute myelogenous leukemia. × *2,000.*

FIGURE 3-31. Inclusions in acute myelocytic leukemia.
Electron micrograph of type of inclusion shown in Figure 3-30. The inclusion has many small virus-like particles (*arrows)* and numerous electron-dense structures (*asterisks*), with some filamentous material as a matrix. Mitochondria (*M*) and the edge of the nucleus (*N*) are also present. × *48,000.*

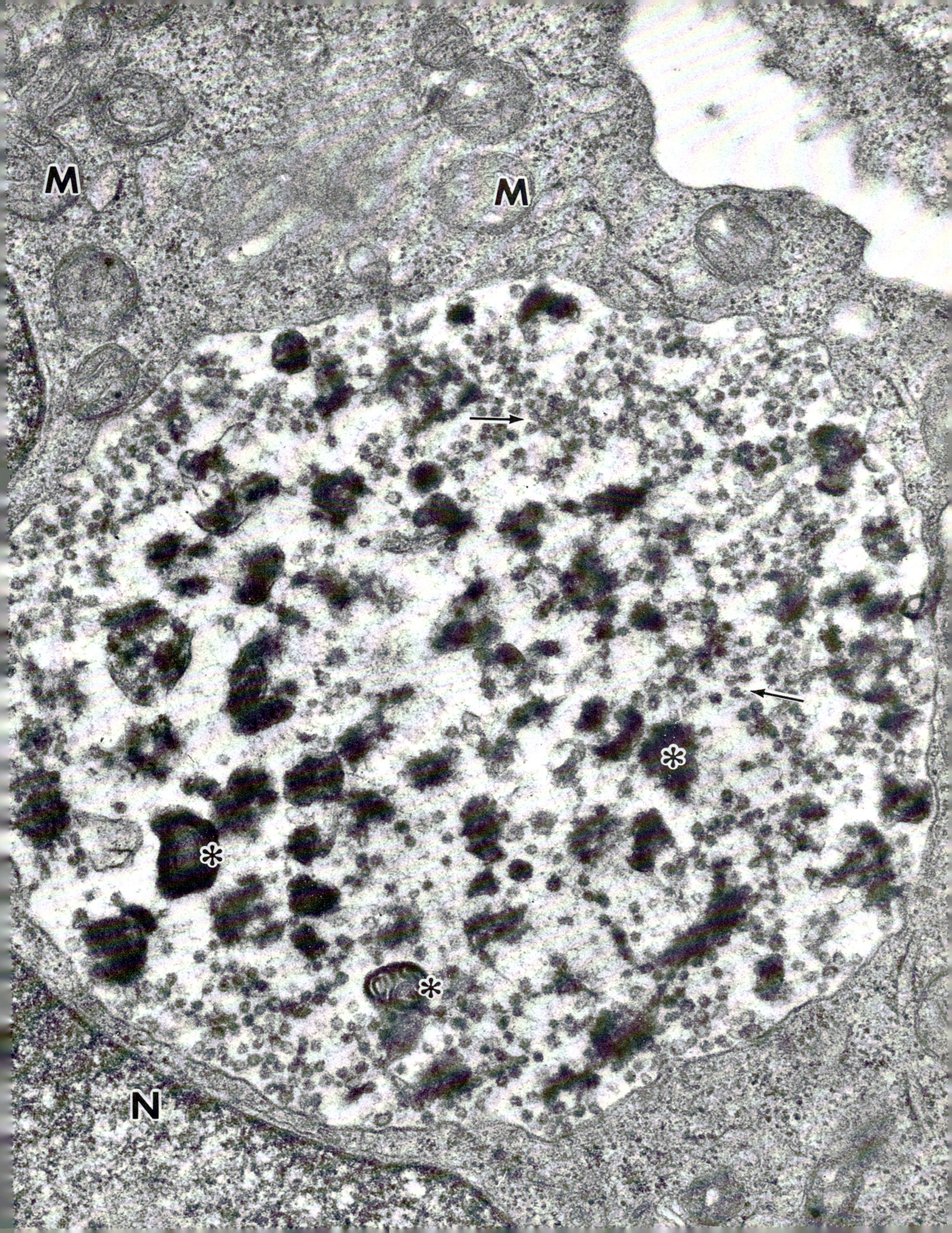
M
M
N

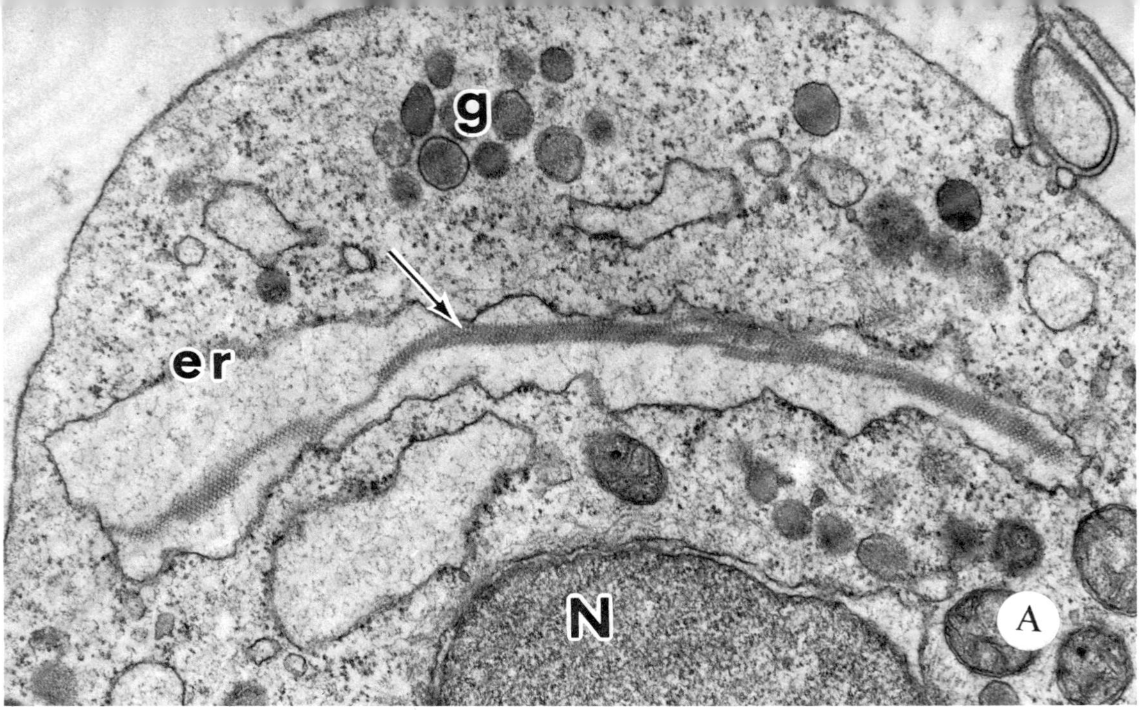

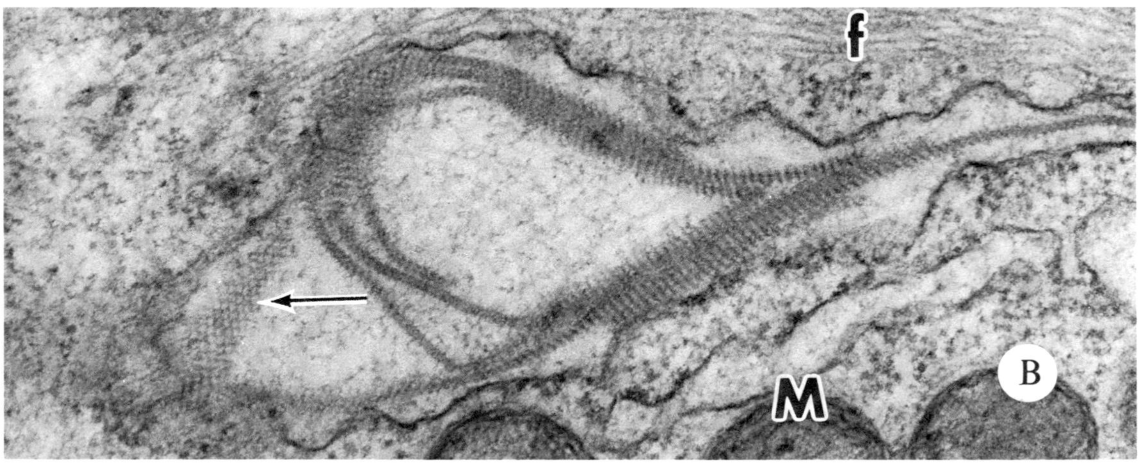

FIGURE 3-32. Cytoplasmic inclusions in acute promyelocytic leukemia.

A. A peculiar cytoplasmic inclusion (*arrow*) in a cell of acute promyelocytic leukemia. The inclusion is in the cisterna of endoplasmic reticulum (*er*). Both periodic and honeycomb structures are clearly discernible. There are a part of the nucleus (*N*), scattered granules (*g*), mitochondria, and ribosomes in the cytoplasm. × *30,000.*

B. Details of an inclusion found in another leukemic cell from the same case as in Figure 3-32**A.** Periodic structure of about 200 Å with associated honeycomb structure (*arrow),* fibrillar (*f*) formation, and tips of scattered, round mitochondria (*M*) are also seen. × *56,000.*

Reprinted with permission from Matsuoka, M., Hattori, A., Mizushina, T., and Jinbo, C. *Acta Med Biol 17:*49, 1969.

FIGURE 3-33. Myelocyte in chronic myelocytic leukemia.

Ultrastructural detail differs little from normal myelocytes, except for asynchronism in the rate of maturation of the nucleus (*N*) and cytoplasmic organelles. The Golgi complex (*G*) lies within nuclear indentation, and granules (*g*) and mitochondria (*M*) are widely scattered. Nuclear chromatin of a normal cell at this stage of cytoplasmic maturation has already developed a fairly heavy marginal pattern. × *20,000.*

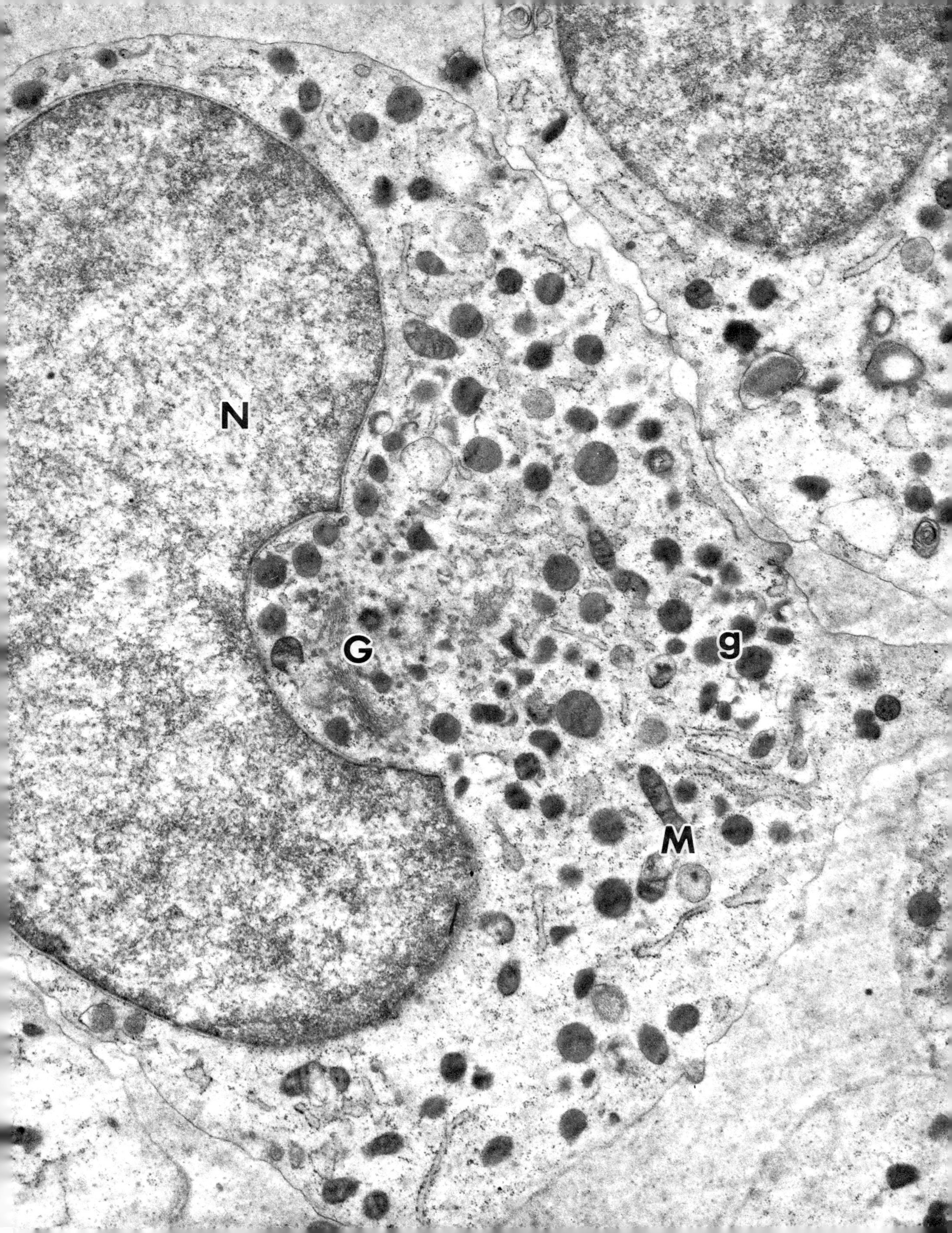
N
G
g
M

of orderly maturation. The diagnosis of chronic myelocytic leukemia may be confirmed in most cases by the negative reaction to alkaline phosphatase and the presence of Ph chromosomes (80 per cent) (Fitzgerald *et al.*, 1963; Ezdinli *et al.*, 1970). Electron microscopy of the cells (Anderson, 1966) shows various forms which are intermediate between blastic and mature granulocytes. These cells do not differ significantly from normal; however, certain asynchronous maturation between the nucleus and the cytoplasm is evident. An example of leukemic cells in this disorder is illustrated in Figure 3-33. No apparent abnormality can be detected.

EOSINOPHILS

MORPHOLOGY AND PHYSIOLOGY

Leukocytes that develop distinctive pinkish-orange granules in their cytoplasm routinely stained for light microscopy are called eosinophils (Fig. 3-34). These elements, detected by Jones (1848) (cited by Vaughn, 1953), compose only a small minority of circulating leukocytes. However, eosinophils are noted commonly in peripheral tissues and have led some to consider them as primarily tissue elements (Bessis, 1956).

The immature eosinophils are believed to share a common ancestor with other granulocytes. It is not well established how and when the eosinophil differentiation commences in the blastic form. This is due partly to the absence of clear criteria for stages of maturation. The only reliable criterion of eosinophil differentiation is the nuclear appearance and shape; however, eosinophils rarely show much nuclear segmentation, usually not more than three segments, even in mature forms. If one assumes that classes of granulocytes could be identified by the presence of specific granulation, eosinophils would not be detectable before the myelocyte stage, since no specific granulation would form at the promyelocyte stage (Spicer and Hardin, 1969). It is unknown whether eosinophils share the same promyelocyte precursor with neutrophils. Eosinophil myelocytes in bone marrow are about 15μ with a round nucleus and a rudimentary nucleolus (Fig. 3-35). The cytoplasm has large granules of about 0.5μ without internal structures or crystals, and a developed endoplasmic reticulum. Internal dense structures become apparent during maturation (Fig. 3-36); however, the contribution of the Golgi apparatus in elaboration of the granules is unclear. Occasionally, immature granules of human eosinophilic myelocytes show ring structure (Fig. 3-37*A*) and degeneration and degranulation to the exterior of the cells (Fig. 3-37*B*). In rabbit eosinophilic myelocytes, peroxidase has been identified in specific granules, endoplasmic reticulum, the Golgi apparatus, and the nuclear envelope (Bainton and Farquhar, 1970). This finding suggests that the segregation and packaging of enzymes in the granules is a function of the Golgi apparatus.

As the cells mature, more granules can be seen in individual cells, and internal opaque structures become more distinctive (Figs. 3-38 and 3-39). These are called "crystalloid" or "internum" structures and are considered to be a unique element, distinctive of mature eosinophilic granules. The "internum" is embedded in an amorphous, less electron-opaque material called "externum." In smears, most eosinophils in the circulation are about 13 to 18μ and have large granules. Mature eosinophils are known to be motile and phagocytize foreign material. Histochemically, granules react positively in peroxidase (Bainton and Farquhar, 1970), in acid phosphatase (Ghidoni and Goldberg, 1966; Seeman and Palade, 1967), and in ATPase (Ackerman, 1964), and they are rich in arginine (Ackerman, 1964). The granules react positively to PAS after saliva digestion (Ackerman, 1964). Biochemically, eosinophilic granules have enzymes similar to those of neutrophils except for the high content of peroxidase and the absence of lysozymes and phagocytin (Archer and Hirsch, 1963a).

Crystalloid structures unique for eosinophilic granules are observed in various animal species, including man, rabbit, horse, monkey, rat and mouse; in cats, there are concentrically arranged lamellated structures (Osako, 1959). Human eosinophils of reactive bone marrows may have more than one internal crystalloid structure. Their morphology is heterogeneous, including needle-shapes, large squares, triangles, rhomboid tetrahedrons or a combination of all these structures (Fig. 3-30). Under high magnification, a periodic array of about 30 to 40 Å (Breton-Gorius, 1966; Miller *et al.,* 1966) is discernible in granules of man, rats, mice, and guinea pigs. These central cores have been analyzed and appear to be phospholipids, mostly unsaturated fatty acids (Faller, 1966) or peroxidase (Miller, *et al.,* 1966). The internal discs appear to remain unchanged while the externum is dissolved in reactive states. The formation of characteristic structures, called Charcot-Lyden crystals, are noted regularly in areas where many eosinophils are being broken down. These inclusions may be composed of the dense internal structures of degraded granules which are left to combine and form the larger crystalloid structure (Welsh, 1959) or possibly from cytoplasmic protein (Archer and Blackwood, 1965).

No thorough kinetic studies on eosinophils have been done; it is not clear whether values proposed for granulocytes may also be applicable. Murakami *et al.* (1969), using radioactive thymidine, estimated the eosinophil kinetics in two humans and proposed the transit times of 1 to 1.5 days for band forms in bone marrow and 2.5 to 3 days for peripheral blood eosinophils. Foot (1965) estimated the appearance of "daughter" eosinophils in rat blood from DNA synthesis by an eosinophil myelocyte at 60 to 73 hours, transit time in blood as 8 to 12 hours, and in tissue at 22 hours.

FUNCTION

Functions of eosinophils and their granules are not clearly known, but they are thought to be vehicles for transport of various materials, including antigen (Speirs, 1958), histamine (Vaughn, 1953; Archer, 1960), and profibrinolysin (Barnhart and Riddle, 1963). They may be utilized or decomposed in the peripheral tissues. Eosinophils have been recognized in foci of allergy and parasitic infection. Antigen-antibody complex attracts eosinophils to local sites and may be the primary mechanism of local eosinocytosis in allergic reactions. Eosinophils reportedly take up yeast cell wall actively (Archer and Hirsch, 1963b); however, such phagocytic activity is believed to be insignificant when styrene particles, *Escherichia coli,*

(*text continues on page 146*)

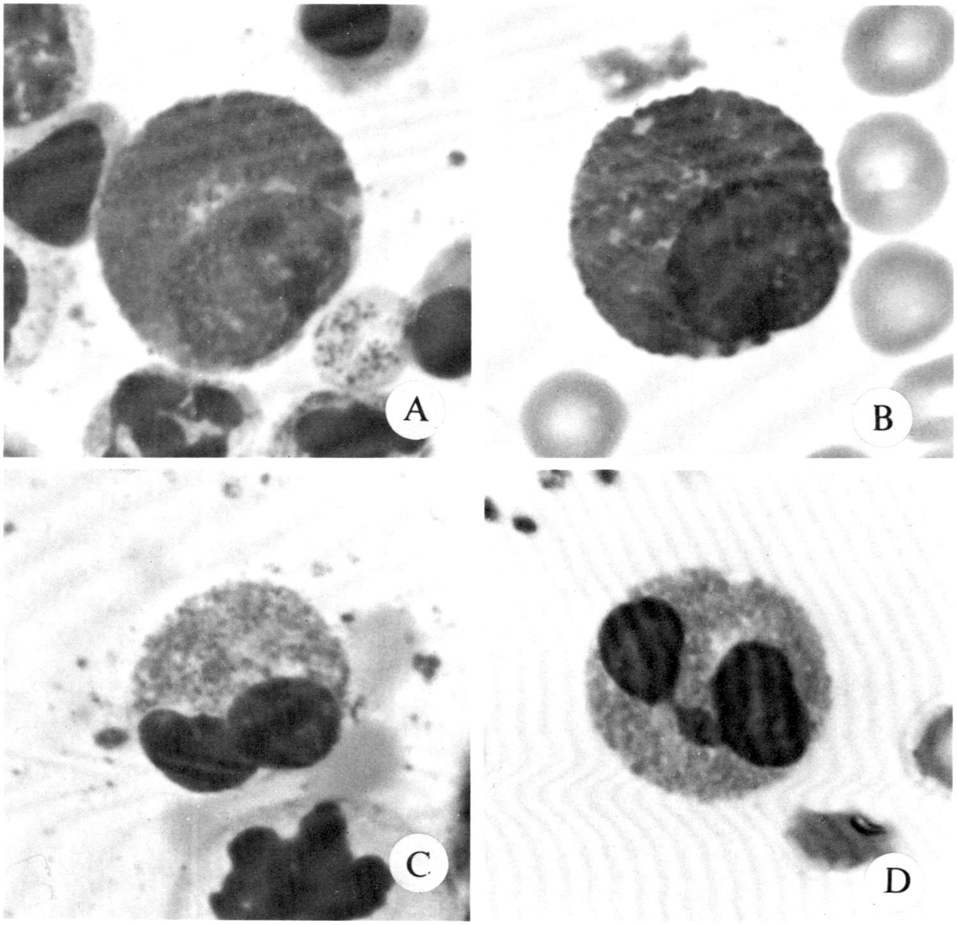

FIGURE 3-34. Light micrographs of eosinophils at various stages of maturation.
A. Early myelocyte from bone marrow. × *2,000.*
B. Myelocyte from bone marrow. × *2,000.*
C. Binucleated form from bone marrow. × *2,000.*
D. Mature eosinophil from peripheral blood. × *2,000.*

FIGURE 3-35. Eosiniphilic myelocyte from bone marrow.
Several large granules (*g*) have not developed crystalloid inclusions; their lack of internal pattern (see Figs. 3-45 and 3-46) suggest that they are not basophilic granules. Chromatin in nucleus (*N*) has started to condense, and cytoplasm, with a few mitochondria (*M*), has developed endoplasmic reticulum (*er*). Note absence of granules commonly found in promyelocytes or myelocytes. × *26,300.*

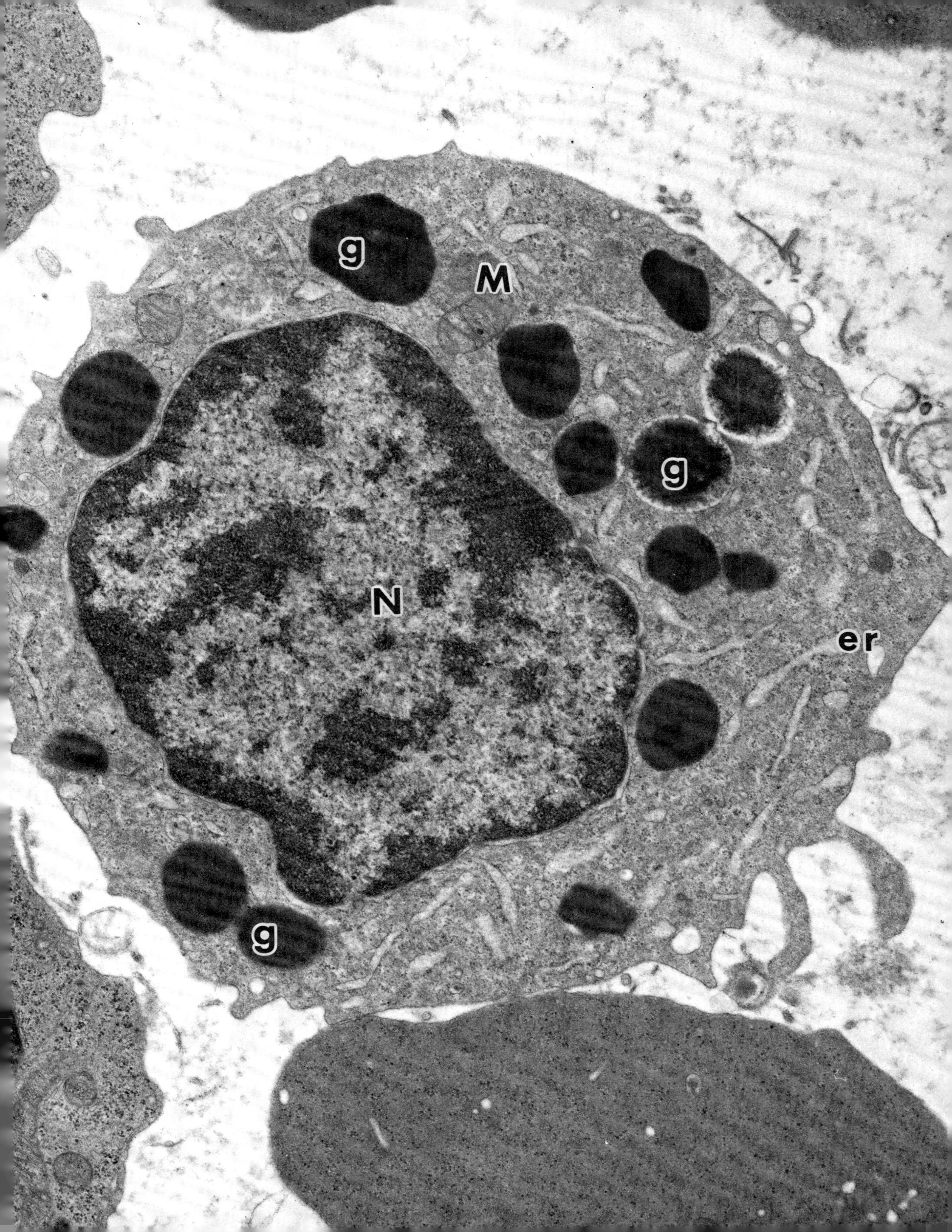
g
M
g
N
er
g

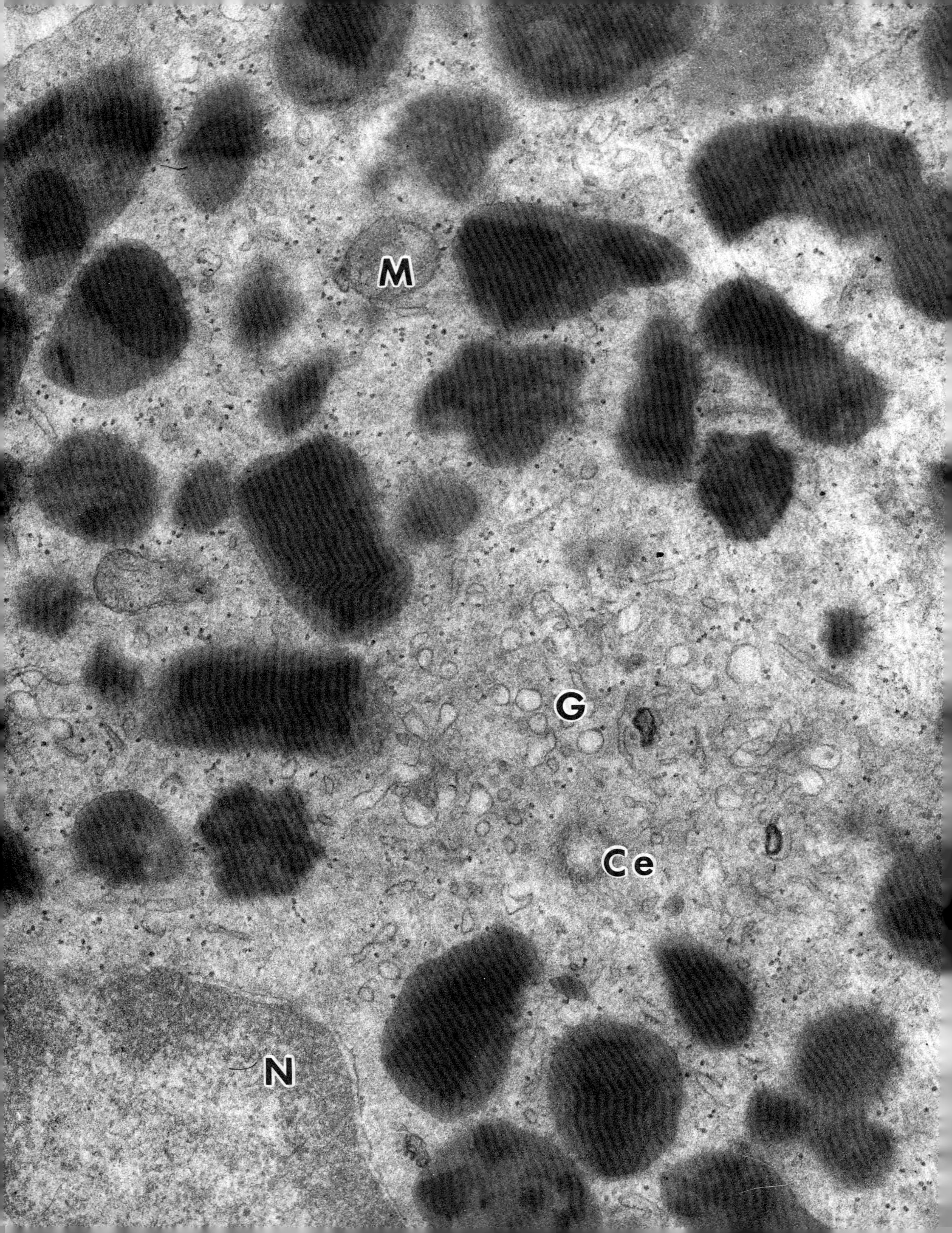
M
G
Ce
N

FIGURE 3-36. Eosinophilic myelocyte.
Cytoplasm of eosinophilic myelocyte with Golgi complex (*G*), a centriole (*Ce*) surrounded by many eosinophilic granules, and internal structures of granules beginning to appear. There is no clear indication of the role of the Golgi apparatus in granular formation in this cell. There are some mitochondria (*M*), and the edge of the nucleus (*N*) can be seen. Scattered dense particles are glycogen. × *49,500.*

Figures 3-37 and 3-38 appear on the following pages

FIGURE 3-37. Eosinophils.
A. Eosinophilic myelocyte with ring-shaped densities in the granules (*g*), some distended endoplasmic reticulum (*er*), and a portion of the nucleus (*N*). × *42,000.*
B. Immature bone marrow eosinophil with degeneration of granules; some appear to be leaving the cell (*arrows*). This process of degranulation is thought to take place in the mature eosinophil in peripheral circulation or in situ in tissues. Its significance in an immature eosinophil in the bone marrow is not understood. × *42,000.*

FIGURE 3-38. Normal mature eosinophil from peripheral blood.
Cytoplasm has many eosinophilic granules with dense internal structures in a variety of shapes. There are a few well-preserved mitochondria (*M*) and a fat vacuole (*asterisk*); two lobes of the nucleus (*N*) are transected. × *19,500.*

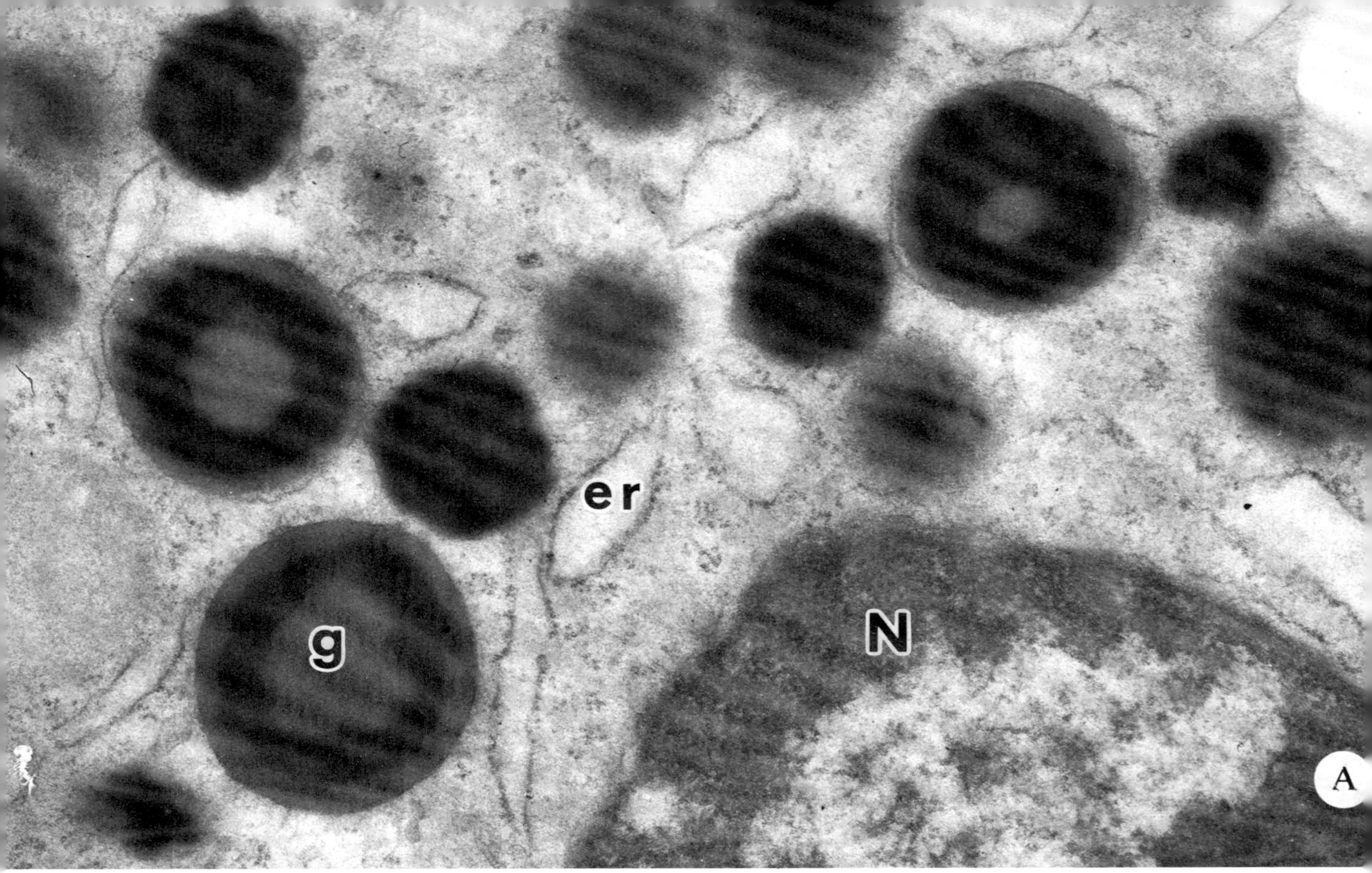
er
g
N
A

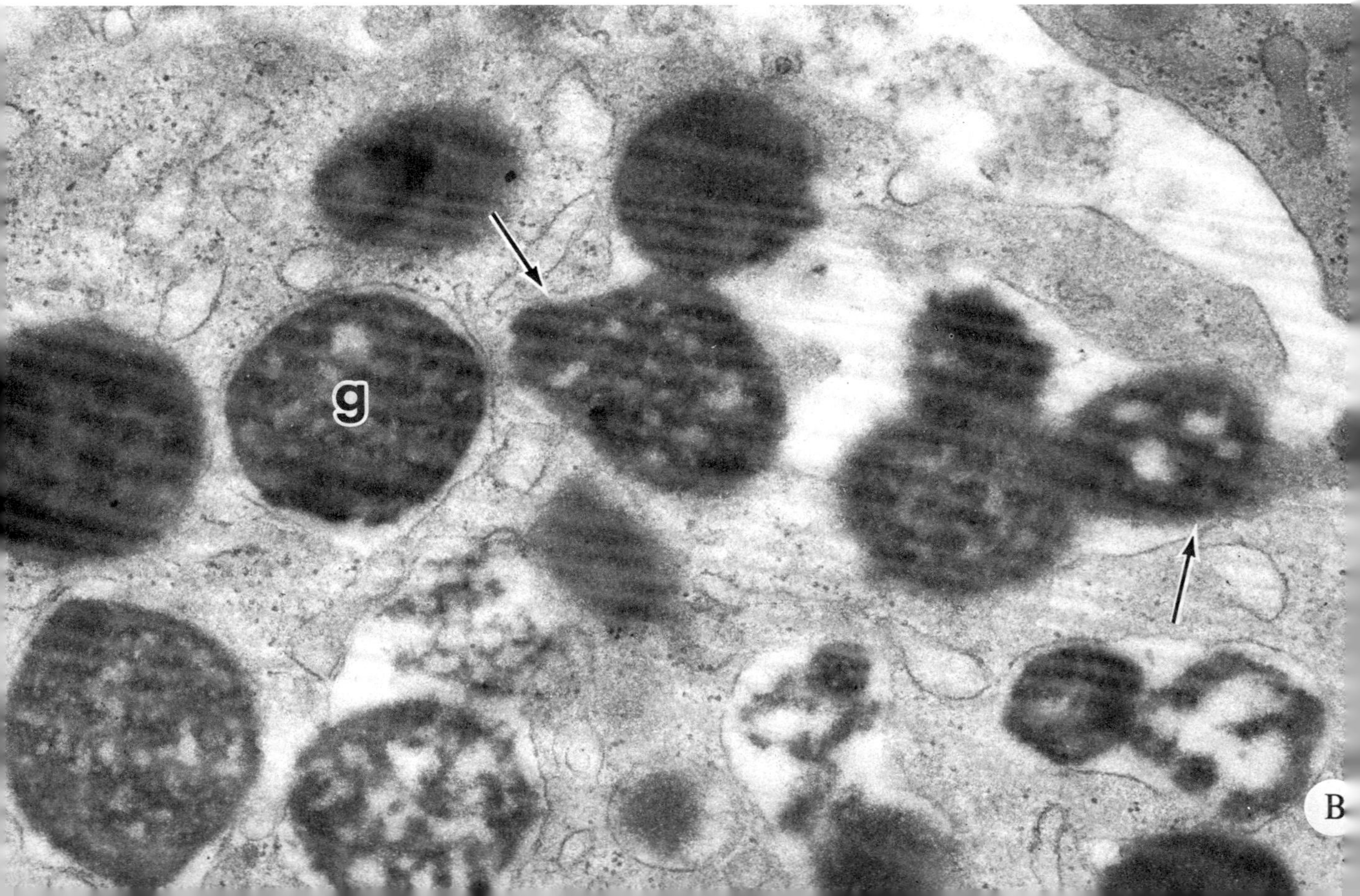
g
B

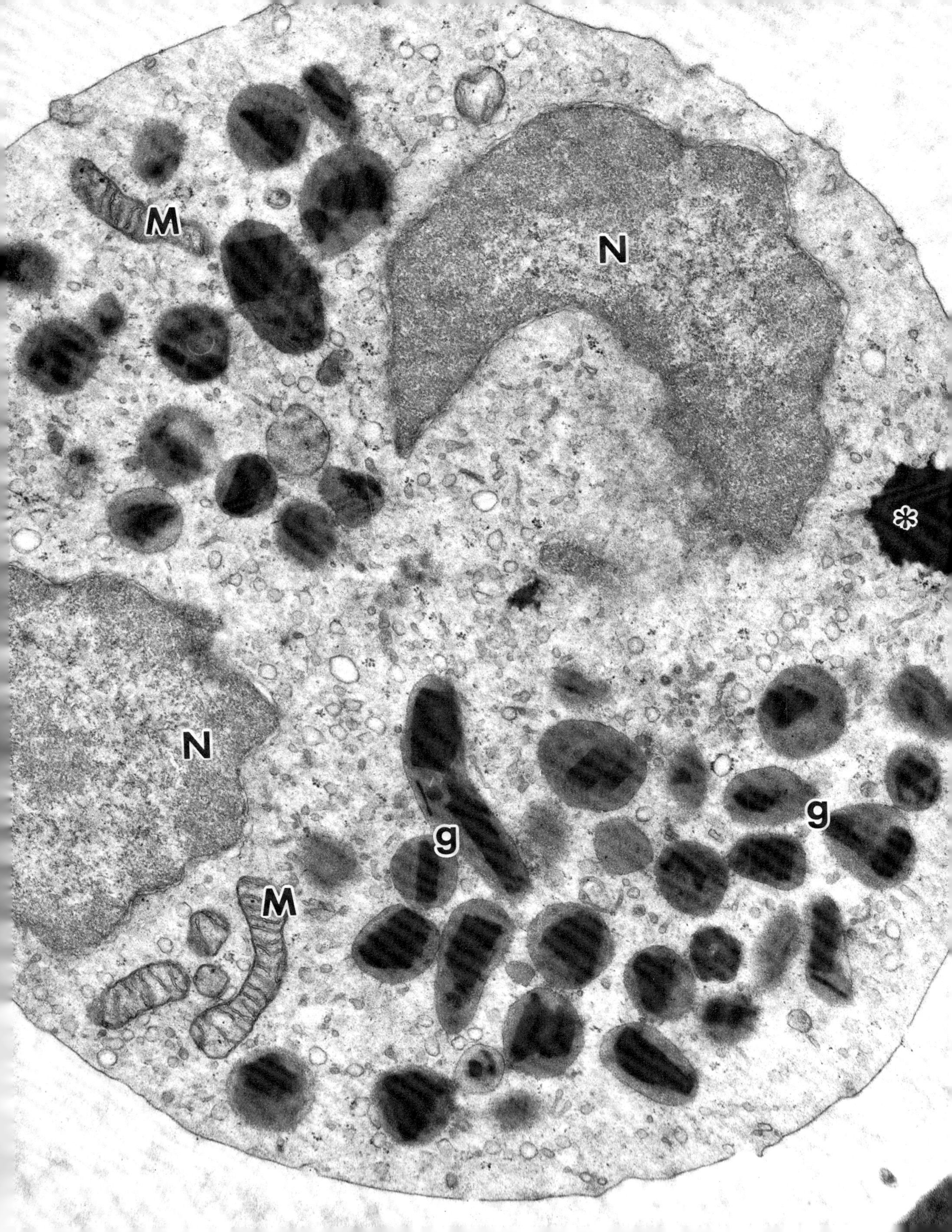
M
N
*
N
g
g
M

Staphylococcus aureus 502A, and *Candida albicans* (Cline *et al.*, 1968) are used as foreign bodies. During phagocytosis, eosinophils ingest insoluble antigen and antibodies (Litt, 1964), antigen-antibody complex (Sabesin, 1963), aggregated gamma globulin (Zucker-Franklin, 1966), and sensitized erythrocytes (Archer and Hirsch, 1963b). During phagocytosis, the disintegration of granules and the release of their enzymes have been demonstrated histochemically (Cotran and Litt, 1969).

PATHOLOGY

Leukemic manifestations of either eosinophils or basophils are reported infrequently. An extensive discussion on this topic is available (Dameshek and Gunz, 1964), but we include an electron micrograph of cells from a case of eosinophilic leukemia (Fig. 3-40). Note the distinctive intragranular discs in each granule. There is no abnormality in the morphology of proliferating cells and no judgment is made of the stage of cell maturation.

BASOPHILS (MASTOCYTES)

Granulated cells known now as mast cells were discovered by Recklinghausen (1863) and Waldeyer (1875) before Ehrlich (1879b) defined them by their metachromatic granules. The term "mast cell" originated from the overladen granules which make the cells appear as if they are overfed. Mastocytosis in skin in urticaria pigmentosa was reported by Unna (1894). Since then, significant inflammatory, hemodynamic, and hemostatic activities of mast cells have been explored extensively.

Blood basophils, found in peripheral blood by Ehrlich (1879a), were called "blood mast cells" because they contained metachromatic granules similar to those in tissue mast cells. He suggested that their origin was in bone marrow. Because of the rarity of basophils in blood-forming organs and peripheral blood, studies on "blood mast cells" are more limited than on "tissue mast cells." Nevertheless, the presence of similar chemicals in both mast cells and basophils helps to confirm their similarity. These two cell types are regarded as functionally similar and can be categorized as the "basomastocyte system" (Selye, 1965) despite some differences in morphology and their distinctive locations. Details of their morphology and pathophysiology are available in monographs (Riley, 1959; Selye, 1965).

MAST CELLS

Mast cells are primarily tissue cells observed near the perivascular location of many organs, a location favoring the release of their granular content to the blood. Though they are considered to be normal constituents in human bone marrow, their significance in disease is unclear (Werner and Krause, 1965). The cells appear as elongated forms with slender cytoplasmic projections or as small round forms containing a single nucleus, oc-

(text continues on page 152)

FIGURE 3-39. Eosinophil cytoplasm.
The cytoplasm of this eosinophil demonstrates the heterogeneous character of the dense internal structures in granules (*g*) of normal human eosinophils. A few mitochondria (*M*) are also present. × *49,500.*

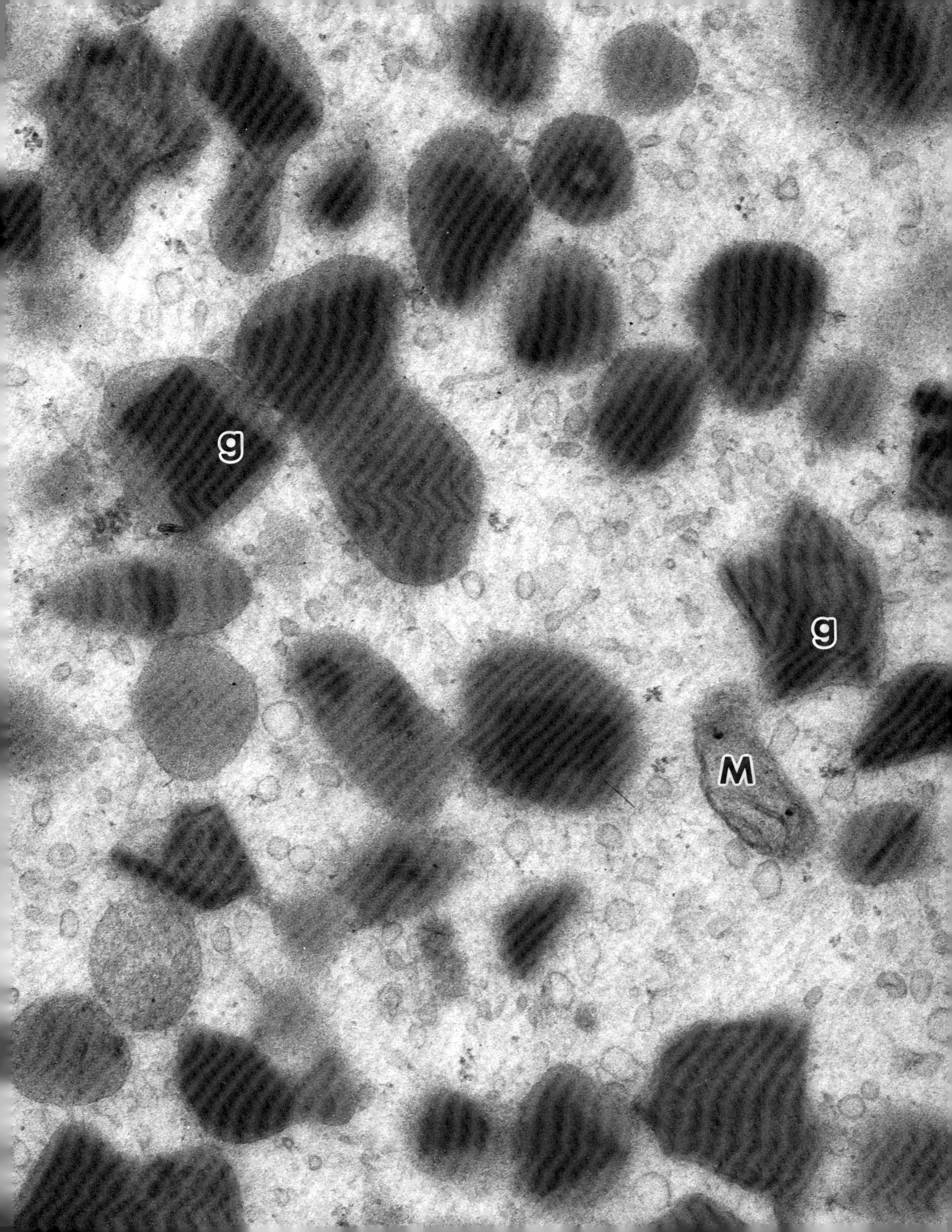
g
g
M

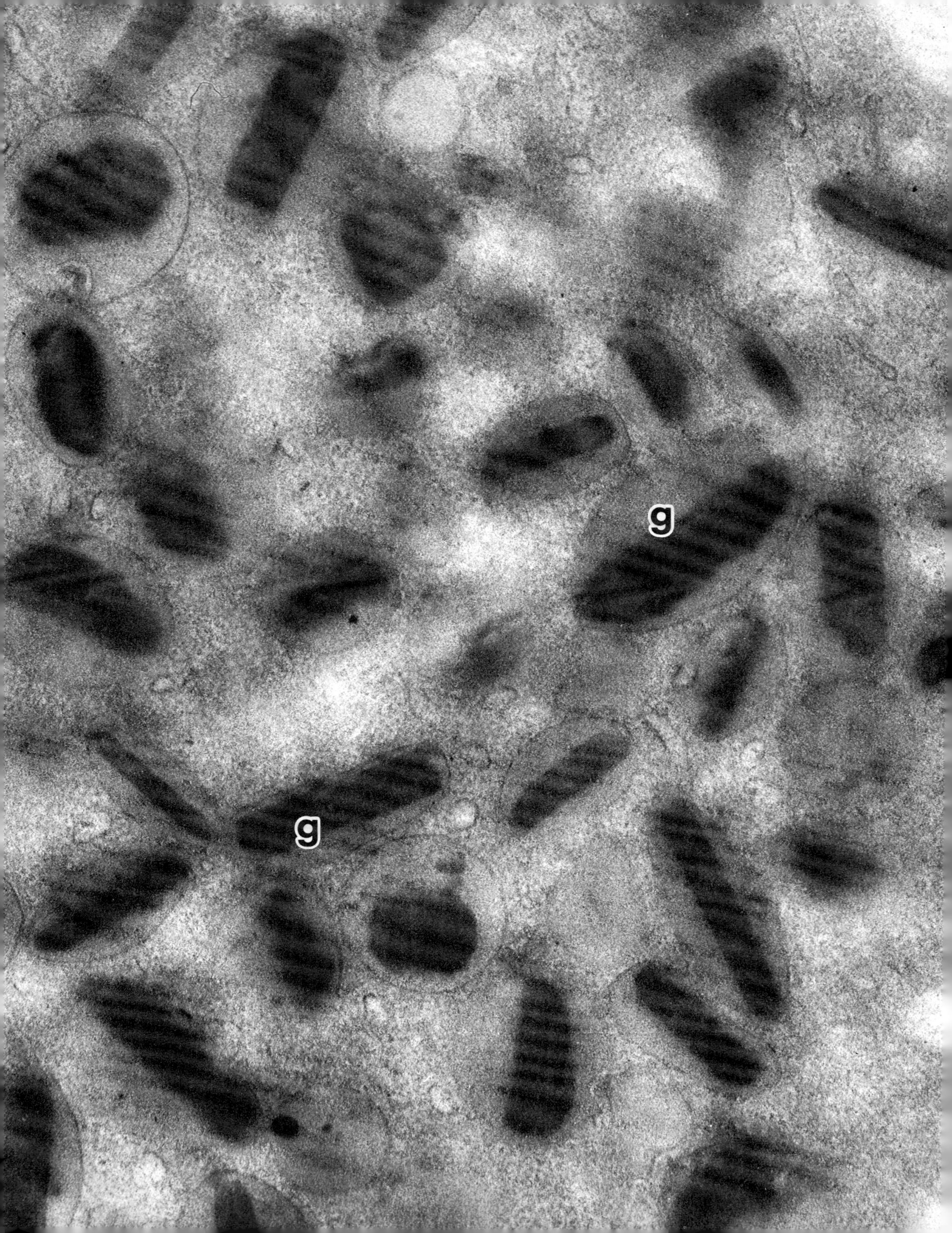
g
g

FIGURE 3-40. Eosinophilic leukemia.
Eosinophil cytoplasm from case of eosinophilic leukemia. There is greater consistency in the shape of internal structures of the granules (*g*), reflecting more typical inclusions usually seen in other animal species. × *66,000.*

Figures 3-41 and 3-42 appear on the following pages

FIGURE 3-41. Round form of mast cell.
In this mast cell from human lymph node, the granules are immature and contain no internal structures. There are slender cytoplasmic projections (*arrows*), and chromatin of the nucleus (*N*) is condensed. The Golgi complex (*G*) is well developed, and ribosomes are scattered throughout the cytoplasm. A few fat (F) vacuoles are also present. × *29,000.*

FIGURE 3-42. Elongated form of mast cell.
This mast cell from human bone marrow has cytoplasmic projections (*arrows*), numerous granules (*g*) containing heterogeneous internal structures, and several mitochondria (*M*). The nucleus (*N*) contains no nucleolus. × *19,700.*

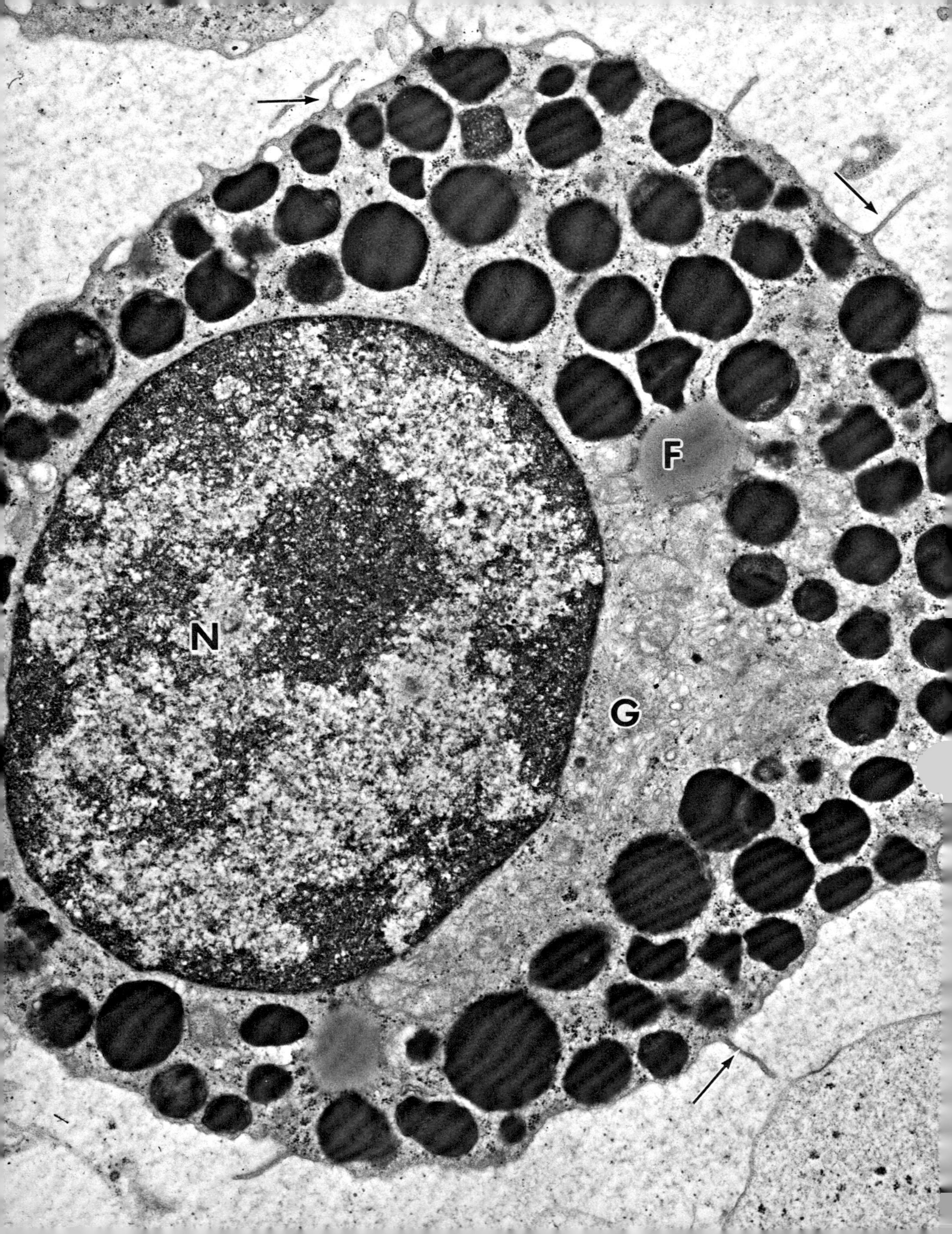
F
N
G

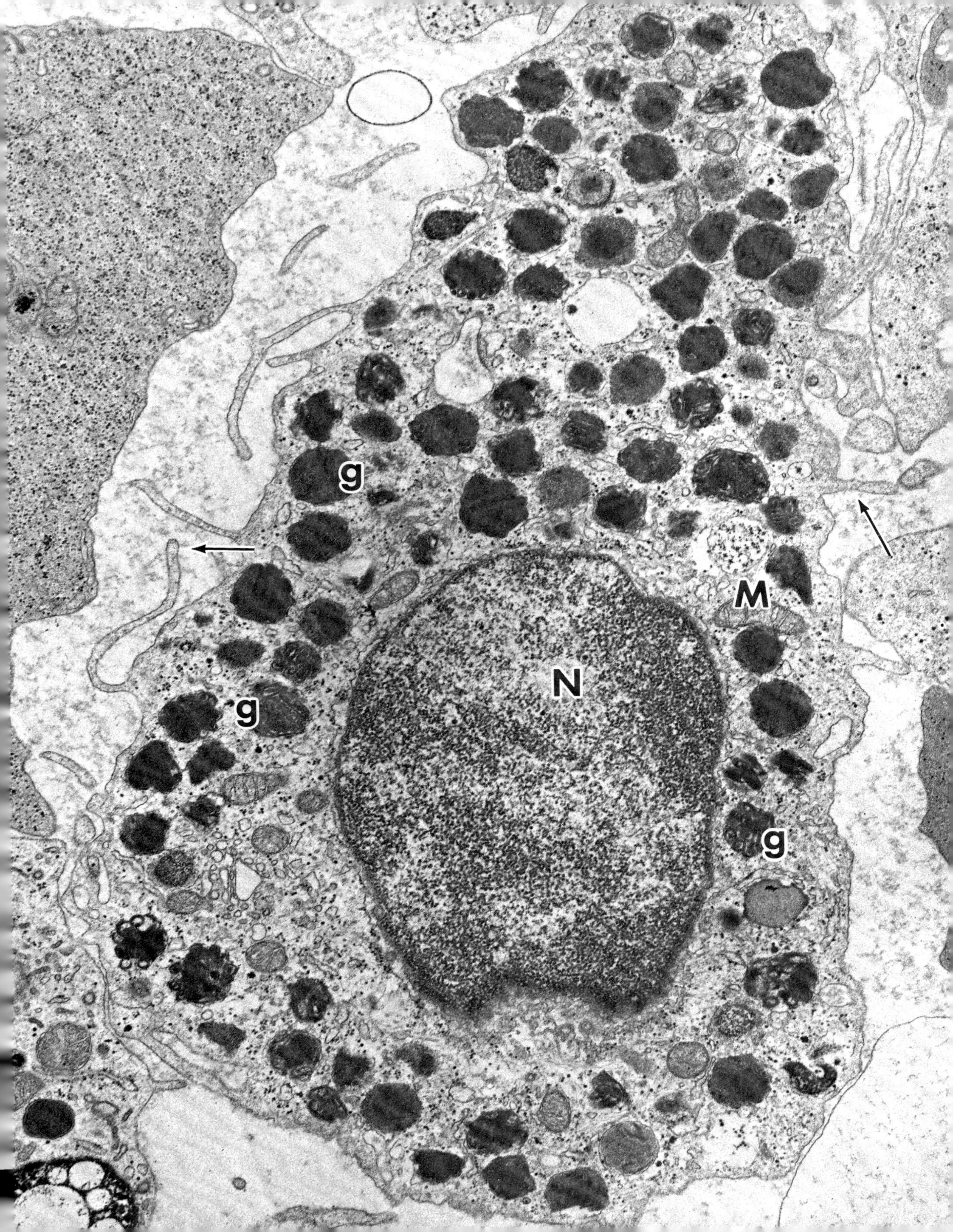
g
g
N
M
g

casionally bilobulated; however, the nucleus may be indistinct because of the many granules covering it. Specific granules of mast cells in man, rabbits, birds, and fish are highly water soluble, in contrast to granules of the rat, hamster, mouse, and dog (Selye, 1965). Selye recommended alcohol formol as the best fixative for these granules. Specific granules of mast cells appear metachromatic when stained by basic aniline dyes, such as methylene blue, toluidine blue, cresyl violet, etc. This characteristic is due to the strongly negative charge of such chemicals as sulfuric acid within the granules. The positive staining of the granules with the PAS reaction, alcian blue (Gomori, 1941), astra-blue (Pioch, 1957), and colloidal iron (Fullmer, 1959) suggests the presence of acid mucopolysaccharides. These histochemical characteristics could be explained by the large amounts of heparin in the granules (Holmgren and Wilander, 1937; Jorpes *et al.,* 1937). The failure of granules in individual mast cells or those in one tissue to show similar reaction to others with the above stains suggests a heterogeneity of chemical constituents in each granule. Some pharmacologically important agents, such as histamine (Schauer and Werle, 1959; Lagunoff *et al.,* 1961) and 5-hydroxytryptamine (5-HT) (Benditt *et al.,* 1955), have also been demonstrated in basophil or mast cell granules. The presence of these chemicals has also been confirmed by biochemical methods on separated granules (Hagen *et al.,* 1959; Sampson and Archer, 1967). Various important enzymes, such as acid phosphatase (Schauer and Eder, 1962), ATPase (Eder and Schauer, 1961), beta glucuronidase (Schauer and Eder, 1962), and protease (Glenner *et al.,* 1962), have also been demonstrated. The basis for the affinity of silver salts to the mast cell granules is less clear.

Ultrastructural studies on normal human mast cells have been reported (Stoekenius, 1956; Fedorko and Hirsch, 1965; Weinstock and Albright, 1965; Kobayashi *et al.,* 1968). Mast cells in human blood-forming organs and other connective tissues are round (Fig. 3-41) to elongated in shape (Fig. 3-42), with electron-dense granules up to 0.7μ. Projections from the cell membrane of many pseudopodia or microvilli are observed (Figs. 3-41 and 3-42). This is highly characteristic and not seen in other granulated blood cells. A single nucleus is in somewhat eccentric position (Figs. 3-41 and 3-42). The chromatin is usually condensed and no nucleolus is found, an indication of their mature nature. The nuclear margin is at times somewhat irregular, a deformation produced by the presence of nearby granules. Poorly to well-developed Golgi apparatuses and modest numbers of smooth endoplasmic reticulum are also seen in the cytoplasm (Figs. 3-41 and 3-42), as well as diffusely distributed ribosomes, scattered glycogen particles (Fig. 3-42), and fibrillar structures (Weinstock and Albright, 1965). Specific granules in human mast cells vary from those that are homogeneously dense (Fig. 3-41) to those which contain various crystalline material, including "scrolls" (Fig. 3-43) (Weinstock and Albright, 1965). These latter structures represent a highly or-

(text continues on page 158)

FIGURE 3-43. Mast cell granules.
Details of some mast cell granules show a predominance of scroll forms. Dense particles in cytoplasm are glycogen (*arrow*). Mitochondria (*M*) and a portion of the nucleus (*N*) are at left border. × *85,000.*

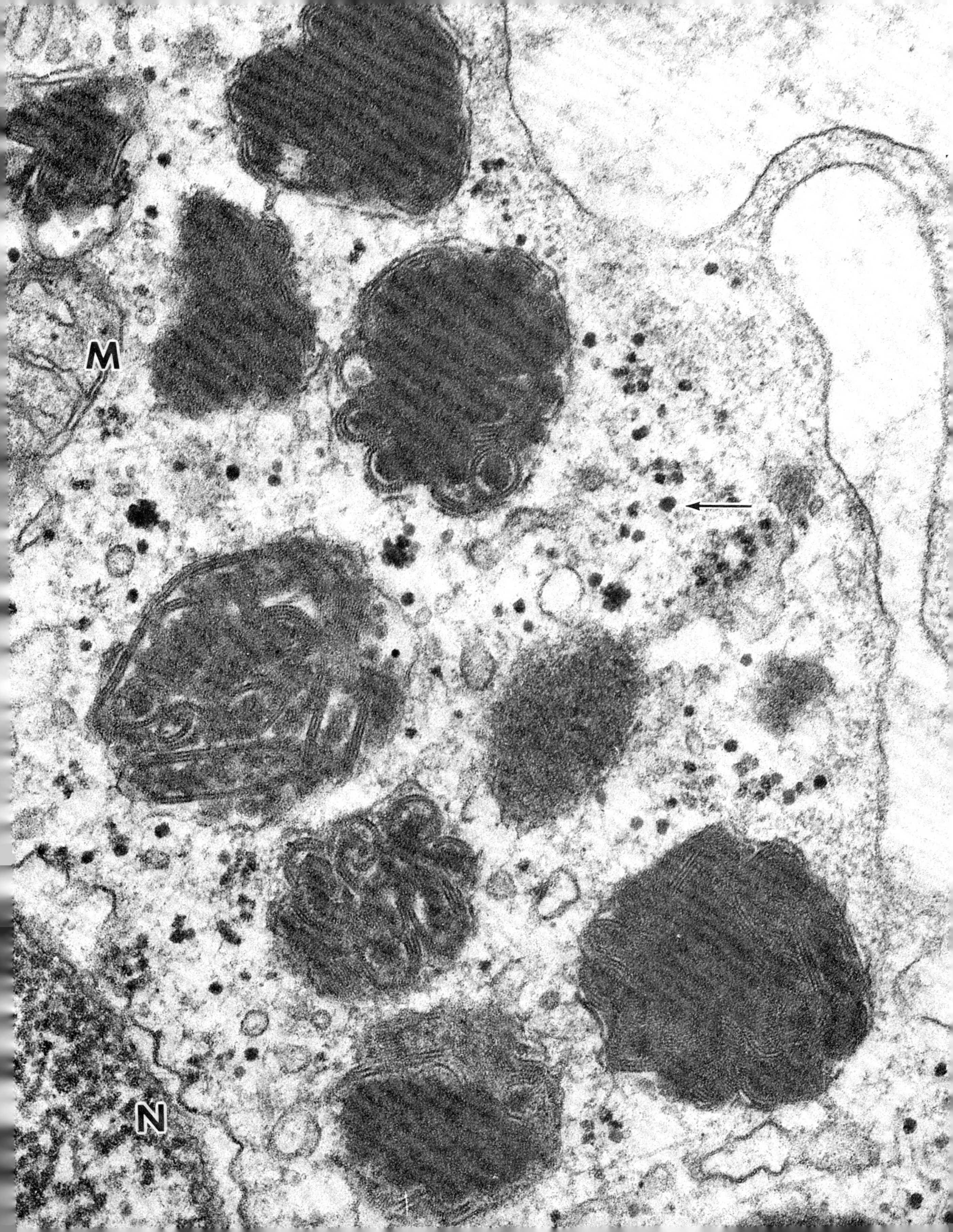
M
N

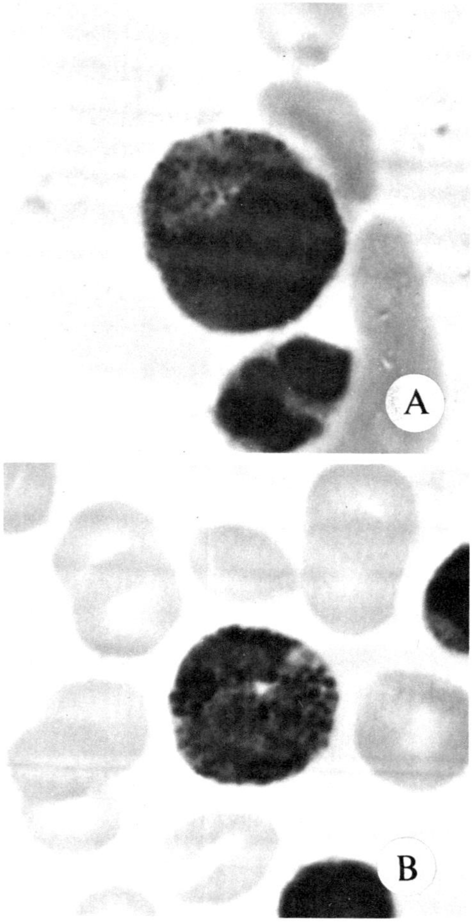

Figure 3-44. Light micrographs of basophils.
A. Basophilic myelocyte from bone marrow. × *2,000.*
B. Basophil from peripheral blood. × *2,000.*

FIGURE 3-45. Basophilic myelocyte.
Basophil at myelocyte stage in human bone marrow contains large cytoplasmic granules (*g*) with many dense particles near the Golgi apparatus (*G*) and centriole (*Ce*). Some of the vacuolated-appearing granules (*arrow*) may be a fixation artifact. Chromatin in the nucleus (*N*) is condensed. There are a few mitochondria (*M*). × *25,200.*

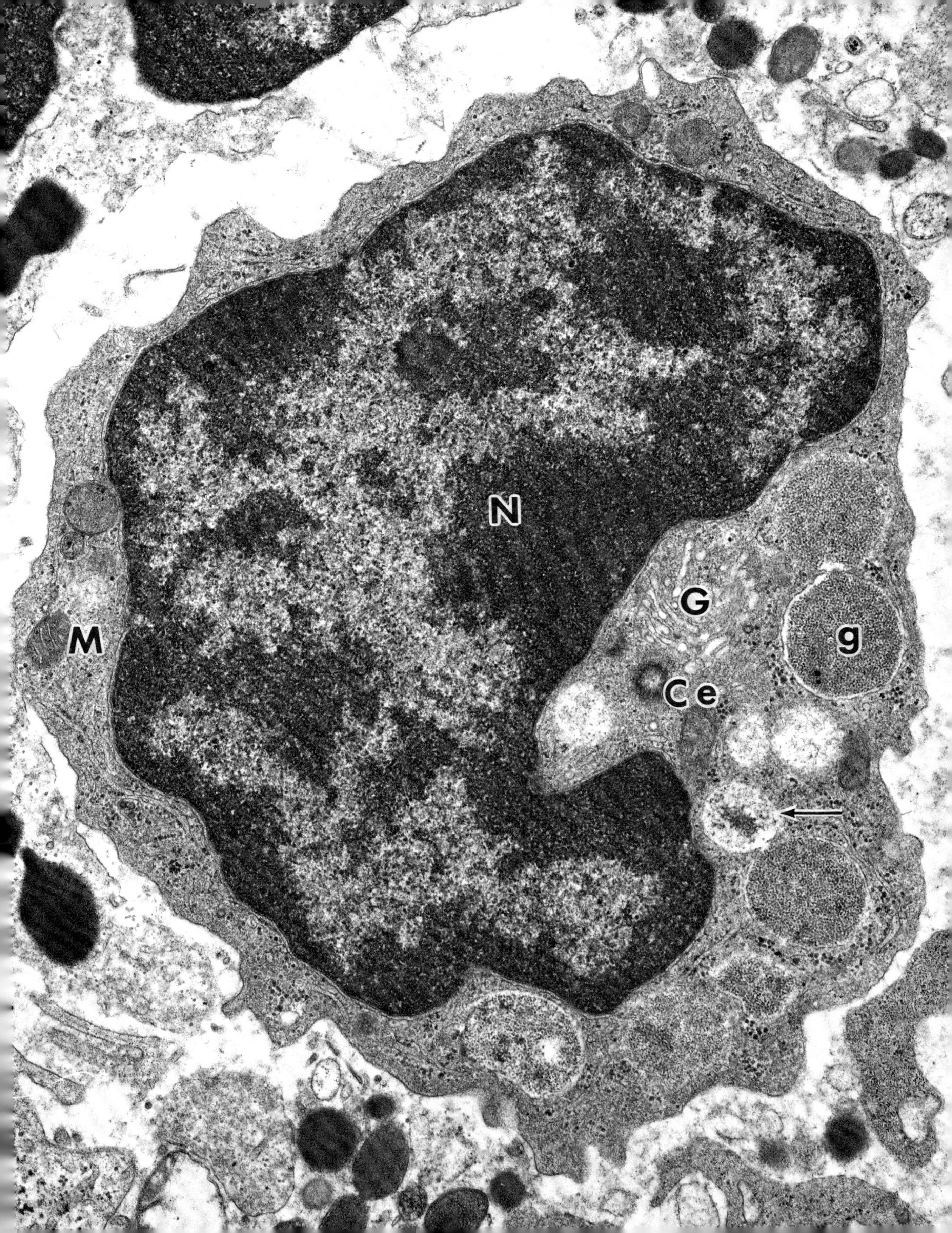
N
G
g
M
Ce

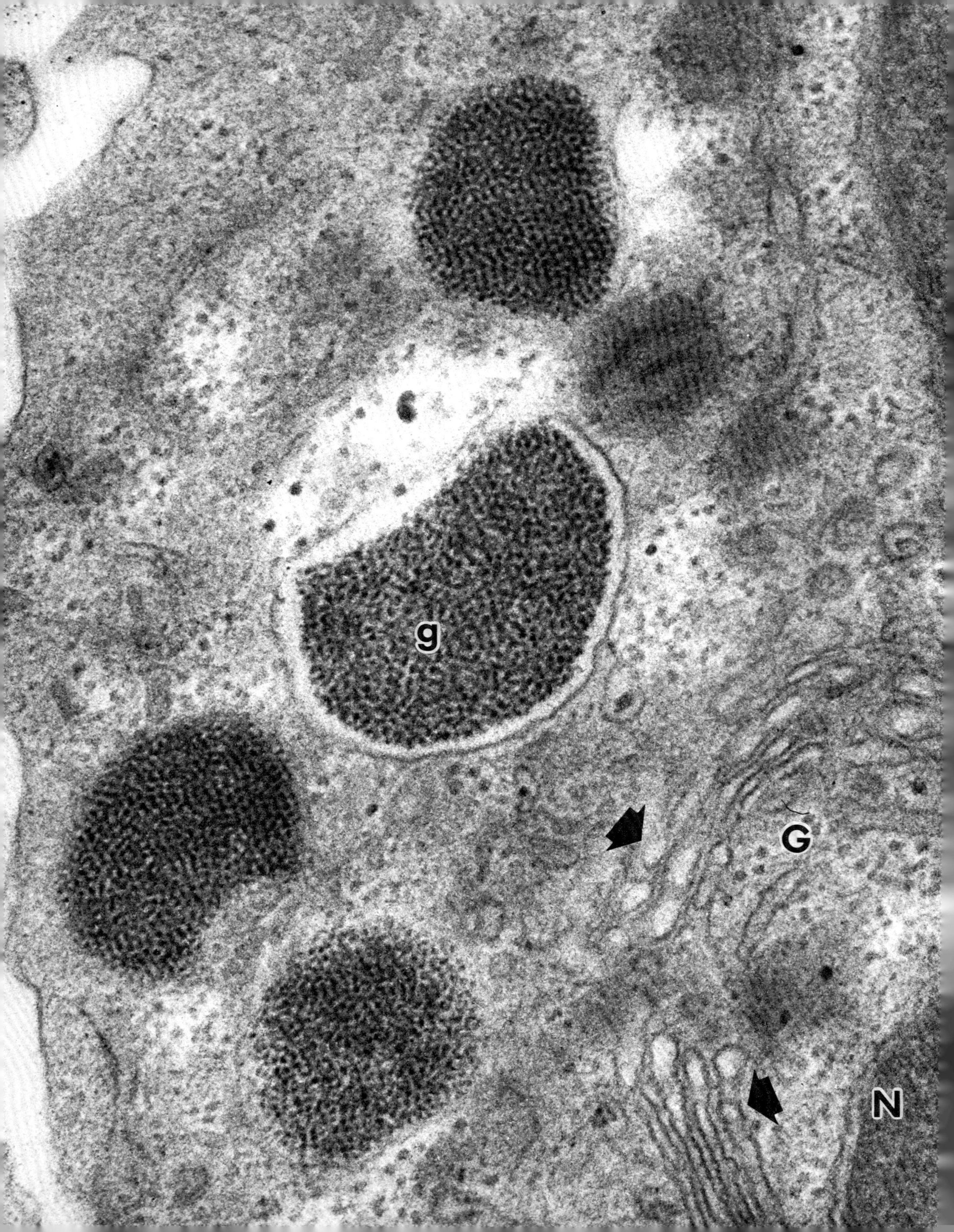
g
G
N

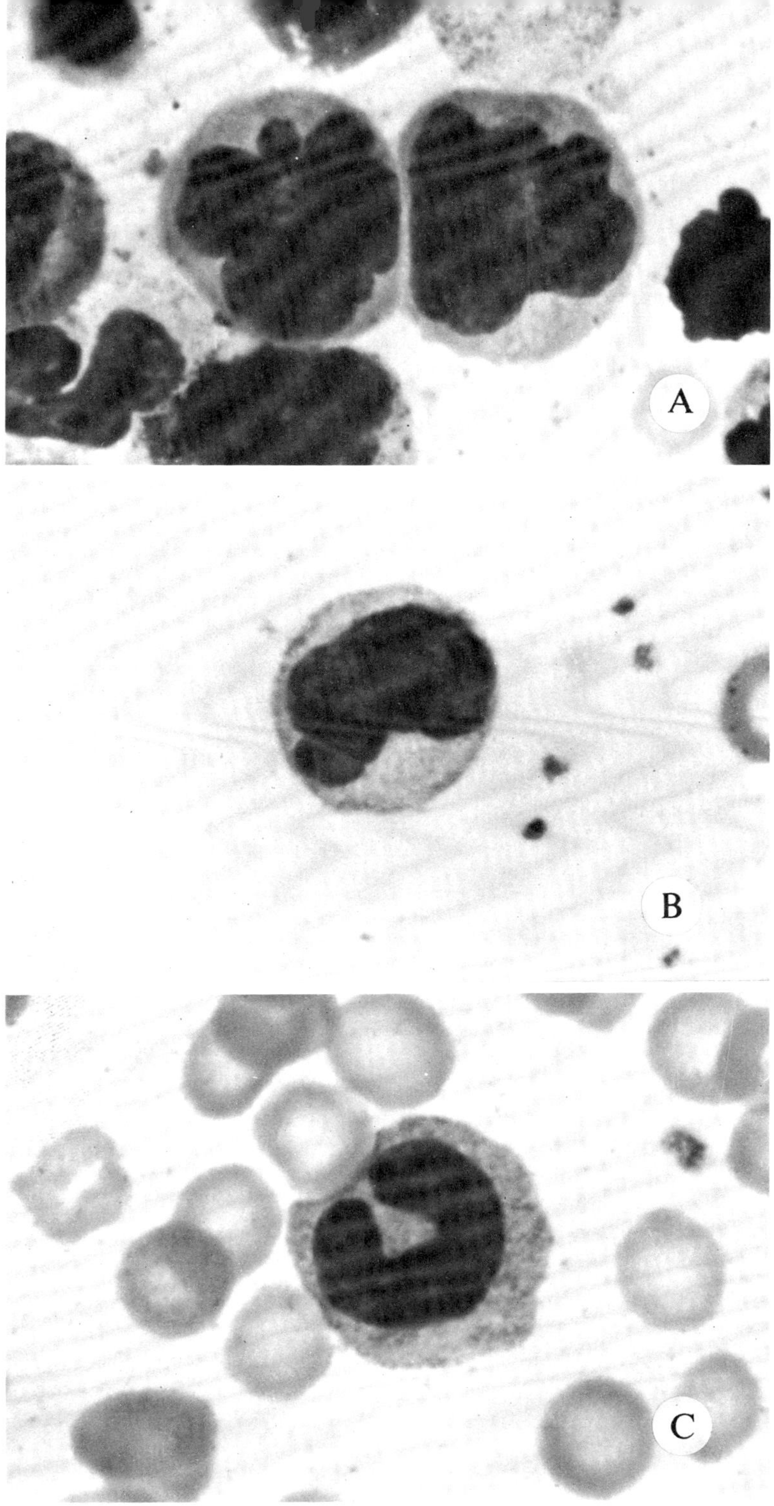

FIGURE 3-47. Light micrographs of monocytes and their precursors.
A. In the monoblast or promonocyte in bone marrow, there is a near absence of granules and a highly lobulated nucleus. × *2,000.*
B, C. Monocytes from peripheral blood show two different nuclear shapes. × *2,000.*

FIGURE 3-46. Basophil granules.
These basophil granules (*g*) contain electron-dense particles. The lamellar structures of the Golgi apparatus (*G*) terminate in vesicular shapes (*arrows*). A portion of the nucleus (*N*) is visible. × *95,000.*

dered array of parallel dense and less dense lines with a periodicity of about 70 Å. Occasionally, hexagonal or honeycomb lattices are evident (Weinstock and Albright, 1965).

These two types of granules are seen in both elongated and oval shaped-cells. Similar observations have been made on specific granules of other animal species (Fernando and Movat, 1963; Combs, 1966; Takeoka *et al.,* 1966), and in granules of transplantable murine mastocytoma (Christensen *et al.,* 1963). The formation of these granules has been proposed as occurring in the Golgi apparatus (Combs, 1966), by pinocytosis (Burton and Bensley, 1958), from mitochondria (Gusek, 1961), or by endoplasmic reticulum (Sellyei and David, 1963). However, if their formation is consistent with that observed in other granulated cells, it is probably a function of the Golgi apparatus, with the collaborating activity of endoplasmic reticulum.

Mast cells in vivo discharge granules from cell surface (Thiéry, 1963), a phenomenon which is considered to be important in releasing pharmacological agents to local tissues. The edematous skin reaction in urticaria pigmentosa is generally regarded as due to the discharged granules from the local mast cells (Kobayashi *et al.,* 1968). When degranulation and release of 5-HT from the rat mast cell was studied in an in-vivo system, a correlation between degranulation and increase in 5-HT content was demonstrated (Jansson and Penttilä, 1969). The mechanisms by which the cell is stimulated to discharge granules is not understood clearly. The granule discharge in vivo may be triggered by various exogenous or intrinsic stimulants, including trauma, as well as by injection of various pharmacological drugs. Soluble chemical substances may also be released from the cell in the absence of accompanying granule discharge per se. Discharged granules may be eliminated from the tissues by phagocytosis. Eosinophils, or other phagocytic interstitial elements may thus create cells resembling the original mast cells. These cells should be distinguished from true mast cells and the term "pseudo-mast cells" may be applicable (Selye, 1965).

BASOPHILIC GRANULOCYTES

Basophilic granulocytes differ morphologically and cytogenically from mast cells. In humans, basophils are a distinct minority of the granulocyte population (about 0.5 per cent in the peripheral blood). In smears, they are about 10μ in diameter and have characteristic metachromatic granules (Fig. 3-44). The nucleus is somewhat lobulated, resembling that of mature neutrophils. Similar to eosinophils, basophils are formed in the bone marrow and are believed to share a common ancestor with neutrophils. No reliable kinetic study is available on this cell at this time. The granules of basophils are known to contain heparin (Laves and Thoma, 1950) and histamine embedded in a framework of lipoprotein (Ackerman, 1963). The basophils also contain glycogen particles which are not related to the specific granules (Kaung, 1969). These cells appear to be positive in peroxidase reaction (Lennert and Schubert, 1961); however, neither extensive cytochemistry nor biochemical analyses on the specific granules of basophils are available.

Electron microscopy on the human basophils, presented by several investigators (Anderson, 1966; Watanabe *et al.,* 1967; Zucker-Franklin, 1967), shows a lobulated nucleus in the middle of the cytoplasm, which contains a rudimentary Golgi apparatus, modest numbers of endoplasmic reticulum, and dispersed as well as clustered glycogen particles (Fig. 3-45). The granules of basophils are about 0.1 to 0.4μ in diameter, and in thin sections consist of an orderly arrangement of granulofilamentous structures of about 100 to 200 Å within a single membrane (Fig. 3-46). Granules also contain either thick subunits of high electron density or thinner subunits of less electron opacity, which may be immature forms of the dense granules or artifacts produced by poor fixation. A protein core with periodical arrays of about 40 Å has also been reported (Watanabe *et al.,* 1967). Myelin figures may be seen in some granules (Anderson, 1966; Watanabe *et al.,* 1967; Zucker-Franklin, 1967).

Basophilic granules in some animals may differ from those in man. Lamellated (132 to 140 Å) or hexagonal lattices may be seen in guinea-pig cells (Winquist, 1963; Fedorko and Hirsch, 1965; Terry *et al.,* 1969). The basic units of the lattices are composed of a 50 Å three-layered structure with 15 Å dense outer layers, separated by a 20 Å lighter area. Formation of immature granules by the Golgi apparatus is suggested.

MONOCYTES

MORPHOLOGY AND PHYSIOLOGY

Intermediate forms between polymorphonuclear leukocytes and lymphocytes were described by Ehrlich in 1891. These "transitional forms" were assumed to be between lymphocytes and granulocytes. These elements were subsequently distinguished clearly from lymphocytes by Pappenheim and Ferrata (1910) and Schilling-Torgau (1912).

The origin of monocytes is highly controversial. The classic view that monocytes originate independently from cells of the reticuloendothelial system, particularly sinus endothelium and young mesenchyma of the spleen, has been supported by many leading morphologists particularly in Europe (Aschoff, 1924; Bessis, 1956). In this concept, monocytes are blood histiocytes. Others hold that monocytes are formed in bone marrow (Rohr, 1960) and are members of the myeloid cell series originating from a specific blastic compartment, monoblasts found in both spleen and bone marrow (Cunningham *et al.,* 1925). Still others believe they are formed from promyelocytes (Leder, 1967), or share the stem cell with granulocytes (Downey, 1938; Bakalos, 1949). Though the concept of their origin in marrow has become more popular and is now experimentally supported, the idea of dualistic source may be convenient to explain the origin of these cells in both physiological and pathological conditions. Problems relating to the origin of malignant monocytes will be discussed.

Blood monocytes in stained smears (Fig. 3-47) appear similar to large or atypical lymphocytes except that they have a pleomorphic nuclear pattern with a coarse chromatin distribution, and the cytoplasm contains a number of azurophilic granules known to be peroxidase-positive, although agranulated forms may be observed by light microscopy. Careful examination under phase microscopy reveals the peculiar plasma membrane which is characteristic of phagocytic cells. The cells are easily distinguished from lymphocytes as they tend to adhere more to glass surfaces and can be separated from the nonadhering lymphocytes.

Electron microscopically, monocytes in the peripheral blood can be distinguished easily from both granulocytes and typical lymphocytes (Tanaka, 1958) (Fig. 3-48). They are of medium size, with an indented nucleus. The cytoplasm contains small vesicular elements, both agranular and granular, as well as several electron-opaque granules similar to the few seen in granulocytes (Figs. 3-48 and 3-49). However, the mitochondria appear larger than those of neutrophils, more like those in lymphocytes. Intracytoplasmic fibrils are observed frequently (dePetris *et al.*, 1962; Tanaka, 1964) (Fig. 3-50*A*), and, occasionally, other peculiar inclusion bodies are seen (Fig. 3-50*B*). Peripheral monocytes have been observed to transform gradually into large mononuclear cells and epithelioid cells in vitro (Sutton and Weiss, 1966). Cultures of monocytes in skin chambers also show transformation into large, elongated mononuclear cells which can hardly be distinguished from fibroblasts.

Recently, Fedorko and Hirsch (1970) described the ultrastructure of both monoblasts and promonocytes of the mouse bone marrow after separating them in vitro from myelocytic series. In smears, the monoblasts are cells of about 20μ in diameter with no cytoplasmic granules. The cells show active phagocytosis but not as pronounced as that in mature forms. Ultrastructurally, the monoblast is a cell of 5 to 10μ in size with minimum nuclear indentation. The chromatin net is dispersed loosely in the nucleus, and there is a prominent nucleolus. The Golgi area is rather small and granules are observed in the cytoplasm. Large amounts of polyribosomes and tubular endoplasmic reticulum are also present; the many vesicles near the cell surface suggest an active endocytosis. The promonocyte is a cell of about 10 to 20μ in diameter and shows cytoplasmic structures resembling those of mature monocytes, except for the presence of many polyribosomes.

A search for immature monocytes in human bone marrow reveals some immature forms which we think are distinguishable from myeloblasts (Fig. 3-51). Unlike myeloblasts, the immature monocytes show an indented nucleus, with early signs of chromatin clumping. The cytoplasm develops tubular endoplasmic reticulum; small vesicles and various sizes of dense granules, presumably azurophilic granules, are evident. The more mature cells (Figs. 3-52 and 3-53) have a nucleus with a clear indentation, the start of chromatin clumping, and development of many azurophilic granules and membrane systems. Active movement from the bone marrow (Fig. 3-54) is shown by the progression of the cell through a capillary wall.

Kinetic studies on monocytes indicate an intravascular half-life of about 3 days in rats (Whitelaw, 1966) and 32 hours in mice (van Furth and Cohn, 1968). Three generations are estimated between primitive precursors and the mature cells

(text continues on page 169)

FIGURE 3-48. Monocyte from peripheral blood.
This monocyte has characteristic features of scattered dense granules (*g*), vesicular system, rounded, moderately large mitochondria (*M*), and some endoplasmic reticulum. The irregular cellular surface and numerous vacuoles (*arrows*), particularly near periphery, suggest active endocytosis. Two lobes of the nucleus (*N*) are present. × *19,500.*

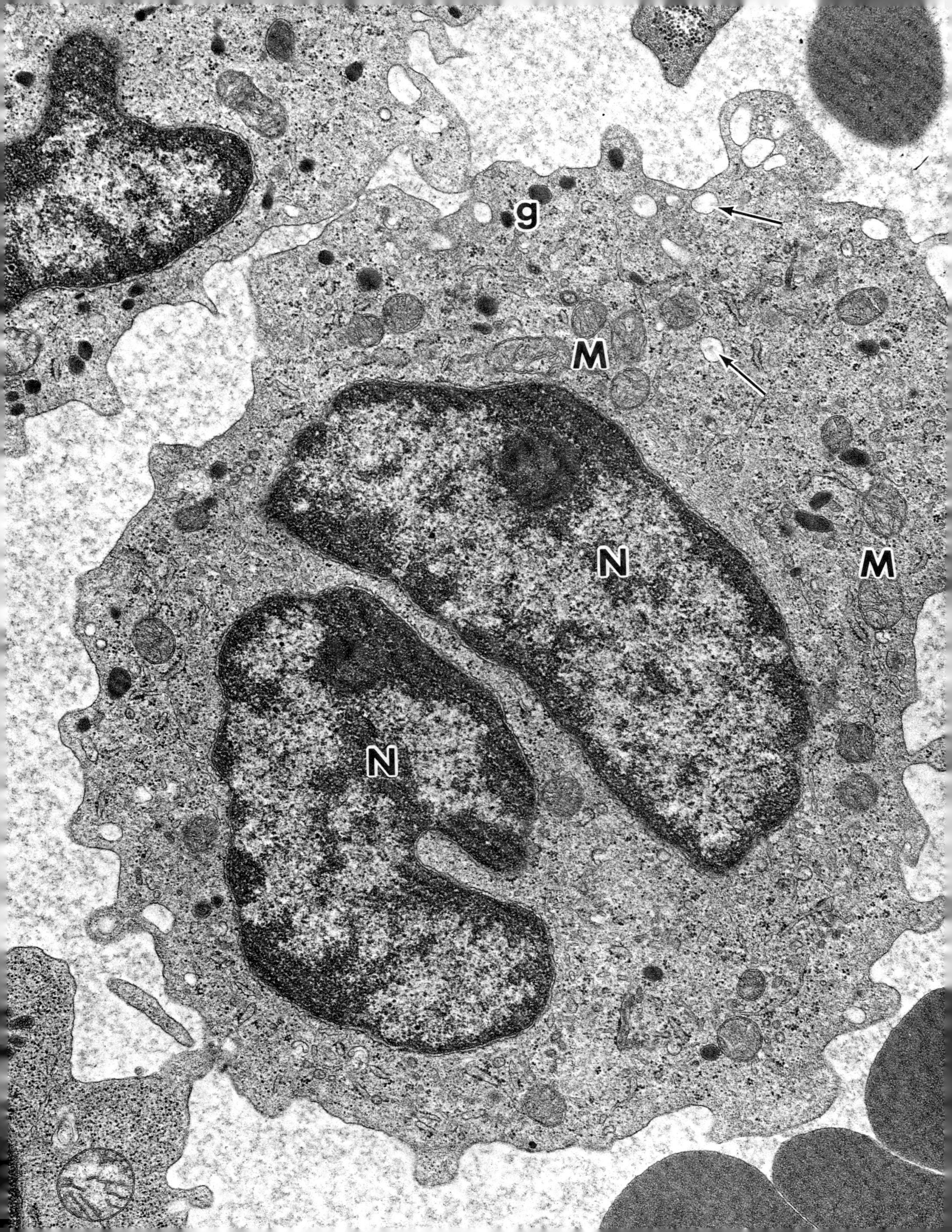
g
M
M
N
N

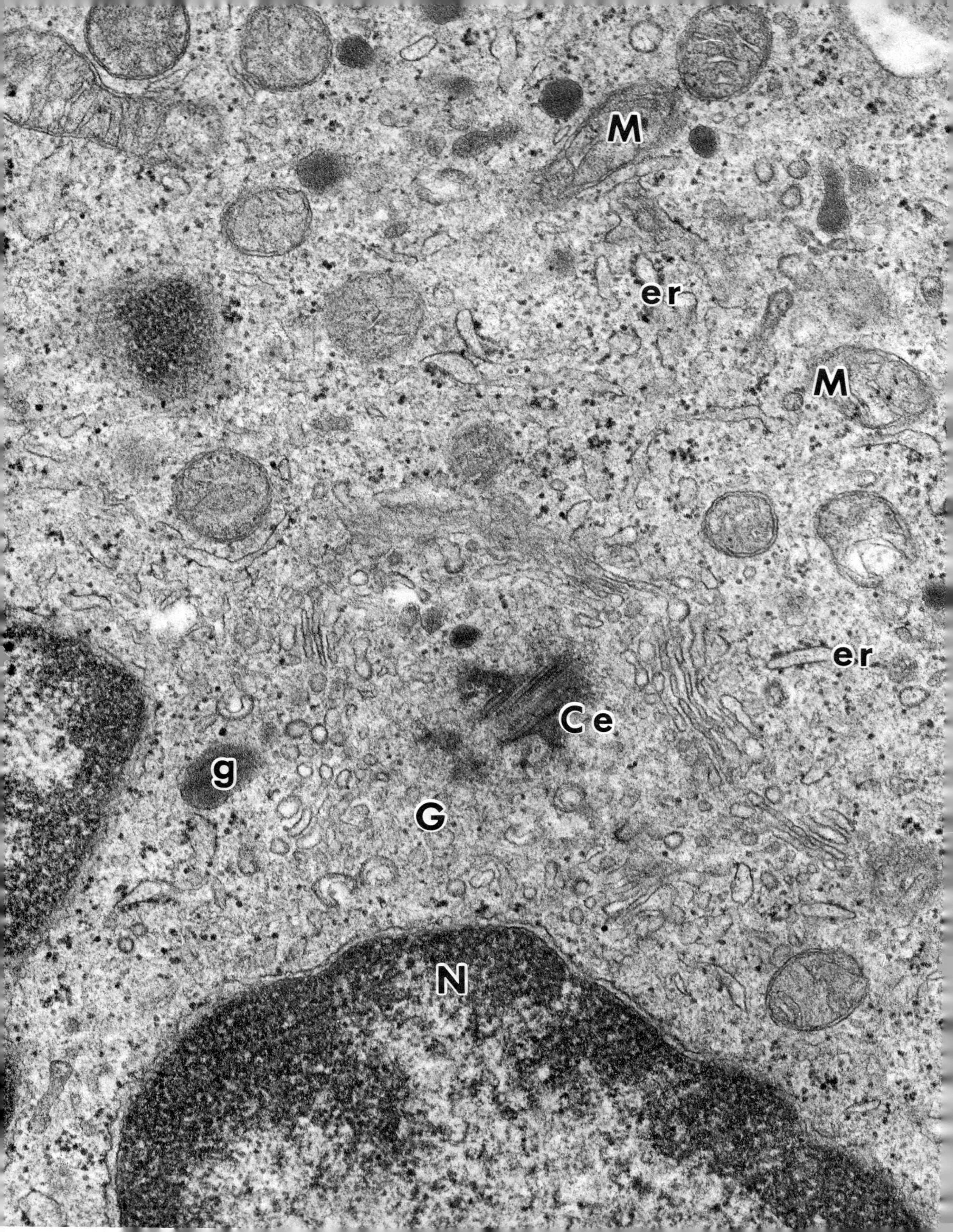
M
er
M
er
Ce
g
G
N

FIGURE 3-49. Monocyte from peripheral blood.
In the Golgi (*G*) area of a monocyte from peripheral blood are numerous small vesicles and some rough endoplasmic reticulum (*er*) that may be involved in granule formation. The centriole (*Ce*), several mitochondria (*M*), and the edge of the nucleus (*N*) are present. × *45,000.*

Figures 3-50 through 3-53 appear on the following pages

FIGURE 3-50. Cytoplasmic detail of monocytes.
A. Free fibrillar formation (*arrows*) is fairly common; granules (*g*) and a mitochondria (*M*) are also present. × *81,000.*
B. This unusual cytoplasmic inclusion (*arrow*) is uncommon and of unknown significance. Small scattered dense particles are glycogen. Some endoplasmic reticulum (*er*) and a portion of a mitochondrion (*M*) are visible. × *66,500.*

FIGURE 3-51. Immature monocytes.
Two immature cells in human bone marrow differ from typical myeloblasts in two characteristics: (1) the nucleus (*N*) has early condensation of chromatin and cells are developing nuclear invagination; (2) cytoplasmic generation of granules differs from that seen in myelocytes (see Figs. 3-6 through 3-8) and promyelocytes and generally indicates the probable classification of these cells in the monocytic series. The Golgi complex (*G*) and several mitochondria (*M*) are apparent in the lower cell. × *16,600.*

FIGURE 3-52. Maturing monocyte.
Large mononuclear cell with deeply indented nucleus (*N*) from human bone marrow has cytoplasmic characteristics similar to those seen in Figure 3-51. Only a few dense granules (*g*) and profiles of tubular endoplasmic reticulum are present. This distinguishes these cells from promyelocytes. There are numerous rounded mitochondria (*M*) and the Golgi complex (*G*). × *15,500.*

FIGURE 3-53. A monocyte in bone marrow.
Medium-sized human bone marrow cell with characteristics of a monocyte contains an indented nucleus (*N*), dense granules (*g*), ovoid mitochondria (*M*), and scattered vesicular and endoplasmic reticular systems. × *28,500.*

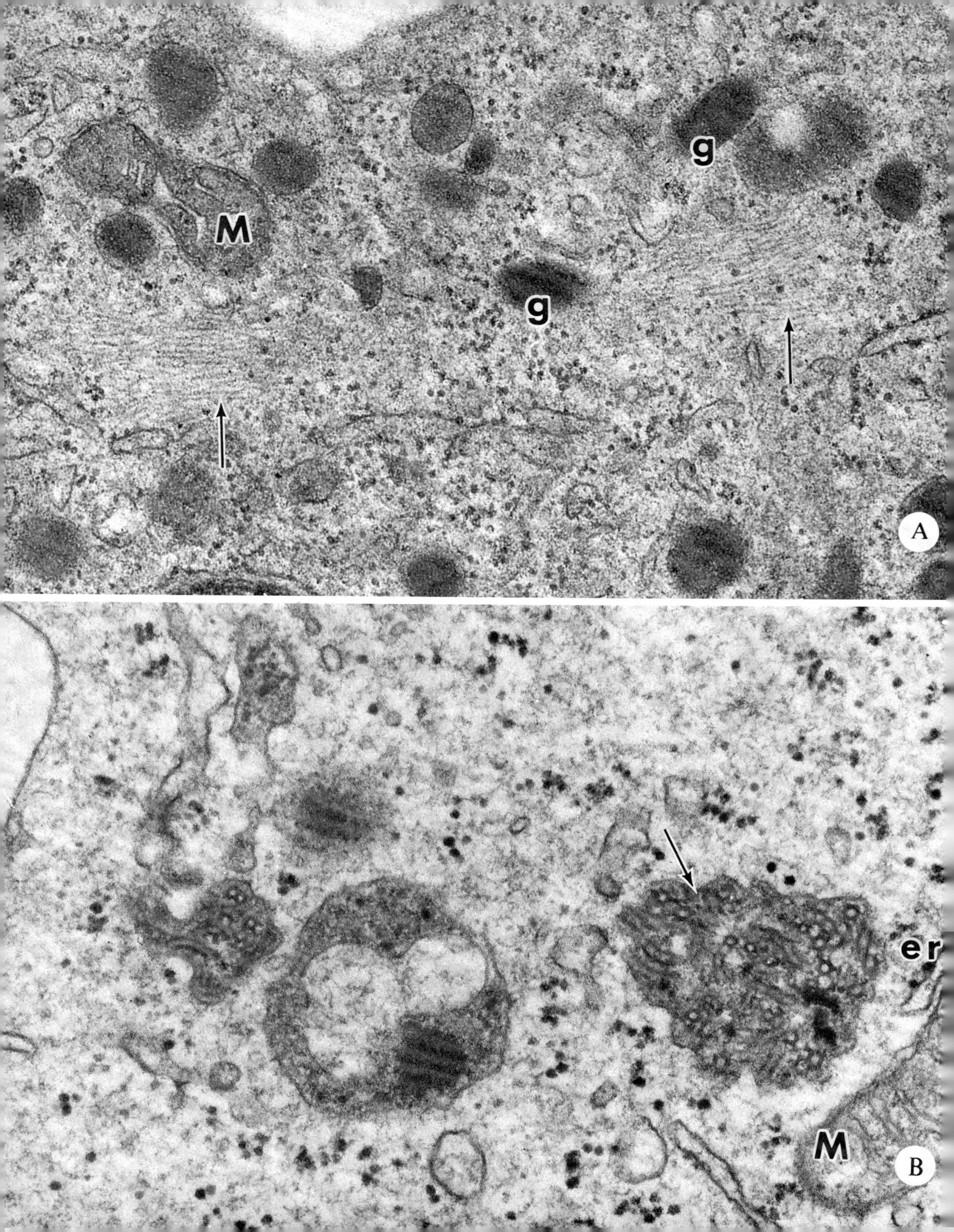
g
M
g
A
er
M
B

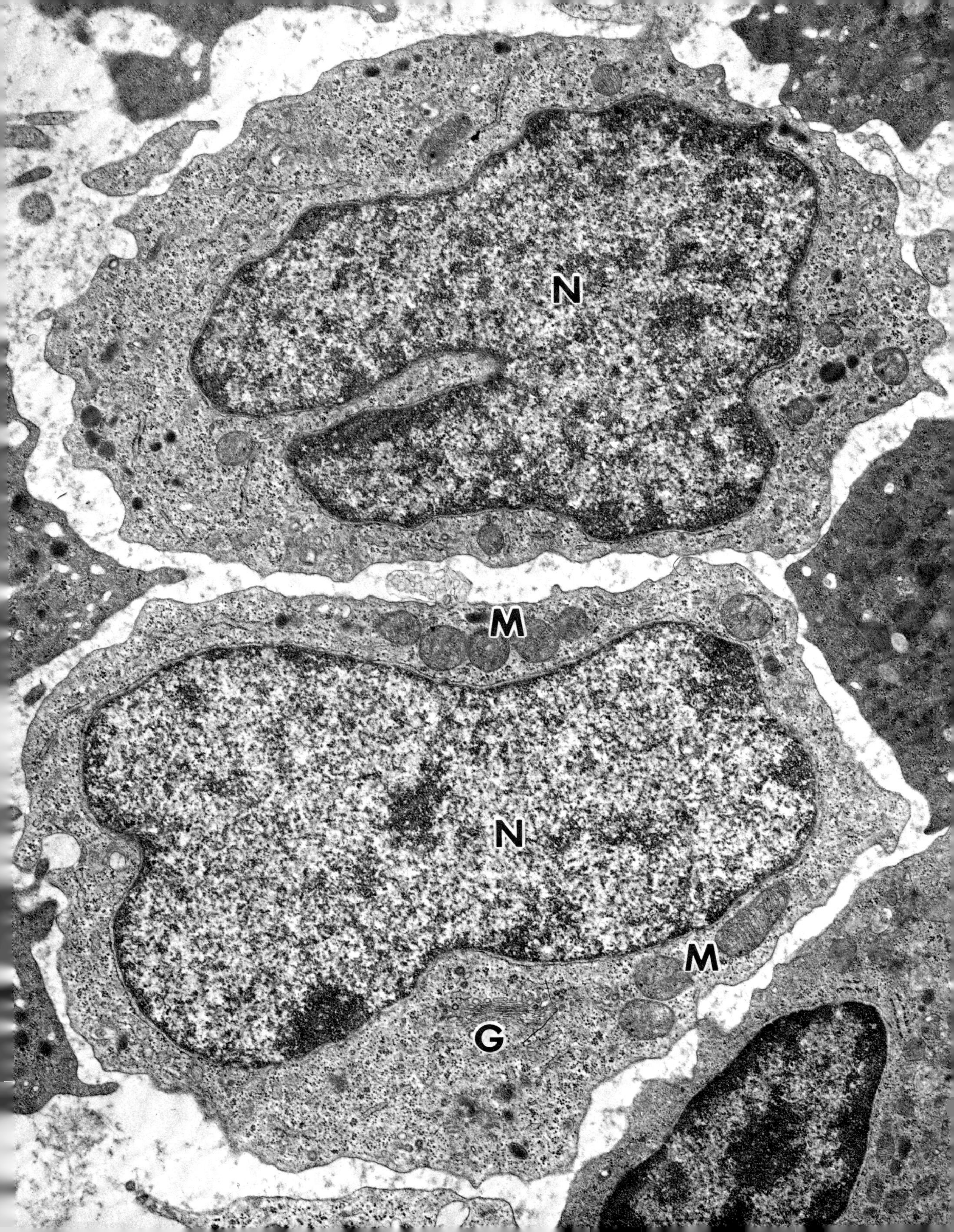
N
M
N
M
G

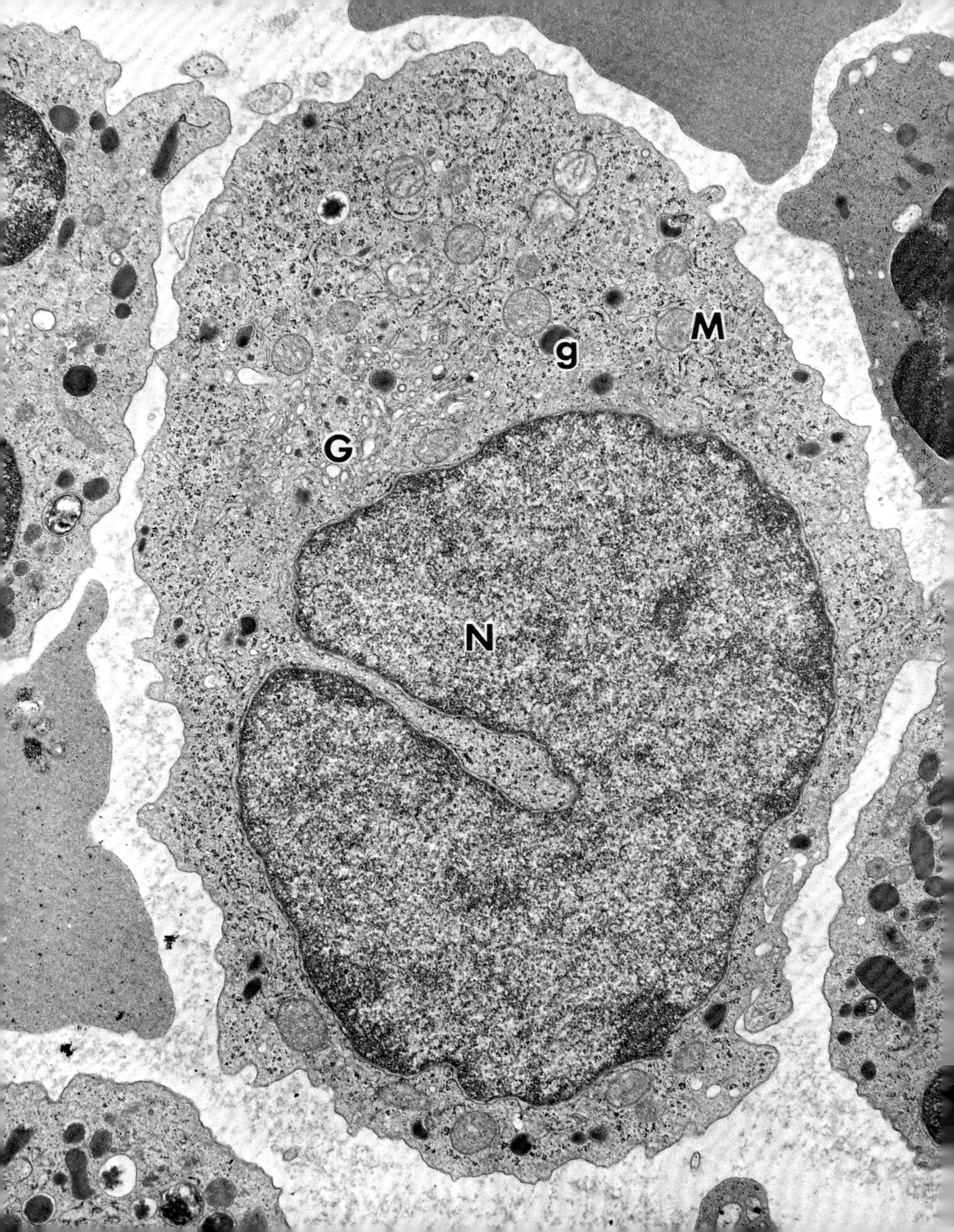
M
g
G
N

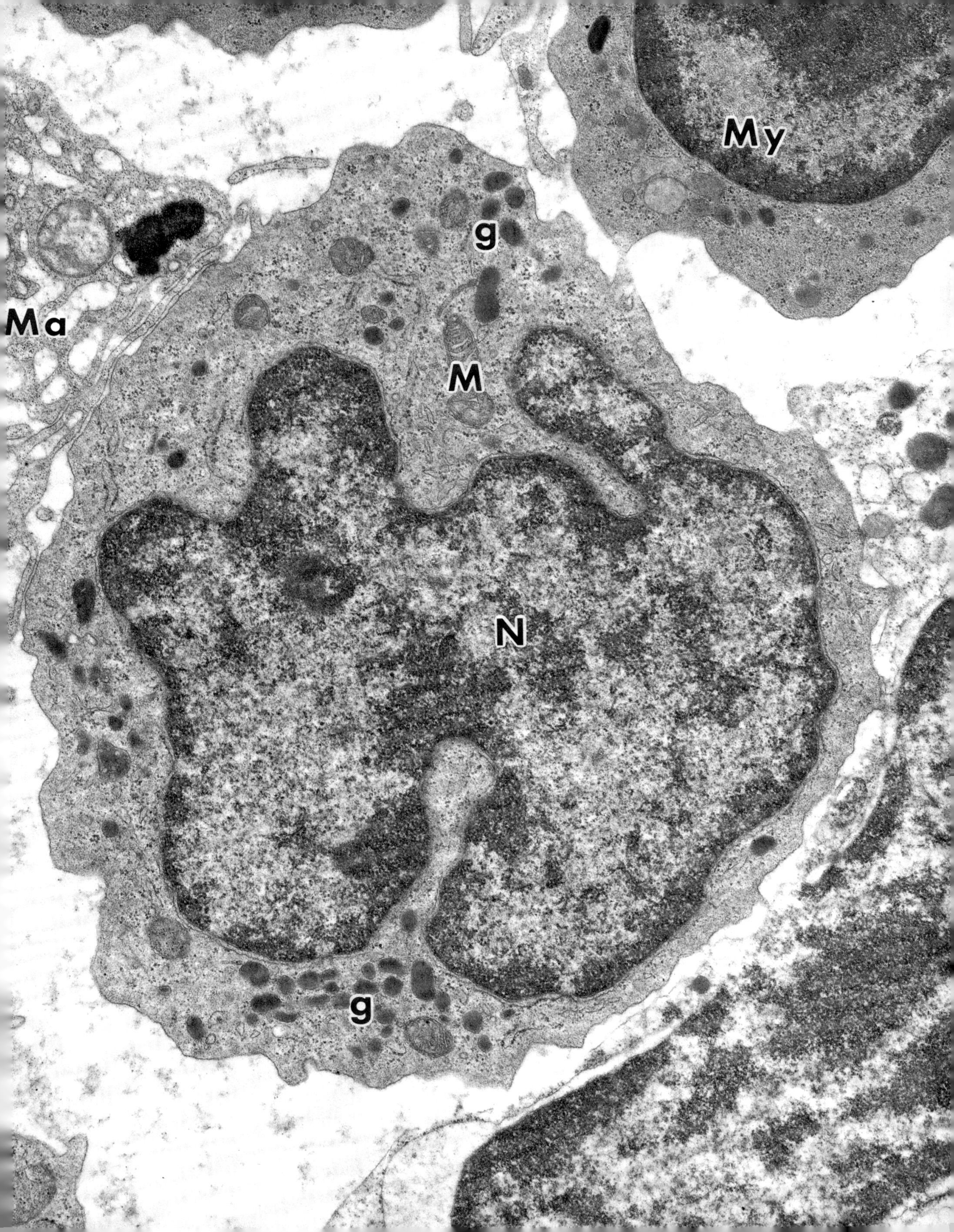
My
g
Ma
M
N
g

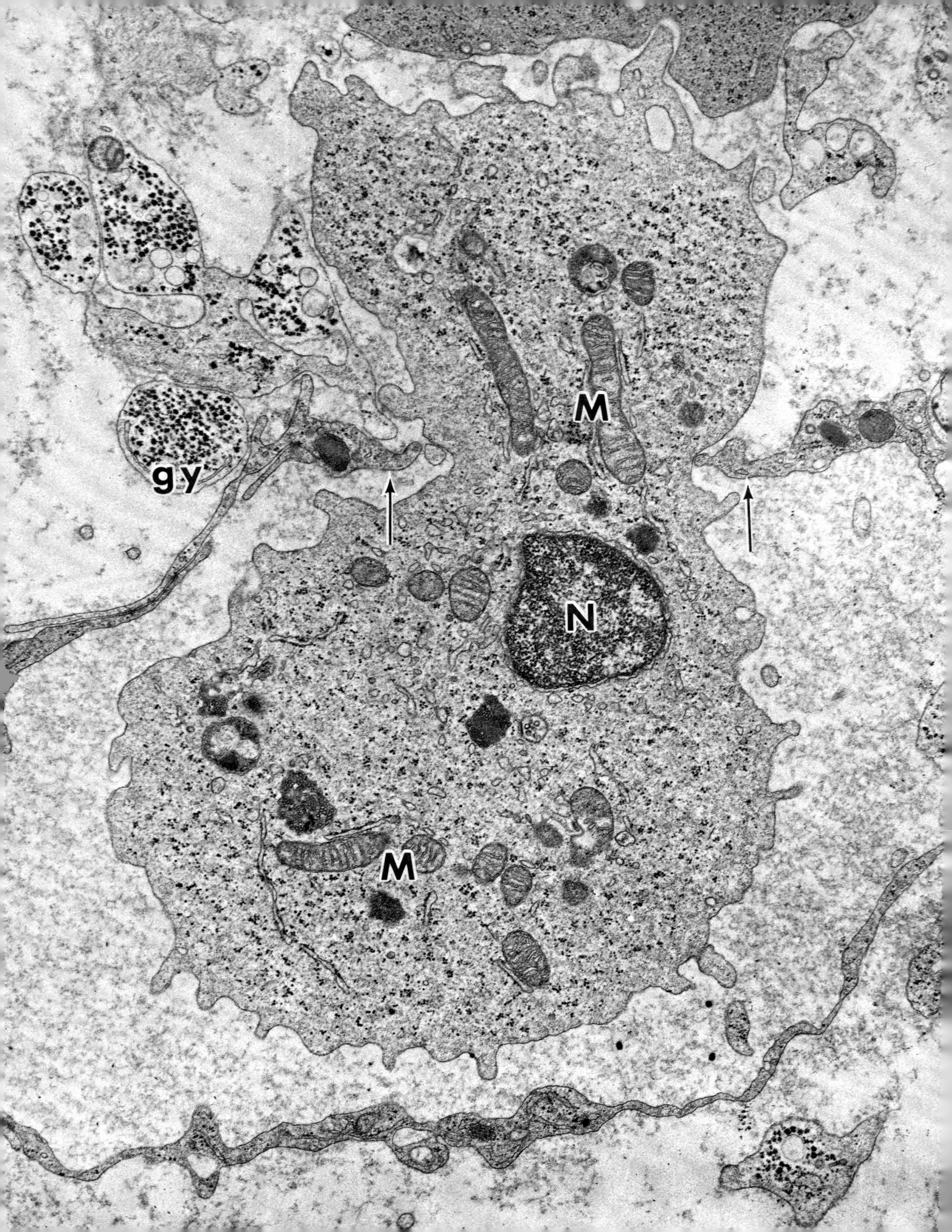
gy
M
N
M

(Whitelaw, 1966). Unlike granulocytes, immature monocytes do not stay in a maturation pool for any length of time (van Furth, 1970). Blood monocytes leave the circulation at a random rate (Whitelaw, 1966; van Furth, 1970) and stay in tissues for a long time (van Furth, 1970).

FUNCTION

The phagocytic activity of these cells has been well established. Earlier extensive studies of Sabin and associates (1930) stressed the significance of blood monocytes as the origin of tissue macrophages and epithelioid cells. This classic concept of monocyte function has been confirmed by many recent publications on the development of monocytes into macrophages in subcutaneous tissues, serosal cavities, and pulmonary spaces (van Furth, 1970) (see Chap. 7). Monocytes are mobile and represent a readily available macrophage compartment. In irradiated parabiotic rats (Caffrey-Tyler and Everett, 1966) mononuclear cells which resemble monocytes are suggested as pluripotential stem cells capable of repopulation.

PATHOLOGY

Although there is much information favorable to the marrow origin of blood monocytes, the origin of leukemic monocytes is still controversial. Malignant proliferation of monocytes (transitional forms) was first described by Reschad and Schilling-Torgau in 1913, and leukemic manifestation of cells of the reticuloendothelial system was introduced by Ewald (1923). Downey (1938) distinguished two types of cells in monocytic leukemia—the Schilling (histiocytic) and Naegeli (monocytic) types—and left them in the category of monocytic leukemia though he considered the two forms to be of different origin. Two types of monocytic leukemia were clearly distinguished by Belding *et al.* (1955). The histiocytic type was regarded as a manifestation of malignant reticuloendotheliosis, and the term was used to define the monocytic type. More recently, the term monocytic leukemia has been used to define leukemia of the histiocytic type (Dameshek and Gunz, 1964; Rappaport, 1966), and leukemia of the blood monocytic type has been classed as an acute granulocytic leukemia (Rappaport, 1966) or its variant (Dameshek and Gunz, 1964; Leder, 1967). Since recent experimental data favor the marrow origin of blood monocytes, it is convenient to retain the category of blood monocytic leukemia.

The difficulty of recognition by light microscopy lies in the indistinguishable characteristics of the monocyte and its precursors from immature granulocytes. The close relationship or possible common origin of myelocytic and monocytic cell lines makes the distinction between their leukemic states difficult. A similar problem has been discussed on the differentiation between early erythroid and

FIGURE 3-54. Migrating monocyte.
The peculiar inclusions in Figure 3-50**B** were found in this monocyte, which is passing through endothelial lining (*arrows*) of a small vessel or sinusoid. Only the tip of the nucleus (*N*) is present, along with mitochondria (*M*) and other cytoplasmic organelles. Small structures containing many glycogen (*gy*) particles are probably blebs released from a megakaryocyte. × *18,000.*

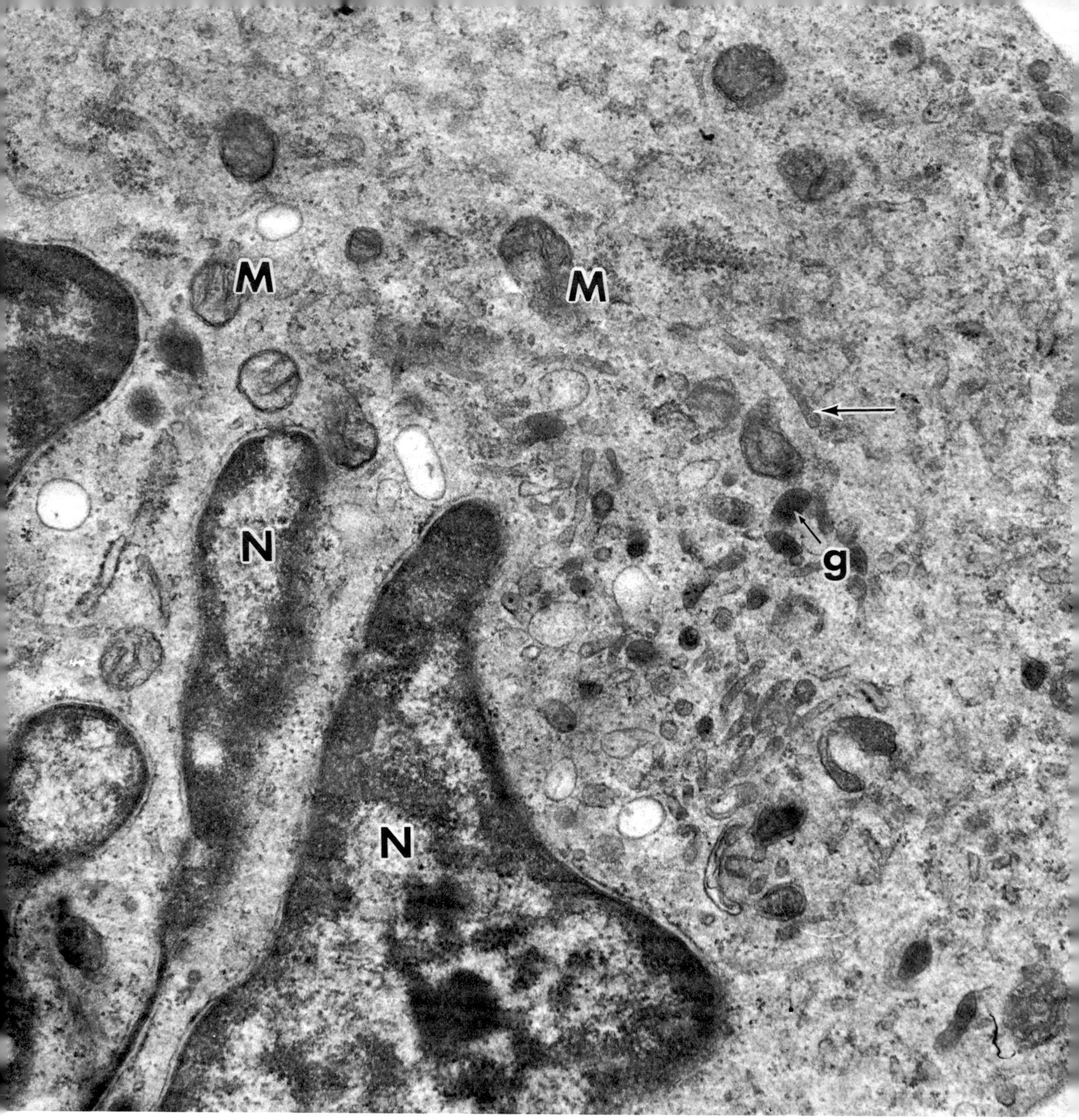

FIGURE 3-55. Monocytic leukemia.
Portion of cell from case of monocytic leukemia with cytoplasmic characteristics similar to typical monocytes. There is a well-developed vesicular system (*arrow*) and numerous small granules (*g*). Mitochondria (*M*) appear to be smaller than usual and nucleus (*N*) has numerous deep invaginations. × *30,000.*

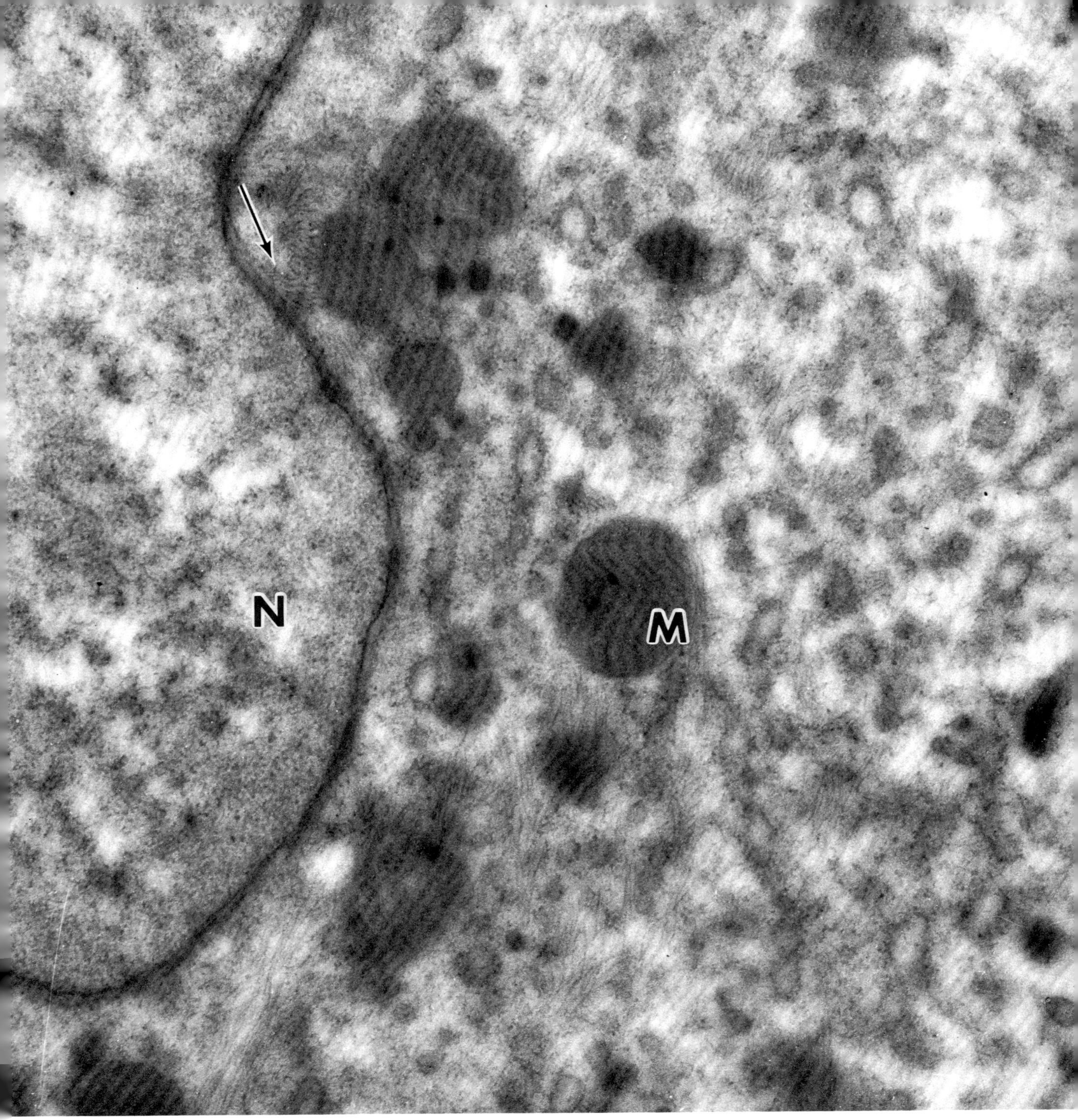

FIGURE 3-56. Monocytic leukemia.
Cytoplasm of cell from case of monocytic leukemia demonstrates that this "histiocytic" type differs significantly from the "monocytic" type in Figure 3-55. Although cytoplasm has a vesicular appearance, there is an unusual mitochondrion (*M*) and many scattered fine fibrils, some of which seem to be associated with the nuclear (*N*) membrane (*arrow*). × *42,000.*
Reprinted with permission from Tanaka, Y. *J Nat Cancer Inst 33:*467, 1964.

myeloid leukemia forms (Chap. 2). Differential electron microscopic studies on cells of both types of monocytic leukemia are rare. The confusion in classification may become clarified when distinctions of the two monocytic cell origins are understood.

We studied one case of each by electron microscopy and found significant differences in their ultrastructure. A part of a monocytic leukemia cell of the typical monocytic type is shown in Figure 3-55, and can be distinguished easily from immature granulocytes. Figure 3-56 illustrates a part of a leukemic cell of histiocytic type; note its significant difference from the cell in Figure 3-55. The case used in Figure 3-40*B* was originally diagnosed as acute myelocytic leukemia; however, the spleen showed systemic proliferation of endothelial cells without signs of leukemic infiltration. These two figures show the difference in the two types of leukemic cells and suggest the potential of electron microscopy in establishing the identity of monocytic leukemia of the monocytic type.

REFERENCES

Ackerman, G. A., Grasso, J. A., and Knouff, R. A. Morphological and histochemical studies of the leukemic cells from a patient with atypical myeloblastic leukemia with special reference to intracytoplasmic mucopolysaccharide vacuoles and fibrillar formation. *Blood 16*:1253, 1960.

Ackerman, G. A. Cytochemical properties of the blood basophilic granulocyte. *Ann NY Acad Sci 103*:376, 1963.

Ackerman, G. A. Histochemical differentiation during neutrophil development and maturation. *Ann NY Acad Sci 113*:537, 1964.

Ackerman, G. A. Ultrastructure and cytochemistry of the developing neutrophil. *Lab Invest 19*:290, 1968.

Akasaka, K. An electron microscopic study of blood cells. Ultrastructure of leukemic cells. *Acta Haemat Jap 26*:193, 1963.

Anderson, D. R. Ultrastructure of normal and leukemic leukocytes in human peripheral blood. *J Ultrastruct Res Suppl 9,* 1966.

Archer, G. T., and Hirsch, J. G. Isolation of granules from eosinophil leucocytes and study of their enzyme content. *J Exp Med 118*:277, 1963a.

Archer, G. T., and Hirsch, J. G. Motion picture studies on degranulation of horse eosinophils during phagocytosis. *J Exp Med 118*:287, 1963b.

Archer, G. T., and Blackwood, A. Formation of Charcot-Leyden crystals in human eosinophils and basophils and study of the composition of isolated crystals. *J Exp Med 122*:173, 1965.

Archer, R. K. Studies with eosinophil leucocytes isolated from the blood of the horse. *Brit J Haemat 6*:299, 1960.

Aschoff, L. Das reticulo-endotheliale system. *Ergeb Inn Med Kinderheilk 26*:1, 1924.

Athens, J. W., Mauer, A. M., Ashenbucker, H., Cartwright, G. E., and Wintrobe, M. M. Leukokinetic studies, I. A method for labeling leukocytes with diisopropyl fluorophosphate (DFP^{32}). Blood *14*:303, 1959.

Athens, J. W. Granulocyte Kinetics in Health and Disease. In *Human Tumor Cell Kinetics.* Nat Cancer Inst Monogr *30*:135, 1969.

Baggiolini, M., Hirsch, J. G., and deDuve, C. Resolution of granules from rabbit heterophil leukocytes into distinct populations by zonal sedimentation. *J Cell Biol 40*:529, 1969.

Baggiolini, M., Hirsch, J. G., and deDuve, C. Further biochemical and morphological studies of granule fractions from rabbit heterophil leukocytes. *J Cell Biol 45*:586, 1970.

Bainton, D. F., and Farquhar, M. G. Origin of granules in polymorphonuclear leukocytes. Two types derived from opposite faces of the Golgi complex in developing granulocytes. *J Cell Biol 28*:277, 1966.

Bainton, D. F., and Farquhar, M. G. Differences in enzyme content of azurophil and specific granules of polymorphonuclear leukocytes. 1. Histochemical staining of bone marrow smears. *J Cell Biol 39*:286, 1968a.

Bainton, D. F., and Farquhar, M. G. Differences in enzyme content in azurophil and specific granules of polymorphonuclear leukocytes. II. Cytochemistry and electron microscopy of bone marrow cells. *J Cell Biol 39*:299, 1968b.

Bainton, D. F., and Farquhar, M. G. Segregation

and packaging of granule enzymes in eosinophilic leukocytes. *J Cell Biol 45*:54, 1970.

Bakalos, D. On the precursors and the reactive and hyperplastic process of the blood cells. *Acta Med Scand 135*:99, 1949.

Barnhart, M., and Riddle, J. M. Cellular localization of profibrinolysin (plasminogen). *Blood 21*:306, 1963.

Barr, M. L., and Bertram, E. G. A morphological distinction between neurones of the male and female and the behaviour of the nucleolar satellite during accelerated nucleoprotein synthesis. *Nature* (*London*) *163*:676, 1949.

Belding, H. W., Daland, G. A., and Parker, F., Jr. Histiocytic and monocytic leukemia. A clinical, hematological and pathological differentiation. *Cancer 8*:237, 1955.

Benditt, E. P., Wong, R. L., Arase, M., and Roeper, E. 5-hydroxy-tryptamine in mast cells. *Proc Soc Exp Biol Med 90*:303, 1955.

Bernhard, W. The detection and study of tumor viruses with the electron microscope. *Cancer Res 20*:712, 1960.

Bessis, M., and Breton-Gorius, J. Examen des cellules leucémiques au microscope électronique par la methode des coupes, *Presse Med 63*:189, 1955.

Bessis, M. *Cytology of the Blood and Blood-forming Organs* (Ponder, E., transl.). Grune & Stratton, New York, 1956.

Bessis, M., Bernard, J., and Seligmann, M. Étude cytologique d'un cas de maladie de Chediak. *Nouv Rev Franc Hemat 1*:422, 1961.

Bessis, M., and Thiéry, J. P. Electron microscopy of human white blood cells and their stem cells. *Int Rev Cytol 12*:199, 1961a.

Bessis, M., and Thiéry, J. P. Étude au microscope électronique sur les leucémies humaines. 1. Les leucémies granulocytaires, *Nouv Rev Franc Hemat 1*:703, 1961b.

Bessis, M., and Breton-Gorius, J. Pathologie et asynchromisme de développement des organelles cellulaires au corps des leucémies agués granulocytaires. Étude au microscope électronique. *Nouv Rev Franc Hemat 9*:245, 1969.

Bierman, H. R., Kelly, K. H., Byron, R. L., Jr., and Marshall, G. J. Leucophoresis in man. I. Haematological observations following leucocyte withdrawal in patients with non-haematological disorders. *Brit J Haemat 7*:51, 1961.

Boll, I. Morphologische Studien zum Verhalten von Knochenmarkzellen in vitro. Granuloblastenmitosen. *Folia Haemat 3*:58, 1958.

Bornstein, D. L., and Woods, J. W. Species specialty of leukocytic pyrogens. *J Exp Med 130*:707, 1969.

Braunsteiner, H., and Pakesch, F. Electron microscopic observations on leukemic cells. *Acta Haemat 24*:64, 1960.

Breton-Gorius, J. Structures périodiques dan les granulations éosinophiles et neutrophiles des leucocytes polynucléaires du sang de l'homme. *Nouv Rev Franc Hemat 6*:195, 1966.

Burton, A. L., and Bensley, S. H. The finer structure of developing mast cells. *Anat Rec 130*:280, 1958.

Caffrey-Tyler, R. W., and Everett, N. B. A radioautographic study of hemopoietic repopulation using irradiated parabiotic rats. Relation to the stem cell problem. *Blood 28*:873, 1966.

Capone, R. J., Weinreb, E. L., and Chapman, G. B. Electron microscope studies on normal human myeloid elements. *Blood 23*:300, 1964.

Cartwright, G. E., Athens, J. W., and Wintrobe, M. M. The kinetics of granulopoiesis in normal man. *Blood 24*:780, 1964.

Caspersson, T., Zech, L., and Johansson, C. Differential binding of alkylating fluorochromes in human chromosomes. *Exp Cell Res 60*:315, 1970.

Chediak, M. M. Nouvelle anomalie leucocytaire de caractère constitutionnel et familial. *Rev Hemat 7*:362, 1952.

Christensen, H. E., Iversen, O. H., and Rask-Nielsen, R. Studies on a transplantable mastocytoma in mice. II. Electron microscopic observations. *J Nat Cancer Inst 30*:763, 1963.

Clausen, K. P., and von Hamm, E. Fine structure of malignancy-associated change (MAc) in peripheral human leucocytes. *Acta Cytol 13*:435, 1969.

Cline, M. J., Hanifin, J., and Lehrer, R. I. Phagocytosis by human eosinophils. *Blood 32*:922, 1968.

Cohn, Z. A., and Hirsch, J. G. The isolation and properties of the specific cytoplasm granules of rabbit polymorphonuclear leucocytes. *J Exp Med 118*:983, 1960.

Combs, J. W. Maturation of rat mast cells. An electron microscope study. *J Cell Biol 31*:563, 1966.

Cotran, R. S., and Litt, M. The entry of granule-associated peroxidase into the phagocytic vacuoles of eosinophils. *J Exp Med 129*:1291, 1969.

Cowdry, E. V. The vital staining of mitochondria

with Janus green and dimethylsafranin in human blood cells. *Int Mschr Anal Physiol 31*:267, 1915.

Craddock, C. G., Jr., Adams, W. S., Perry, S., Skoog, W. A., and Laurence, J. S. Studies of leukopoiesis: Technique of leukophoresis and response of myeloid tissue in normal and irradiated dogs. *J Lab Clin Med 45*:881, 1955.

Cronkite, E. P., and Fliedner, T. M. Granulocytopoiesis. *New Eng J Med 270*:1347, 1964.

Cronkite, E. P. Kinetics of Granulocytopoiesis. In *Human Tumor Cell Kinetics.* Nat Cancer Inst Monogr *30*:51, 1969.

Cunningham, R. S., Sabin, F. R., and Doan, C. A. Development of leucocytes, lymphocytes and monocytes from a specific stem cell in adult tissues. *Contrib Embryol 84*:227, 1925.

Dameshek, W., and Gunz, F. *Leukemia* (2nd ed.). Grune & Stratton, New York, 1964.

Davidson, W. M., and Smith, D. R. A morphological sex difference in the polymorphonuclear neutrophil leucocytes. *Brit MJ 2*:6, 1954.

Davidson, W. M. Inherited variations in leukocytes. *Seminars Hemat 5*:255, 1968.

dePetris, S., Karlsbad, G., and Pernis, B. Filamentous structures in the cytoplasm of normal mononuclear phagocytes. *J Ultrastruct Res 7*:39, 1962.

Döhle, H. Leukocyteneinschlüsse bei Scharlach. *Zbl Bakt 61*:63, 1911.

Dorr, A. D., and Moloney, W. C. Acquired pseudo-Pelger anomaly of granulocytic leukocytes. *New Eng J Med 261*:742, 1959.

Douglas, S. D., Blume, R. B., and Wolff, S. M. Fine structural studies of leukocytes from patients and heterozygotes with the Chediak-Higashi syndrome. *Blood 33*:527, 1969.

Downey, H. Monocytic leukemia and leukemic reticulo-endotheliosis. *Handbook Hemat 2*:1275, 1938.

Dunn, W. B., Hardin, J. H., and Spicer, S. S. Ultrastructural localization of myeloperoxidase in human neutrophil and rabbit heterophil and eosinophil leucocytes. *Blood 32*:935, 1968.

Dunn, W. B., and Spicer, S. S. Histochemical demonstration of sulfated mucosubstances and cationic proteins in human granulocytes and platelets. *J Histochem Cytochem 17*:668, 1969.

Duplan, J. F., Bessis, M., and Breton-Gorius, J. Les appendices nucléaires (caryoschizes) des granulocytes. XIV. Après irradiation générale. Étude au microscope électronique. *Nouv Rev Hemat 9*:205, 1969.

Eder, M., and Schauer, A. Fermenthistochemische und experimentelle untersuchungen an Gewebsmastzellen. *Beitr Path Anat 124*:251, 1961.

Ehrlich, P. Uber die specifischen Granulationen des Blutes. *Arch Anat Physiol* (*Physiol Abtl*) *3*:571, 1879a.

Ehrlich, P. Beitrag zur Kenntnis der granulierten Bindegewebszellen und der eosinophilen Leukocyten. *Arch Anat Physiol* (*Physiol Abtl*) *3*:166, 1879b.

Ehrlich, P. *Farbenanalytische Untersuchungen zur Histologie und Klinik des Blutes.* Hirchwald, Berlin, 1891.

Ehrlich, P. Die Anämie. In *Spezielle Pathologie und Therapie* (Northnagel, H., ed.) Holder, Wien, 1898, vol. 8.

Ewald, O. Die leukämische Retikuloendotheliose, *Deutsch Arch Klin Med 142*:222, 1923.

Ezdinli, E. Z., Sokal, J. E., Crosswhite, L., and Sandberg, A. A. Philadelphia chromosome-positive and -negative chronic myelocytic leukemia. *Ann Intern Med 72*:175, 1970.

Faller, A. Zur Frage von Struktur und Aufbau der eosinohilen Granula. *Z Zellforsch 69*:551, 1966.

Fedorko, M. E., and Hirsch, J. G. Crystalloid structure in granules of guinea pig basophils and human mast cells. *J Cell Biol 26*:973, 1965.

Fedorko, M. E. Effect of chloroquine on morphology of cytoplasmic granules in maturing human leukocytes. An ultrastructural study. *J Clin Invest 46*:1932, 1967.

Fedorko, M. E., and Hirsch, J. G. Structure of monocytes and macrophages. *Seminars Hemat 7*:109, 1970.

Fernando, N. V. P., and Movat, H. Z. The fine structure of connective tissue. III. The mast cell. *Exp Molec Path 2*:450, 1963.

Fitzgerald, P. H., Adams, A., and Gunz, F. W. Chronic granulocytic leukemia and the Philadelphia chromosome. *Blood 21*:183, 1963.

Foot, E. C. Eosinophil turnover in the normal rat. *Brit J Haemat 11*:439, 1965.

Freeman, J. A., and Samuels, M. S. The ultrastructure of a "fibrillar formation" of leukemic human blood. *Blood 13*:725, 1958.

Freeman, J. A. The ultrastructure and genesis of Auer bodies. *Blood 15*:449, 1960.

Freeman, J. A. Origin of Auer bodies. *Blood 27*:499, 1966.

Fullmer, H. M. Differences in mechanism in staining reactions for mast cells. *Nature* (*London*) *183*:1274, 1959.

Ghidoni, J. J., and Goldberg, A. F. Light and electron microscopic localization of acid phosphatase activity in human eosinophils. *Amer J Clin Path 45*:402, 1966.

Giemsa, G. Ein Vereinfachung und Vervollkommnung meiner Methylenazur-Methylenblau-Eosin-Färbenmethode zur Erzielung der Romanowsky-Nochtschen Chromatinfärbung. *Zbl Bakt 37*: 308, 1904.

Giemsa, G. Ueber eine neue Schnellfärbung mit meiner Azureosinlösung. *München Med Wschr 57*:2476, 1910.

Glenner, G. G., Hopsu, V. K., and Cohen, L. A. Histochemical demonstration of a trypsin-like esterase activity in mast cells. *J Histochem Cytochem 10*:109, 1962.

Gomori, G. Distribution of acid phosphatase in the tissues under normal and under pathologic conditions. *Arch Path 32*:189, 1941.

Goodman, J. R., and Moore, R. E. Electron microscopic study of phagocytosis of staphylococcus by human leukocytes. *J Bact 71*:547, 1956.

Graham, G. S. The oxidizing ferment of the myelocyte series of cells and its demonstration by an alpha-naphthol-pyronin method. *J Med Res 35*: 231, 1916.

Graham, G. S. Benzidine as a peroxidase reagent for blood smears and tissues. *J Med Res 39*:15, 1919.

Gusek, W. Elektronenoptische Untersuchungen über die Ultrastruktur von Mastzellen. *Arch Klin Exp Derm 213*:573, 1961.

Hagen, P., Barnett, R. J., and Lee, F. Biochemical and electron microscopic study of particles isolated from mastocytoma cells. *J Pharmacol Exp Ther 126*:91, 1959.

Harm, H. Beinflussung das weissen Blutbilder von Pelger-und Nicht Pelger-Kanichen durch colchicin. *Acta Haemat 10*:95, 1953.

Hegglin, R. Gleichzeitige Konstitutionelle Veränderungen an Neutrophilen und Thrombozyten. *Helv Med Acta 12*:439, 1945.

Higashi, O. Congenital abnormality of peroxidase granules—a case of "congenital gigantism of peroxidase granules"; preliminary report. *Tohoku J Exp Med 58*:246, 1953.

Hirsch, J. G., and Cohn, Z. A. Degranulation of polymorphonuclear leucocytes following phagocytosis of microorganisms. *J Exp Med 112*: 1005, 1960.

Hirsch, J. G. Cinemicrophotographic observations on granule lysis in polymorphonuclear leucocyte during phagocytosis. *J Exp Med 116*:827, 1962.

Hirschhorn, R., and Weissmann, G. Isolation and properties of human leukocyte lysosomes *in vitro*. *Proc Soc Exp Biol Med 119*:36, 1965.

Holmgren, H., and Wilander, O. Beitrag zur kenntnis der Chemie und Funktion der Ehrlichschen Mastzellen. *Z Mik Anat Forsch 42*:242, 1937.

Horn, R. G., and Spicer, S. S. Sulfated mucopolysaccharide and basic protein in certain granules of rabbit leukocytes. *Lab Invest 13*:1, 1964.

Huehns, E. R., Lutzner, M., and Hecht, F. Nuclear abnormalities of the neutrophils in D_1 (13–15) trisomy syndrome. *Lancet 1*:589, 1964.

Huët, G. J. Über eine bisher unbekannte familiäre Anomalie der Leukocyten. *Klin Wschr 11*:1264, 1932.

Ito, S. Electron microscopic study of the leukemic cells in the bone marrow. *Acta Haemat Jap 29*: 22, 1966.

Janoff, A., and Zweifach, B. W. Production of inflammatory changes in the microcirculation by cationic proteins extracted from lysosomes. *J Exp Med 120*:747, 1964.

Jansson, S. E., and Penttilä, A. Effect of pH, temperature, osmolarity and drugs on 5-hydroxytryptamine content and light and electron microscopic structure of rat mast cells in vitro. *Exp Cell Res 54*:367, 1969.

Jordan, S. W., and Larsen, W. E. Ultrastructural studies of the May-Hegglin anomaly. *Blood 25*: 921, 1965.

Jorpes, E., Holmgren, H., and Wilander, O. Über das Vorkommen von Heparin in den Gefässwänden und in den Angen, Ein Beitrag zur Physiologie der Ehrlichschen Mastzellen. *Z Mikr Anat Forsch 42*:279, 1937.

Kaplow, L. S., and Burstone, M. S. Cytochemical demonstration of acid phosphatase in hematopoietic cells in health and in various hematological disorders using azo dye techniques. *J Histochem Cytochem 12*:805, 1964.

Kaplow, L. S. Simplified myeloperoxidase stain using benzidine dihydrochloride. *Blood 26*:215, 1965.

Kaung, D. T. Periodic acid-Schiff reaction in human basophilic leucocytes. *Acta Haemat 42*:269, 1969.

Killmann, S. A., Cronkite, E. P., Fliedner, T. M., and Bond, V. P. Mitotic indices of human bone marrow cells. III. Duration of some phases of erythrocytic and granulocytic proliferation computed from mitotic indices. *Blood 24*:267, 1964.

Kobayashi, T., Midtgord, K., and Asboe-Hansen, G. Ultrastructure of human mast-cell granules. *J Ultrastruct Res 23*:153, 1968.

Kondo, K., Yoshitake, J., and Takemura, K. The fine structure of Auer bodies. *J Electron Micr (Tokyo) 15*:237, 1966.

Kosenow, W., and Scupin, R. Geschlechtsbestimmung auf Grand morphologischer Leukocytenmerkmale. *Klin Wschr 34*:51, 1956.

Koszewski, B. J., Vahabzabeh, H., and Willrodt, S. Hemosiderin content of leukocytes in animals and man and its significance in the physiology of granulocyte. *Amer J Clin Path 48*:474, 1967.

Kundel, D. W., Tanaka, Y., Tijo, J. H., Whang, J., and Fishbein, W. N. Chromosome Philadelphia inclusions filamenteuses et corps d'Auer dans un cas de transformation aiguë de leucémie myéloideth chronique. *Nouv Rev Franc Hemat 3*:844, 1963.

Lagunoff, D., Philips, M., and Benditt, E. P. The histochemical demonstration of histamine in mast cells. *J Histochem Cytochem 9*:534, 1961.

Laves, W., and Thoma, K. Histoencymatische Untersuchungen an den Mastzellen des Blutes. *Klin Wschr 28*:95, 1950.

Leader, R. W., Padgett, G. A., and Gorham, J. R. Studies of abnormal leukocyte bodies in the mink. *Blood 22*:477, 1963.

Leder, L. D. Der Nachweis der Naphthol-As-D-chloracetate-esterase und seine Bedeutung für die histologische Diagnostik. *Deutsch Ges Path Verh 48*:317, 1964.

Leder, L. D. *Die Herkunst der Blutmonozyten und Beziehungen zur den sog Histiozyten in der monozyt.* Springer, Berlin, 1967.

Lennert, K. and Schubert, J. C. F. Zur Cytochemie der Blut und Gewebsmastzellen. *Verh. Deutsch Ges Inn Med* 66th Kongr Wiesbaden, 1960, *p. 1061, 1961.*

Litt, M. Studies in experimental eosinophilia. VI. Uptake of immune complexes by eosinophils. *J Cell Biol 23*:355, 1964.

Lockwood, W. R., and Allison, F. Electron micrographic studies of phagocytic cells. I. Morphological changes of the cytoplasm and granules of rabbit granulocytes associated with ingestion of rough pneumococcus. *Brit J Exp Path 54*: 593, 1963.

Low, F. N., and Freeman, J. A. *Electron Microscopic Atlas of Normal and Leukemic Blood.* McGraw Hill, New York, 1958.

Lusher, J. M., Schneider, J., Mizukami, I., and Evans, R. K. The May-Hegglin Anomaly: Platelet function, ultrastructure and chromosome studies. *Blood 32*:950, 1968.

Lutzner, M. A., and Hecht, F. Nuclear anomalies of the neutrophil in a chromosomal triplication: The D_1 (13–15) trisomy syndrome. An electron microscopic study. *Lab Invest 15*:597, 1966.

Lutzner, M. A., Lowrie, C. T., and Jordan, H. W. Giant granules in leukocytes of the beige mouse. *J Hered 58*:299, 1967.

Marchal, G., Bessis, M., and Thiéry, J. P. Ultrastructure des corps d'Auer. *Rev Hemat 14*:413, 1959.

Matsuoka, M., Hattori, A., Mizushina, T., and Jinbo, C. The ultrastructure of the cryofibrinogen in acute promyelocytic leukemia displaying the defibrination syndrome and fibrillar inclusions in promyelocytes. *Acta Med Biol 17*:49, 1969.

May, R., and Grünwald, L. Ueber Blutfärbingen. *Zbl Inn Med 23*:265, 1902.

May, R. Leukocyteneinschlüsse. *Deutsch Arch Klin Med 96*:1, 1909.

McCall, C. E., Katayama, I., Cotran, R. S., and Finland, M. Lysosomal and ultrastructural changes in human "toxic" neutrophils during bacterial infection. *J Exp Med 129*:267, 1969.

McDuffie, N. G. Crystalline patterns in Auer bodies and specific granules of human leukocytes. *J Microscopie 6*:321, 1967a.

McDuffie, N. G. Nuclear blebs in human leukemia cells. *Nature (London) 214*:1341, 1967b.

Mehes, K. Nuclear projections in neutrophils. *Blood 28*:598, 1966.

Melmonk, K. L., and Cline, M. J. The interaction of leukocytes and the kinin system. *Biochem Pharmacol 17* (suppl):271, 1968.

Metchnikoff, E. Ueber ein Sprcsspilzkaukheit des Daphnien. Beitrag zur Lehre über den Kampf der Phagocyten gegen Krankheitserreger. *Virchow Arch Path Anat 96*:177, 1884.

Miller, F., DeHarven, E., and Palade, G. D. The structure of eosinophil leukocyte granules in rodents and in man. *J Cell Biol 31*:349, 1966.

Moore, K. L., Graham, M. A., and Baar, M. L. The detection of chromosomal sex in hermaphrodites from a skin biopsy. *Surg Gynec Obstet 96*:641, 1953.

Morley, A. A. A neutrophil cycle in healthy individuals. *Lancet 2*:1220, 1966.

Murakami, I., Ogawa, M., Amo, H., and Ota, K. Studies on kinetics of human leucocytes in vivo with ^{3}H-thymidine autoradiography. II.

Eosinophils and basophils. *Acta Haemat Jap 32*:384, 1969.

Naegeli, O. Uebes rothes knochenmark und Myeloblasten. *Deutsch Med Wschr 26*:287, 1900.

Neumann, E. Ueber die Bedeutung des Knochenmarks für die Blutbildung, *Zbl Med Wiss 6*: 689, 1868.

Neumann, E. Ein Fall von Leukamie mit Erkrankung des Knochenmarks. *Arch Heilk 11*:1, 1870.

Ogawa, T. Electron microscopic observation of leukemic cells in six cases of so-called acute promyelocytic leukemia. *J Electronmicr 17*: 260, 1968.

Ohota, H. A biochemical study on the neutrophilic granules isolated in a pure state from leukocyte homogenate. *Acta Haemat Jap 27*:555, 1964.

Olsson, I. Isolation of human leucocyte granules using colloidal silica-polysaccharide density gradients. *Exp Cell Res 54*:352, 1969.

Osaka, R. An electron microscopic observation on the specific granules of eosinophil leukocytes of vertebrates. *Acta Haemat Jap 22*:134, 1959.

Padgett, G. A., Leader, R. W., Gorham, J. R., and O'Mary, C. C. The familial occurrence of the Chediak-Higashi syndrome in mink and cattle. *Genetics 49*:505, 1964.

Pappenheim, A., and Ferrata, A. Ueber die Verschiedenen lymphoiden Zellformen des normalen und pathologisches Blutes. *Folia Haemat 10*:78, 1910.

Pioch, W. Über die Darstellung saurer Mucopolysaccharide mit dem Kupferphthalocyaninfarbstoff Astrablau. *Virchow Arch Path Anat 330*: 337, 1957.

Pelger, K. Demonstratie van een paar zeldzaam voorkomende typen van bloodlichaampjes en bespreking der patienten. *Ned T Jdchr Geneesk 72*:1178, 1928. (Cited by Davidson, 1968.)

Pruzansky, J. J., and Patterson, R. Subcellular distribution of histamine in human leucocytes. *Proc Soc Exp Biol Med 124*:56, 1967.

Rappaport, H. Tumors of the Hematopoietic System. In *Atlas of Tumor Pathology, Section III, Fascicle 8.* Armed Forces Institute of Pathology, Washington, 1966.

Rebuck, J. W., Barth, C. L., and Petz, A. M. New leukocytic dysfunction at the inflammatory sites in Hegglin's, Hurler's and Pelger-Huët anomalous states. *Fed Proc 22*:427, 1963.

Recklinghausen, F. von. Ueber Eiter- und Bindgewebskörperchen. *Virchow Arch Path Anat 28*: 157, 1863.

Reschad, H., Schilling-Torgau, Ueber eine neue Leukämie durch echte Uebergangsformen (Splenozytenleukämie) und ihre Bedeutung für die Selbständigkeit dieser Zellen. *Munchen Med Wschr 60*:1981, 1913.

Rich, A. R., Wintrobe, M. M., and Lewis, M. R. The differentiation of myeloblasts from lymphoblasts by their manner of locomotion. *Bull Hopkins Hosp 65*:291, 1939.

Riley, J. F. *The Mast Cells.* Livingstone, Edinburgh, 1959.

Rohr, K. *Das Menschliche Knochenmark.* Thieme, Stuttgart, 1960.

Rosse, W. F., and Gurney, C. W. The Pelger-Huët anomaly in three families and its use in determining the disappearance of transfused neutrophils from the peripheral blood. *Blood 14*: 170, 1959.

Saba, H. I., Roberts, H. R., and Herion, J. C. The anticoagulant activity of lysosomal cationic proteins from polymorphonuclear leukocytes. *J Clin Incest 46*:580, 1967.

Sabesin, S. M. A function of the eosinophil: Phagocytosis of antigen-antibody complexes. *Proc Soc Exp Biol Med 112*:667, 1963.

Sabin, F. R., Doan, C. A., and Forkner, C. F. Studies in tuberculosis. *J Exp Med 52* (Suppl 3):1 1930.

Sampson, D., and Archer, G. J. Release of histamine from human basophils. *Blood 29*:722, 1967.

Schauer, A., and Werle, E. Zur histochemischen Darstellung des Histamins der Mastzellen. *Ges Exp Med 131*:100, 1959.

Schauer, A., and Eder, M. Die Entwicklung von Mucopolysacchariden und Bildung histochemisch nachweisbarerer Enzyme währen der Mastzellreifung. *Virchow Arch Path Anat 335*:72, 1962.

Schilling-Torgau, V. *Das Blutbild und seine Klinische Verwertung (mit Einschluss der Tropfenkrankheiten). Kurzgefasste technische, theoretische und praktische Anleitung zur mikroskopischen Blutuntersuchung.* Fischer, Jena, 1912.

Seeman, P. M., and Palade, G. E. Acid phosphatase localization in rabbit eosinophils. *J Cell Biol 34*:745, 1967.

Sellyei, M., and David, H. Untersuchungen über die Ultrastruktur einer Variante des Furthschen Mäusen mastozytoms. *Z Mikr Anat Forsch 70*: 103, 1963.

Selye, H. *The Mast Cells.* Butterworth, Washington, 1965.

Seman, G., and Seman, C. Electron-microscopic search for virus particles in patients with leukemia and lymphoma. *Cancer 22*:1033, 1968.

Smetana, K., Gyorkey, F., Gyorkey, P., and Busch, H. On the ultrastructure of nucleoli in human leukemia myeloblasts. *Exp Cell Res 58*:303, 1969.

Sorenson, G. D. Electron microscopic observations of viral particles within myeloma cells of man. *Exp Cell Res 24*:219, 1961.

Speirs, R. S. A theory of antibody formation involving eosinophils and reticuloendothelial cells. *Nature* (*London*) *181:* 681, 1958.

Spicer, S. S., and Hardin, J. H. Ultrastructure, cytochemistry, and function of neutrophil leukocyte granules. *Lab Invest 20*:488, 1969.

Steinbrinck, W. Uber ein neue granulationsanomalie der Leukocyten. *Deutsch Arch Klin Med 193*:577, 1948.

Stoekenius, W. Zur Feinstruktur der granula menschlicher gewebsmastzellen. *Exp Cell Res 11*: 656, 1956.

Sutton, J. S., and Weiss, L. Transformation of monocytes in tissue culture into macrophages, epitheloid cells and multinucleated giant cells. *J Cell Biol 28*:303, 1966.

Takeoka, O., Matsui, S., and Ashihara, T. Electron-microscopic observations on the fine structure of basophilic granulocytes of newt (Triturus pyrrhogaster). *Acta Haemat 35*:344, 1966.

Takeuchi, T., and Utsunomiya, S. Sensitivity of cytochemical demonstration of alkaline and acid phosphatase in blood cells. *Acta Path Jap 2*:57, 1952.

Tanaka, H. Comparative cytologic studies by means of an electron microscope on monocytes, subcutaneous histiocytes, reticulum cells in the lymph nodes and peritoneal macrophages. *Ann Rep Inst Virus Res Kyoto Univ* (Series A) *1*:87, 1958.

Tanaka, Y. Fibrillar structures in the cells of blood-forming organs. *J Nat Cancer Inst 33*: 467, 1964.

Tanaka, Y., Bell, W. R., and Brindley, D. Pseudoviral inclusion bodies in acute leukemia. A report of two cases, *J Nat Cancer Inst 38*:629, 1967.

Terrasse, J., Cararoc, M., and Bessis, M. Un cas de leucémie avec inclusions sphériques. *Rev Hemat 13*:331, 1958.

Terry, R. W., Bainton, D. F., and Farquhar, M. G. Formation and structure of specific granules in basophilic leukocytes of the guinea pig. *Lab Invest 21*:65, 1969.

Thiéry, J. P. Étude au microscope électronique de la maturation et de l'excrétion des granules des mastocytes. *J Microscopie 2*:549, 1963.

Unna, P. G. *Histopathologie der Hautkrankheiten* (*Neurofibrom, Urticaria pigmentosa, milaria, syphilide*). Leopold Voss, Hamburg, 1894.

van Furth, R., and Cohn, Z. A. The origin and kinetics of mononuclear phagocytes. *J Exp Med 128*:415, 1968.

van Furth, R. Origin and kinetics of monocytes and macrophages. *Seminars Hemat 7*:125, 1970.

Vaughn, J. The function of the eosinophile leukocyte. *Blood 8*:1, 1953.

Waldeyer, W. Ueber Bindegewebszellen. *Arch Mikr Anat 11*:176, 1875.

Wassmuth, D. R., Hamilton, H. E., and Sheets, R. F. May-Hegglin anomaly, Hereditary affection of granulocytes and platelets. *JAMA 183*:737, 1963.

Watanabe, I., Donahue, S., and Hoggatt, N. Method for electron microscopic studies of circulating human leukocytes and observation of their fine structure. *J Ultrastruct Res 20*:336, 1967.

Weinstock, A., and Albright, J. T. The fine structure of mast cells in normal human gingiva. *J Ultrastruct Res 17*:245, 1965.

Weissmann, G. Lysosomes. *Blood 24*:594, 1964.

Welsh, R. A. The genesis of the Charcot-Lyden crystal in the eosinophilic leukocyte of man. *Amer J Path 35*:1091, 1959.

Werner, W., and Krause, A. R. Die Gewebsmastzellen in menschlichen Knochenmark. *Frankfurt Z Path 74*:651, 1965.

Wetzel, B. K., Horn, R. G., and Spicer, S. S. Fine structural studies on the development of heterophil, eosinophil, and basophil granulocytes in rabbits. *Lab Invest 16*:349, 1967a.

Wetzel, B. K., Spicer, S. S., and Horn, R. G. Fine structural localization of acid and alkaline phosphatases in cells of rabbit blood and bone marrow. *J Histochem Cytochem 15*:311, 1967b.

White, J. G. The Chediak-Higashi syndrome: a possible lysosomal disease. *Blood 28*:143, 1966a.

White, J. G. Virus-like particles in the peripheral blood cells of two patients with Chediak-Higashi syndrome. *Cancer 19*:877, 1966b.

Whitelaw, D. W. The intravascular lifespan of monocytes. *Blood 28*:455, 1966.

Windhorst, D. B., Zelickson, A. S., and Good, R. A. Chediak-Higashi syndrome: Hereditary gigantism of cytoplasmic organelles. *Science 151*: 81, 1966.

Winquist, G. Electron microscopy of the basophilic granulocyte. *Ann NY Acad Sci 103*:352, 1963.

Zucker-Franklin, D., and Hirsch, J. G. Electron microscope studies on the degranulation of rabbit peritoneal leukocytes during phagocytosis. *J Exp Med 120*:569, 1964.

Zucker-Franklin, D. The phagosomes in rheumatoid synovial fluid leukocytes: a light fluorescence, and electron microscope study. *Arthritis Rheum 9*:24, 1966.

Zucker-Franklin, D. Electron microscopic study of human basophils. *Blood 29*:878, 1967.

Zucker-Franklin, D. Electron microscopic studies of human granulocytes. Structural variations related to function. *Seminars Hemat 5*:109, 1968.

chapter 4

MEGAKARYOCYTES AND PLATELETS

Detailed reviews on the historical background of megakaryocyte and platelet discovery have been published by Tocantins (1948) and Robb-Smith (1967). They describe the discovery by Robin (1849) of megakaryocytes, multilobated nuclear giant cells of the bone marrow, which was followed by more precise descriptions by Koelliker (1867), Hoffman and Langerhause (1869), and Heidenhein (1890). The term megakaryocyte was introduced by Howell in 1890 to distinguish this cell from an osteoclast.

Platelets were noticed in peripheral blood by many investigators before Bizzozero (1882) described their role in thrombus formation in rabbits and guinea pigs. Wright (1906), in studying both platelets and megakaryocytes, proposed that platelets were produced by these giant cells in the marrow, a concept confirmed by many investigators and no longer disputed.

MORPHOLOGY

MEGAKARYOCYTES

In man megakaryocytes are found predominantly in the bone marrow and are observed rarely in other blood-forming organs; other species may show megakaryocytes in spleen, liver, and lungs. These cells contain multiple nuclei and are notable for their size, frequently over 100μ in the mature cell (Fig. 4-1). The cytoplasm stains blue and contains a very large number of azurophilic granules. The density of the cytoplasmic stain and number of granules may vary as the cell matures. The granules appear as small refractile spheres in the phase microscope and the frequent accumulation of glycogen gives a strong PAS reaction.

Several stages of maturation can be identified in stained marrow preparations. The immature megakaryoblast is distinguished from other immature elements by

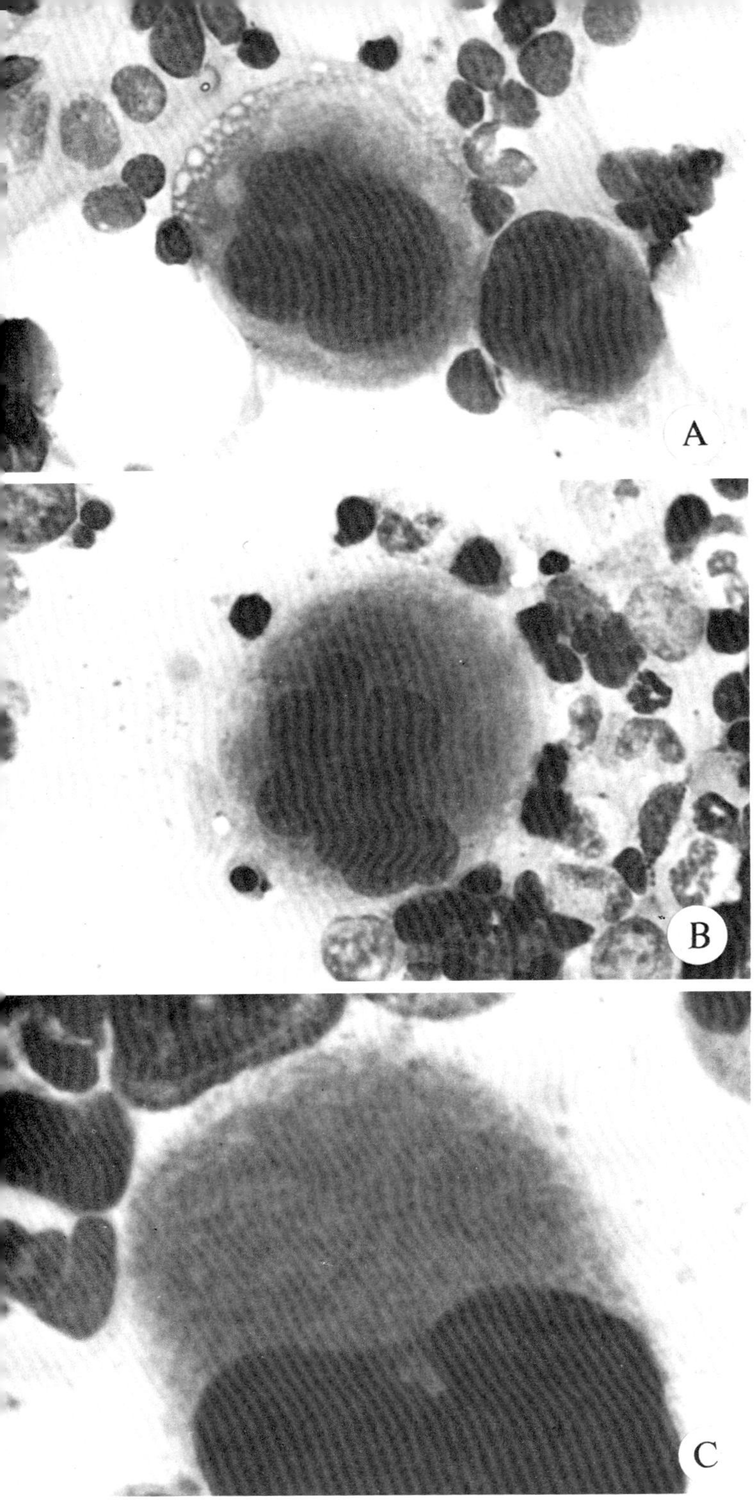

FIGURE 4-1. Light micrographs of megakarocytes.
A. Multinucleated cell with basophilic cytoplasm containing some granulation and vacuoles. × *1,000.*
B. Mature cell showing some evidence of cytoplasmic changes prior to platelet release. × *1,000.*
C. Details of cytoplasmic granular network in a mature cell. × *2,000.*

FIGURE 4-2. Megakaryoblast from bone marrow.
Binucleated (*N*) megakaryoblast from hyperplastic bone marrow has a large Golgi area (*G*) with signs of granule formation. The vesicular system (*arrows*) and other organelles such as endoplasmic reticulum and mitochondria (*M*) have started to develop. The maturation of this cytoplasm can be contrasted with the minimal structures seen in hemocytoblasts. × *16,500.*

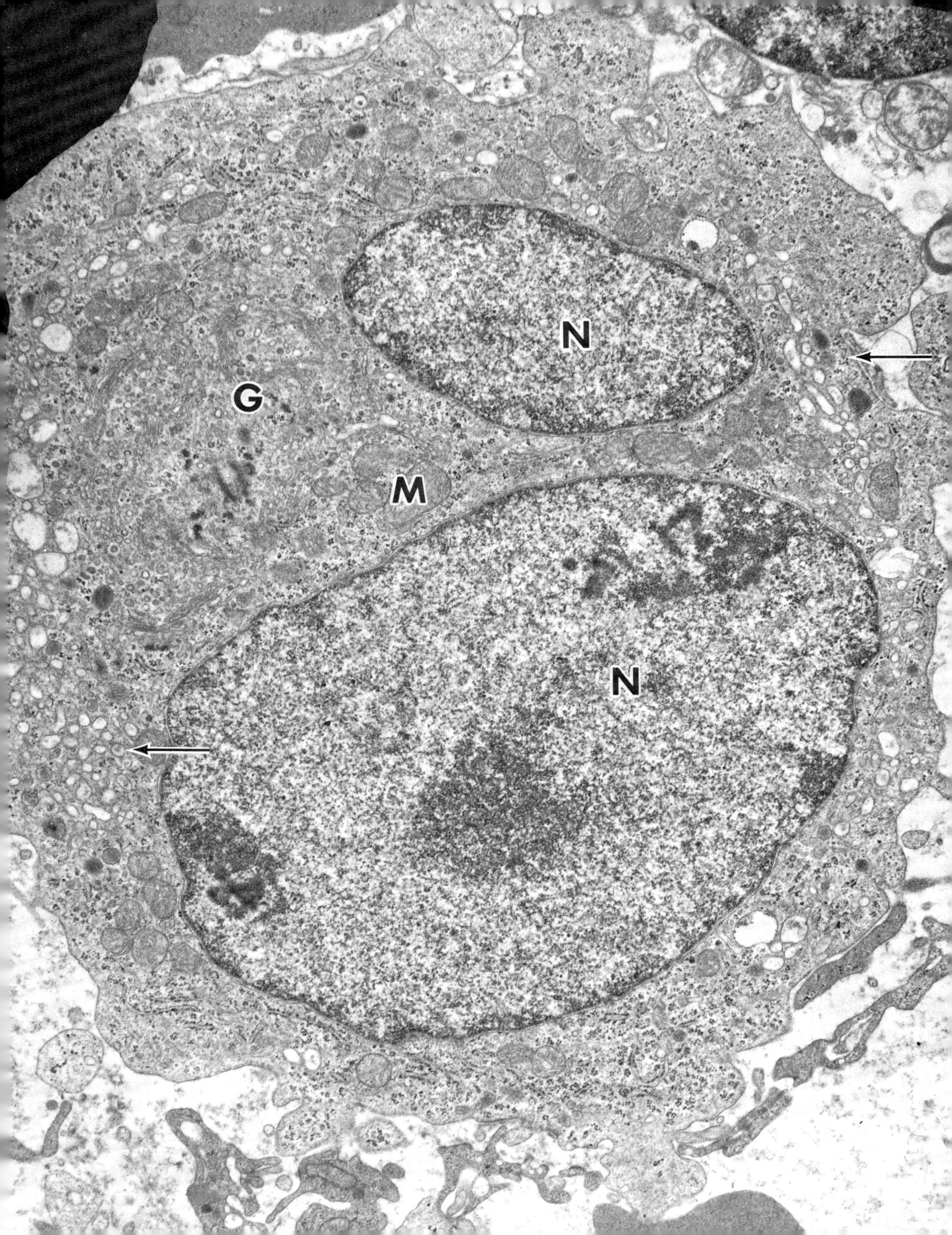
N
G
M
N

its larger size and multilobular nucleus with distinctive nucleoli. This young form, "the megakaryoblast," was identified in electron micrographs by Zamboni (1965) in fetal hepatic hematopoiesis. Electron micrographs of these immature cells from human bone marrow (Fig. 4-2) resemble hemocytoblasts, except for a larger Golgi area with some initial granule formation.

The next stage of maturation discernible by light microscopy is the "basophilic megakaryocyte." The strong basophilic stain indicates the abundant polyribosomal content of the cytoplasm (Fig. 4-3). This cell shows the early granule formation in the cytoplasm near the nucleus and the Golgi area, a stage of development identified easily in human bone marrow preparations. This develops into the "granular megakaryocyte," with the production of many small azurophilic granules (Figs. 4-4 through 4-9). Electron micrographs of granular megakaryocytes were published by Pease (1955) and Kautz and deMarsh (1955). In these multinucleated cells, more than one pair of centrioles is usually seen (Figs. 4-4 and 4-5); this is related to the replication of the nucleus without cell division. Formation of azurophilic granules is seen frequently in or near the Golgi apparatus (Fig. 4-6) (Jones, 1960). The granules are scattered throughout the cytoplasm and some show dense cores (nucleoids) (Figs. 4-5 through 4-7) and are called "bull's-eye" granules. These dense cores are reported to contain mucopolysaccharides (Spicer *et al.*, 1969). Microtubules, microvesicles, and aggregates of glycogen particles are common (Fig. 4-9); many small round mitochondria are scattered throughout the extensive cytoplasm. Profiles of tubular endoplasmic reticulum are commonly noted in basophilic megakaryocytes and in the early stages of granulated megakaryocytes (Figs. 4-3 through 4-5).

During the later stage of differentiation, smooth membrane becomes predominant in the cytoplasm (Figs. 4-7 through 4-9). These giant cells are occasionally seen with a narrow rim of agranular cytoplasm which appears to form blebs (Fig. 4-8) and may represent one mechanism of platelet formation from the cytoplasm of megakaryocytes which produces "platelets" with only a few granules and, in some instances, no apparent granules.

The more characteristic mechanism for platelet formation by fragmentation was demonstrated by Yamada (1957) in rat spleen and later confirmed by many (Behnke, 1969). The mature megakaryocyte forms "platelet demarcation vesicles" or a network of vesicles within the dense granular cytoplasm (Figs. 4-7 and 4-8). These segregate pieces of cytoplasm and become fracture lines or planes of rupture, which release the pieces of cytoplasm that then become platelets for entrance into the circulation (Fig. 4-10). Giant complex nuclei with a narrow rim of cytoplasm are seen occasionally in the bone marrow (Fig. 4-11*A*). These structures are considered to be the nuclear residue of a megakaryocyte after it has released its cytoplasm as platelets. Clustered platelets in sinusoids may be seen in bone marrow (Fig. 4-11*B*), and they are considered to be recently released platelets.

(text continues on page 196)

FIGURE 4-3. Maturing megakaryocyte.
In this young megakaryocyte, at completion of mitosis, the chromosomes (*Ch*) have coalesced and developed a new nuclear membrane. The wide cytoplasm has few granules, many mitochondria, ribosomes and endoplasmic reticulum. A Golgi area (*G*) is present on each side of the new nucleus. × *14,500.*

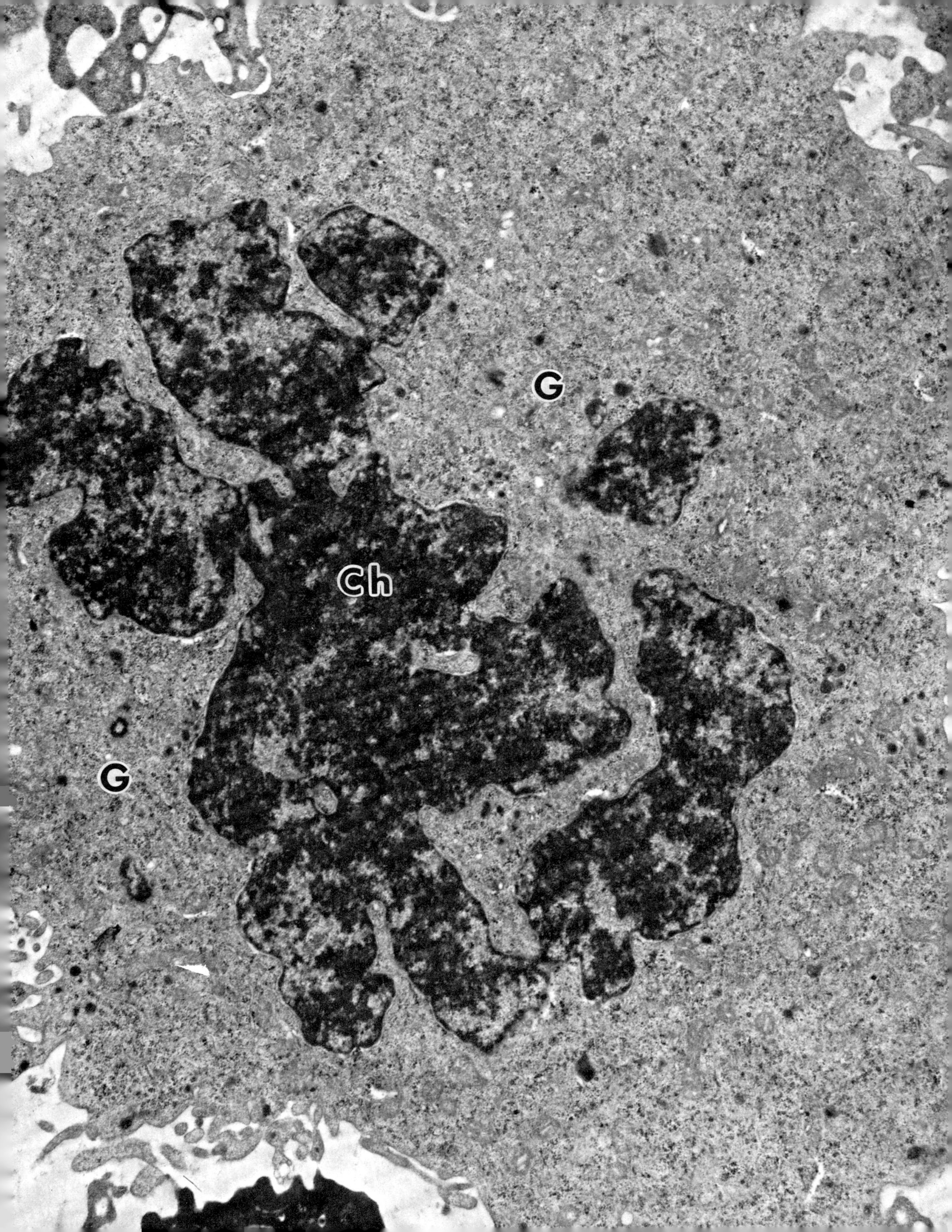
G
Ch
G

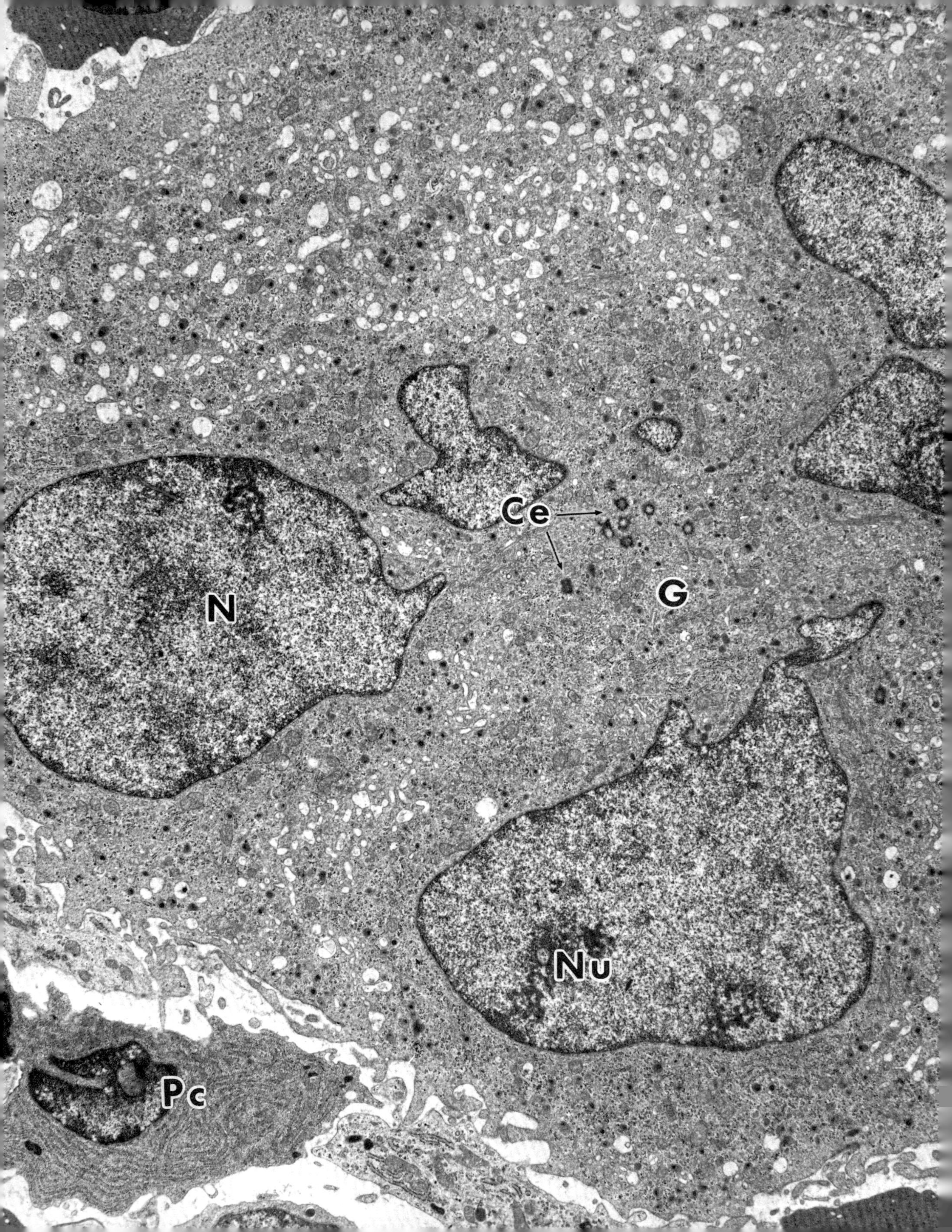
Ce
N
G
Nu
Pc

FIGURE 4-4. Maturing megakaryocyte.
Multinucleated megakaryocyte shows evidence of increased maturation. The cytoplasm contains numerous specific granules, vesicles, and tubular endoplasmic reticulum. The many mitochondria are smaller than those seen in the megakaryoblast stage. Several centrioles (*Ce*) are in the Golgi area (*G*). Prominent nucleoli (*Nu*) are in three of the nuclei (*N*). A portion of a plasma cell (*Pc*) is in the lower left corner. × *19,200.*

Figures 4-5 through 4-8 appear on the following pages ⇨

FIGURE 4-5. Maturing megakaryocyte.
Details of centrioles (*Ce*) and portion of the Golgi area of Figure 4-4. The numerous centrioles (*Ce*) are consistent with the polyploid character of megakaryocytes that have several mitoses without cellular division. There are portions of the lamellar (*s*) and vesicular (*v*) parts of the Golgi apparatus. Cytoplasm contains numerous granules (*g*), small mitochondria (*M*), some rough endoplasmic reticulum (*er*), microtubules (*mt*), and two parts of nuclei (*N*). × *35,000.*

FIGURE 4-6. Granular megakaryocyte.
Golgi vesicles involved in formation of granules (*arrows*), apparently at various stages of maturation. Several mitochondria (*M*) and edge of a nucleus (*N*) are present. × *66,500.*

FIGURE 4-7. Mature megakaryocyte.
In mature megakaryocyte, cytoplasm has developed a vesicle system—smooth endoplasmic reticulum (*ser*)—leading to formation of platelets. Note numerous granules (*g*), very small round mitochondria (*M*), and part of a nucleus (*N*). × *21,000.*

FIGURE 4-8. Mature megakaryocyte.
Approximately one-third of the cut area of a whole megakaryocyte shows two nuclei (*N*) and a migrant lymphocyte (L) within the cytoplasm. The many granules and vesicles of this mature cell cytoplasm resemble structures seen in mature platelets. There are also large projections (*B*) of agranular cytoplasm on cell surface. × *10,000.*

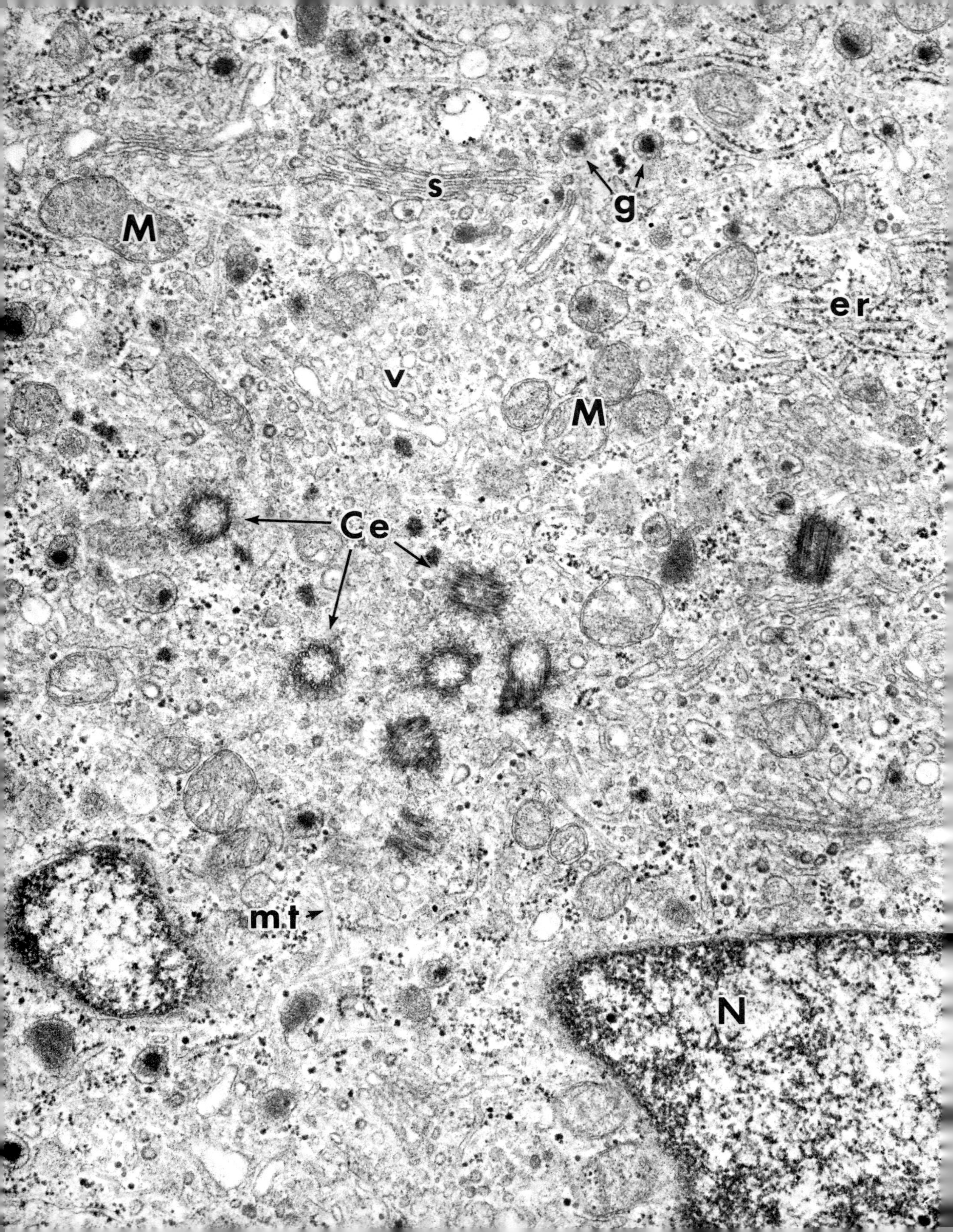

s
g
M
er
v
M
Ce
mt
N

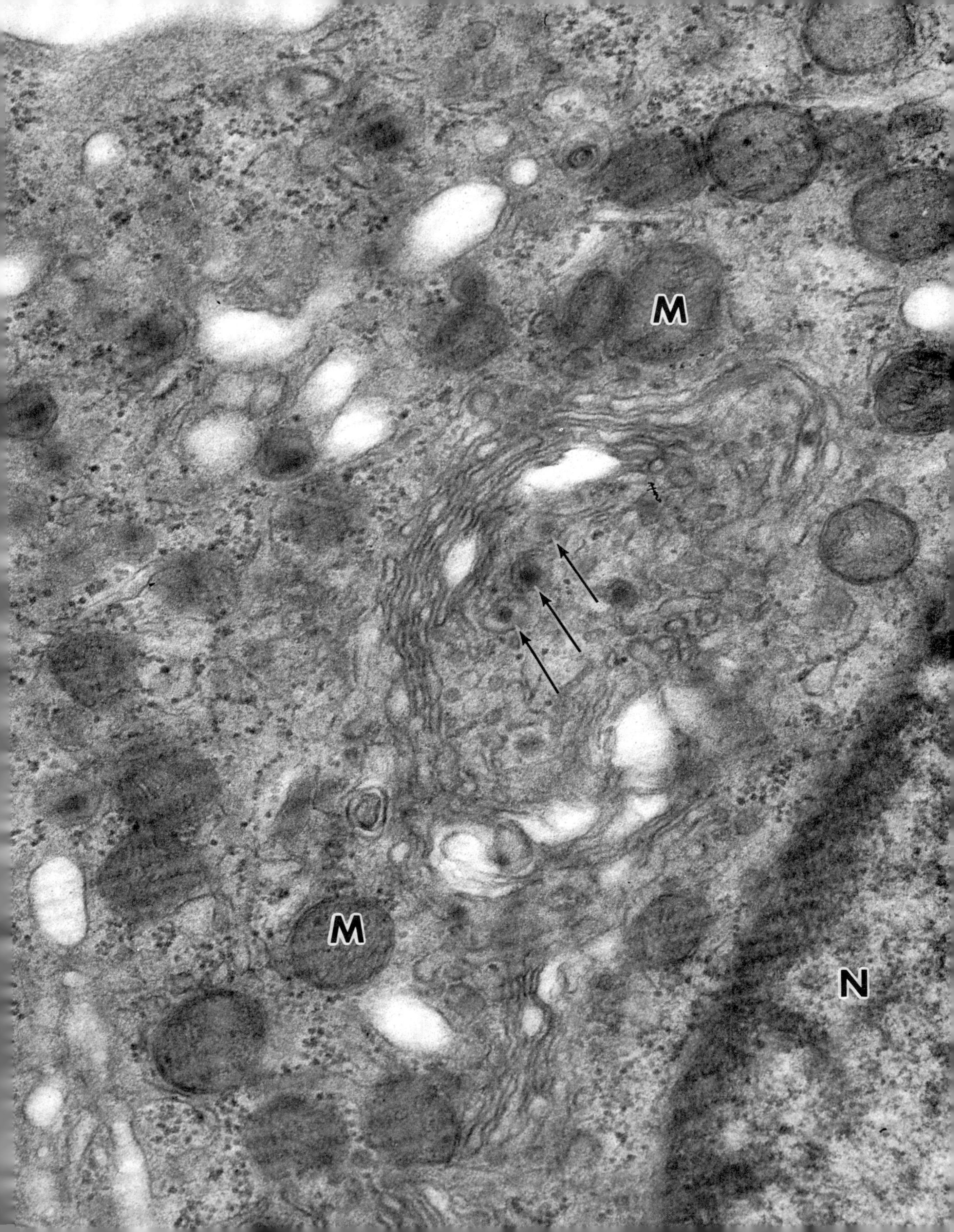
M
M
N

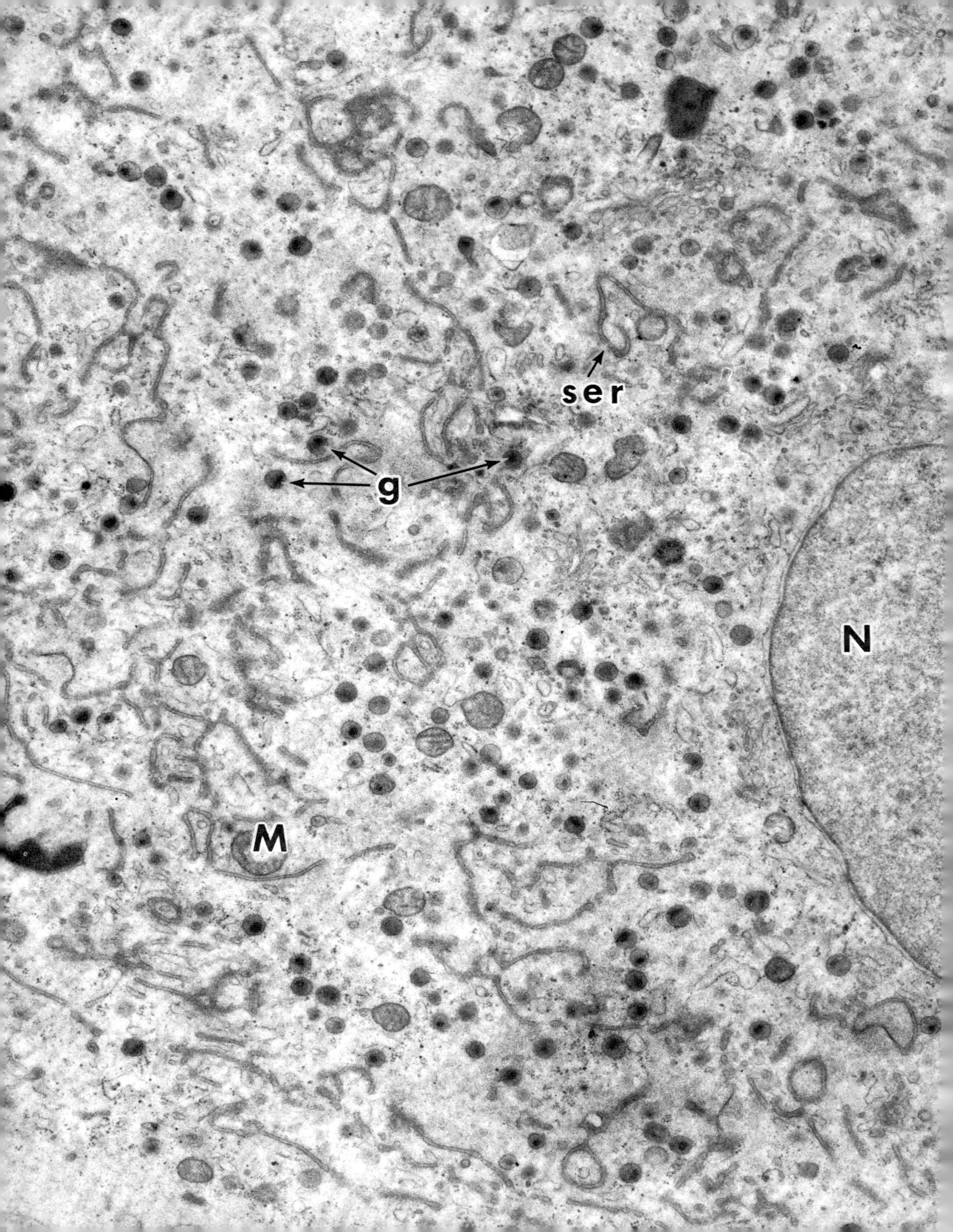
ser
g
N
M

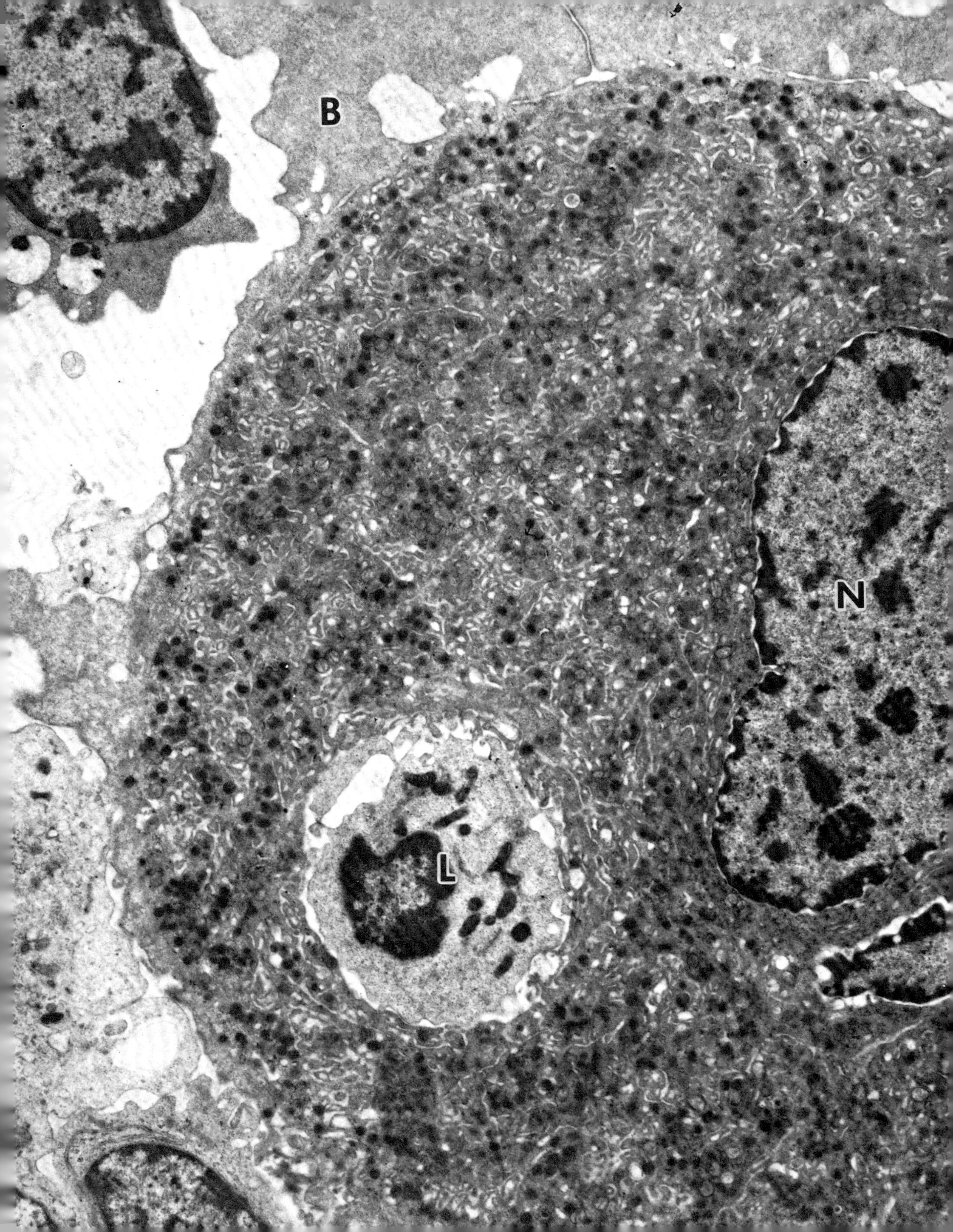
B
N
L

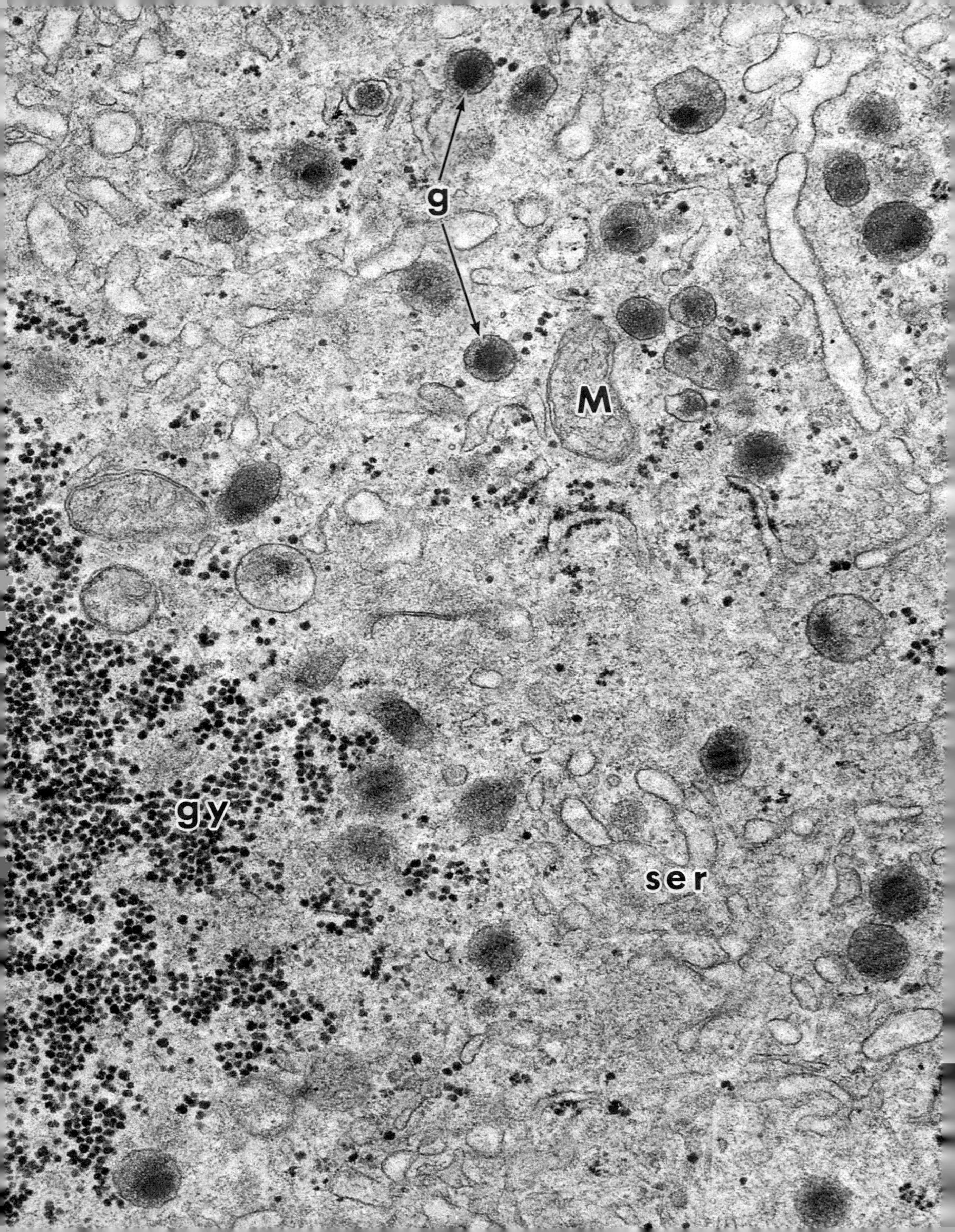

g
M
gy
ser

FIGURE 4-9. Mature megakaryocyte.
Cytoplasm of well-differentiated megakaryocyte contains many granules, some with dense bull's eye (*g*), mitochondria (*M*), tubular endoplasmic reticulum (*ser*), and glycogen granules (*gy*). × *40,000.*

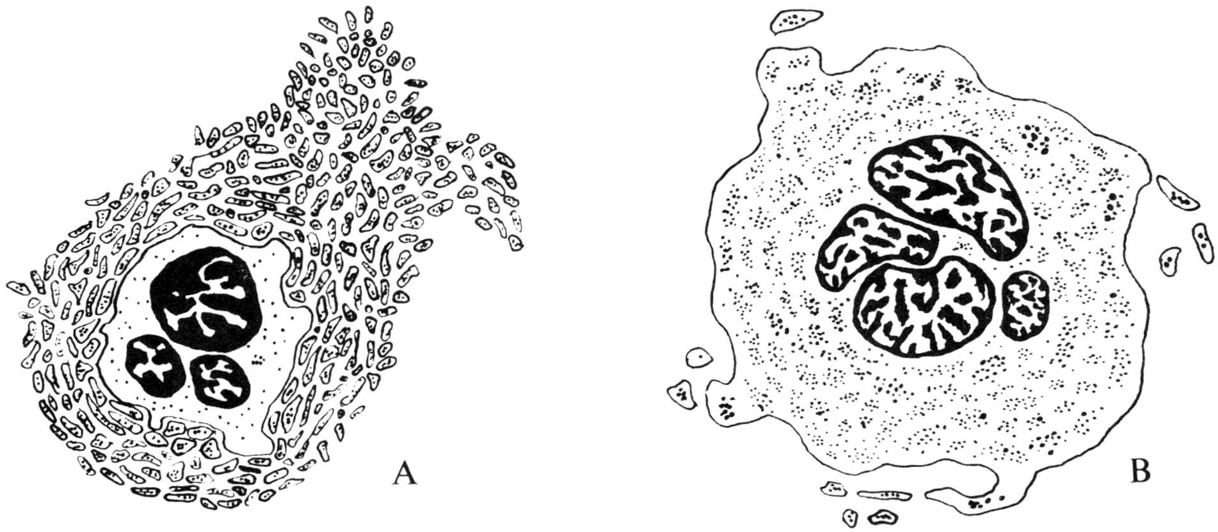

FIGURE 4-10. Two mechanisms of platelet release.
A. Disintegration of entire cytoplasm occurs along cleavage planes set up by tubular system.
B. Blebs form from surface of cell.

Figures 4-11 through 4-12 appear on the following pages

FIGURE 4-11. Events in platelet release.
A. A large invaginated nuclear complex (*N*) is probably several nuclei of a megakaryocyte, with only a rim and small entrapped masses of cytoplasm containing granules (*arrows*) like those found in megakaryocyte and platelets. × *6,200.*
B. Platelets cluster in lumen of marrow sinus after release from a megakaryocyte. They are adjacent to an endothelial cell (*En*). × *4,500.*

FIGURE 4-12. Normal platelets in peripheral blood.
The platelets contain numerous alpha granules (*g*), some with dense bull's eye (*arrow*) and occasionally very dense ones (*asterisk*). Small round mitochondria (*M*), vesicles (*v*), glycogen (*gy*), and microtubules (*mt*) are also present. × *30,000.*

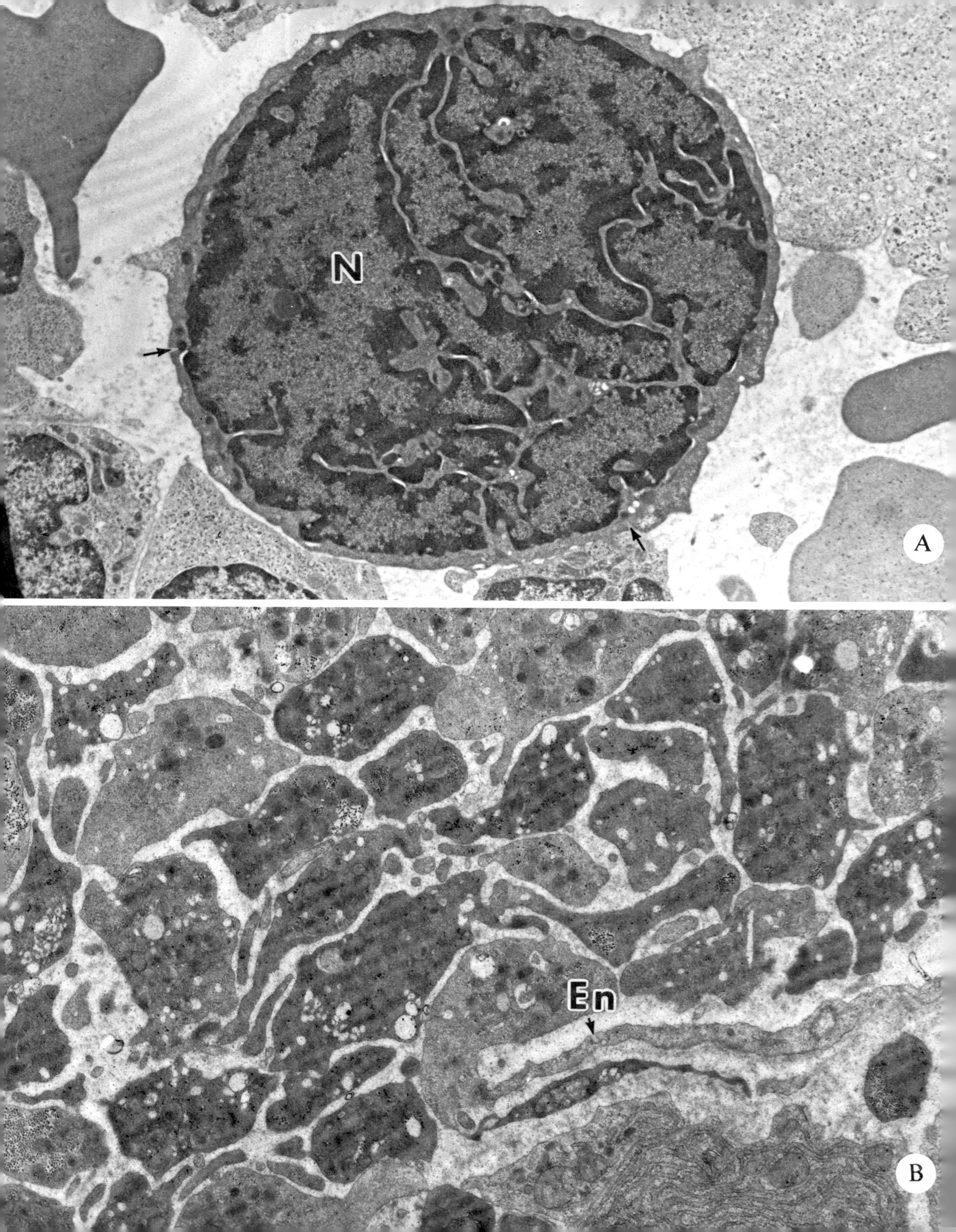
N
A
En
B

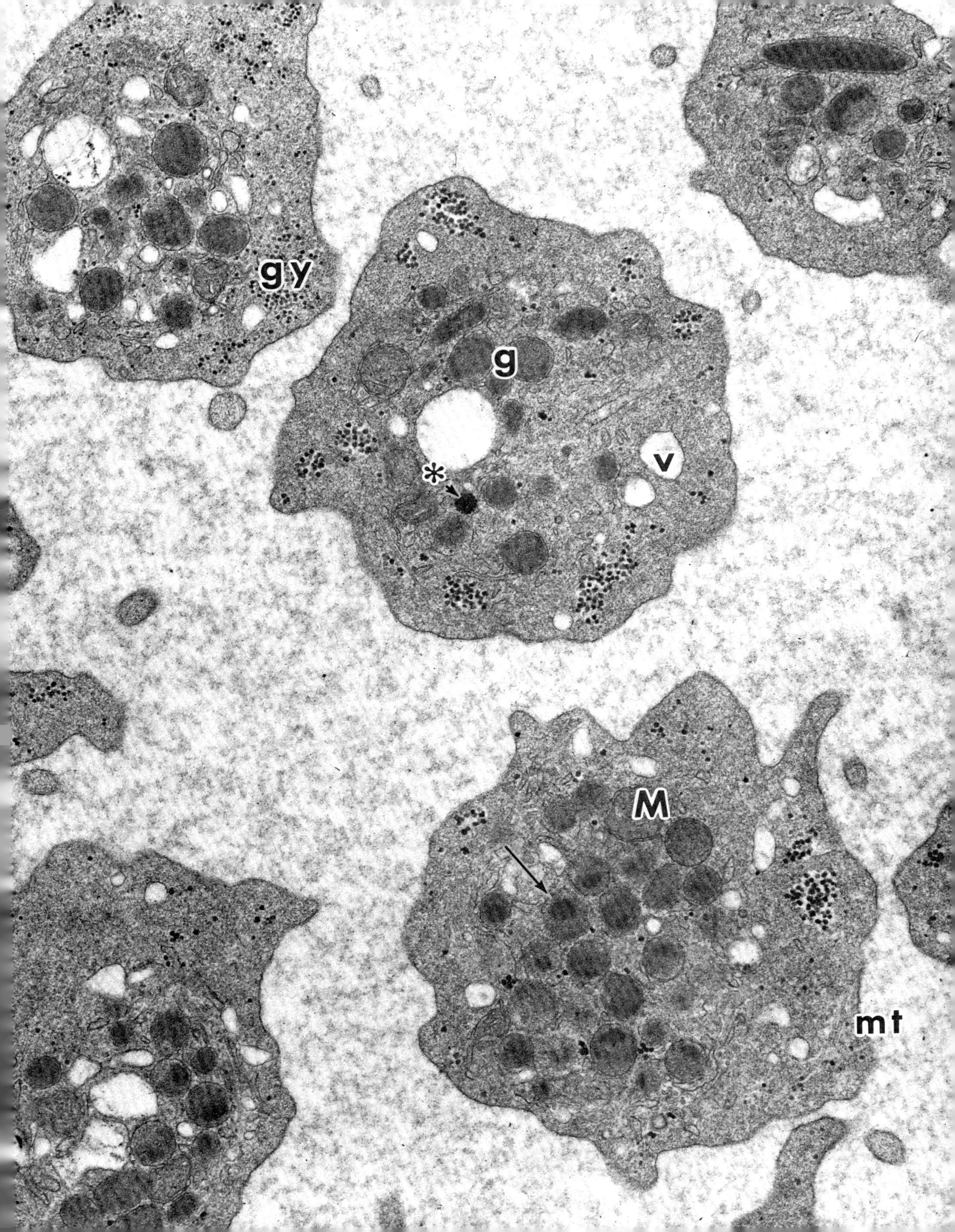
gy
g
v
*
M
mt

PLATELETS

Platelets, also called thrombocytes, are fragments of megakaryocyte cytoplasm. Nonmammalian species have blood elements that perform the clot formation function but contain a nucleus. Detailed morphological studies of platelets by light microscopy are limited by their small size (2 to 4μ). Platelet size and shape vary depending upon the manner of preparation; however, both stained blood smears and wet preparations clearly reveal small granules and PAS-positive material, possibly glycogen.

Platelets were first studied with the electron microscope by Wolpers and Ruska (1939), using a spreading whole-cell preparation technic. Similar technics were used by several other early investigators (Bessis and Burstein, 1948; Braunsteiner *et al.,* 1953); however, clear cytoplasmic details (Rinehart, 1955; DeRobertis, 1955; Goodman *et al.,* 1957) were not apparent until thin-section technics were introduced. Electron micrographs of thin sections show a round or rod-shaped mass of cytoplasm with a few thin projections or spicules extending from the surface (Fig. 4-12). The cytoplasm has several different organelles, including various granules, glycogen, small round mitochondria, a system of vesicles or reticulum, and some microtubules (Fig. 4-13*A*). The latter appear as a bundle in the margin of circulating mammalian platelets. The very dense granules (Fig. 4-13*B*) were thought to contain serotonin (5-hydroxytryptamine) (Tranzer *et al.,* 1966); however, this substance is extrinsic and is absorbed from the plasma rather than being synthesized by platelets. Greek symbols have been used to designate some of the platelet organelles (Schulz and Hiepler, 1959). The alpha granulomeres have a distinctive border and usually an amorphous, moderately opaque content, and they are the most prevalent granule in normal platelets. The beta granulomeres are mitochondria; the gamma granulomeres are the microvesicles; and the delta granulomeres are the vacuoles or reticulum.

Platelet aggregation and clot formation involve a series of morphological transformations. There is an increase in microprojections or spicules from the surface, enhancing the adherence and aggregation of groups of platelets. Initially, the granules tend to centralize while the nongranular cytoplasm and microtubules occupy the more peripheral areas, forming the "hyalomere" or clear zone (Rodman *et al.,* 1962, 1963). The aggregate of platelets leads to a coalescence of the outer membrane along areas of contact, leading to further centralization of granules. As the aggregates form, fibrin appears and the alpha granulomeres disintegrate (White *et al.,* 1965) and produce platelet thrombus. Clot retraction occurs after coagulation of blood is completed.

The search for contractile material led to the discovery of fibrils in platelets. These intracellular microfibrils have been found in platelets treated by osmotic shock, brief sonication, pressure homogenization, or by the addition of ADP

FIGURE 4-13. Platelet details.

A. There are a marginal array of microtubules (*mt*), some glycogen granules (*gy*), and some alpha granules (*g*). × *75,000.*

B. An electron-dense granule (*asterisk*) in a platelet is thought to contain 5-hydroxytryptamine. × *139,000.*

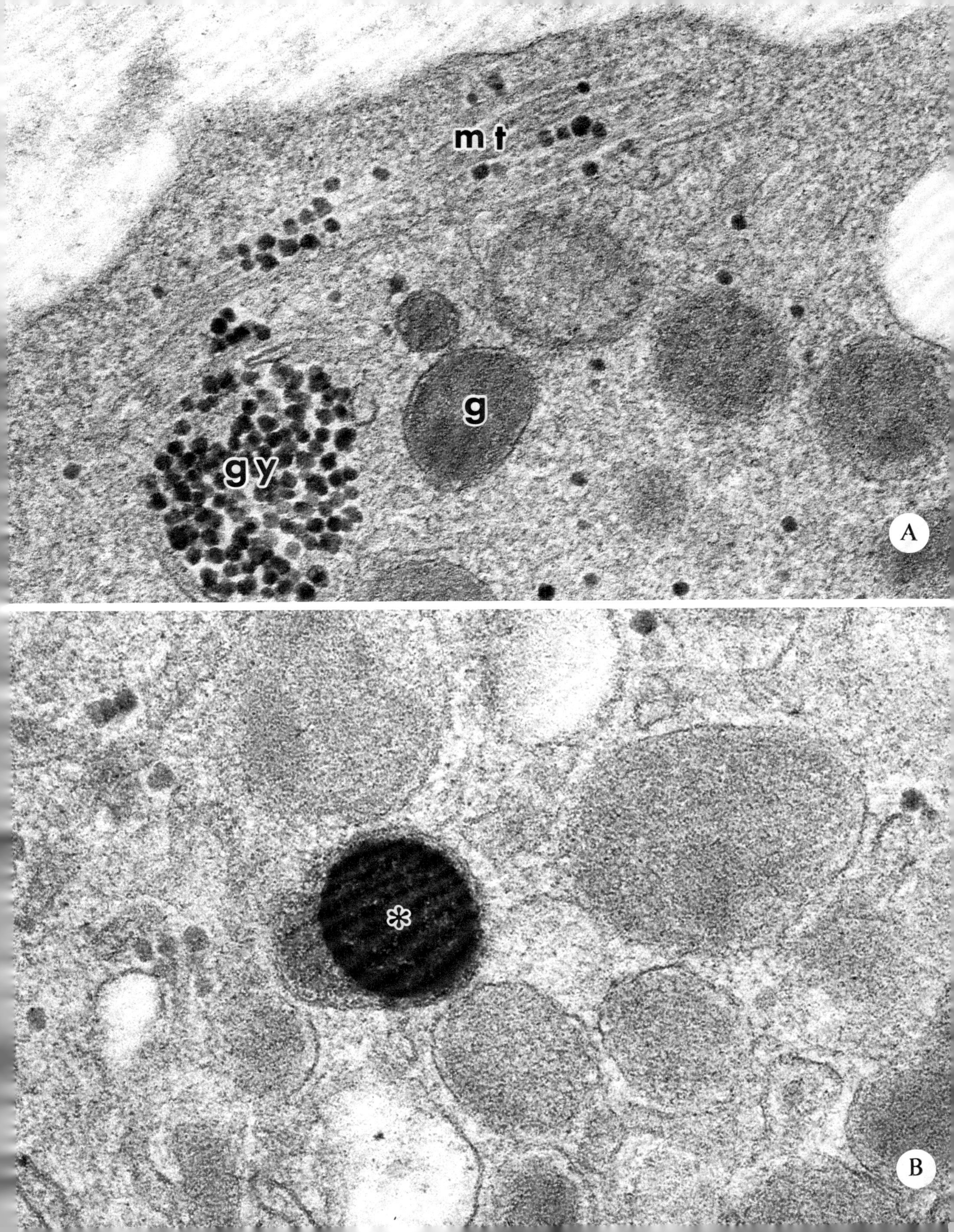
mt
g
gy
A
B

(Zucker-Franklin, 1969). The similarity of these fibrils to actin and myosin of muscle suggested that they may be the thrombasthenin, a contractile protein extracted from platelets by Bettex-Galland and Lüscher (1961). Hovig (1968) reported microtubules which may also be related to this protein and involved in clot retraction.

Easy induction of adhesion of platelets is the important first step in initiation of thrombi. This has stimulated interest in the surface characteristic of platelets (White and Krivit, 1965; Bull, 1966; Behnke, 1968). The surface of megakaryocytes and platelets has been shown to be coated with acid mucosubstances, most probably sialomucin (Spicer *et al.,* 1969), and have ATPase activity (White and Krivit, 1965). The adhesion of platelets to nonplatelet surfaces is induced in vitro by ADP and in vivo by trauma (tissue thromboplastin and/or collagen) (Ashford and Freiman, 1967). This adhesion phenomenon leads to platelet aggregation (clumping) in loco, and the formation of platelet thrombi. When platelets contact the surface of foreign material, they also tend to entrap the object within the resulting platelet aggregate (Schulz, 1961; Movat *et al.,* 1965).

CYTOGENESIS

The origin of megakaryocytes is not well established. Although immature forms have been described by both light and electron microscopy, the nature of their precursors is uncertain. One concept is that they have a mutual stem cell with other myeloid cell types; another separates them from erythromyelocytic precursors (Morse and Stohlman, 1966).

Cell division may occur only during the committed blastic cell state, although DNA synthesis may continue in cells that are no longer dividing. This DNA synthesis during maturation of the megakaryocyte may be in mononuclear cells and produce quantitative chromatin values that exceed the amounts in diploid forms. These polyploid precursors (Ebbe, 1970) may mature to form various multinucleated polyploid cells. The development of giant cells with multiple nuclei and polyploid forms is usually associated with impaired cytoplasmic division. Histochemical analysis of DNA content of megakaryocytes presents polyploid forms of 8N, 16N, 32N, and 64N (representing multiples of unit amounts of DNA, 2N in a diploid cell). Multinucleated cells with 4N polyploid state were not found (Odell and Jackson, 1970). The high polyploid forms are noted in cells at higher states of differentiation (deLaval and Paulus, 1969; Odell and Jackson, 1970). The initial labeling index of rat multinucleated megakaryocytes 30 minutes after injection of ^{3}H-thymidine shows that cells with low ploidy have high values, indicating active DNA synthesis (Odell and Jackson, 1970). This observation is in conflict with that of deLaval and Paulus (1969) who claimed that ^{3}H-thymidine is incorporated only into nonsegmented megakaryocytes in guinea pigs. Nothing is known about the regulation of megakaryocytopoiesis, which maintains the steady flow of platelets into the circulation. The estimated transit time of each stage of developing megakaryocytes in rats is 8 to 14 hours for megakaryoblast, 11 to 19 hours for basophilic megakaryocyte, and 24 to 42 hours for granulated megakaryocyte (Ebbe and Stohlman, 1965).

The life span of circulating platelets in humans has been determined by labeling technics to range from 9.2 to 11.2 days. This may be altered in hematological disorders and is subject to some variation by daily production rate and other factors (Paulus and Thompson, 1969). Aged platelets are removed from the circulation by the reticuloendothelial system; normally, about one-third are removed in the spleen and two-thirds in the liver (Aster, 1969).

The release of megakarycyte cytoplasm to form platelets usually takes place in both inter- and intrasinusoidal areas of bone marrow (Wright, 1906; Behnke, 1969). Two mechanisms may be considered for platelet formation: (1) complete simultaneous fragmentation of cytoplasm, and (2) pinching-off of megakaryocyte cytoplasm (Fig. 4-10). Kaufman *et al.* (1965b) estimated that one megakaryocyte produces approximately 4,000 platelets. It has been reported that 24 to 68 per cent of mature megakaryocytes that leave the blood-forming organs are trapped in passage through pulmonary capillaries (Kaufman *et al.,* 1965a,b). These trapped megakaryocytes continue to release platelets from nonhematopoietic locations and may contribute to 30 per cent of the circulating platelets. The fate of the residual megakaryocyte nucleus after the release of platelets is not known. Yamada (1957) speculated that they may either disintegrate or regenerate new cytoplasm and form more platelets.

FUNCTION

The primary role of circulating platelets is to prevent blood loss after vascular rupture by contributing to clot formation. Clot formation is a complicated process which involves platelets, endothelium of blood vessels, and a series of plasma factors reacting in sequence. This topic has been reviewed by Lüscher (1967). This series of reactions is initiated immediately following injury to a blood vessel. Platelets adhere to collagen fibers or react to ruptured tissue cells. The adhesion is followed by release of serotonin, ADP, and other active agents which increase platelet aggregation and initiate the series of enzymatic and biochemical reactions of plasma clot formation.

Platelets contain several intrinsic clotting factors involved in clot formation. The presence of the platelet factors and a variety of organelles led to attempts to correlate specific factors to a given organelle. Schulz and Hiepler (1959) suggested that a group of platelet enzymes, thrombokinases, were in the alpha granules (granulomeres). White and Krivit (1965) attributed fibrinogen to these same granules. These alpha granules were apparently positive for acid phosphatase (Marcus and Zucker-Franklin, 1964) and ATPase (White and Krivit, 1965), which are also found on plasma membranes. This same organelle has also been credited with beta glucuronidase (Dohrmann and Klesper, 1960), cathepsin (Marcus and Zucker, 1965), and thromboplastic platelet factor III (Johnson *et al.,* 1959; White and Krivit, 1966). This last material is a lipoprotein (molecular weight about 1 million) and is released from platelets early in their metamorphosis after adhesion and aggregation (White and Krivit, 1966). The difficulties of platelet particle separation have led to uncertainties in these correlations. The vesicular system of the platelet is also considered to be an intrinsic prothrombin activator able to trigger clot formation (Marcus *et al.,* 1966). Very recently, Day *et al.* (1969) compared three methods of particle separation, and their best separations suggested that only acid hydrolytic enzymes were present in alpha granules, while a second group of more dense granules were nonlysosomal and contained serotonin (5-hydroxytryptamine) (Fig. 4-13*B*) and metabolically inactive ATP and ADP. This is consistent with the earlier re-

(*text continues on page 204*)

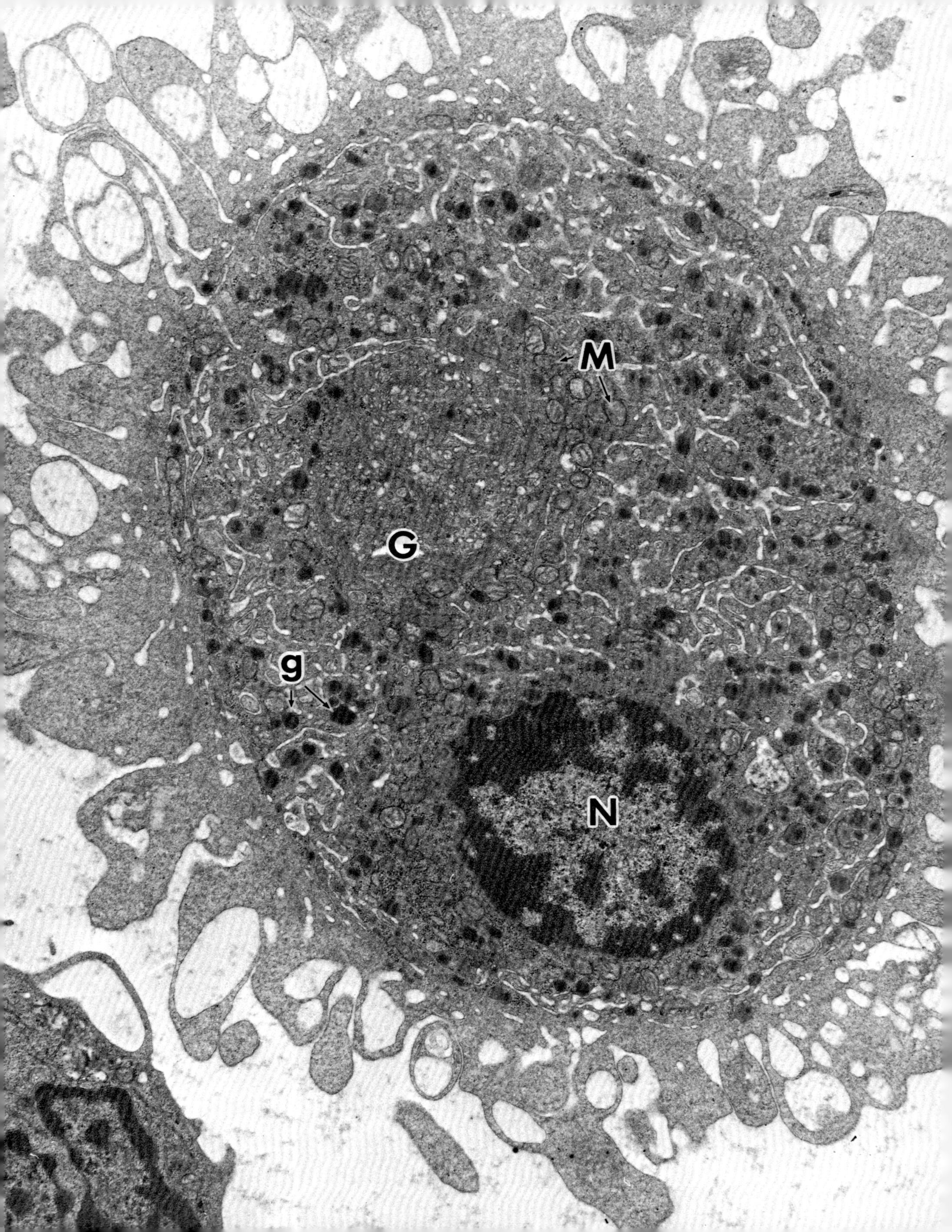
M
G
g
N

FIGURE 4-14. Atypical megarkaryocyte.
This small atypical megakaryocyte is representative of those found in bone marrow of myelocytic leukemic patient. (Nearly all megakaryocytes in this marrow had only one or two nuclei.) This cell has a highly irregular surface with active bleb formation, a relatively large Golgi apparatus (*G*), normal-appearing granules (*g*), mitochondria (*M*), a single nucleus (*N*), and vesicles. × *11,000.*

Figures 4-15 and 4-16 appear on the following pages

FIGURE 4-15. Atypical megakaryocyte.
Cytoplasm of atypical megakaryocyte, from a different leukemic patient than the cell shown in Figure 4-14, is highly vesicular, (*v*), without much evidence of demarcation vesicles for platelet formation. There are a Golgi complex (*G*), small mitochondria (*M*), and the edge of a nucleus *(N)*. × *22,500.*

FIGURE 4-16. Giant platelets.
These giant platelets from peripheral blood of a young girl are comparable in size to the neutrophil (*Ne*) and contain many granules (*g*) and many vesicular areas (*ser*). *Plastic: Maraglas.* × *21,600.*

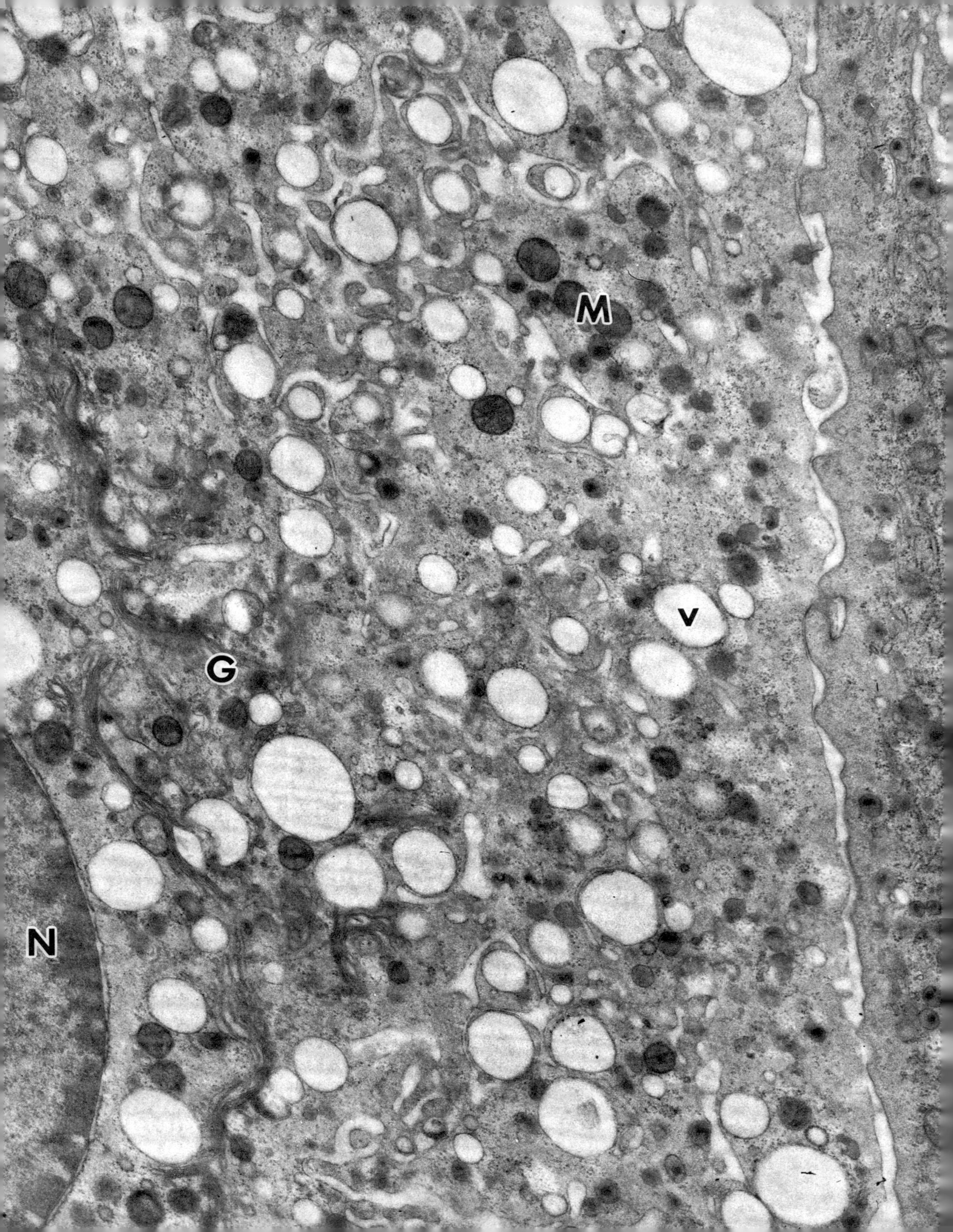
M
V
G
N

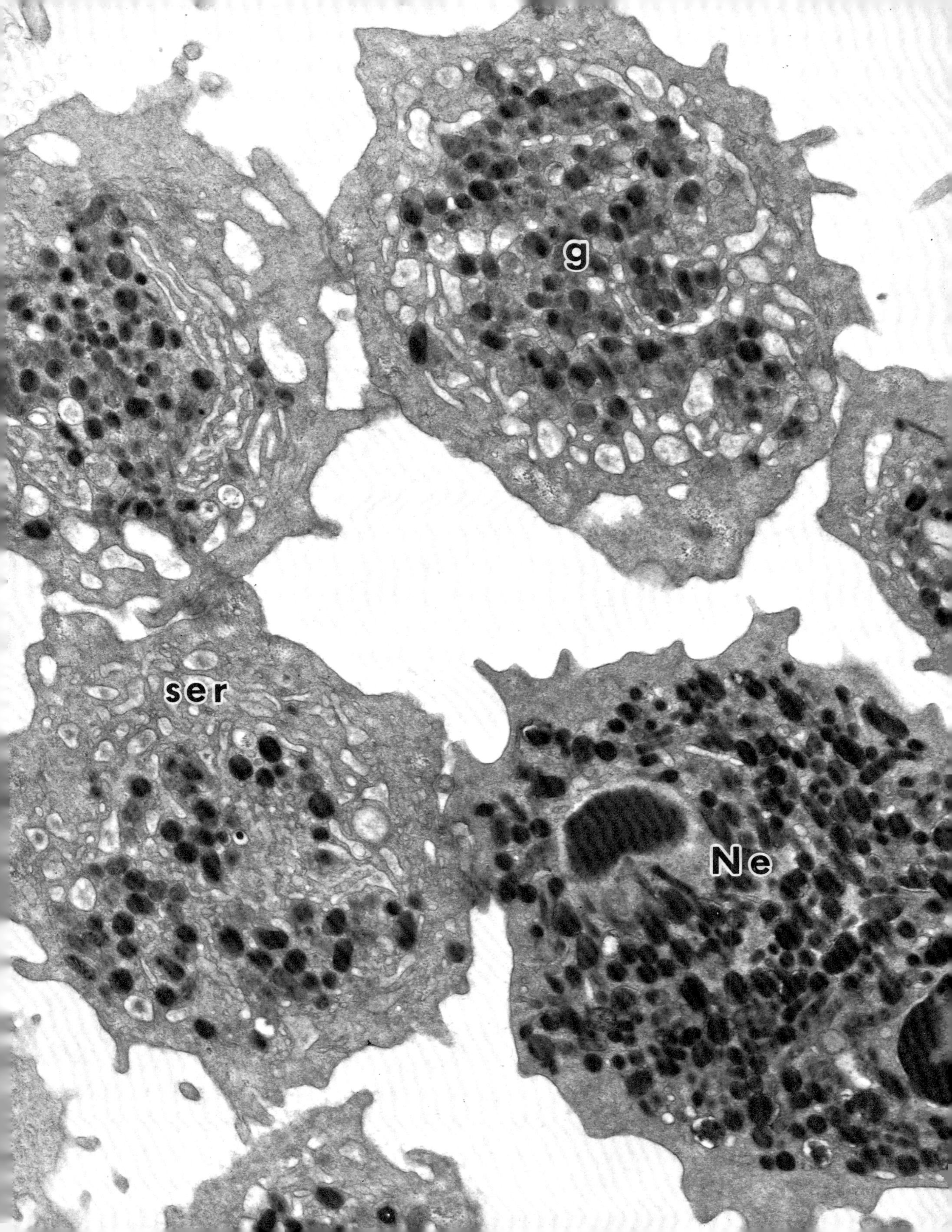
g
ser
Ne

port of Tranzer *et al.* (1966) on serotonin. The careful analysis and yet rather inconclusive results of Day *et al.* (1969) emphasize the difficulty of assigning a specific clotting role to a specific platelet structure.

Platelet absorption of plasma clotting factors include factors V, VII, XI, XII, XIII and fibrinogen. These are also present in the plasma, and deficiency or impaired function of any one or several of these plasma factors or platelet components can produce severe hemorrhagic conditions.

PATHOLOGY

Most pathological conditions primarily involved in platelet production are associated with impaired hemostasis, but some do not appear to have a morphological abnormality in platelets. Reports concerned with electron microscopic examination of platelets in these conditions are limited. Though some have claimed certain abnormalities in both megakaryocytes and platelets, such observations are rather inconclusive and still need future verification.

MYELOPROLIFERATIVE DISORDERS

Megakaryocytosis in association with significant thrombocytosis is seen frequently in various forms of myeloproliferative disorders, particularly in chronic myelocytic leukemia and polycythemia vera. In these conditions, production of the small megakaryocytes, about 25μ in diameter, has been reported. These cells are usually mono- or binuclear, and lobulation or indentation of the nucleus is insignificant (Fig. 4-14). The cytoplasm is usually modest in volume, and a moderate number of azurophilic granules is evident. Examination of bone marrow from some leukemic cases shows atypical megakaryocytes. These cells show some granule formation in or near the Golgi apparatus; however, the formation of the demarcation vesicles or membranes may be insufficient (Fig. 4-15). The significance of these cells is unknown and no abnormality in blood coagulation is usually reported in these cases. Studies on peripheral blood in leukemia show considerable variation in size and morphology of circulating platelets (Haguenau *et al.,* 1963). The most interesting finding is, perhaps, the presence of a large population of abnormal platelets which contain only a few or no granules in the cytoplasm. These abnormal features of circulating platelets in leukemia may be reflected in abnormal coagulation, as occasionally reported in leukemia.

INHERITED TISSUE DEFECTS

Giant platelets are frequently seen in combination with inborn abnormalities of other cells and tissues. They are found in association with May-Hegglin abnormality (Jordan and Larsen, 1965; Lechner *et al.,* 1969), where no specific ultrastructural anomaly is detected and there is no sig-

FIGURE 4-17. Giant platelets from same patient as in Figure 4-16.
A. In addition to granules (g) and usual vesicles (*ser*), there is a peculiar, tight multitubular structure (*asterisk*). *× 45,600.*
B. Same type of multitubular structure (*asterisk*) is seen here as in Figure 4-17**A,** but in a megakaryocyte of the same patient. *Plastic: Maraglas. × 38,600.*

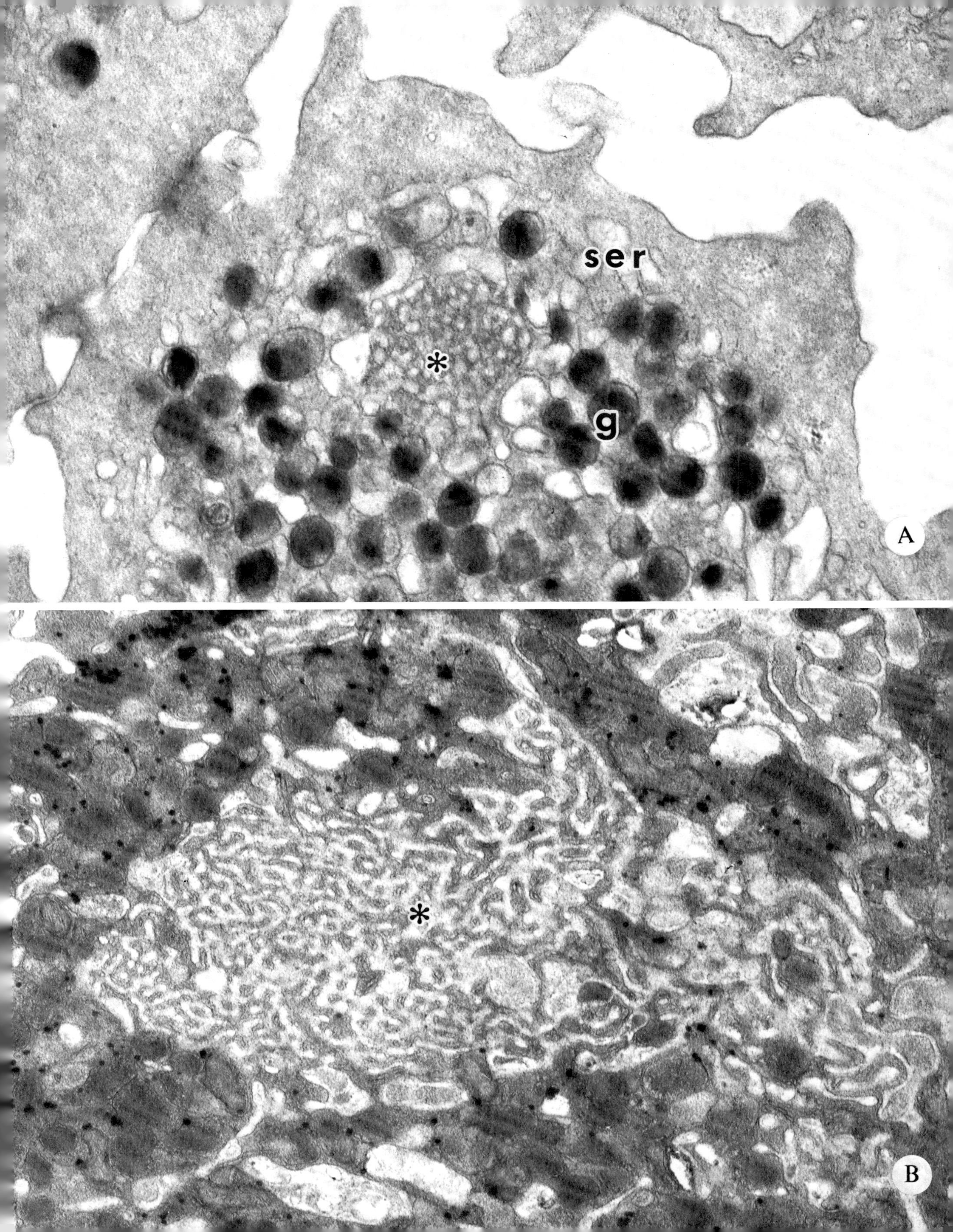
ser
*
g
A
*
B

nificant malfunction of the platelets which might contribute to clot formation or retraction.

Congenital giant platelets have been detected in hemostasis, in which impairment of platelet thromboplastic activity has been claimed (Revol, 1944; Bernard and Soulier, 1948), but the platelets were not studied by electron microscopy.

Giant platelets have been found in children suffering from renal insufficiency, hearing loss, and hemorrhagic tendencies (Epstein *et al.,* 1971). In addition to being large (Fig. 4-16) the platelets often contain large masses of vesicular structures (Fig. 4-17*A*), show a decrease of alpha granules per volume of cytoplasm (Fig. 4-16), and exhibit defective ADP platelet adhesiveness during in vitro tests. The vesicular structures are strikingly similar to those found in peritoneal macrophages by Brederoo (1971). He has called this collection of vesicles "labyrinths" and has found that they are strongly positive in peroxidase activity. Abnormal megacaryocytes are also seen in the bone marrow of children whose giant platelets contained these structures. (Figs. 4-17*B* and 4-18).

IDIOPATHIC THROMBOCYTOPENIC PURPURA

Platelets in this condition have been investigated by Falcão *et al.* (1969) and Falcão and Gautier (1969) in several cases, one case before and after splenectomy. The bleeding tendency is thought to be due to the thrombopenic condition rather than to malfunction of the platelets. Ultrastructural study on the platelets reveals some abnormalities. According to Falcão and Gautier (1969), platelets show fewer membrane structures, possibly because of the poor development of the demarcation membranes in megakaryocytes, which might reflect the reported 8- to 12-hour life span of platelets instead of the normal 8 to 10 days. It is unclear how ultrastructural abnormalities relate to the thrombopenic condition. No abnormality is found in the cytoplasmic organelles.

THROMBASTHENIA

Hemorrhagic diathesis associated with congenital malfunction of platelets is called thrombasthenia, and the lesion is consistent with heterogenic abnormalities of platelet function. Hellem (1960) and Gaarder *et al.* (1961) demonstrated that platelets from thrombasthenic patients were defective in adhesiveness as a result of reduced activity in response to ADP treatment. Hardisty *et al.* (1964) defined thrombasthenia as a congenital bleeding disorder characterized by a normal platelet count, a long bleeding time, and a complete failure of platelet aggregation by ADP treatment. Although the release of intrinsic ADP is normal, there is an impaired clot retraction. They concluded that the primary defect of this disorder is the abnormality of the platelet membrane. Heterozygotes may have impaired clot retraction but platelet aggregation is normal. Ultrastructurally, a size abnormality of platelet granules has been reported (Nakajima and Kono, 1968).

FIGURE 4-18. Megakaryocyte.
Megakaryocyte from same patient as that in Figures 4-16 and 4-17 has a very large nucleus (*N*), atypical cytoplasm with grossly uneven distribution of granules, and large areas containing mostly vesicles (*ser*). There are cytoplasmic blebs on the surface (*arrow*) with few or no granules. *Plastic: Maraglas.* × *9,600.*

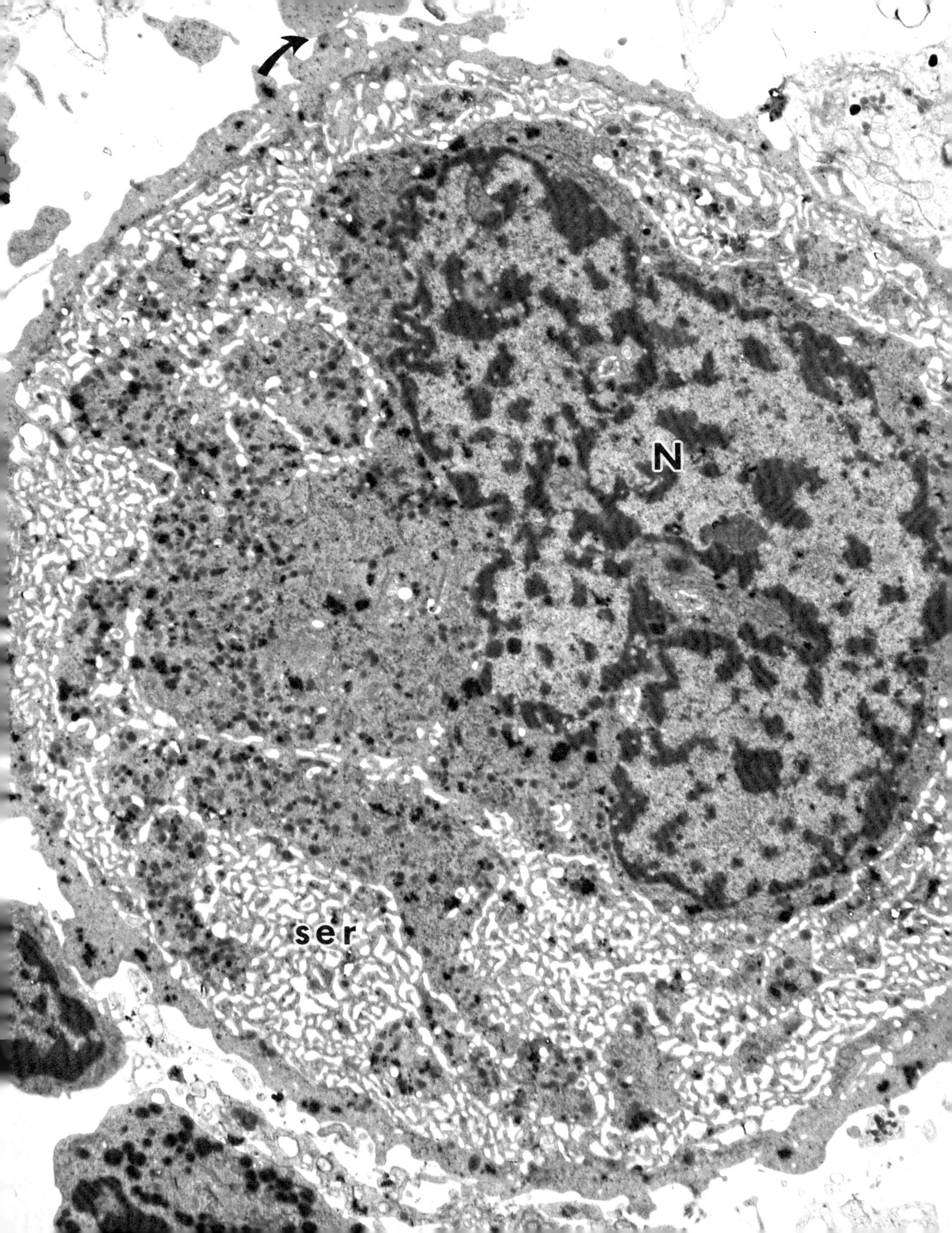
N
ser

THROMBOCYTHEMIA

A hemorrhagic phenomenon is occasionally found in cases with very high platelet counts. The disease is called "hemorrhagic thrombocythemia" (Gunz, 1960). The clinical manifestations include spontaneous bleeding and splenomegaly, and the disorder occurs in both sexes. Extremely high platelet counts and various defective functions of the platelet have been reported; however, no etiological factor has been disclosed.

Though malfunction of platelets has been speculated, no morphological abnormality of either platelet or megakaryocyte has been detected by routine light microscopy, except for variations in size and shapes. Earlier, Rebuck *et al.* (1961) reported no ultrastructural abnormality in platelets of this condition. Later, Jean *et al.* (1966) reported abnormal granules of the platelets in four cases of primary thrombocythemia. This observation is further confirmed by Schulz and Pottel (1969) and Simar and Hugues (1969). According to Schulz and Pottel (1969) atypical granules—such as drumstick-shaped, bull's-eye, and giant granules—may constitute up to 18 per cent of the total granules.

The presence of such granulation in addition to impaired demarcation tubules is also noted in proliferating megakaryocytes. All the observed abnormalities in this condition are nonpathognomonic since similar abnormalities have been reported in other conditions.

VON WILLEBRAND'S DISEASE

von Willebrand's disease has been characterized by a tendency to bleed from mucous membranes, a prolonged bleeding time, moderately reduced plasma level of factor VIII, and an autosomal-dominant mode of inheritance (Strauss and Bloom, 1965). Earlier possible qualitative abnormality of platelets was considered to be the primary factor and was called a constitutional thrombopathy (von Willebrand and Jürgens, 1933). The platelet defect originally proposed and the deficiency of platelet factor VIII are now denied. Ultrastructurally, granular abnormalities in circulating platelets were reported by several (Eriksson *et al.,* 1961; Jean *et al.,* 1963; Marx and Jean, 1964); however, these are regarded as nonspecific to this disorder (David-Ferreira, 1964).

REFERENCES

Ashford, T. P., and Freiman, D. G. The role of the endothelium in the initial phases of thrombosis; an electron microscopic study. *Amer J Path 50*:257, 1967.

Aster, R. H. Studies of the fate of platelets in rats and man. *Blood 34*:117, 1969.

Behnke, O. Electron microscopical observations on the surface coating of human blood platelets. *J Ultrastruct Res 24*:51, 1968.

Behnke, O. An electron microscopic study of rat megacaryocyte. II. Some aspects of p'atelet release and microtubules. *J Ultrastruct Res 26*:111, 1969.

Bernard, J., and Soulier, J. P. Sur une nouvelle variété de dystrophie thrombocytaire hémorragipare congénitale. *Sem Hop Paris 24*:3217, 1948.

Bessis, M., and Burstein, M. Études sur les thrombocytes au microscope électronique. *Rev hemat 3*:48, 1948.

Bettex-Galland, M., and Lüscher, E. F. Thrombosthenin—a contractile protein from thrombocytes. Its extraction from human blood platelets and some of its properties. *Biochim Biophys Acta 49*:536, 1961.

Braunsteiner, H., Fellinger, K., and Pakesch, F.

Elektron mikroskopische Beobachtungen der Blutplättchen bei Thrombasthenie. *Klin Wschr 31*:21, 1953.

Brederoo, P. Personal Communication, 1971.

Bull, B. S. The ultrastructure of negatively stained platelets. Some physiologic implications. *Blood 28*:901, 1966.

David-Ferreira, J. F. The blood platelet; Electron microscopic studies. *Int Rev Cytol 17*:99, 1964.

Day, H. J., Holmsen, H., and Hovig, T. Subcellular particles of human platelets. A biochemical and electron microscopic study with particular reference to the influence of fractionation techniques. *Scand J Haemat Suppl 7,* 1969.

deLeval, M., and Paulus, J. M. Nuclear maturation and cytoplasmic organelles and antigens in guinea pig and human megakaryocytes. *Blood 34*:529, 1969.

DeRobertis, E. Electron microscopic observations of the platelet-fibrin relationship in blood clotting. *Blood 10*:528, 1955.

Dohrmann, R., and Klesper, R. Untersuchungen zur β-Glucuronidase-aktivität menschlicher Thrombocyten. *Klin Wschr 38*:595, 1960.

Ebbe, S., and Stohlman, F., Jr. Megakaryocytopoiesis in the rat. *Blood 26*:20, 1965.

Ebbe, S. Responses of the Thrombocytopoietic System to Platelet Depletion and Irradiation. In *Hemopoietic Cellular Proliferation* (Stohlman, F., Jr., ed.). Grune & Stratton, New York, 1970, p. 285.

Epstein, C. J., Sahud, M., Piel, C. F., Goodman, J. R., and Bernfeld, M. Hereditary macrothrombocytopathia, nephritis and deafness. *Amer J Med* (in press).

Eriksson, A. W., Hiepler, E., Jürgens, R., Lehmann, W., and Schulz, H. Untersuchungen zur Thrombopathie (v. Willerbrand-Jürgens). *Klin Wschr 39*:32, 1961.

Falcão, L., Caen, J., and Gautier, A. Étude évolutive de l'ultrastructure des mégacaryocytes dans un cas de purpura thrombopénique idiopathique avant 12 jours et 5 mois après splénectomie. *Blut 19*:156, 1969.

Falcão, L., and Gautier, A. Ultrastrukturelle Veranderungen menschlicher Megakaryozyten bei Blutkrankeiten 1969. Der Thrombozyt (Marx, R., ed.). *Verh 12 Kongress Deutsche Ges Hamat* 1969.

Gaarder, A., Jonsen, J., Laland, S., Hellen, A., and Owren, P. A. Adenosine diphosphate in red cells as a factor in the adhesiveness of human blood platelets. *Nature* (*London*) *192*:531, 1961.

Goodman, J. R., Reilly, E. G., and Moore, R. E. Electron microscopy of formed elements of normal human blood. *Blood 12*:428, 1957.

Gunz, F. W. Hemorrhagic thrombocythemia: a critical review. *Blood 15*:706, 1960.

Haguenau, F., Hollmann, K. H., Levy, J. P., and Boiron, M. Étude au microscope électronique des plaquettes sanguines dan les leucémies humaines. *J. Microscopie 2*:529, 1963.

Hardisty, R. M., Dormandy, K. M., and Hutton, R. A. Thrombasthenia. Studies of three cases. *Brit J Haemat 10*:371, 1964.

Hellem, A. J. The adhesiveness of human blood platelets in vitro. *Scand J Clin Lab Invest 12* (suppl. 51), 1960.

Hovig, T. The ultrastructure of blood platelets in normal and abnormal states. *Ser Haemat 1*:3, 1968.

Jean, G., Racine, L., Gautier, A., and Marx, R. Granulations denses anomales dans les thrombocytes humains. *Thromb Diath Haemorrh 10*: 42, 1963.

Jean, G., Marx, R., and Gautier, A. Applications de la recherche ultrastructurale à l'étude des thrombocythémies. *Nouv Rev Franc Hémat 6*: 591, 1966.

Johnson, S. A., Sturrock, R. M., and Rebuck, J. W. Morphological Localization of Platelet Factor 3 Activity in Normal Platelet. In *Blood Clotting Factors* (Deutsch, E., ed.). Pergamon, New York, p. 105.

Jones, O. P. Origin of megakaryocyte granules from Golgi vesicles. *Anat. Rec. 138*:105, 1960.

Jordan, S. W., and Larsen, W. E. Ultrastructural studies of the May-Hegglin anomaly. *Blood 25*: 921, 1965.

Kaufman, R. M., Airo, R., Pollack, S., and Crosby, W. H. Pulmonary megakaryocytes: their origin and significance. *J Clin Invest 44*:1063, 1965a.

Kaufman, R. M., Airo, R., Pollack, S., and Crosby, W. H. Circulating megakaryocytes and platelet release in the lung. *Blood 26*:720, 1965b.

Kautz, J., and deMarsh, Q. B. Electron microscopy of sectioned blood and bone marrow elements. *Rev Hémat 10*:314, 1955.

Lechner, K., Breddin, K., Moser, K., Stockinger, L., and Wenzel, E. May-Hegglinsche Anomalie. *Acta Haemat 42*:303, 1969.

Lüscher, E. F. Platelets in haemostasis and thrombosis. *Brit J Haemat 13*:1, 1967.

Marcus, A. J., and Zucker-Franklin, D. Enzyme and

coagulation activity of subcellular platelet fractions. *J Clin Invest 43*:1241, 1964.

Marcus, A. J., and Zucker, M. B. *The Physiology of Blood Platelets.* Grune & Stratton, New York, 1965.

Marcus, A. J., Zucker-Franklin, D., Safier, L. B., and Ullman, H. L. Studies on human platelet granules and membranes. *J Clin Invest 45*:14, 1966.

Marx, R., and Jean, G. Zur Pathogenese der v. Willebrand-Jürgens-Syndrome: Eine klinische und submikroskopische Studie. *Klin Wschr 42*: 491, 1964.

Morse, B. S., and Stohlman, F., Jr. Regulation of erythropoiesis. XVIII. The effect of vincristine and erythropoietin on bone marrow. *J Clin Invest 45*:1241, 1966.

Movat, H. Z., Weiser, W. J., Glynn, M. F. and Mustard, J. F. Platelet phagocytosis and aggregation. *J Cell Biol 27*:531, 1965.

Nakajima, M., and Kono, K. Studies on the ultrastructure of platelets of hemophiliacs. *Acta Haemat Jap 31*:71, 1968.

Odell, T. T., Jr., and Jackson, C. W. Megakaryocytopoiesis. In *Hemopoietic Cellular Proliferation* (Stohlman, F., Jr., ed.). Grune & Stratton, New York, 1970, p. 278.

Paulus, J. M., and Thompson, K. H. Computer analysis of platelet survival curves. *Blood 34*: 529, 1969.

Pease, D. C. Marrow cells seen with the electron microscope after ultrathin sectioning. *Rev Hemat 10*:300, 1955.

Rebuck, J. W., Riddle, J. M., Brown, M. G., Johnson, S. D., and Monto, R. W. Volumetric and Ultrastructural Studies of Abnormal Platelets. In *Blood Platelet. International Symposium,* Henry Ford Hospital. Little, Brown, Boston, 1961.

Revol, L. Diathèse hémorragique avec grosses anomalies morphologiques des plaquettes. Étude critique des divers syndromes hémogénique. *Sang 16*:176, 1944.

Rinehart, J. F. Electron microscopic studies of sectioned white blood cells and platelets, with observations on the derivation of specific granules from mitochondria. *Amer J Clin Path 24*: 605, 1955.

Robb-Smith, A. H. T. Why the platelets were discovered. *Brit J Haemat 13*:618, 1967.

Rodman, N. F., Jr., Mason, R. G., McDevitt, N. B., and Brinkhous, K. M. Morphologic alterations of human blood platelets during early phases of clotting. Electron microscopic observations of thin sections. *Amer J Path 40*:271, 1962.

Rodman, N. F., Jr., Painter, J. C., and Mcdevitt, N. B. Platelet disintegration during clotting. *J Cell Biol 16*:225, 1963.

Schulz, H., and Hiepler, E. Über die Lokalisierung von gerinnungsphysiologischen Aktivitäten in submikroskopischen Struktren der Thrombocyten. *Klin Wschr 37*:273, 1959.

Schulz, H. Über die Phagozytose von kolloidalen Siliziumdioxyd durch Thrombozyten mit Bemerkungeu zur submikroskopischen Struktur der Thromboxytenmembran. *Folia Haemat (NF) 5*: 195, 1961.

Schulz, H., and Pottel, A. Elektronenmikroskopische Untersuchungen der Megakaryozyten und Thrombozyten eines Falles von primär hämorrhagischer Thrombozythämie. *Blut 19*:208, 1969.

Simar, L. J., and Hugues, J. Ultrastructure des plaquettes dans deux cas de thrombocythémie. *Acta Haemat 41*:33, 1969.

Spicer, S. S., Green, W. B., and Hardin, J. H. Ultrastructural localization of acid mucosubstance and antimonate-precipitable action in human and rabbit platelets and megakaryocytes. *J Histochem Cytochem 17*:781, 1969.

Strauss, H. S., and Bloom, G. E. von Willebrand's disease: Use of a platelet-adhesiveness test in diagnosis and family investigation. *New Eng J Med 273*:171, 1965.

Tranzer, J. P., DaPrada, M., and Pletscher, A. Ultrastructural localization of 5-hydroxytryptamine in blood platelets. *Nature (London) 212*:1574, 1966.

Tocantins, L. M. Historical notes on blood platelets. *Blood 3*:1073, 1948.

von Willebrand, E. A., and Jürgens, R. Uber eine neue Bluterkrankheit, die konstitutionelle Thrombopathie. *Klin Wschr 12*:414, 1933.

White, J. G., Krivit, W., and Vernier, R. L. The platelet-fibrin relationship in human blood clots: An ultrastructural study utilizing ferritin-conjugated anti-human fibrinogen antibody. *Blood 25*:241, 1965.

White, J. G., and Krivit, W. Fine structural localization of adenosine triphosphatase in human platelets and other blood cells. *Blood 26*:554, 1965.

White, J. G., and Krivit, W. The ultrastructural localization and release of platelet lipids. *Blood 27*:167, 1966.

Wolpers, C., and Ruska, H. Strukturuntersuchungen zur Blutgerinnung. *Klin Wschr 18*:1077, 1939.

Wright, J. H. Die Entstehung der Blutplättchen. *Virchow Arch Path Anat 186*:55, 1906.

Yamada, E. The fine structure of the megakaryocyte in the mouse spleen. *Acta Anat 29*:267, 1957.

Zamboni, L. Electron microscopic studies of blood embryogenesis in humans. II. The hemopoietic activity in the fetal liver. *J Ultrastruct Res 12*: 525, 1965.

Zucker-Franklin, D. Microfibrils of blood platelets: Their relationship to microtubules and the contractile protein. *J Clin Invest 48*:165, 1969.

chapter 5
LYMPHOCYTES

Lymphocytes are major formed elements of lymph nodes; they constitute the dominant cells in lymph of lymphatic vessels and about one-fourth the leukocytes in peripheral blood. The lymphatic vessels had been observed by Greek scientists in 300 to 250 B.C. A careful description of the system was first made by Aselli* from his study of the mesentery of dogs. He called them canaliculae of lacteal vessels, and associated them with mesenteric lymph nodes. The discovery of the cisterna chyli, the thoracic duct, and its communication to the vena cava was made by Pecquet* in 1651. The term "lymphatics" was introduced by Bartholin* to describe this canalicular system and to distinguish it from blood vessels. The presence of formed elements in lymph was acknowledged by Virchow† in 1851 before the precise description of lymphocytes by Ehrlich in 1891, by which time these elements had been called "Lymphkörperchen" or "Lymphzellen"; the term "lymphocyte" evolved around 1890.

The role of lymph nodes in the formation of Lymphkörperchen was described by the middle of the nineteenth century, and was variously called cytogenes Gewebe (Kölliker, 1852),** adenoides Gewebe (His, 1860),** a konglobierte Drüsensubstanz (Henle, 1843),** retikuläres Gewebe (Frey, 1861),** cytoblastisches Gewebe (Ellenberger, 1906).** However, the term "lymphoid" tissues (Waldeyer)** has been used consistently since the introduction of the term. The concept of lymphoid tissues distributed in various organs under a single tissue system was suggested by Henle (1861).** The production of the small lymphocyte was predicted from the Keimzentrum by Flemming (1885), and the concept was held by many until recently.

* Cited by Yoffey & Courtice (1956).

† Cronkite et al. (1964).

** Cited by Hellman (1930).

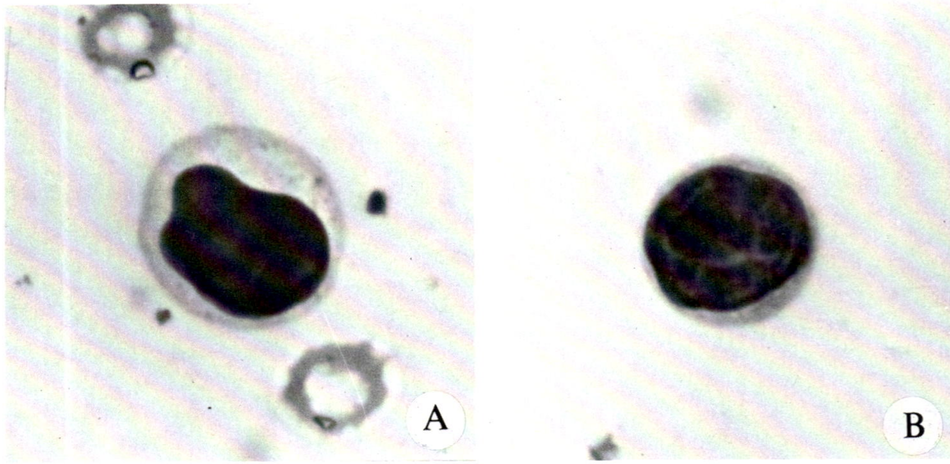

FIGURE 5-1. Lymphocytes from normal blood.
A. Large lymphocyte with abundant cytoplasm containing a few small granules. Nucleus has typical clumping of chromatin. × *2,000.*
B. Small lymphocyte with narrow rim of cytoplasm and condensed chromatin in the nucleus. × *2,000.*

FIGURE 5-2. Lymphocytes from normal human peripheral blood.
These show typical clumping of chromatin in nuclei (*N*). Lower cell has what appears to be residual density from a nucleolus (*Nu*). All cells contain several large ovoid mitochondria (*M*), some scattered endoplasmic reticulum, and innumerable single ribosomes in the cytoplasm. Cell at upper right has a dense inclusion (*arrow*). A platelet (*P*) is also present. × *17,400.*

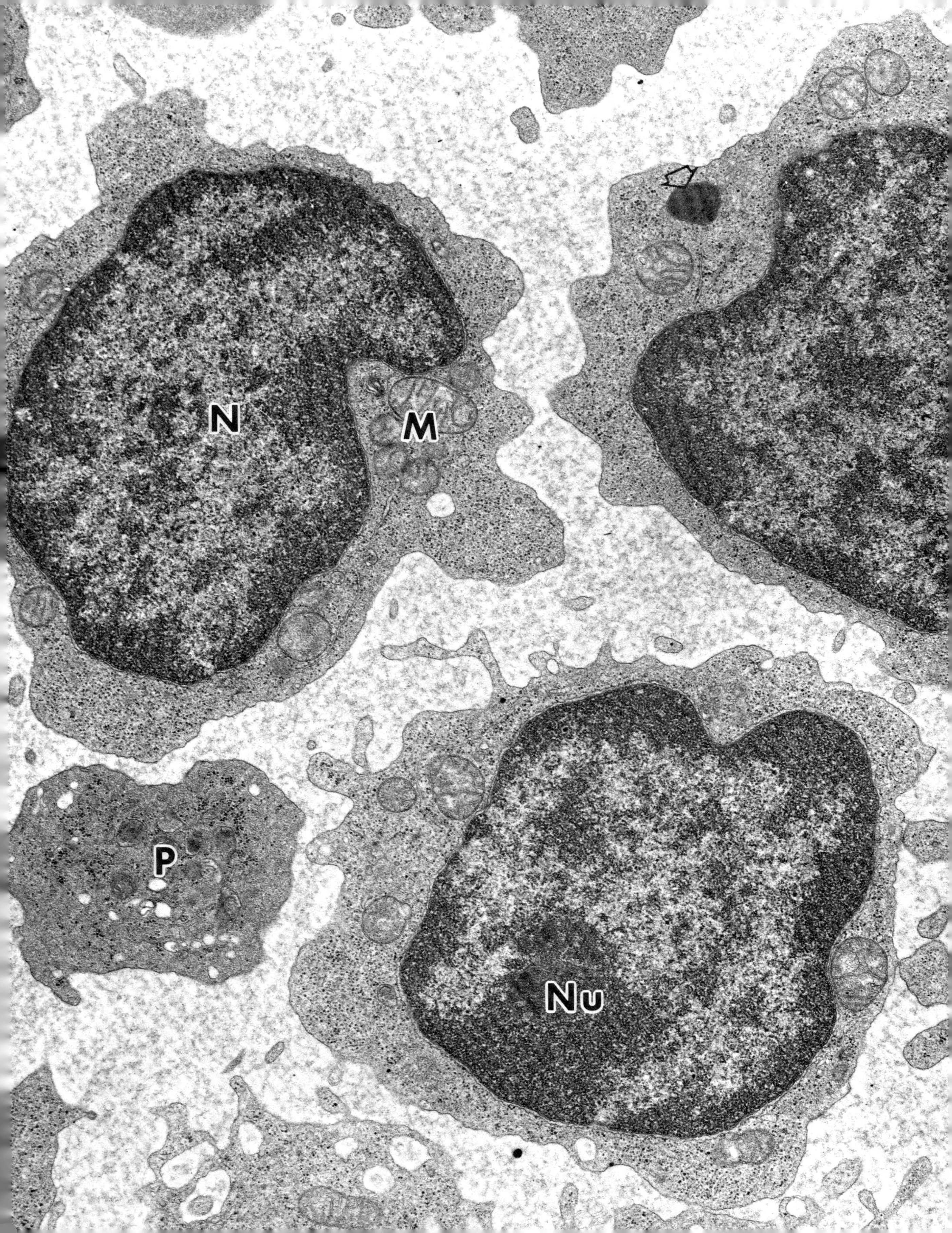
N
M
P
Nu

The currently accepted anatomy of the lymph nodes was posed by Huedorfer in 1921,** but because lymphocytes have little to characterize their morphology and are in an apparently static state, very little was known about their function before 1950. Since then, many important discoveries have been made relating to the wide range in life span of lymphocytes, their role in the body defense mechanisms, their relation to cell generation, etc. Some concepts are still evolving, and there is a need for more information and experimentation to understand fully the origin and function of these cells.

MORPHOLOGY

The typical morphology is best seen in small lymphocytes of the peripheral blood (Fig. 5-1). Although the cells categorized as "lymphocytes" have been accepted as a functionally uniform group, comparable to erythroid or myeloid cells, there is serious doubt whether this is a homogeneous population.

One difficulty in the study of lymphocytes lies in the absence of any distinctive marker by which one can identify them at the single-cell level. Consequently, such vague terms as "lymphoid cells" or "atypical lymphocytes" have been used to describe lymphocyte-like cells with some uncommon characteristics. Unfortunately, these terms only create more confusion, since the "lymphoid cell" may or may not be a lymphocyte. The term "lymphoid cell" which is used extensively at present may mean different things to different investigators.

The introduction of the electron microscope was expected to help differentiate the lymphocytes from lymphoid cells, but the fine structural detail of lymphoid cells has not led to a clear categorization of the lymphocyte. The small, inactive lymphocytes are fairly distinctive, but the medium or large ones, which may be "stimulated" lymphocytes or lymphoid cells, also have fairly well-defined characteristics. Figures 5-2 and 5-3 are examples of sections containing normal lymphocytes in both peripheral blood and lymph nodes.

In contrast to other types of blood cells, morphological alterations in the process of lymphocyte maturation are modest, and immature lymphocytes are not easily distinguished from mature ones. The most reliable distinction is perhaps the difference in size rather than specific cytoplasmic characteristics. Many mitoses were postulated as taking place between the primitive reticulum cell stage and mature lymphocytes (Grundmann, 1958), but there are few clues as to the gradation of maturity.

The problem of defining the steps in maturation is also complicated by the suggestion that lymphocytes from different tissues may have different functions but appear morphologically identical—e.g., lymphocytes from the thymus may have different roles in immune response from those from the bone marrow. Furthermore, the small lymphocyte, which is considered to be the mature form, is ap-

** Cited by Hellman (1930).

FIGURE 5-3. Normal lymphocytes in lymph node.
Three of these small lymphocytes have denser cytoplasm. These are essentially identical to the small circulating lymphocytes shown in Figure 5-2; however, others have less electron-dense cytoplasm. The inclusion (*arrow*) in lower left cell is a "Gall" body. The cell also contains numerous mitochondria (*M*). × *14,500.*

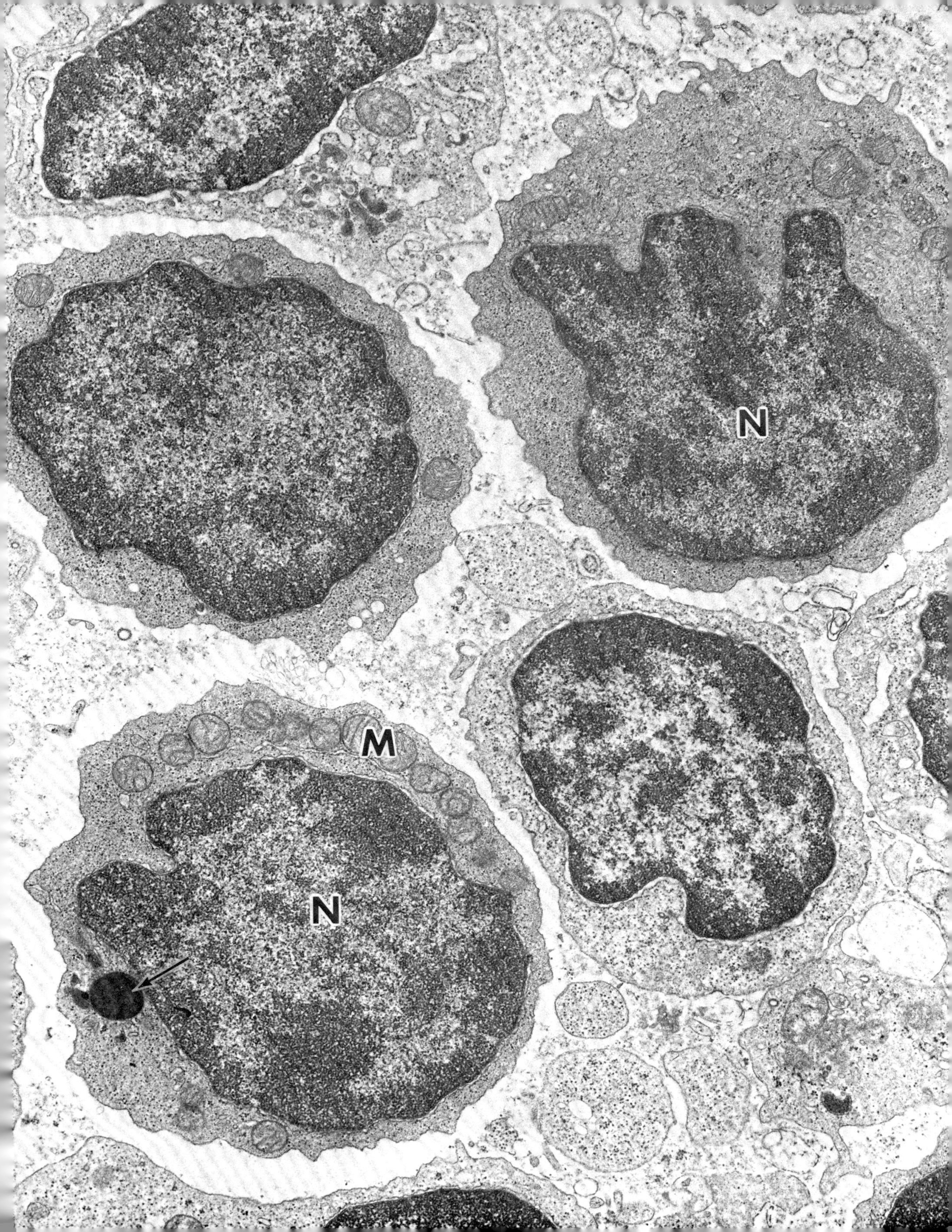
N
M
N

parently a dormant or resting cell and may circulate in the body for months or years, but, on stimulation, it may change into an active cell that is morphologically indistinguishable from similar apparently immature cells freshly produced in lymph nodes.

IMMATURE CELLS

Lymph nodes stimulated by antigens produce large ameboid cells with a distinctive nucleolus and highly basophilic cytoplasm near the germinal center. These cells are particularly predominant after an immunological challenge and may be the blastic forms of both lymphocyte and plasma cell. Various names have been given to them, including (in relation to lymphocytogenesis): large lymphocyte (Maximow, 1927a; Bloom and Fawcett, 1968); large lymphoid cell (Heilmeyer and Begemann, 1955); hemopoietic reticulum cell (Sundberg, 1955); lymphogonia (Benda, 1896; Amano *et al.,* 1951); lymphoblast (a term used by many investigators); basophilic stem cell or large germinoblast (Lennert, 1961); hemocytoblast or prolymphoblast (Bessis, 1956); and hemocytoblast (Bernhard and Leplus, 1964). In relation to plasmocytogenesis, the names used are: transitional cell (Fagraeus, 1948); and large hyperbasophilic or pyroninocyte cell (Policard, 1963). At present, no distinction is possible between the mother cells of lymphocytes and of plasma cells. Dameshek (1963) proposed the term "immunoblast" since cells of this group may be the mother cells of all immunologically competent cells. In smears, the cells are large, about 20 to 25μ, and have a round or oval nucleus which stains a transparent rose color. The chromatin of the nucleus is evenly distributed, with consistently distinct nucleoli. The cytoplasm is strongly basophilic, without granulation except for a few occasional azurophilic granules. Histochemically, the cells show strong pyroninophilia, suggesting abundant RNA.

Their structural appearance is quite characteristic and easily distinguishable from lymphocytes and lymphoblasts. Their ultrastructural morphology was first described by Tanaka (1957) and confirmed by many. Bernhard and Leplus (1964) suggested that the large nucleolus and polyribosomes were the unique structures which distinguished them from the lymphoblast.

The cell is large and has an ameboid appearance (Fig. 5-4). The nucleus is usually oval with slight indentation. The chromatin network is coarse but distributed evenly in the nucleus. The nucleolus is large and quite distinctive. The cytoplasm is moderately wide and contains a moderately developed Golgi apparatus, many polyribosomes, and, at times, a modest amount of endoplasmic reticulum. The plasma membrane may show a number of micropinocytotic processes. Several types of hemocytoblasts, intermediate to lymphoplasma cells, have been distinguished in reactive lymph nodes responding to homografts (André-Schwartz, 1964). Ferritin-conjugated antibody technics have demonstrated antibodies in the endoplas-

FIGURE 5-4. Hemocytoblast.
Hemocytoblast (*center*) from human lymph node has a large reticular nucleus (*N*) with irregular outline and a nucleolus (*Nu*). The cytoplasm has many polyribosomes, moderately large Golgi apparatus (*G*), some endoplasmic reticulum (*er*) and mitochondria (*M*). A portion of a second hemocytoblast (*Hyb*) is at upper left. × *13,000.*

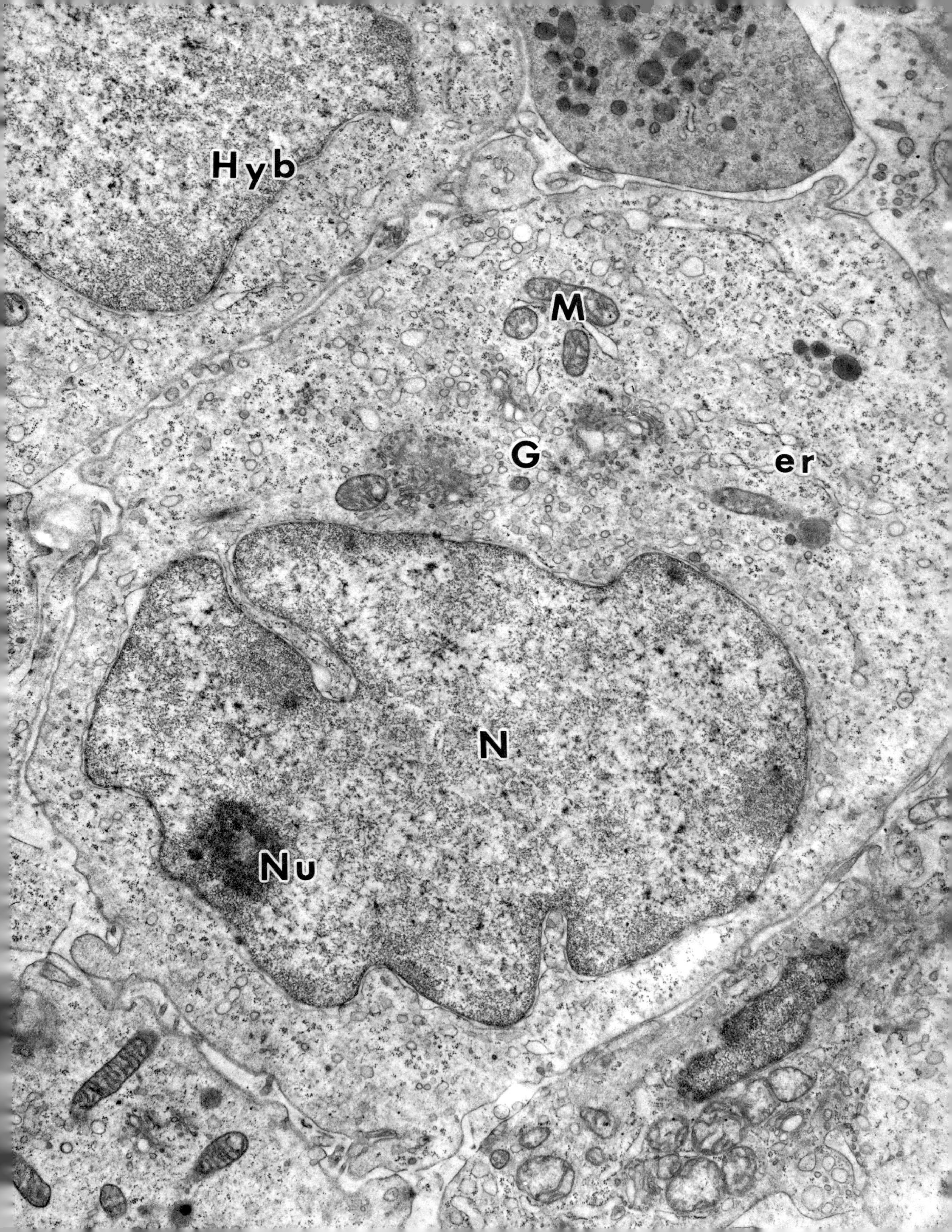
Hyb
M
G
er
N
Nu

mic reticulum of similar cells proliferating in the secondary immunological response (de Petris, and Karlsbad, 1965). The origin of this stimulated cell is not clearly established; however, immature mesenchymal compartments of lymph nodes, or self-production of similar cells and transformation from small lymphocytes, are all possible sources.

LYMPHOBLASTS

Medium-sized cells with vesicular nucleus and a nucleolus are commonly seen in histological sections of stimulated lymph nodes. These have been called medium lymphocytes (Bloom and Fawcett, 1968) or lymphoblasts (Bessis, 1956; Bernhard and Leplus, 1964) and are generally accepted as the committed blastic form of the lymphocytic line. These round cells are 9 to 13μ in diameter, and the nucleus stains a deeper rose color than more immature cells. In smears, the chromatin tends to show more coarse flocculation but is less prominent than that in small lymphocytes. One or two nucleoli can be clearly recognized in phase microscopy.

Electron microscopic descriptions of lymphoblasts have been reported by many investigators. Bernhard and Leplus (1964) describe two major characteristics in cells of the lymphocytic series: (1) a few large and clear mitochondria which tend to be grouped at one pole of the cell, and (2) an almost complete lack of endoplasmic reticulum. In studies of large numbers of lymphocytes in lymph nodes and peripheral blood, we found it difficult to distinguish lymphoblasts from small lymphocytes, except for the difference in size (Fig. 5-5). The chromatin pattern, the nuclear shape, and the amount of ribosomes and other cytoplasmic structures, including endoplasmic reticulum, vary considerably in individual cells. It is not clear whether this variation indicates the heterogeneity of lymphocyte population, a morphological alteration which occurs during the cell maturation, or a change of function.

LYMPHOCYTES IN PERIPHERAL BLOOD

Circulating Cells

Most lymphocytes in the peripheral blood are considered to be mature forms. Two groups are generally distinguished by their size: those with small cells of 6 to 8μ by light microscopy, and larger cells about 9 to 16μ (Fig. 5-1). Some investigators place an intermediate group of medium-sized cells between the two. In normal individuals, 10 per cent are larger lymphocytes, the rest are smaller. The term "large lymphocyte" should not be confused with the same term introduced by Maximow (1927a) who used it for the cell now designated as "hemocytoblast." The proportion of large lymphocytes may increase in the circulation in infants. However, it is not clear whether these large lymphocytes in the peripheral blood are immature forms of small lymphocytes,

(*text continues on page 226*)

FIGURE 5-5. Lymphocyte.
This large lymphocyte with wide cytoplasm contains a well-developed Golgi complex (*G*), centrioles (*Ce*), and several mitochondria (*M*). Single ribosomes are widely scattered throughout. The primary distinguishing characteristic of this cell from an erythroblast is the shape of the nucleus (*N*), single ribosomes as compared to polyribosomes, and size of Golgi apparatus. × *26,000.*

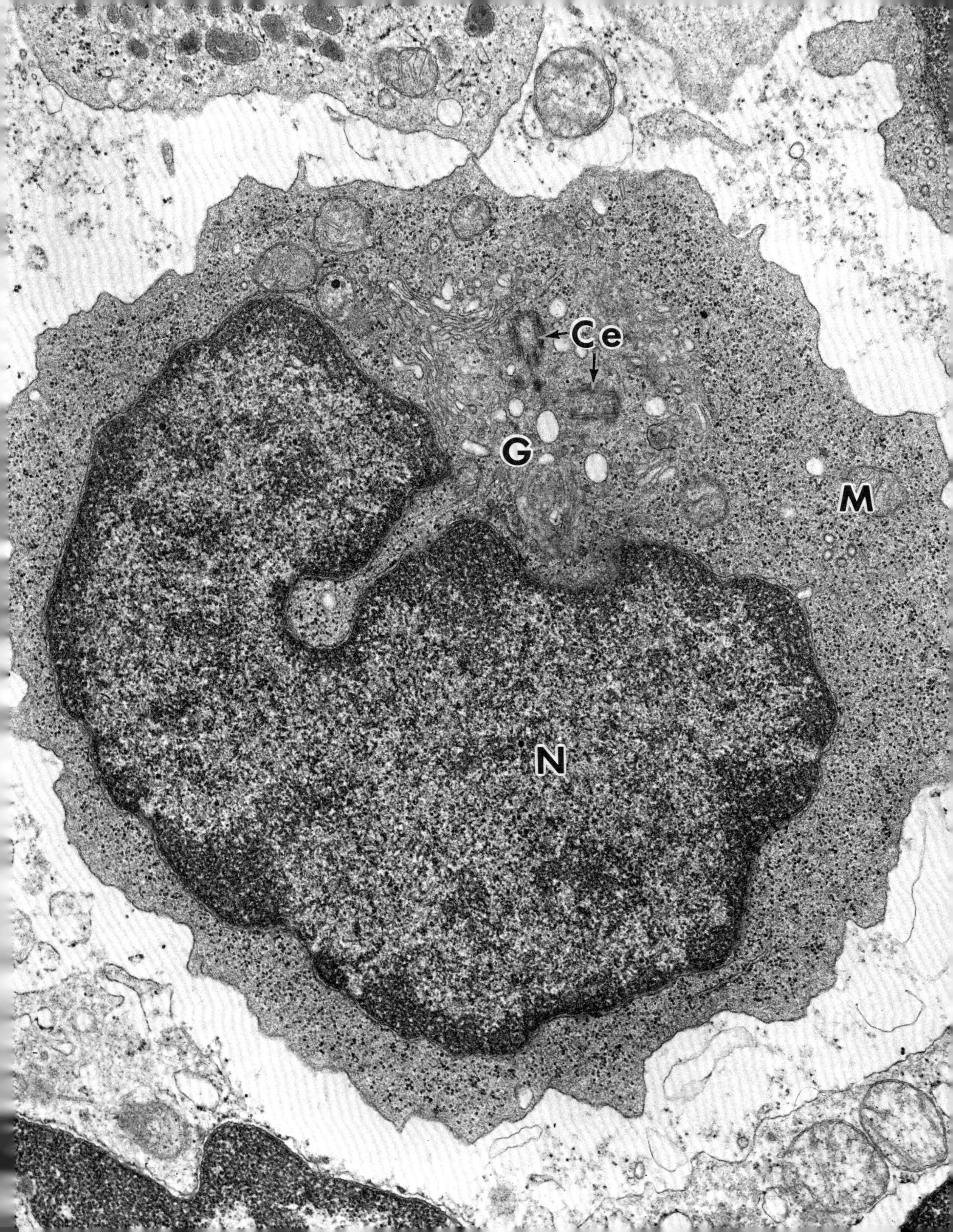
Ce
G
M
N

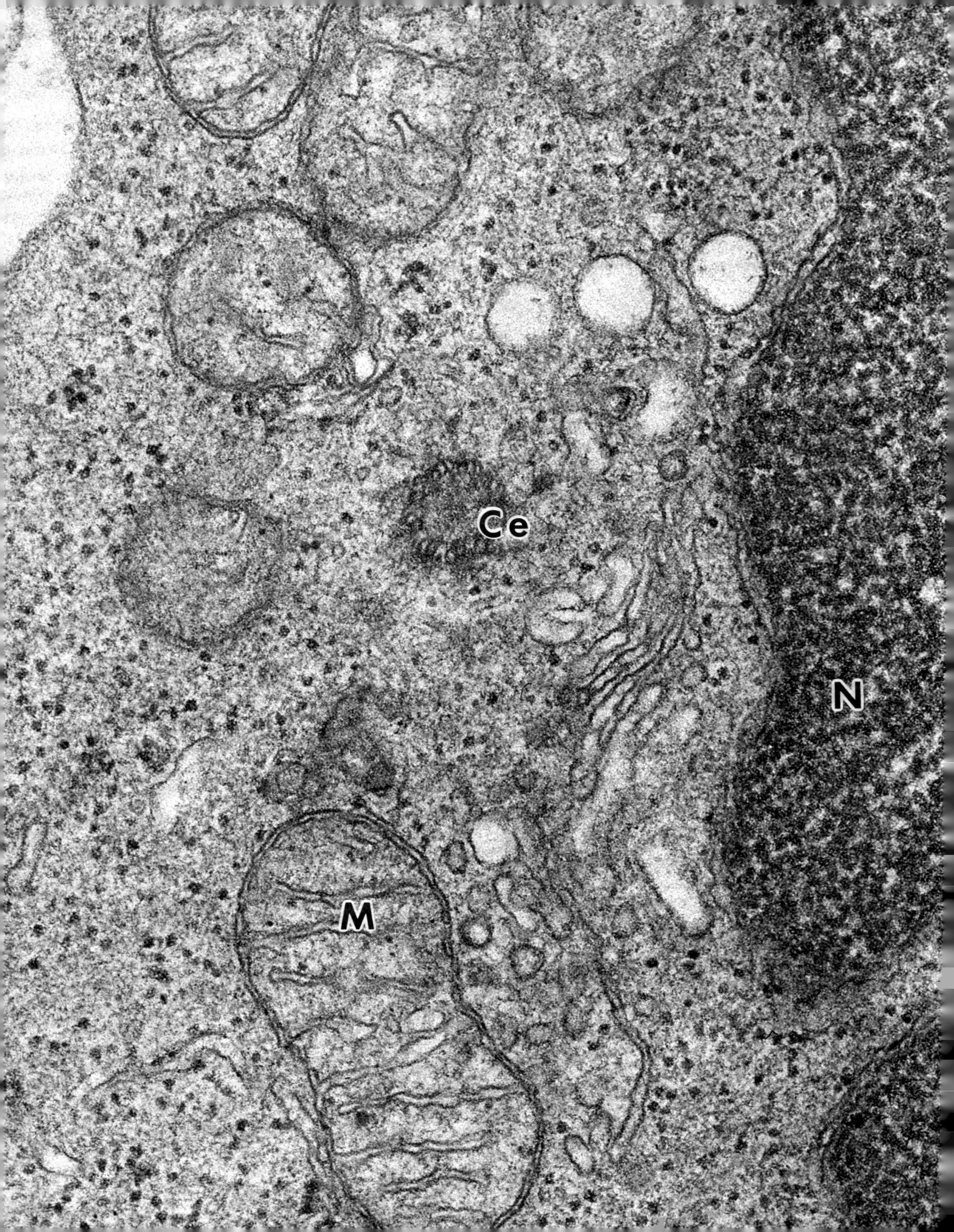
Ce
N
M

FIGURE 5-6. Portion of a lymphocyte.
Adjacent to the Golgi complex of this medium-sized lymphocyte are a centriole (*Ce*), mitochondria (*M*), and nucleus (*N*). × *89,000.*

Figures 5-7 and 5-8 appear on the following pages

FIGURE 5-7. Inclusions in a lymphocyte.
A. Two round inclusions (*in*) contain some electron-dense material. One has several small particles; the other is completely filled with structure interpreted as "Gall" body (*arrow*). A mitrochondrion (*M*) is near by, and a portion of the nucleus (*N*) shows. *Fixation: Osmium.* × *57,000.*
B. Similar structures (*arrow*) may be the same type but appear different because of the different fixation. A fat vacuole (*F*) is also present. × *53,000.*
C. This cytoplasmic inclusion (*in*) is filled with some flocculated material. × *53,000.*

FIGURE 5-8. Small lymphocytes.
These lymphocytes in a lymph node show variation in cytoplasmic density. Portion of cell at upper right corner and cell at lower left have essentially the same electron density. The central cell and one in upper left corner are more electron-lucent. There is no other significant difference in their morphology. The nuclei (*N*) and mitochondria (*M*) are similar, as are the Golgi complexes (*G*). × *16,500.*

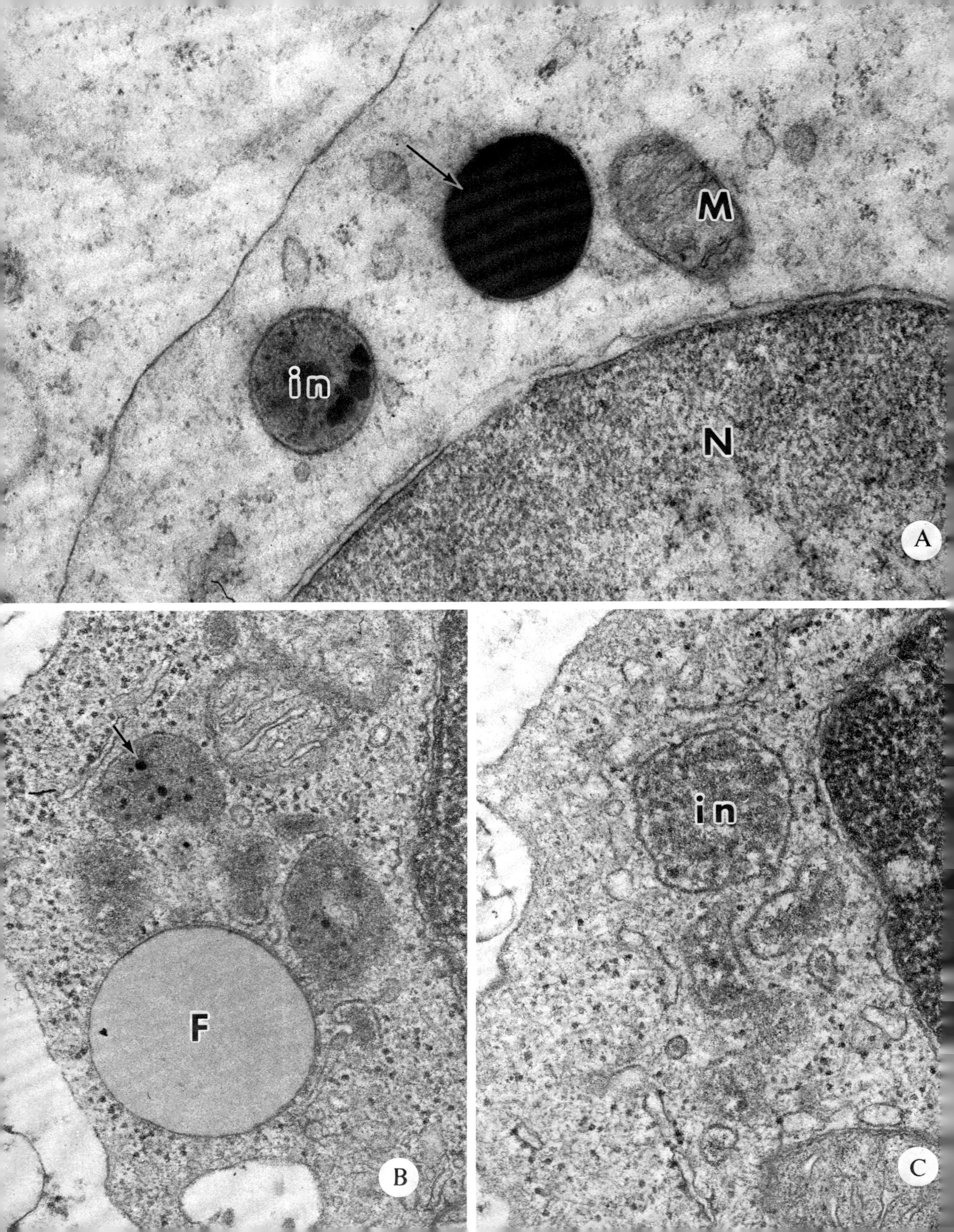

M
in
N
A
F
B
in
C

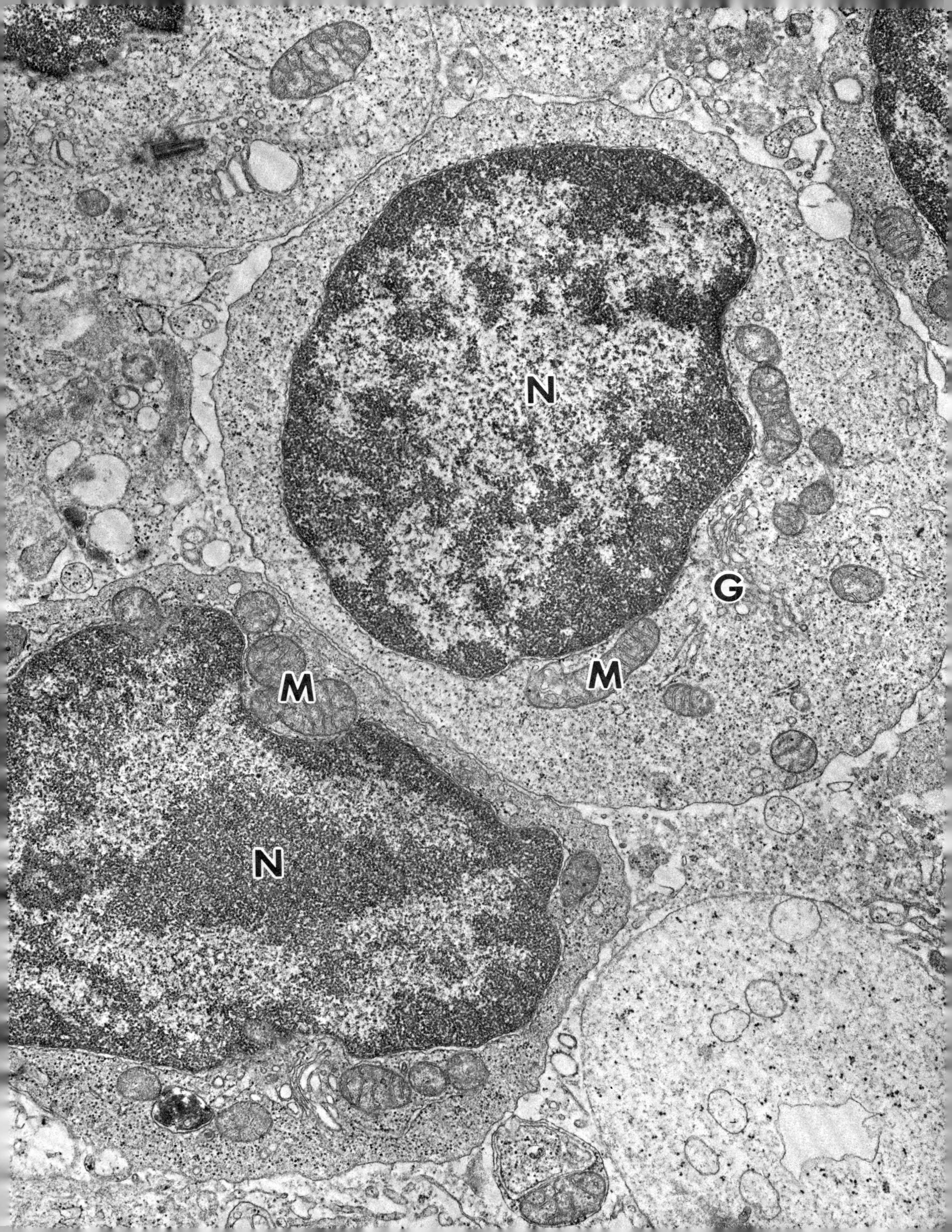
N
G
M
M
N

lymphoblasts, or are nonlymphatic mononuclear cells.

In stained smears the nuclei of small lymphocytes appear round; those of the larger lymphocytes are frequently indented. The chromatin shows a dense but coarse flocculation and is more reticular in larger cells, which occasionally show one nucleolus. The cytoplasm is a sky-blue color and granules are usually absent except for a few azurophilic types. These granules have a negative reaction in peroxidase but are positive in acid phosphatase. In supravital preparation, the cell is motile and moves in a characteristic "hand-mirror" manner. Phase microscopy of living lymphocytes confirms all the characteristics of cells in smear preparation—e.g., the large nucleus with dense chromatin aggregation and clear cytoplasm. Frequently, refractile granules called Gall's bodies can be observed.

Small lymphocytes have few ultrastructural characteristics which distinguish them from lymphoblasts (Figs. 5-2 and 5-3) other than their smaller size. The nucleus is generally round but frequently indented; the chromatin is condensed in the middle of the nucleus and commonly resembles a nucleolus. The narrow rim of the cytoplasm has a few large mitochondria and a poorly developed Golgi area (Figs. 5-2, 5-3, and 5-6). Endoplasmic reticulum is rarely seen. Single ribosomes are generally small and suggest an inactive state. Infrequently, glycogen granules and various cytoplasmic inclusions (Figs. 5-2, 5-3, and 5-7) can be observed in the cytoplasm; intranuclear fibrils (Stefani and Tonaki, 1970) and peculiar cytoplasmic inclusions (Hovig *et al.,* 1968) have also been reported.

Tissue-Infiltrating Cells

Various forms of lymphocyte-like cells are found by ultrastructural study of lymphoid tissues. Except for a few modifications, the structures of these cells are similar to those of the typical circulating lymphocytes (Fig. 5-8). These cells are frequently observed in the peripheral blood, compose a minority of the small lymphocyte population, and may be observed more frequently in tissues where lymphoid infiltration has taken place. Their functional significance is unknown. They may be a variant of typical small blood lymphocytes or lymphocytes with different activities. This observation fits the modern concept of lymphocyte physiology in that they are heterogeneous in function and life span.

Another type of lymphocyte-like cells is that which has developed an endoplasmic reticulum (Fig. 5-9). However, the development of endoplasmic reticulum is insufficient for them to be defined as plasma cells, and their state of maturation is too advanced for them to qualify as plasma cell precursors. Their nature or function is not clear. In lymphoid organs and many other connective tissues, occasional cells are observed with all the lymphocyte characteristics, but with a highly indented nucleus similar to nuclei seen in Sézary cells (Fig. 5-27*C,D.*). The morphology resembles that of graft-rejecting cells (Wiener *et al.,* 1964). Brief descriptions of both types are given in subsequent sections.

Two functionally different types of lymphoid cells are present in chickens (thymus- and bursa-derived) (Good *et al.,* 1966). Attempts to delineate the ultrastructural difference of lymphocytes in two different organ systems show only differences in cell size and polyribosome content (Clawson *et al.,* 1967; Heiniger *et al.,* 1967). These morphological markers are nonspecific and vary considerably during cell differentiation or active proliferation and thus would not be useful in determining the lymphocyte identity in different organs.

THORACIC DUCT LYMPHOCYTES

Thoracic duct lymph has been used to study lymphocyte physiology because large amounts are easily available in experimental animals and its cellular content is almost exclusively lymphocytic. Stained smears show a wide variation in lymphocyte size. They are generally classified as large, medium, and small types, on the basis of morphological characteristics, the nuclear index, or the relative ratio of the nuclear to cytoplasmic diameters. In guinea pigs, approximate percentages of each group are 2.7 per cent for the large cells and 97 per cent for the small lymphocytes (Reinhardt and Yoffey, 1957). This figure may not be correct since the cells classified as small lymphocytes may contain large numbers of medium-sized lymphocytes (Everett *et al.,* 1960). Many large lymphocytes of thoracic duct lymph incorporate radioactive thymidine, suggesting that they are capable of mitosis (Gowans, 1959; Everett, *et al.,* 1960). The predominant group of small lymphocytes is considered to be a nondividing population, since most of the cells do not incorporate tritiated thymidine (Gowans, 1959; Everett *et al.,* 1960). The ratio of these forms varies both with species and age, and is affected by hormonal and nutritional conditions: The large lymphocytes are 2.7 per cent of the cells in the adult guinea pig lymph (Reinhardt and Yoffey, 1957), 25 to 35 per cent in the dog (Perry *et al.,* 1959), and 2 to 15 per cent in sheep and lambs.

Electron microscopic study on the human thoracic lymphocytes made by Zucker-Franklin (1963a) stressed the heterogeneity of collected cells. The published pictures demonstrate that the major formed elements of thoracic duct lymph are small lymphocytes with variations. The latter include nuclear indentation and a chromatin condensation in the middle of the nucleus which resembles the nucleolus. The cytoplasm of these elements frequently contains multivesicular bodies and fibrillar structures. A few large cells appear to be hemocytoblasts, and a larger number, immature lymphocytes. Also, 1 to 2 per cent of these thoracic duct cells have endoplasmic reticulum which resembles that seen in cells in macroglobulinemia or the blastic forms classified by Hall *et al.,* (1967). These cells should not be regarded as lymphocytes at the ultrastructural level. A study of thoracic duct lymph of calves has demonstrated a high population (10 per cent) of plasma cells and their precursors (Weber and Joel, 1966). In mice, developing and mature plasma cells comprise 1.4 per cent of the total thoracic duct lymph cells, and the percentage increases slightly during prolonged lymph drainage (Wivel *et al.,* 1970). Heterogeneity of thoracic duct lymph cells could be expected to be greater after antigens or infections had stimulated regional lymph nodes, as the variation of formed elements in the lymph fluid should reflect the variation in cell stimulation of the supplying lymph nodes. This problem was investigated by Feldman and Nordquist (1967) in rats, but surprisingly, the population of lymphocytes did not change significantly in immunized animals. According to their observation on the stimulated animals, 94 to 96 per cent of thoracic duct cells are lymphocytes, and only 4 to 5 per cent comprise cells of other types. Morse and Reister (1967) compared blood lymphocytosis to that of thoracic duct lymph after pertussis infection in mice and noted that significant lymphocytosis in the blood

(text continues on page 232)

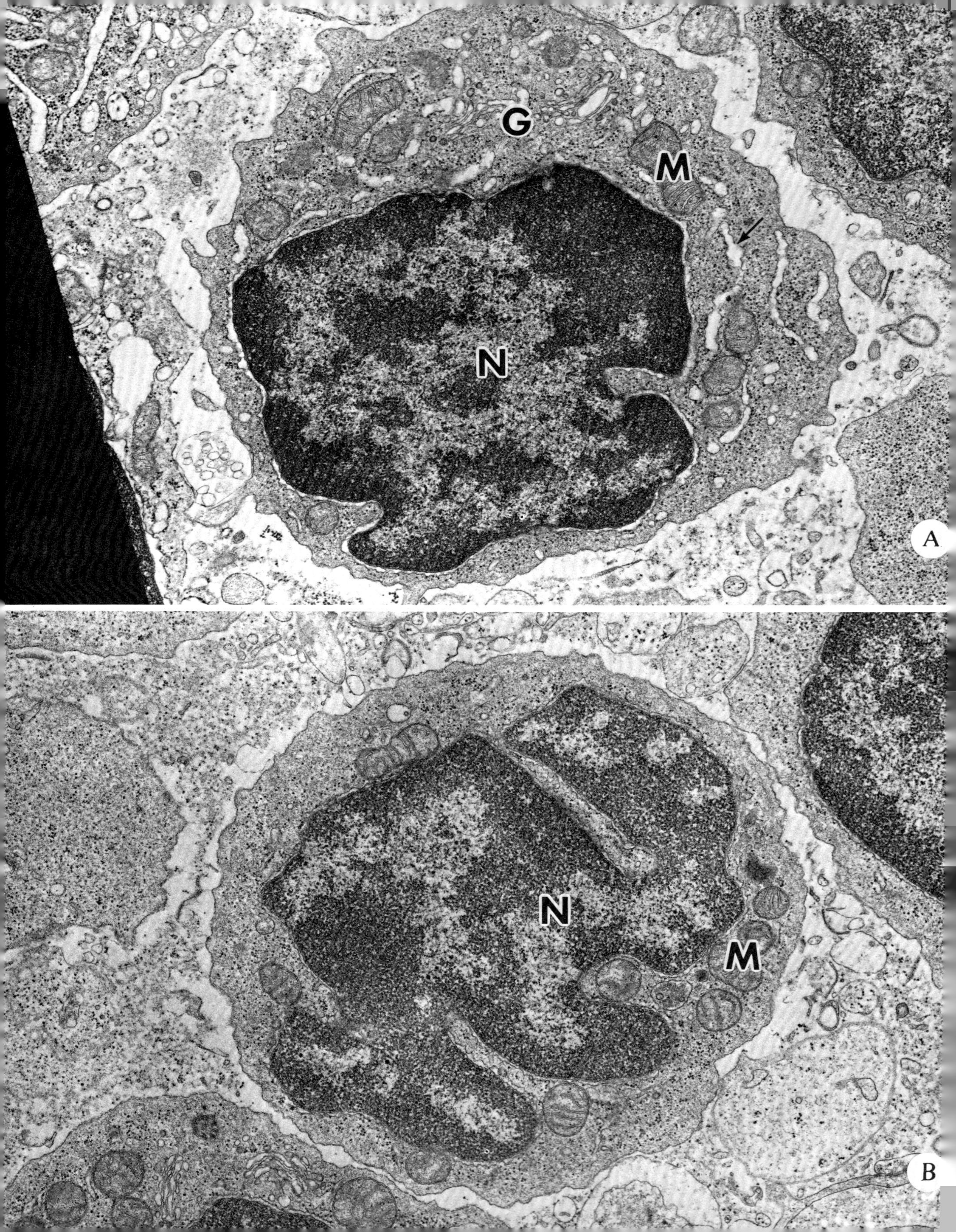
G
M
N
A
N
M
B

FIGURE 5-9. Occasional atypical lymphocytes in lymph nodes.

A. This larger lymphocyte has considerable distention of endoplasmic reticulum cisternae (*arrow*). Mitochondria (*M*) are prominent and large near the Golgi apparatus (*G*). $\times$ *10,500.*

B. Lymphoid cell with indented nuclear (*N*) margin. Mitochondria (*M*) are prominent. $\times$ *10,500.*

Figures 5-10 and 5-11 appear on the following pages

FIGURE 5-10. Transformed lymphocyte.

This lymphocyte from human peripheral blood was incubated for 72 hours. The cellular margin is highly irregular, with numerous cytoplasmic projections; the nucleus (*N*) has a diffuse pattern of chromatin and a large prominent nucleolus (*Nu*). The extensive cytoplasm has a well-developed Golgi complex (*G*), large mitochondria (*M*), and several profiles of endoplasmic reticulum (*er*). There are many scattered ribosomes and polyribosomes. The spherule (*F*) is probably a fat vacuole. $\times$ *15,000.*

FIGURE 5-11. Golgi area of transformed lymphocyte.

In the vicinity of the Golgi complex are a centriole (*Ce*), many microtubules (*mt*), numerous vesicles (*v*), some with lamellated structures (*arrows*), mitochondria (*M*), and two fat (*F*) droplets. $\times$ *55,000.*

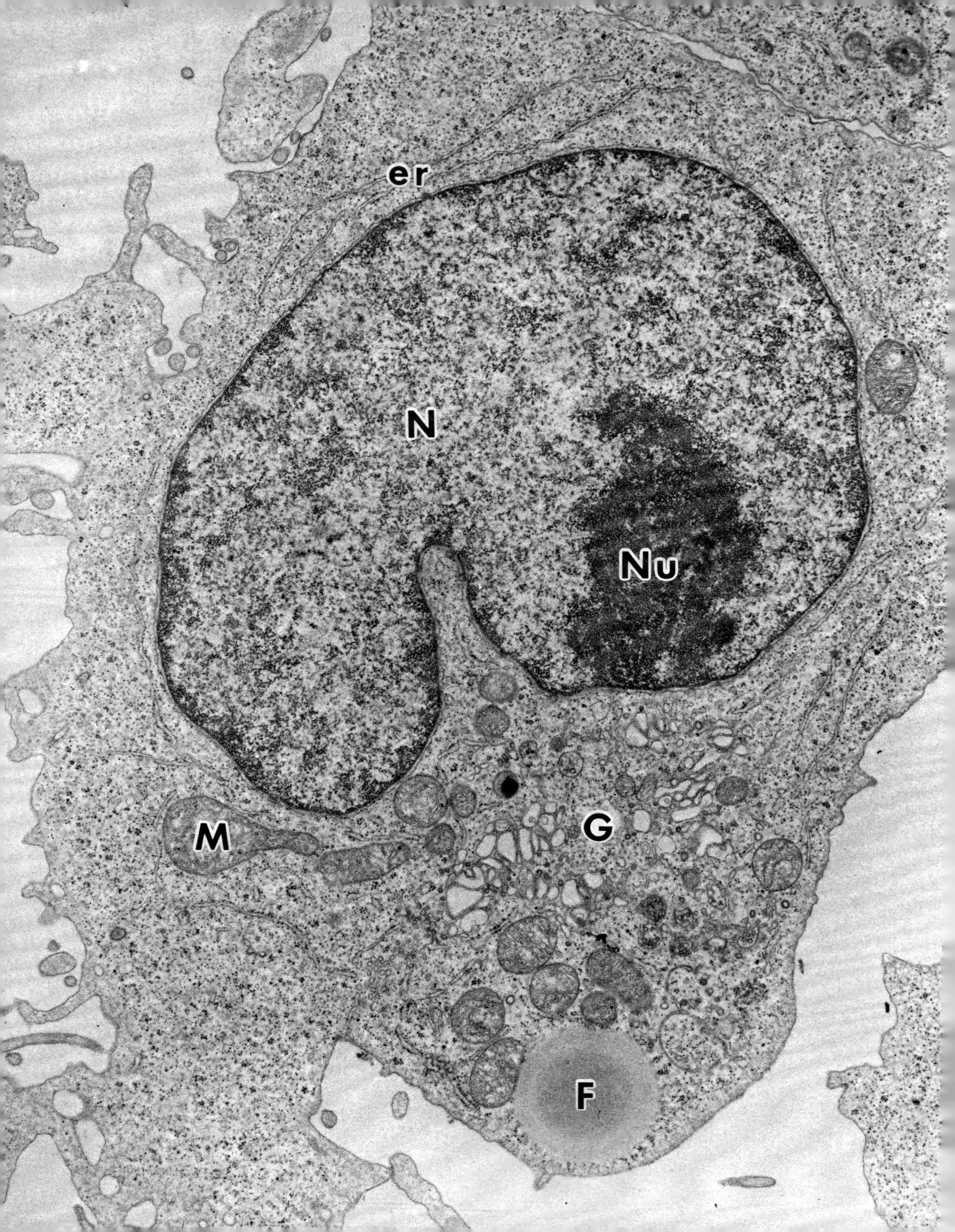
er
N
Nu
M
G
F

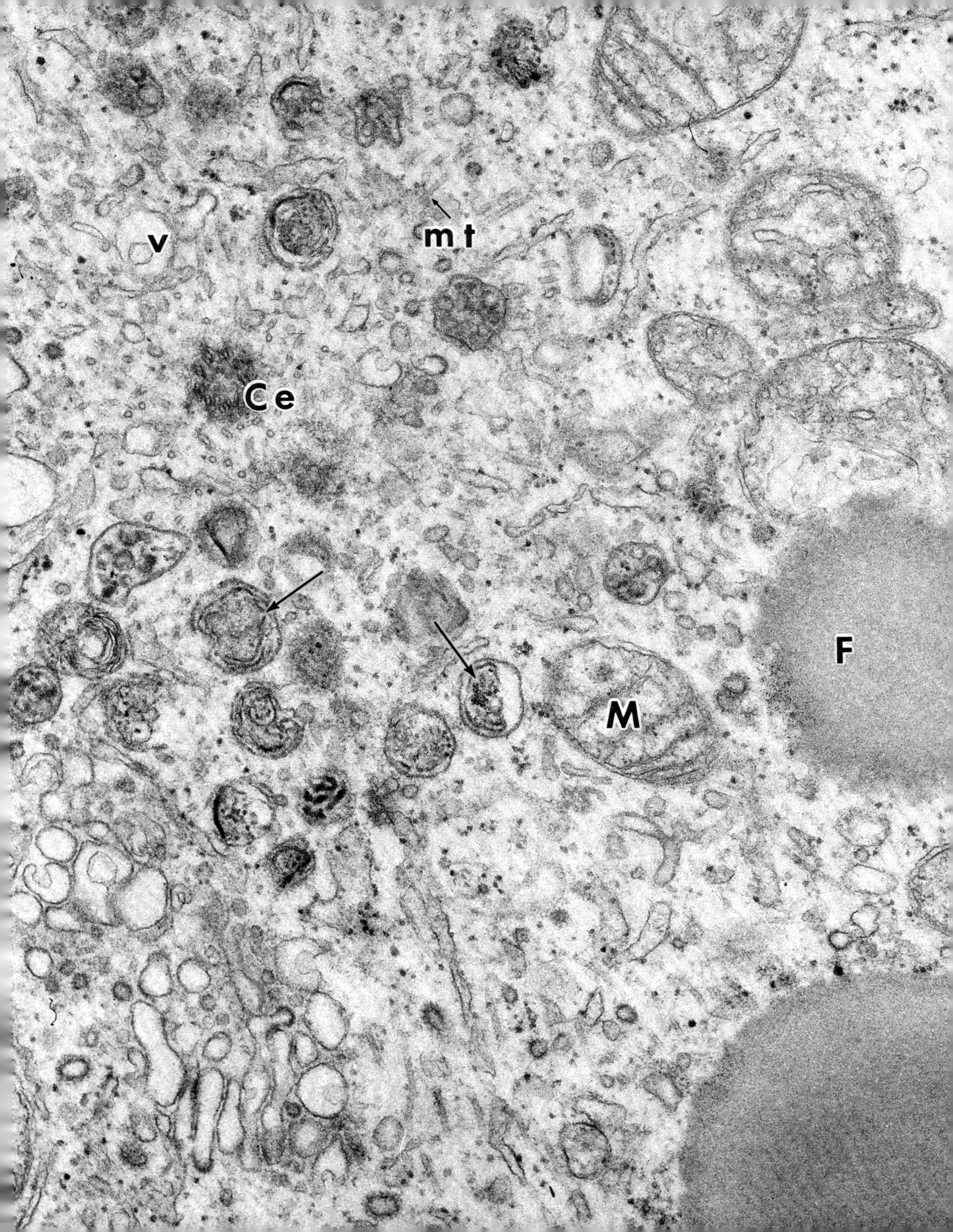

v
mt
Ce
F
M

was produced by the rapid release of preformed lymphocytes into the blood directly from the regional lymph nodes. Total lymphocytosis in the thoracic duct lymph seemed to be decreased. This suggests that the rapid peripheral lymphocytosis is achieved by the mobilization of lymphocytes through nonthoracic duct channels and explains the insignificant alteration of thoracic duct lymphocytes produced by peripheral lymph node infection.

CULTURED LYMPHOCYTES

Proliferation of peripheral blood cells in vitro was first described by Awrorow and Timofejewsky (1914) in a culture of leukemic blood. Maximow (1927b) considered the dividing cells to be lymphocytes or monocytes, on the basis of a smooth sequence of transitional cells from small lymphocytes to macrophages, polyblasts, or fibroblasts. This was not developed further until lymphocytes were identified as proliferating leukocytes, when blood cells were incubated with phytohemagglutinin (Hungerford *et al.*, 1959; MacKinney *et al.*, 1962). Transformation of lymphocytes can be induced by the administration of pokeweed mitogen (Chessin *et al.*, 1966), antigens (Pearmain *et al.*, 1963; Cowling and Quaglino, 1964), mixed leukocyte culture (Bain *et al.*, 1964) and mercury (Schöpf *et al.*, 1967). The technic of stimulating leukocytes is currently used to measure histocompatibility (Bach and Hirschhorn, 1964) and to study the mechanisms of mitosis, as a model for analysis of drug effect and for clinical diagnosis. The topic has been reviewed by Robbins (1964).

Transformation of lymphocytes is first recognized about 24 hours after stimulation with suitable agents. There is a slight morphological alteration as they become larger, with increasing cytoplasmic basophilia. During the first 24 hours, most granulocytes undergo degeneration. Morphological alterations of lymphocytes are more apparent after 48 hours of incubation. The cell alterations and the presence of heterogeneous groups have been clearly defined by light microscopy (Yoffey *et al.*, 1965). By electron microscopy, the proliferating cells show all the characteristics of lymphocytes (Tanaka *et al.*, 1963), and Bernhard and Leplus (1964) have pointed out the striking similarity between transformed cells and hemocytoblasts of lymphoid organs. A typical transformed cell is shown in Figure 5-10. Cells are large, some with diameters of nearly 30μ. They have a large nucleus with indentation and usually a large, distinctive nucleolus. The chromatin network is diffusely reticular. The periphery of these transformed cells is irregular and cytoplasmic projections are commonly seen. A moderately developed Golgi apparatus is seen near the nuclear indentation, with various forms of vesicular elements and granulation in or near this area (Fig. 5-11). These latter structures are rich in acid phosphatase, probably lysosomal in nature (Tanaka and Liddy, 1966).

The extensive cytoplasm has many polyribosomes, large mitochondria, and an occasional neutral fat vacuole; electron-opaque spheres, which probably contain protein, are less common. The tubular endoplasmic reticulum is usually not prevalent in phytohemagglutinin-stimulated lymphocytes. The endoplasmic reticulum is particularly pronounced in the transformed lymphyocytes treated with pokeweed mitogen (Douglas *et al.*, 1967) or antigen (Michalowski *et al.*, 1966). Occasionally, transformed cells have significant amounts of a fibrillar structures (Fig. 5-12), the significance of which is not clear, but similar structures are commonly noted in cells of reticuloendothelial system (Tanaka, 1964).

CELLS IN ANTIBODY FORMATION

At least three groups of cells are considered to be the source of circulating antibody: plasma cells, lymphocytes, and a type of nonphagocytic reticulum cells. A brief description of immunological reactions in tissues will help to elucidate this concept.

A single antigenic stimulus to an animal induces antibody production which lasts for about a month or longer and is usually restricted to the local lymph node. This is called a primary response. A second challenge to the animal with the same antigen will produce a rapid increase in circulating antibody and is a generalized response. This reaction is called a secondary or anamnestic response. The amounts of antibody produced in the secondary response often exceed a few hundred times the level produced in the primary response. During these two responses, high molecular weight, rapidly sedimenting (19S) IgM antibody molecules appear first in the circulation, and are later replaced by (7S) IgG antibody. The increase in IgG coincides with the plasmacytosis that develops in lymph nodes following an antigenic stimulus. Phylogentically, production of IgM antibody has been detected in lower vertebrates, but the production of IgG antibody is limited to more advanced species (Papermaster *et al.,* 1964).

Antibody production in both primary and secondary responses have been studied by Uhr and Finkelstein (1963) and Svehag and Mandel (1964a,b). The anamnestic production of IgG (7S) antibody in the secondary reaction requires the threshold dose of antigen to be about 50 times higher than that needed for induction of IgM antibodies in the primary response. Because of the pronounced differences in antigen-dose requirement for induction and kinetics of IgM and IgG antibody formation, it has been suggested that different cells participate in the formation of the two antibodies. However, they need not be morphologically distinct, since plasma cells have been implicated as the producers of both IgM and IgG specific antibodies.

Although plasma cells have been shown to contribute to circulating IgG (Chap. 6), it is not clear which cells produce IgM antibodies. It has been suggested that cells with a lymphoid appearance may be producing IgM antibodies, on the basis of the histologic observation of the primary macroglobulinemia in which proliferation of lymphoid cells is common. Electron microscopic study of these cells reveals an extensive endoplasmic reticulum closely resembling that of plasma cells (see Figs. 6-31 through 6-35).

Zucker-Franklin (1969) described an intermediate cell between the lymphocyte and plasma cell in her study of peripheral blood from macroglobulinemia. Cells with a similar morphology are seen in lymph nodes after antigenic stimulation and are considered to be precursors of plasma cells. They are observed as transient forms and disappear at a later stage. Many investigators have observed similar cells in efferent lymph after antigenic stimulation in local tissues (Hummeler *et al.,* 1966; Hall *et al.,* 1967; Bosman *et al.,* 1969). Hummeler *et al.* (1966) found that they may contain either IgM or IgG class.

Reticulum cells and their direct descendants have also been suggested as IgM antibody producers. The appearance of a positive reaction for immunoglobulin (IgM), which seems to correspond to mesenchymal elements of the germinal

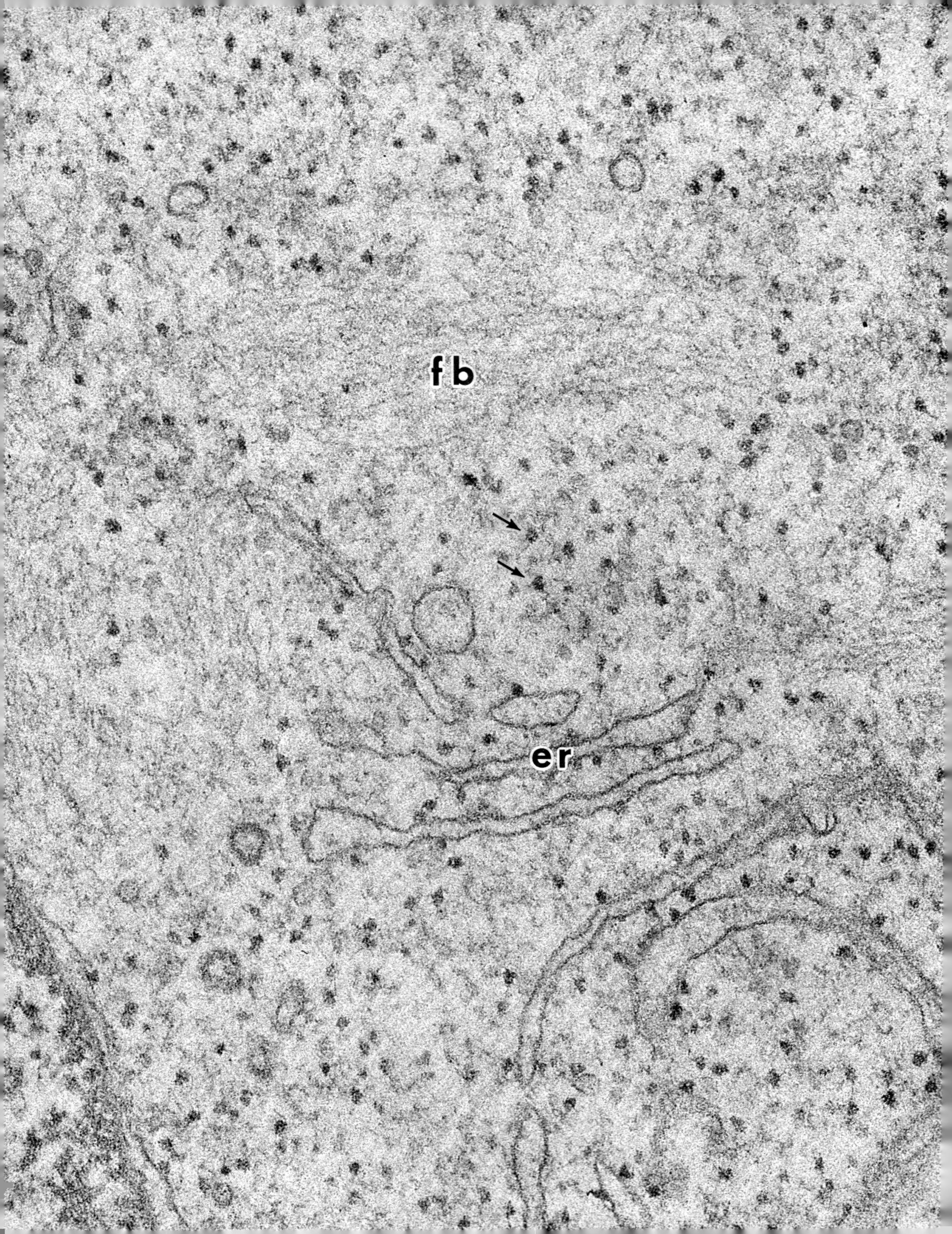
fb
er

center in the primary response (Maruyama and Masuda, 1964) and the presence of macroglobulinemia in reticulum cell malignancies, suggests such activity. Electron microscopically, cells with distended endoplasmic reticulum are noted frequently in such malignancies. There may be a wider spectrum of cells producing IgM molecules than those involved in IgG molecule production.

The presence of two different antibodies in single cells has also been shown both in vivo and in vitro (Mellors and Korngold, 1963; Nossal *et al.,* 1964). Immune cells that might produce more than one class of immunoglobulins were estimated to be as high as 19 per cent in isolated cells (Nossal *et al.,* 1964). However, lymphoid tissues studied by immunofluorescent methods revealed this phenomenon to be rare (Bernier and Cebra, 1965; Cebra *et al.,* 1966) and of doubtful significance in suspended cells analyzed by hemolytic plaque method (Merchant and Brahmi, 1970).

In a study of antibody-forming cells at the single cell level, Harris *et al.* (1966) observed that lymphocytic cells of small size with a small amount of distended endoplasmic reticulum and cells with typical plasma cell morphology, produce IgM antibody. They also detected IgG antibody in the cells of all three morphological types; however, no typical small lymphocytes without endoplasmic reticulum have shown a positive reaction. Cell-bound antibodies have been demonstrated to be closely related to lymphocytes, but it is not clear whether lymphocytes produce this antibody or are only involved in its transport by surface absorption (see section on function).

CYTOGENESIS

CYTOGENESIS IN THE EMBRYO AND CHILD

In man, lymphocytes are not seen in the circulation of the early embryo, and no lymphocytopoiesis occurs in hepatic hematopoiesis. This observation suggests that the genesis of the lymphocytes appears first in embryonal circulation near and after the formation of the thymus, around the third embryonal month; thereafter, lymph nodes develop near the preformed lymph plexus and are completed by the termination of intrauterine life. In rodents, lymphocytogenesis is found only in the thymus before birth, and the formation of spleen and lymph nodes develops after birth.

A thymic role in lymphocytogenesis is generally accepted. In experimental animals, three observations have produced evidence for the thymic contribution: (1) Removal of the thymus within 24 hours after birth results in a significant depression of both lymphoid tissue development and immunological tolerance (Arnason *et al.,* 1962; Waksman *et al.,* 1962). (2) The wasting syndrome of thymectomized newborn may be prevented by the injection of lymphoid cell suspension (Martinez *et al.,* 1964). (3) Migration of labeled lymphocytes can be followed from the thymus to peripheral organs

FIGURE 5-12. Transformed lymphocyte.
Very fine fibrils (*fb*) are found in cytoplasm of a transformed lymphocyte. There is some endoplasmic reticulum (*er*) with only a few attached ribosomes and many freely dispersed single ribosomes (*arrows*). × *120,000.*

(Murray and Woods, 1964; Weissman, 1967). These experiments suggest that the thymus influences the development of lymphoid organs. Aplasia or hypoplasia of thymus in early childhood is frequently associated with impaired immunological reaction (Good *et al.,* 1966), and suggests a similar mechanism in man. In mice, the stem cells for thymic lymphocytes are provided from the circulation at days 10 and 11 of gestation (Owen and Ritter, 1969). The findings in chickens during early embryonal life are similar. The origin of the cells responsible for thymic lymphogenesis is not clearly understood at present (St. Pierre, 1969).

The bursa of Fabricius contributes to the production of antibody-forming cells in chickens (Good *et al.,* 1966). This concept gives the bursa of fowls the progenitory activity of lymphogenesis and provides the mother cells of short-lived lymphocytes which eventually form the antibody-producing cells (plasma cells) in the germinal center of lymph nodes. The thymus provides the progenitors of the long-lived lymphocytes, involved chiefly in cell-mediated immune reactions. Cooper *et al.* (1966) have proposed that the intestinal lymph apparatus (Peyer's patches) is the mammalian equivalent to the bursa of Fabricius of chickens, but there is little experimental support for this idea.

CYTOGENESIS IN THE ADULT

At least four major loci have been proposed for the site of small lymphocyte production in adults; the most popular and classic concept is their origin in generalized lymphatic tissue. It has been accepted for a long time that lymphocytes in man are formed primarily in or near lymph follicles from the immature mesenchymal compartment and mature into small lymphocytes through mitosis. In support of this view are the finding of significant enlargement of lymphocyte cuffs in regional lymph nodes after stimulation by various antigens and the presence of many mitotic cells in these nodes. Newly formed lymphocytes are found in efferent ducts of thymidine-infused nodes. There is not a complete loss of the lymphocyte cuff by elimination of the recirculation or by the absence of other organs which generate lymphocytes. Though there is controversy on the relations between the cells in the germinal center and surrounding follicles (Fliedner *et al.,* 1964; Wakefield and Thorbecke, 1968), it is likely that lymphocyte production is operative in generalized lymph tissue in postnatal life. It is not necessary to conclude that immature compartments of lymph tissues are the only source of new lymphocytes. One can predict that transformation of recirculating lymphocytes occurs in the lymph nodes after they have had contact with suitable antigens.

Three other loci—thymus, bone marrow, and bursa of Fabricius in fowls or intestinal associated lymph tissues (Peyer's patches) in mammals—have been proposed as primary sites of lymphocyte production. The significance of these organs in adult lymphocytogenesis is not easily approached. The thymus in human adults becomes atrophic without a significant effect on lymphocyte production. The thymus in adult rodents decreases in size and activity but does function to produce lymphocytes after a sublethal dose of radiation. Recently, bone marrow control of thymic regeneration was shown in adult rats during the recovery of the organ after irradiation (Takeda *et al.,* 1969). This topic should be reexamined in relation to the stem cell problem, since that concept involves the lymphocyte generation by the bone marrow stem cells. There is very little information on Peyer's patches of the intestines in man, and some of the data from lower mammalian forms may not be applicable.

The heterogeneity of lymphocyte life span has been demonstrated by cytokinetic studies of lymphocyte regeneration. In rats, multiple injections (Caffrey *et al.*, 1962) and continuous infusion of labeled thymidine (Little *et al.*, 1962; Robinson *et al.*, 1965) revealed the presence of two populations of small lymphocytes. One group with a long life span recirculates from blood to lymph and back. From 5 to 8 per cent of circulating small lymphocytes in rats had a life span exceeding 270 days. Two-thirds of the small lymphocytes in the blood, 90 per cent of those in the thoracic duct lymph, and about 20 to 30 per cent of those in the mesenteric lymph nodes are long-lived (Everett *et al.*, 1964). In the second group, studies have shown that all small lymphocytes of bone marrow, 90 per cent of those in the thymus, and most of those in the spleen are of the short-lived type. Most of the short-lived lymphocytes in the thymus disappear from that organ (St. Pierre, 1969), while the few long-lived types emigrate into the circulation (Weissman, 1967).

The total number of thoracic duct lymphocytes delivered during 24 hours is sufficient to replace the total blood lymphocyte population four to five times (Sjövall, 1936). Thus, the recirculation of large numbers of lymphocytes was suspected and verified by Gowans (1959), using labeling technics. Many of the labeled thoracic duct lymphocytes entering the blood escape during the lymph node passage near the postcapillary venules (Marchesi and Gowans, 1964). These recirculating lymphocytes are small, migrate in the lymph nodes around the follicles, and form the so-called lymphocyte cuff. These cells mobilize, upon stimulation, into the efferent lymph and reappear in the general circulation.

Thus, the elimination of a selected population can be accomplished by the combined technic of thoracic duct lymph cannulation and extracorporal irradiation of peripheral blood (Cronkite *et al.*, 1964). By this method, about 90 per cent of small lymphocytes of the peripheral blood and most of those in the thoracic duct are eliminated. The failure to eliminate small lymphocytes from peripheral blood completely suggests that there is a nonrecirculating population in the peripheral blood which may enter the bloodstream through channels other than the thoracic duct. Yoffey (1960) used the term "supplementary lymphocytes" to describe this group. The ratio of supplementary lymphocytes to thoracic duct lymphocytes is surprisingly high, estimated at four to six times in calves (Cronkite *et al.*, 1962).

FUNCTION

Lymphocytes are widely distributed in various organs and are prominent in circulating blood, yet their function has been poorly understood. Many roles have been proposed for these cells. Some of these concepts are summarized here briefly; the basis for them will be found elsewhere. The conclusions may change as more data are obtained.

BODY DEFENSE MECHANISMS

Lymphocytes have long been considered to be involved in body defense mechanisms. Their increased presence in tissue is a common feature of the inflammatory process, particularly in chronic granulomatous infections. However, their limited morphology by light microscopy and uncertain physiological activity have provided little insight about their true activity in inflammation.

Passive transfer studies have shown that lymphocytes can transfer delayed hypersensitivity and "second set" allograft rejection (Chase, 1945; Lawrence, 1949; Wesslen, 1952). Lymphocytes are now known to be directly involved in cell-mediated immune responses, such as delayed hypersensitivity, allograft rejection, graft-versus-host reaction and autoimmunity. An extensive discussion of this subject has been recently presented by Meuwissen *et al.* (1969).

The effects produced in cell-mediated responses progress slowly and are in general pleomorphic. In extreme conditions, a destruction of antigenic host tissues (or cells) can be expected. This phenomenon has been produced experimentally in vitro (Govaerts, 1960; Rosenau and Moon, 1961). The lymphocytes responsible for this reaction are speculated to be the recirculating, long-lived type originating from the thymus, since removal of this organ suppresses the phenomenon (Arnason *et al.,* 1962). By electron microscopy, these cells have been identified as plasma cells (Weiss, 1968), or lymphocytes (Able *et al.,* 1970). The interaction between sensitized lymphocytes and antigenic host tissues (or cells) is highly specific. Many think that sensitized lymphocytes carry specific antibody bound to the cell membrane, but no clear explanation has been given on how the lymphocyte recognizes antigens and forms or absorbs the antibodies matching them.

Other facets of lymphocyte involvement in body defense mechanisms are being investigated. Small lymphocytes are important for immunoglobulin synthesis. They contain the antigen-sensitive cells of a primary response and the carriers of "immunological memory" (Gowans and Uhr, 1966).

CELL GENERATION

The concept of a monophyletic origin of blood-forming organs with "lymphoid cells" as the progenitor of all myelolymphocytic elements was supported by Maximow and his students. Further analysis of the morphology and physiology of lymphoid cells separated the blastic forms of the erythromyelocyte groups from the lymphocytes. This polyphyletic approach considered the small lymphocytes of peripheral blood and lymph nodes as end cell states incapable of division. These small "terminal stage" lymphocytes were thought to represent a differentiated cell line, comparable to the erythrocyte and granulocyte. In 1956, Yoffey and Courtice proposed that these small lymphocytes were a specialized form of primitive mesenchyma in a resting, relatively inactive state. Although this concept was not fully accepted, since the relationship of these cells to other mesenchymal elements was not established, the theory raised enough doubts to challenge the concept that the small lymphocyte was an end cell.

More direct challenge arose from observing the lymphocytic response to phytohemagglutinin (Hungerford *et al.,* 1959) and other cytogenic agents, in which the small lymphocytes in peripheral blood enlarge and proliferate upon stimulation. Studies on the survival of lethally irradiated mice demonstrated that injection of myeloid tissues could prevent radiation death by regeneration of hematopoiesis from transfused donor tissues. However, infusion of lymphoid cells from thoracic duct lymph could not prevent death of the animal (Gesner and Gowans, 1962). Infused donor cells from myeloid tissues proliferated and formed colonies of erythromyelomegakaryocytic variety in the spleen of sublethally irradiated mice (Till and McCulloch, 1961; Becker *et al.,* 1963). Cells from lymph nodes and thymus of both phytohemagglutinin-treated mice (Mekori *et al.,* 1965; Curry *et al.,* 1967) and untreated donor mice (Curry *et al.,* 1967) primarily produced lymphoid colonies. This evidence suggests that the small lymphocytes probably do not function as the pluripotential progenitors in hematopoietic cell generation.

TREPHOCYTES

The role of lymphocytes as trephocytes was suggested almost a century ago, on the basis of the observation that thymic cells contain abundant nucleic acids which are important in nucleoprotein synthesis. Some predicted that nucleic acids released upon lysis of the lymphocytes in peripheral organs were reutilized in new cell production. Therefore, lymphocytes are considered to be storage cells for nucleic acids and to deliver them to the peripheral tissues for nourishment. Lymphocyte DNA was shown to be reutilized in peripheral organs (Bryant, 1963). Since the breakdown of the nuclear DNA and its reutilization could occur in the degeneration processes of any cells, the phenomenon is not considered as the specific function of lymphocytes.

PATHOLOGY

INFECTIOUS MONONUCLEOSIS

This acute infection involving the generalized lymphatic system was described first by Pfeiffer in 1889 under the name of "Drüsenfieber." The presence of many atypical leukocytes in the circulation often led to a misdiagnosis of this condition as leukemia. The term "infectious mononucleosis" was introduced by Sprunt and Evans (1920) to describe an acute illness accompanying an abnormal blood picture. The illness was later identified as the disorder previously known as Drüsenfieber. Detailed morphology of the circulating mononuclear cells was described by Downey and McKinlay (1923). Pathognomonic serological reaction was developed by Paul and Bunnell in 1932. Many causative agents have been suggested, recently herpesvirus (Moses *et al.,* 1968) and Ebstein-Barr virus (Niederman *et al.,* 1968).

Downey and McKinlay (1923) distinguished three types of abnormal mononuclear cells in the circulation and their classification became a standard for describing abnormal lymphocytes in peripheral blood. Type 1 cells, the major form of abnormal cells in this disorder, appear somewhat pleomorphic in shape and size. The nuclear chromatin forms a coarse network, and the nucleus is in a slightly eccentric position. Lobulation of the nucleus is common and has led to the use of the descriptive term "leukocytoid" lymphocytes. The cytoplasm, is vacuolated, foamy, or mottled in appearance and contains azurophilic granules. Type 2 cells are larger, with a more distinctive chromatin pattern. Neither nuclear lobulation nor cytoplasmic vacuolation is common. These cells rarely have azurophilic granules. Type 3 cells are the least common and more closely resemble leukemic cells; this latter interpretation may originate from the atypical nuclear appearance of these cells. The cytoplasm of this group is frequently intensely basophilic, and sometimes leads to their description as lymphoid cells with a plasma cell appearance.

Hematologically, peripheral blood has a mixture of the three types, with a predominance of one type. Many attempts have been made to determine the origin of these cells. These mononuclear cells may originate from infected lymph nodes of the upper respiratory tract since infected lymph nodes show a marked follicular hyperplasia in association with a reticulum cell proliferation. In imprint smears of nodes, primitive cells of 20 to 30μ, with pale basophilic cytoplasm, are seen frequently. Cytochemically, they show similar stain reaction patterns to the infectious mononucleosis cells of peripheral blood. Both lymphocytic and monohistiocytic origins of these atypical cells have been proposed, but there is still no conclusive evidence to determine which is correct. Cytochemical analysis shows them to be intermediate in reaction pattern between lymphocyte and monohistiocyte (Galbraith *et al.,* 1963). One of the more interesting cytochemical reactions is the presence of strong acid phosphatase, considered to be a unique feature of histiocytes. Production of both gamma globulin (van Furth *et al.,* 1966) and heterophil antibody (MacKinney, 1968) has also been demonstrated.

Attempts have been made to describe accurately the three types of cells classified by Downey by electron microscopy (Paegle, 1961; Schumacher *et al.,* 1969). Most of the mononuclear cells show the general characteristics of lymphocytes; however, many are larger and possess more organelles than ordinary lymphocytes and may be immunoblasts (Schumacher *et al.,* 1969). Large lymphoid cells with many polyribosomes, cells with lamellated endoplastic reticulum resembling plasma cells, and others with monohistiocytic characteristics have also been noted (Douglas *et al.,* 1969). Atypical lymphocytes, known as Türk's cells, also appear in peripheral blood in various viral infections and have been considered to be immature or mature plasma cells (Spriggs and Jerrome, 1967). These features indicate an activated condition of infected lymph nodes; however, the many mononuclear lymphoid cells in infectious mononucleosis cannot be interpreted simply as stimulated lymphocytes.

GRAFT REJECTION

Mononuclear cells accumulate around transplanted tissues during the initial stage of tissue rejection and are generally regarded as small lymphocytes. These cells may carry cell-bound antibody which reacts with antigenic host tissue and thus provokes the rejection phenomenon in tissue transplants. An interesting proposal was made by Wiener *et al.* (1964) in an electron microscopic study of skin graft rejection in rabbits. The investigators concluded that the round cells were not lymphocytes but belonged to an unknown cell category, and proposed the term "graft-rejecting cells." This observation is of interest since we have observed similar types of cells in normal and some pathological conditions.

An unidentified cell shown by Feldman and Nordquist (1967) in thoracic duct lymph may correspond to this group. The size of this cell is similar to that of the small lymphocyte, without much condensation of nuclear chromatin. The cytoplasm is less electron-opaque, because background material is absent. There are small vesicles with or without ribosomes in the cytoplasm. According to Wiener *et al.* (1964), these cells resemble the immunologically competent cells described by Binet and Mathé (1961). We have observed this type of cell quite frequently in both benign and malignant proliferation in peripheral organs, examples of which are seen in marrow granuloma and cells in Sézary's syndrome. The forms appear as transitional cells varying from medium to large nonphagocytic mesenchymal cells of the skin; the small type is not easily distinguished from a small lymphocyte. The cells could be activated forms of lymphocytes, but it is not known where they originate and their function is not clearly defined.

MALIGNANCY

Malignant proliferation involving the lymphatic apparatus was recognized by Malpighi (1666) at the middle of the seventeenth century; later, Hodgkin (1832) described similar fatal conditions. At the time when the concept of leukemia was established by Virchow (see Chap. 3) it was generally thought that all leukemic cells originated from lymph nodes or spleen; such a concept was still present at the beginning of the twentieth century. The term "Lymphosarkomatose" was introduced by Kundrat (1893) for the primary malignancy of lymph nodes. He stated that the disease extended chiefly through lymphatic, rather than blood, channels. The close relationship between systemic lymphosarcoma and leukemia was recognized by Türk (1903), who included both lymphocytic leukemia and lymphosarcoma under the present-day category of "lymphosarcoma." Later, Symmers (1918) included lymphocytic leukemia under the general manifestation of lymphosarcoma.

When the present concept of lymphocytic malignancies was developed, there was confusion in understanding the diffuse and tumorous forms of malignancy in blood-forming organs. At present, lymphocytic leukemia and lymphosarcoma are regarded within the same concept—i.e., as malignancy of the lymphocytic system, differing only in the mode of proliferation, whether generalized (leukemia) or localized (lymphosarcoma) or in combination (intermediate). Because of the importance of this malignancy in clinical medicine, extensive studies have been made (Dameshek and Gunz, 1964). Recent studies on lymphocyte physiology show double populations which are determined by the ontogenesis of lymphoid organs. The possibility that various clinical manifestations of lymphoid malignancies, such as leukemic and aleukemic forms, could reflect cytogenetic differences of malignant cells is only a speculation at present.

Lymphocytic Leukemia

This is presently understood to be a generalized form of lymphocyte malignancy which can be divided into two forms: acute and chronic.

Acute Lymphocytic Leukemia. This form is most frequently observed in children within the first 4 years of life. Because it is difficult to distinguish it from the acute form of myelogenous leukemia at the cytological level and because of its unique age distribution in early childhood, the condition is often categorized as acute childhood leukemia (Zuelzer and Flatz, 1960). Its onset is always associated with anemia, a low-grade fever, and enlargement of lymph apparatus in the later stages. Total leukocyte counts vary from slightly elevated to decreased. The presence of abnormal cells in the peripheral blood and bone marrow (Fig. 5-13) establishes the diagnosis. These abnormal cells are frequently indistinguishable from immature myelogenous cells. In

(text continues on page 246)

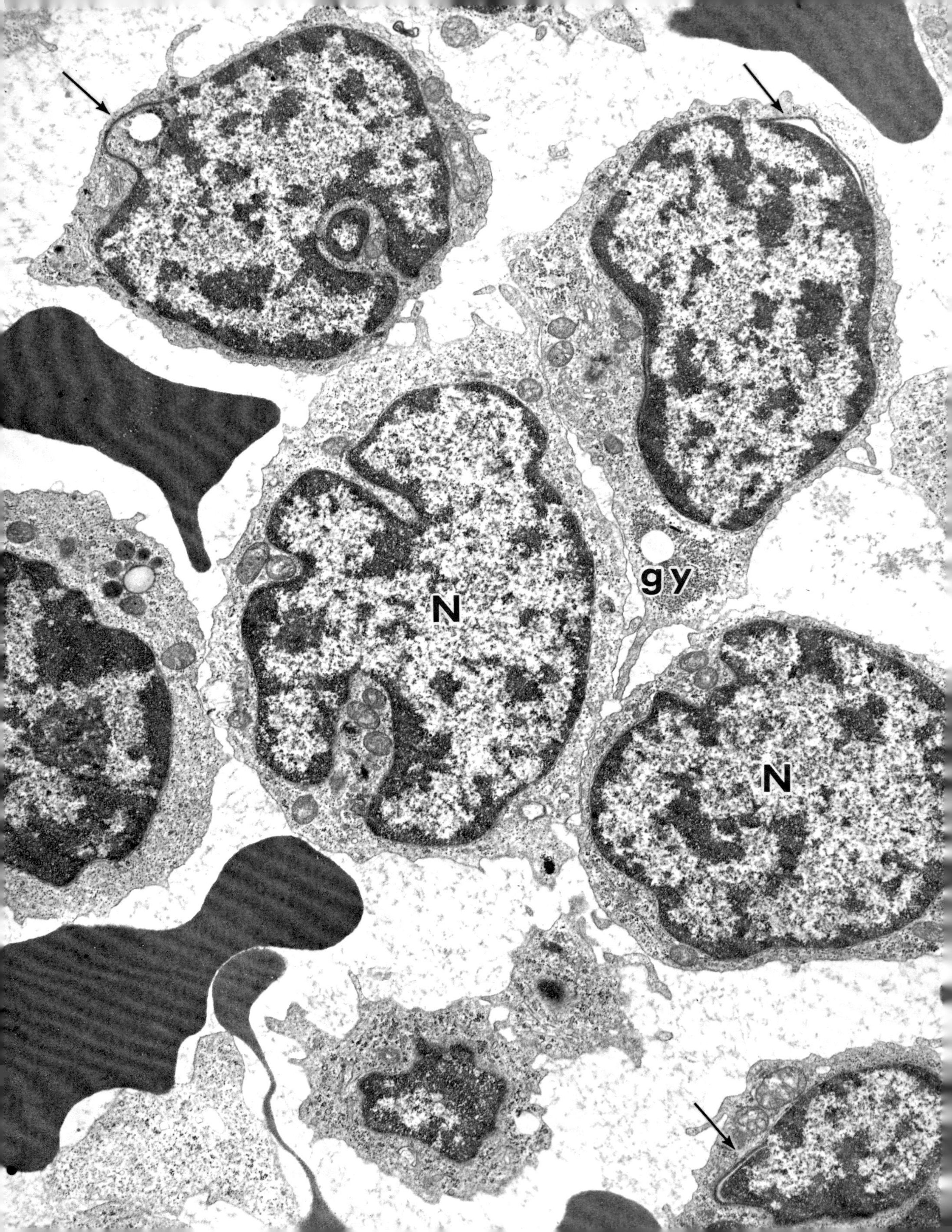
gy
N
N

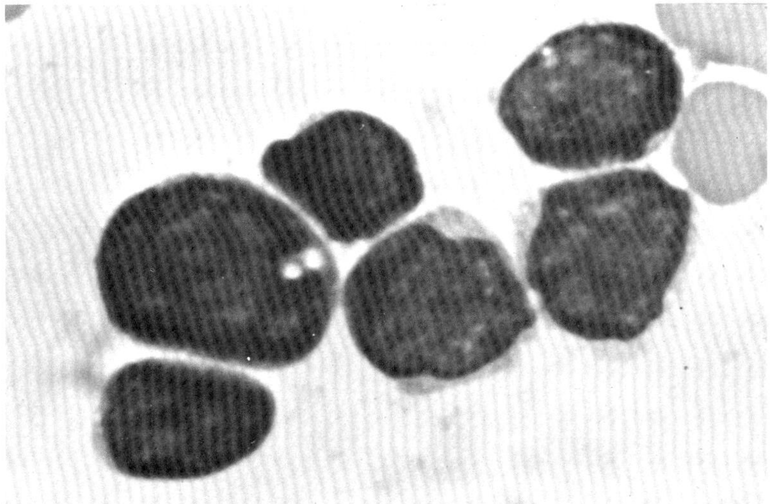

FIGURE 5-13. Leukemic lymphocytes.
These cells are from the bone marrow of a child with acute lymphocytic leukemia. There are four large and two small cells with typical lymphocyte structure. Two vacuoles, presumably fat, appear in one of the large cells. *× 2,000.*

FIGURE 5-14. Typical leukemic lymphocytes.
In these lymphocytes from the bone marrow of a child with acute lymphocytic leukemia (same as in Figure 5-13), the chromatin of the nuclei (*N*) is not as condensed as that in normal subjects. There are several nuclear invaginations and three cells with nuclear envelope projections (*arrows*). Dense particles around vacuole of upper right cell are glycogen (*gy*) granules. *Plastic: Maraglas. × 13,300.*

Figures 5-15 and 5-16 appear on the following pages ⇨

FIGURE 5-15. Leukemic lymphocyte.
This lymphocyte, from same child as represented in Figures 5-13 and 5-14, has less than normal condensation of chromatin in the nucleus (*N*) and two isolated nuclear blebs with lamellar chromatin boundaries (*asterisks*). In the Golgi area (*G*) are two centrioles (*Ce*). Rest of cytoplasm has scattered polyribosomes, small vesicles, and large round mitochondria (*M*). *Plastic: Maraglas. × 35,000.*

FIGURE 5-16. Area of Golgi complex in lymphocytic leukemia.
In this lymphocyte from same child as represented in Figures 5-13 through 5-15 are demonstrated details of the Golgi vesicles, a tangential cut of a centriole (*Ce*), fat (*F*) vacuole, round mitochondria (*M*), and ribosomes. *Plastic: Marglas. × 91,000.*

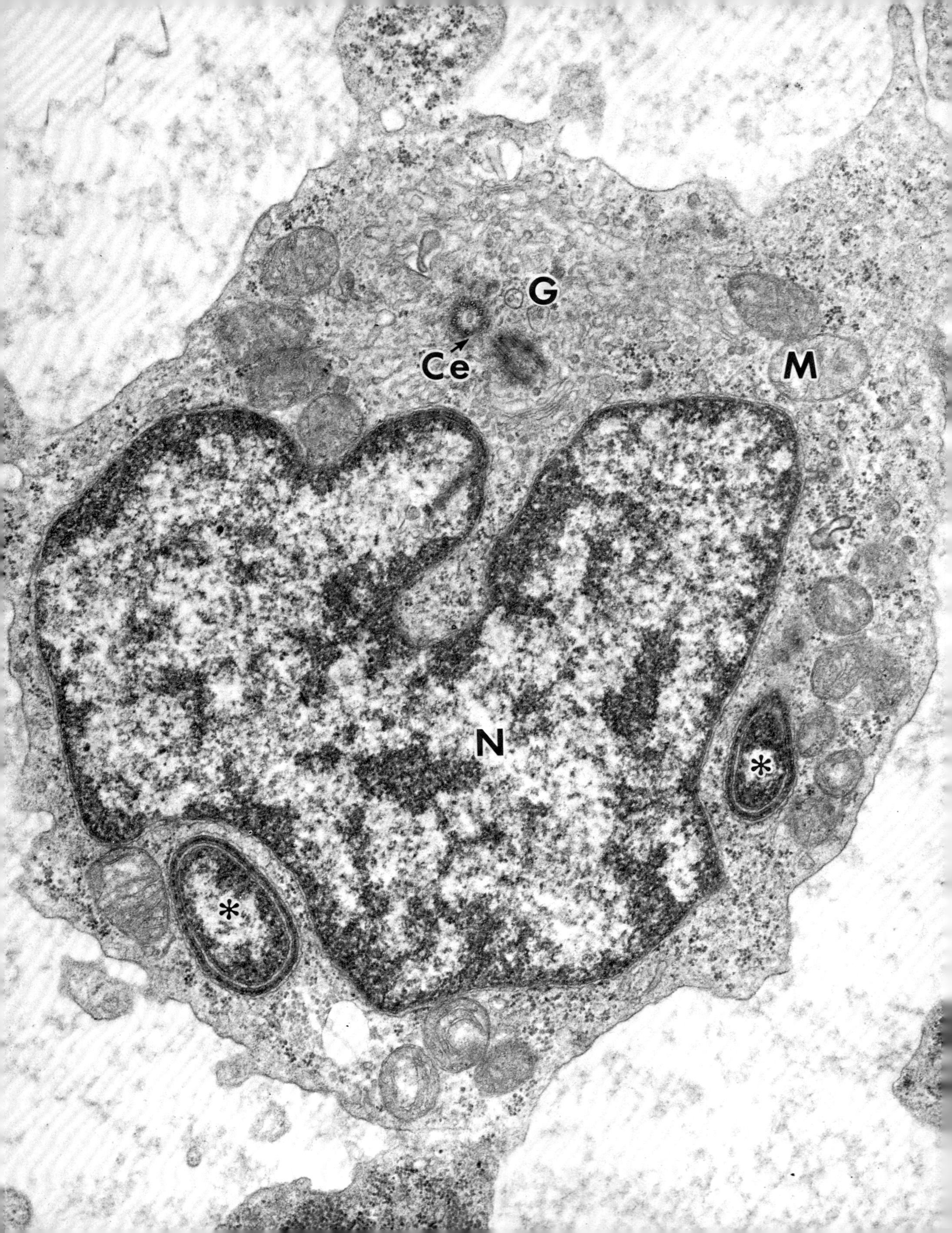
G
Ce
M
N
*
*

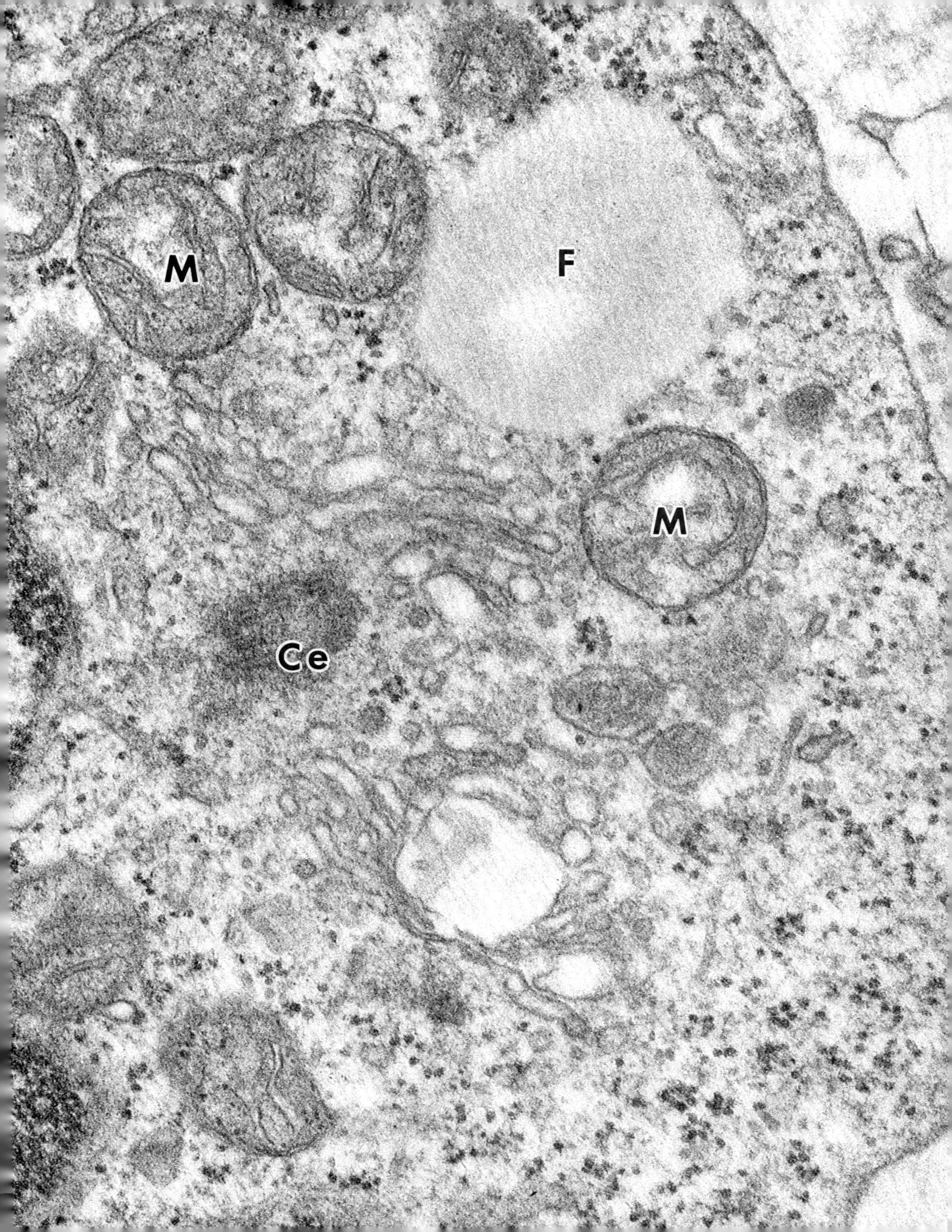
M
F
M
Ce

typical lymphocyte leukemia, cells contain both PAS-positive material (Quaglino and Hayhoe, 1959) and neutral fat vacuoles. Both structures are often recognized in cells of lymphocytic lines (Bennett and Dutcher, 1969).

Electron microscopic features of such proliferating cells favor the conclusion that they are probably lymphocytic cells (Figs. 5-14 through 5-17). Atypical structures include a significant nuclear indentation, large nucleolus, and an excessive number of mitochondria. The nuclear chromatin is less clumped. Leukemic cells possess many polyribosomes and some tubular endoplasmic reticulum. No cytoplasmic granules are observed. The presence of lamellated projections on the margin of the nucleus (Figs. 5-15 and 5-17) is common in Burkitt lymphoma cells (Epstein and Achong, 1965). The vacuoles frequently noted in smears are consistent with amorphous deposits which are probably lipid (Figs. 5-14 and 5-16). Both clusters and dispersed forms of glycogen are seen (Figs. 5-14 and 5-17). Metachromatic inclusions in one case of lymphocytic leukemia appeared to contain mucopolysaccharide and acid phosphatase and, therefore, could be categorized as lysosomes (Tanaka *et al.,* 1967). Electron microscopically many small vesicles of about 50 mμ to 90 mμ were identified within larger vacuoles (see Figs. 3-30 and 3-31).

Chronic Lymphocytic Leukemia. The chronic form usually occurs in individuals between 40 to 60 years of age. The characteristic hematological finding is an increased number of lymphocytes whose morphology is very similar to that of circulating small lymphocytes (Fig. 5-18). The progression of this disease is generally slow, but more than 50 per cent of the patients die during the first 3 years. Electron microscopic examination fails to show any significant subcellular abnormality (Figs. 5-18 and 5-19), although leukemic lymphocytes are usually larger and more immature looking than normal small lymphocytes. Some cells in chronic lymphocytic leukemia have cytoplasmic structures, such as protein crystals (Bernard *et al.,* 1959; de Man and Meiner, 1962), atypical endoplasmic reticulum (Foa *et al.,* 1969), virus-like inclusions (Zucker-Franklin, 1963b), and intranuclear fibrils (Stefani and Tonaki, 1970). The crystalloid structures have been interpreted to reflect the role of lymphocyte in antibody formation.

Malignant Lymphoma

This term is used to define the primary malignancy of lymph nodes and includes heterogeneous histologic entities. Subclassifications are made according to the predominant cell types in a given lesion (Rappaport, 1966). Unlike malignancies of myeloid tissues, the proliferation of free cells is usually associated with mesenchymal growth (reticulum cells). This phenomenon could contribute to the formation of a boundary or cuff of cells that prevents diffusion of malignant cells from the primary locus. There are various in-

FIGURE 5-17. Leukemic lymphocyte.
This cell, from same child as represented in Figures 5-13 through 5-16, shows details of chromatin lamellae (*arrow*) on the edge of the nucleus (*N*), with a cluster of glycogen (*gy*) granules which are larger than the ribosomes (*r*). *Plastic: Maraglas.* × *100,000.*

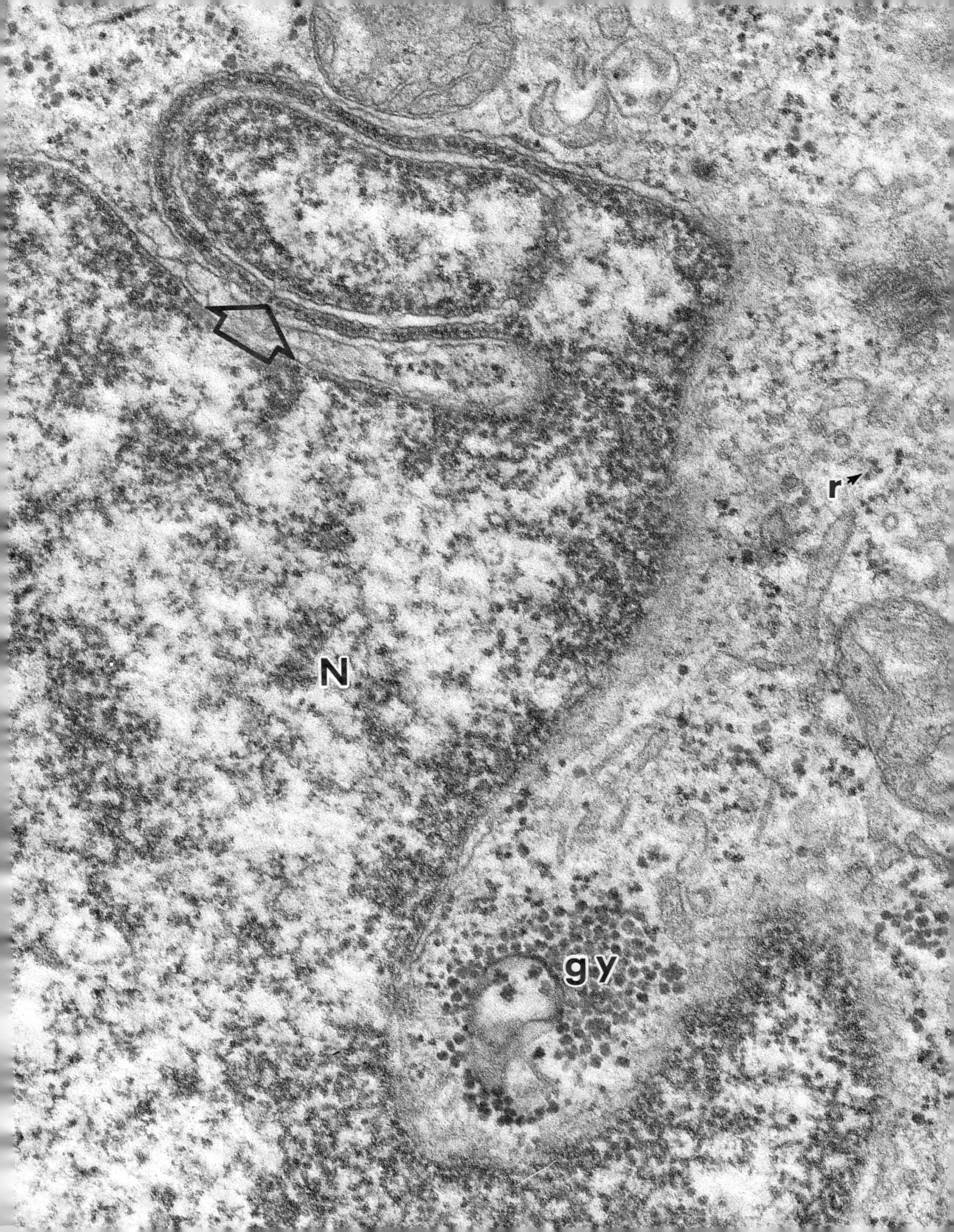
N
gy
r

termediate forms between leukemia and lymphosarcoma. Many electron micrographs of malignant lymphomas were published by Bernhard and Leplus (1964) and by Mori and Lennert (1969), and their cytology is available elsewhere.

Lymphosarcoma. Cells proliferating in lymphosarcoma are ultrastructurally similar to those observed in lymphocytic leukemia. However, there is considerable variation in cell morphology, with deviations of proliferation corresponding to the histologic variation of the disease. Insignificant deviation from leukemia cells may be noted in a well-differentiated form. Undifferentiated forms accompany pleomorphic cell growth, including various intermediates between small lymphocytes and large immature forms—lymphoblasts and hemocytoblasts (Figs. 5-20 through 5-25). Cells from Burkitt lymphoma show typical lymphoblastic forms (Figs. 5-20 and 5-21) proliferating among immature mesenchymal cells. Figures 5-22 and 5-23 illustrate a malignant cell resembling hemocytoblast or a transformed lymphocyte from the pleural effusion of a malignant lymphoma; reticulum cells with intracytoplasmic fibrils are also noted (Fig. 5-24). A variation of circulating malignant cells from a case of malignant lymphoma with invasion into the peripheral blood is illustrated in Figure 5-25; again, the heterogeneity of malignant lymphoid cells is apparent.

A unique histological entity represented by the presence of giant cells (Sternberg-Reed cells) is known as Hodgkin's disease. In this lesion, there is a pleomorphic cell infiltration regarded as a reaction to the neoplastic growth. Ultrastructure of the Sternberg-Reed cells has been reported by Braunsteiner *et al.* (1957), Frajola *et al.* (1958), and Ogawa (1962). The deep invagination and nuclear lobulation with prominent nucleolus and immense size are the most significant features. The significance of the electron-opaque material noted in intrachromatin areas remains unknown. The large cytoplasm contains slight-to-moderate amounts of ribosomes (occasionally, many polyribosomes) and electron-opaque granules. Active phagocytosis by Sternberg-Reed cells has also been reported, a phenomenon which favors the idea that the giant cells are of histiocytic nature.

Sézary's Syndrome. Malignant lymphoreticular proliferation involving primarily the skin is called mycosis fungoides. Its classification with the malignant lymphoma concept is controversial since some consider that it is a distinct clinicopathological entity and different from malignant lymphoma (Bluefarb, 1955; Rappaport, 1966). Abnormal cells in the peripheral blood of erythroderma were noted by Sézary and Bouvrain in 1938; Sézary (1949) summarized his cases within the concept of "cutaneous reticulosis." Sézary's syndrome is regarded as either mycosis fungoides with atypical mononuclear cells (Sézary cells) in the peripheral blood (Clendenning *et al.,* 1964) or a separate abnormality not related to mycosis fungoides (Rappaport, 1966).

(text continues on page 265)

FIGURE 5-18. Chronic lymphocytic leukemia.
Bone marrow leukemic lymphocytes, small and medium-sized, are near a large, more immature form (*asterisk*). A neutrophil (*Ne*) and macrophage (*Ma*) are also present. × *11,000.*

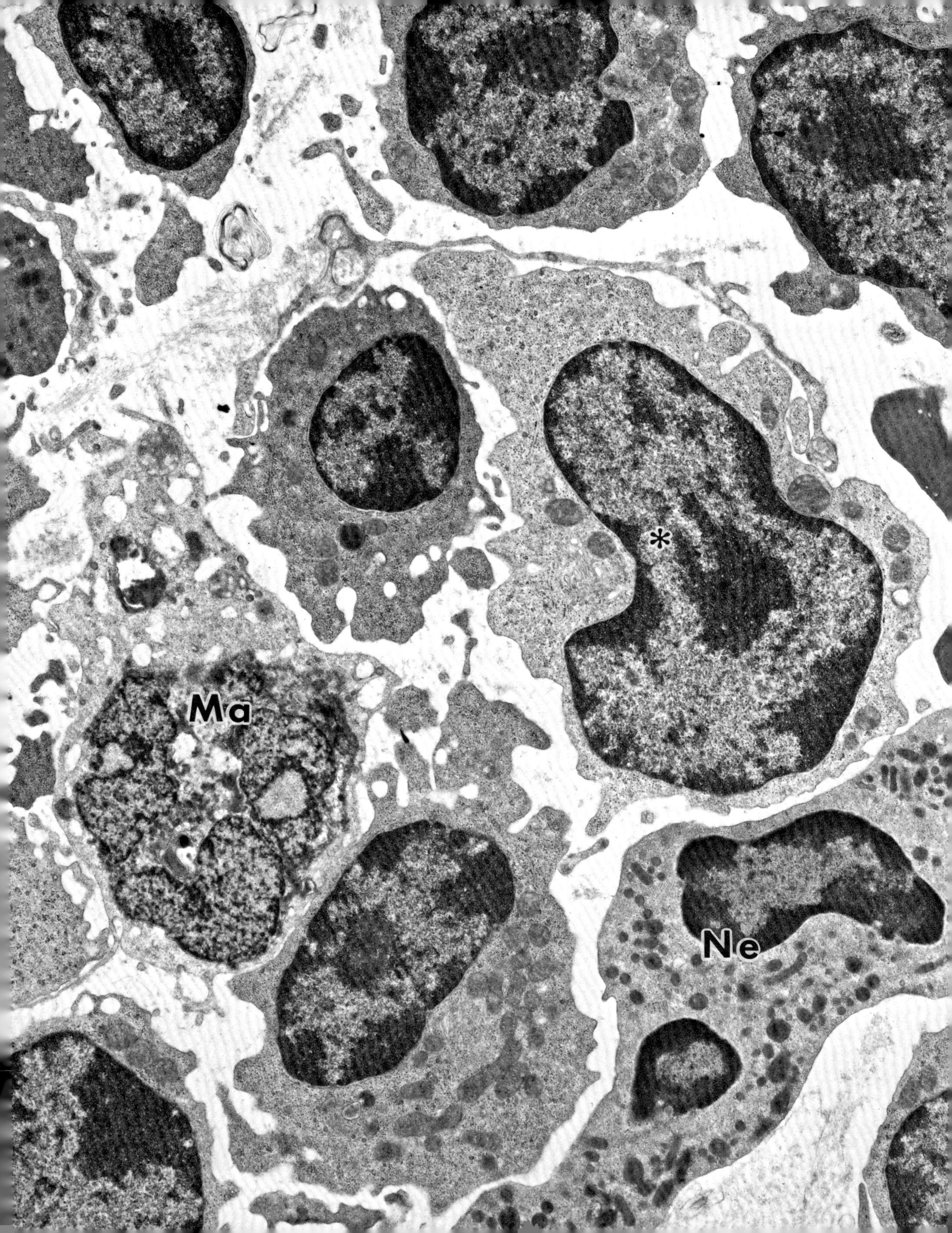
Ma
*
Ne

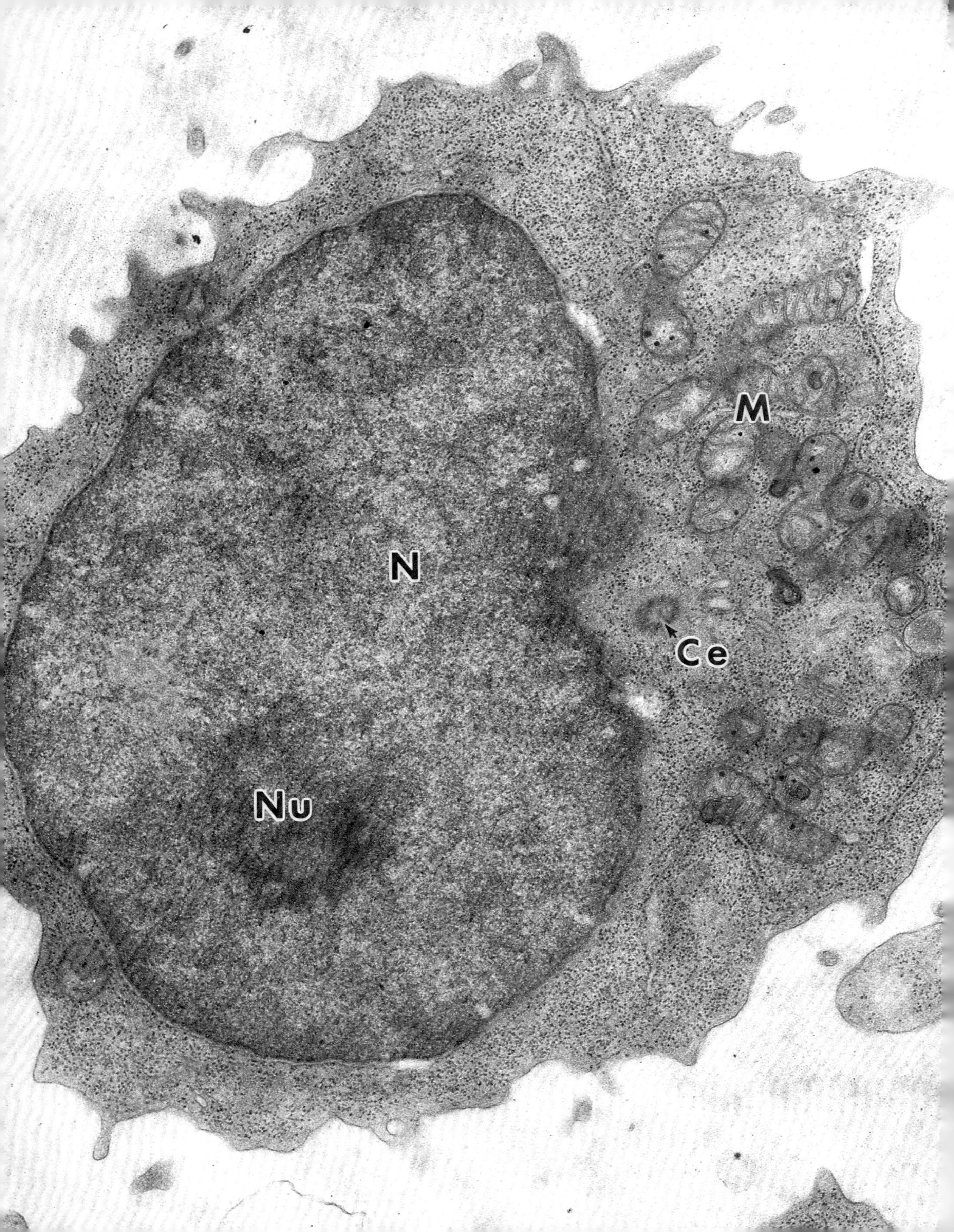
M
N
Ce
Nu

FIGURE 5-19. Chronic lymphocytic leukemia.
This malignant lymphocyte from peripheral blood is moderately large, with increased numbers of mitochondria (*M*), minimal condensation of chromatin in the nucleus (*N*), which has a prominent nucleolus (*Nu*), and a centriole (*Ce*). × *27,000.*

Figures 5-20 and 5-21 appear on the following pages

FIGURE 5-20. Burkitt's lymphoma.
In this section from primary oral lesion in a case of Burkitt's lymphoma are several immature mesenchymal or reticulum cells (*Rc*) and lymphoblasts (*Lb*). The immature reticulum cells have an indistinctive cytoplasmic border, few organelles, and a scattered network of chromatin in their nuclei (*N*). The five lymphoblasts show various stages of chromatin condensation in their nuclei and have fat vacuoles (*arrows*) in their more electron-dense cytoplasm. Two cells (*asterisks*) with fat vocuoles appear to be at an intermediate stage between diffuse reticulum cells and lymphoblasts. × *9,600.*

FIGURE 5-21. Burkitt's lymphoma.
This malignant lymphoblast (*center*) from the same lesion as represented in Figure 5-20, has many polyribosomes, two fat (*F*) vacuoles, a Golgi apparatus (*G*), and several rounded mitochondria (*M*). Some mitochondria are associated with, or have within them, dense lamellar structures (*arrow).* The nucleus (*N*) has scattered loose chromatin and nucleolus (*Nu*). The general appearance is that of immature lymphoblasts seen in normal lymph nodes. Parts of two other lymphoblasts (*Lb*) are also present. × *22,000.*

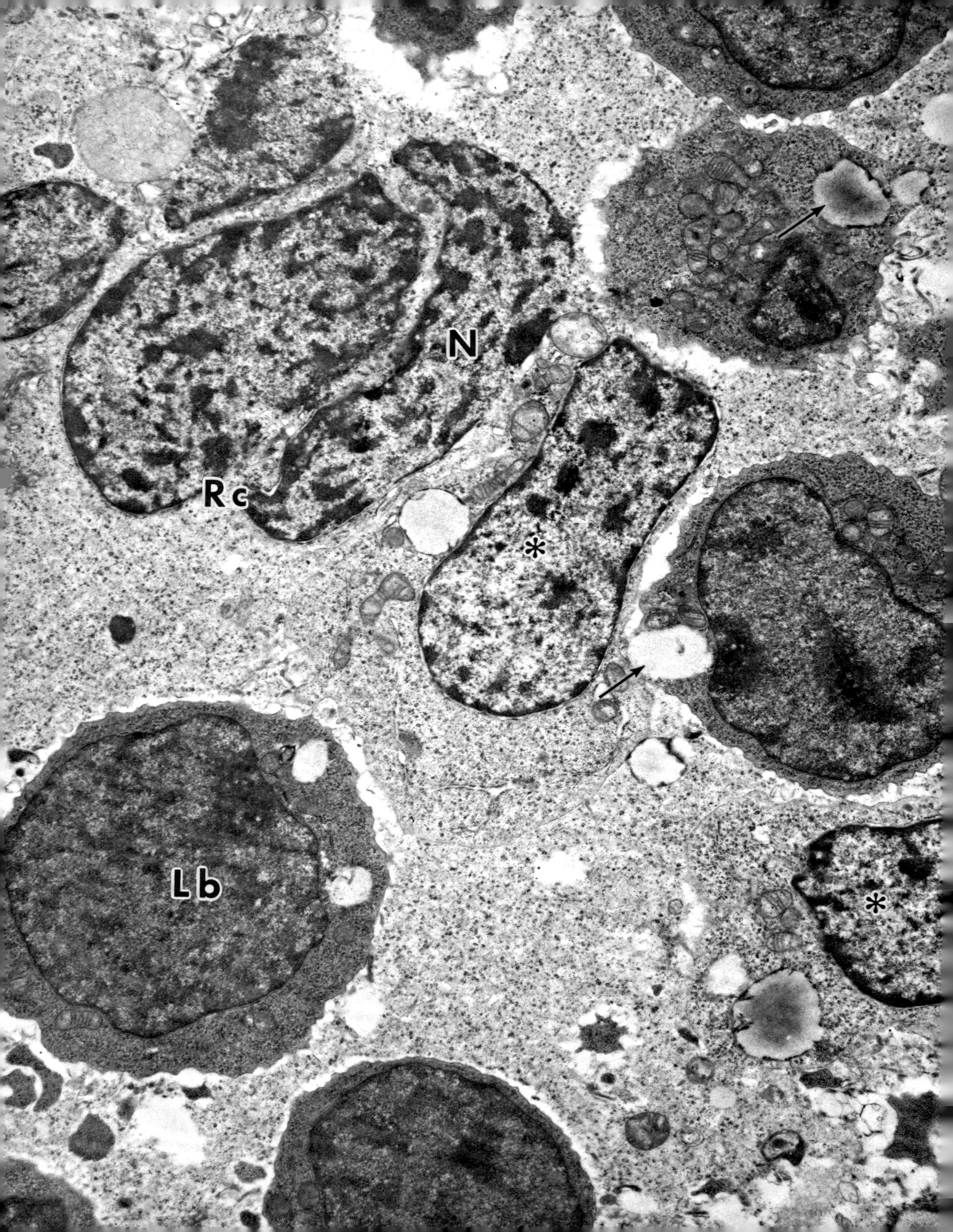
N
Rc
*
Lb
*

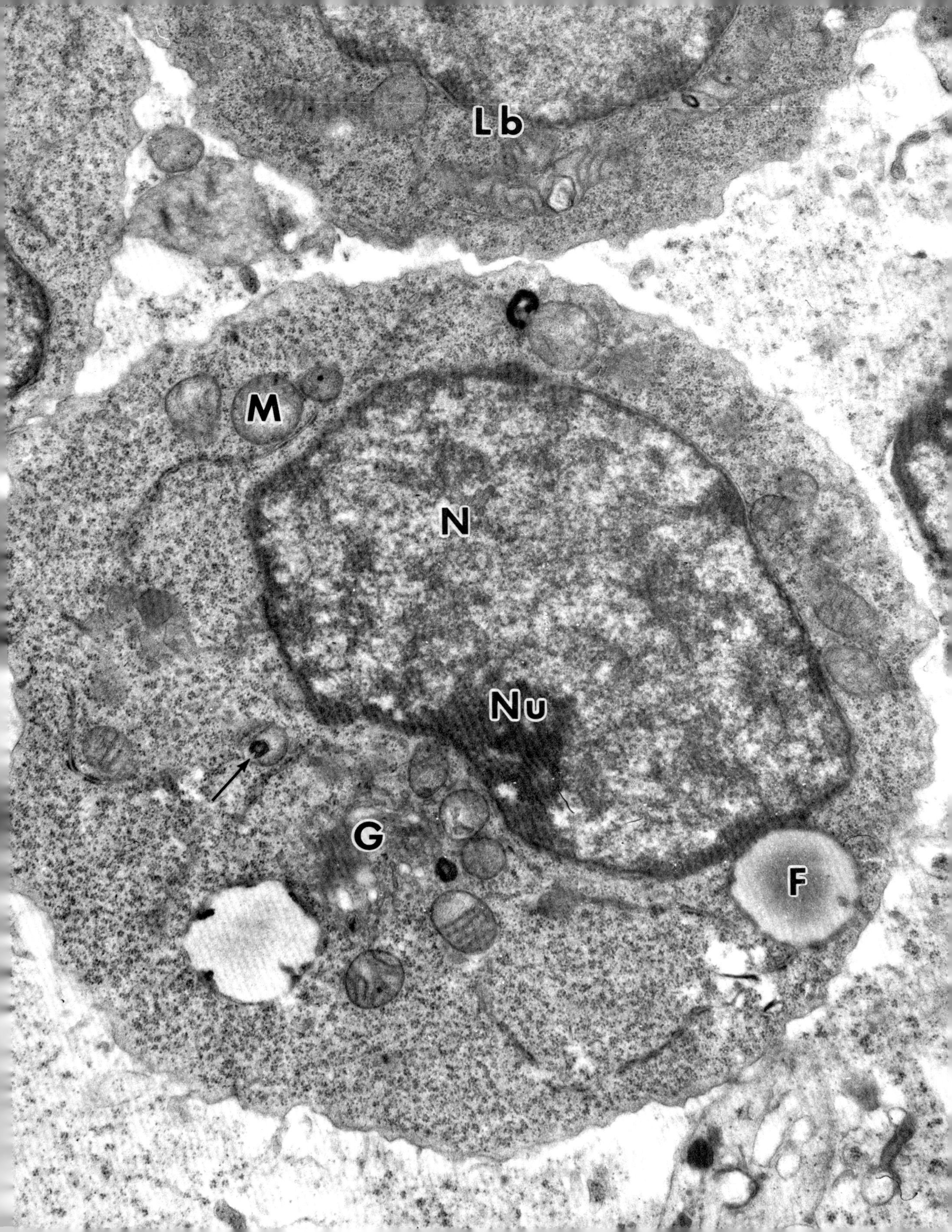
Lb
M
N
Nu
G
F

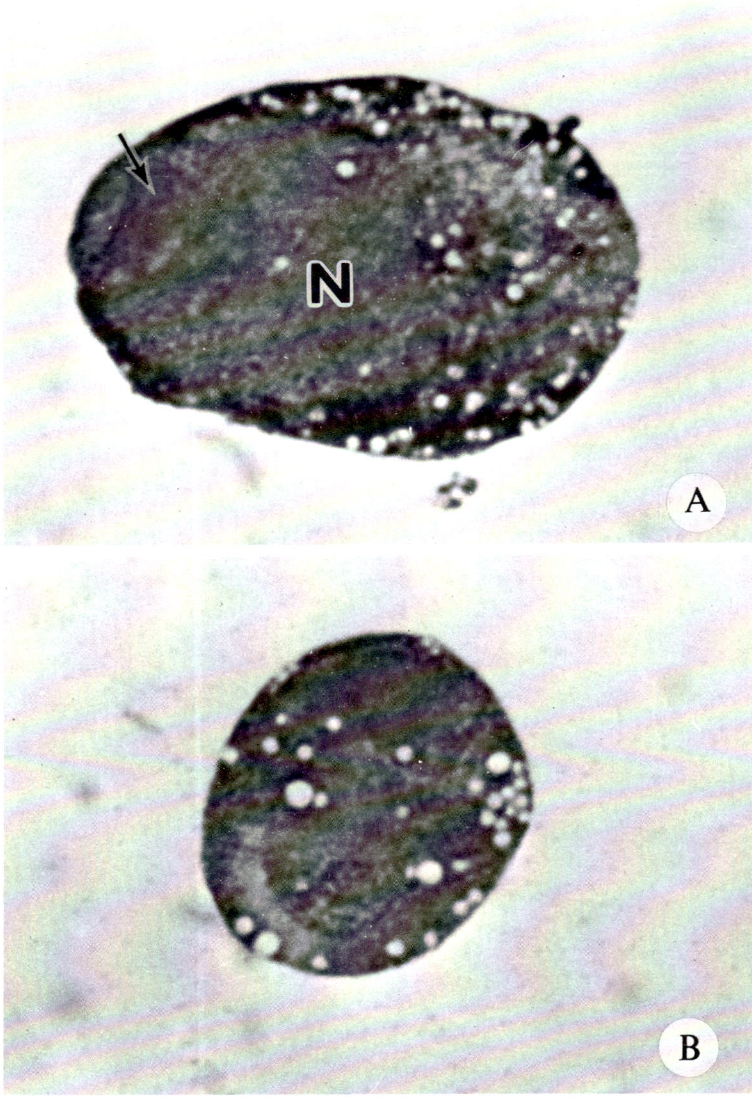

FIGURE 5-22. Cells from pleural effusion in malignant lymphoma.
A. Light micrograph of a very large atypical cell shows large nucleus (*N*), prominent nucleolus (*arrow*), and basophilic cytoplasm, which is heavily vacuolated. *Giemsa stain. × 2,000.*
B. Similar but smaller cell has lobulated nucleus. *Giemsa stain. × 2,000.*

FIGURE 5-23. Cell from pleural effusion in malignant lymphoma.
Immature cell from same case represented in Figure 5-22 has a striking similarity to the transformed lymphocyte (Fig. 5-10). The extensive cytoplasm has many polyribosomes, scattered endoplasmic reticulum (*er*), Golgi apparatus (*G*), large mitochondria (*M*), and fat (*F*) vacuoles. The nucleus (*N*) has a distinct nucleolus (Nu). Dense fibrillar extracellular material (*arrow*) is fibrin. × *16,000.*

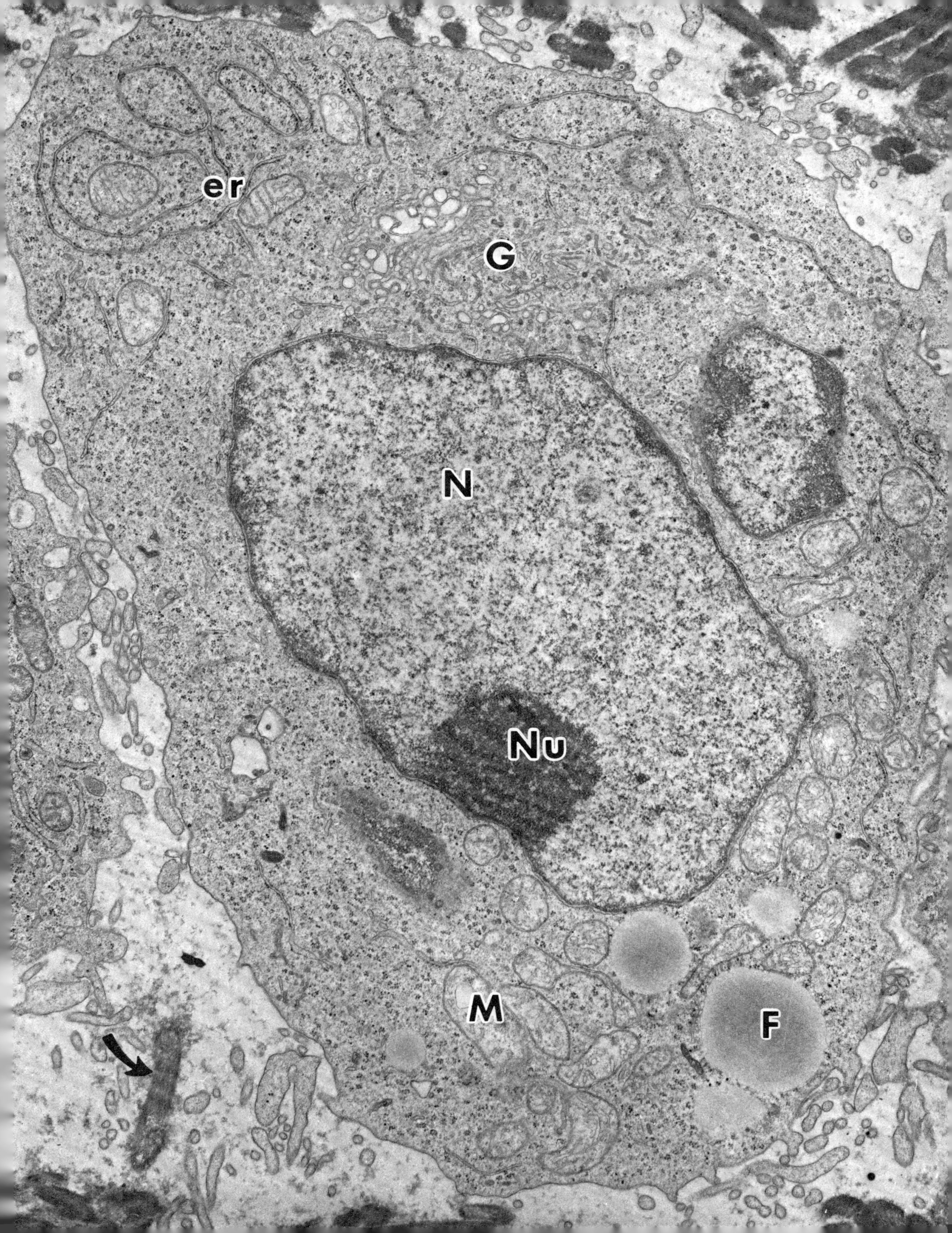
er
G
N
Nu
M
F

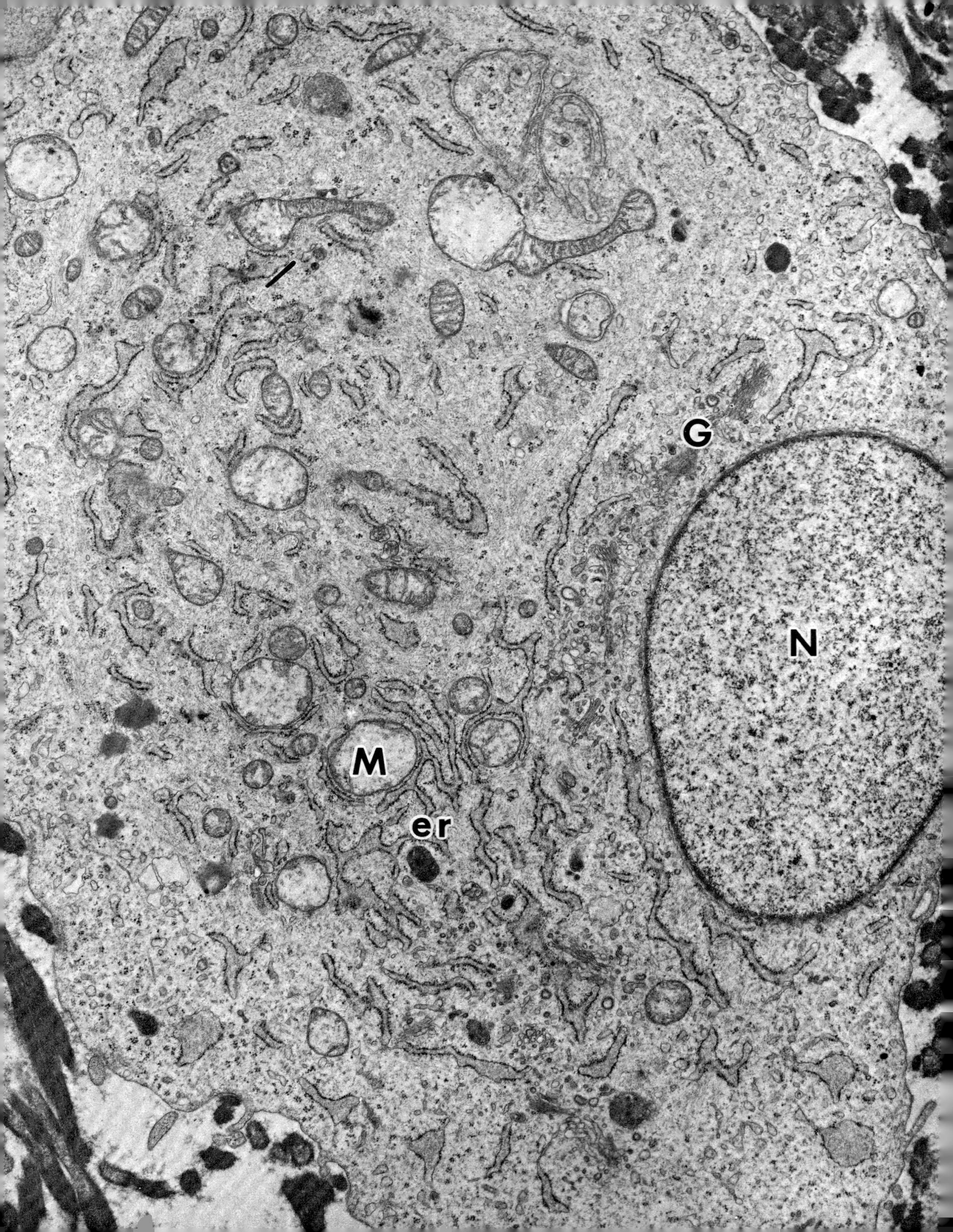
G
N
M
er

FIGURE 5-24. Cell from pleural effusion in malignant lymphoma.
Malignant cell (same case as represented in Figure 5-22 and 5-23) appears more like a reticulum cell than a lymphocyte, with branched form of endoplasmic reticulum (*er*) and fine fibrillar material in its cytoplasm. There are fewer scattered polyribosomes, but mitochondria (M) are present, and a Golgi complex (*G*). The nucleus (*N*) has a pale diffuse chromatin pattern. × *16,000.*

Figures 5-25 and 5-26 appear on the following pages ⇨

FIGURE 5-25. Cells from peripheral blood in malignant lymphoma.
A. In this typical malignant lymphoid cell, the centrally located nucleus (*N*) has patchy condensation of chromatin and distinct indentation. The cytoplasm has many polyribosomes, round mitochondria (*M*), and a very limited amount of endoplasmic reticulum. × *15,800.*
B. This atypical cell, resembling a hemocytoblast, has a round pale nucleus (*N*) with only scattered chromatin, relatively more cytoplasm with round mitochondria (*M*), and slightly distended endoplasmic reticulum (*er*). × *10,000.*
C. Atypical cell has highly indented nucleus (*N*) and cytoplasm with increased amounts of endoplasmic reticulum (*er*). × *12,300.*

FIGURE 5-26. Light micrographs of Sézary cells.
A, B, C. These cells exhibit lymphoid characteristics. × *2,000.*
D, E. These cells are monohistiocytic types. × *2,000.*
F. A bizarre cell contains cytoplasmic vacuoles. × *2,000.*

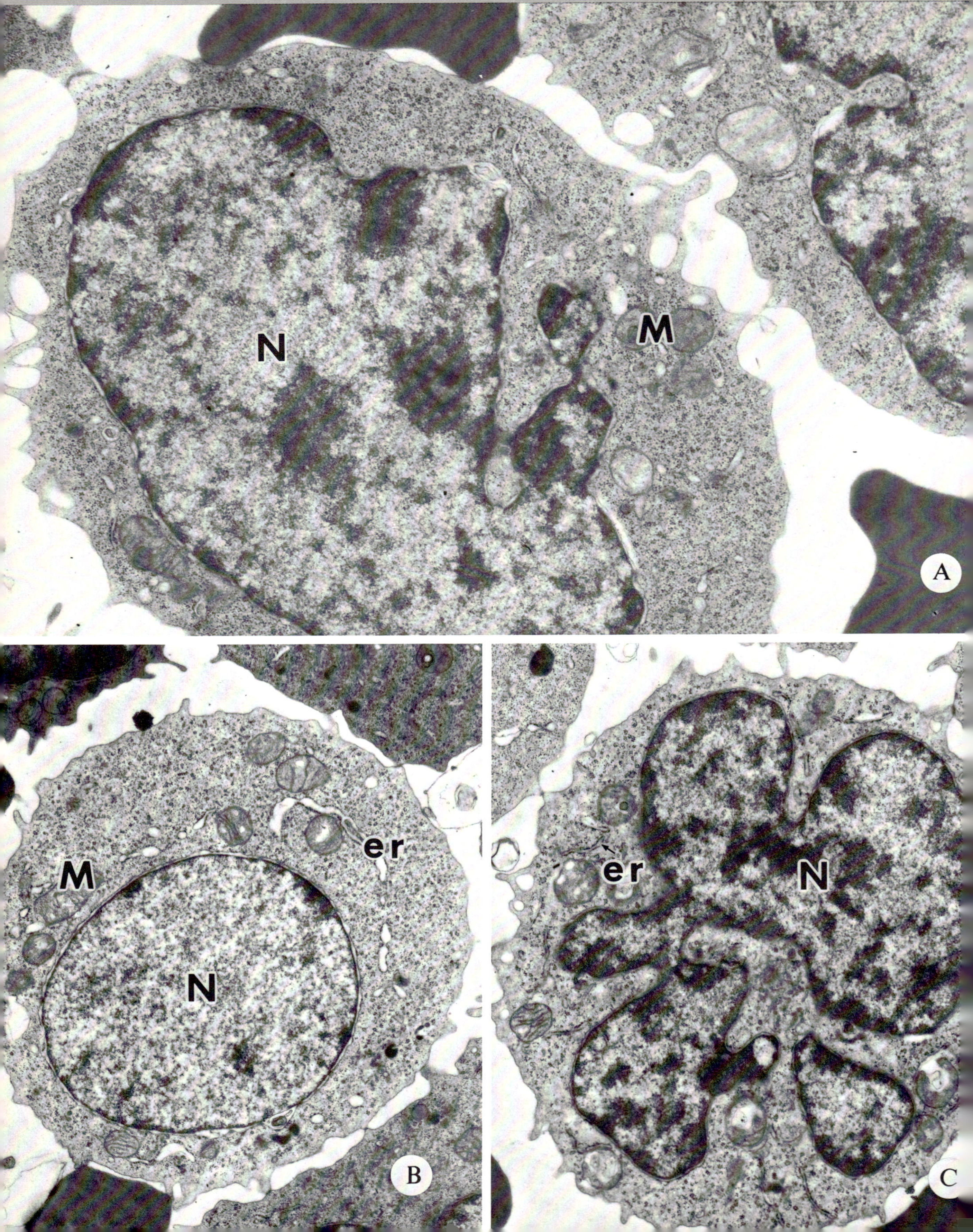
N
M
A
M
er
N
B
er
N
C

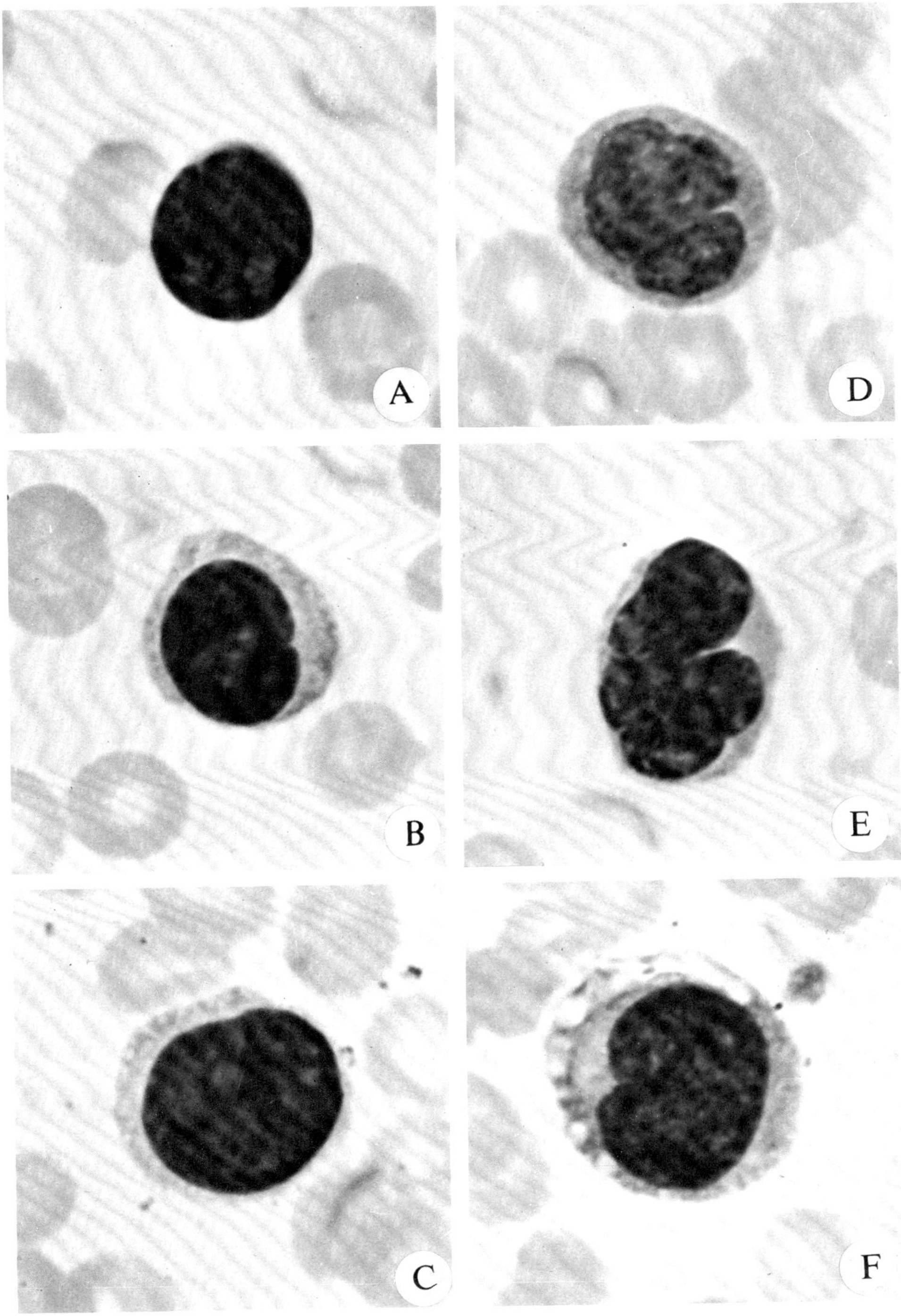
A
D
B
E
C
F

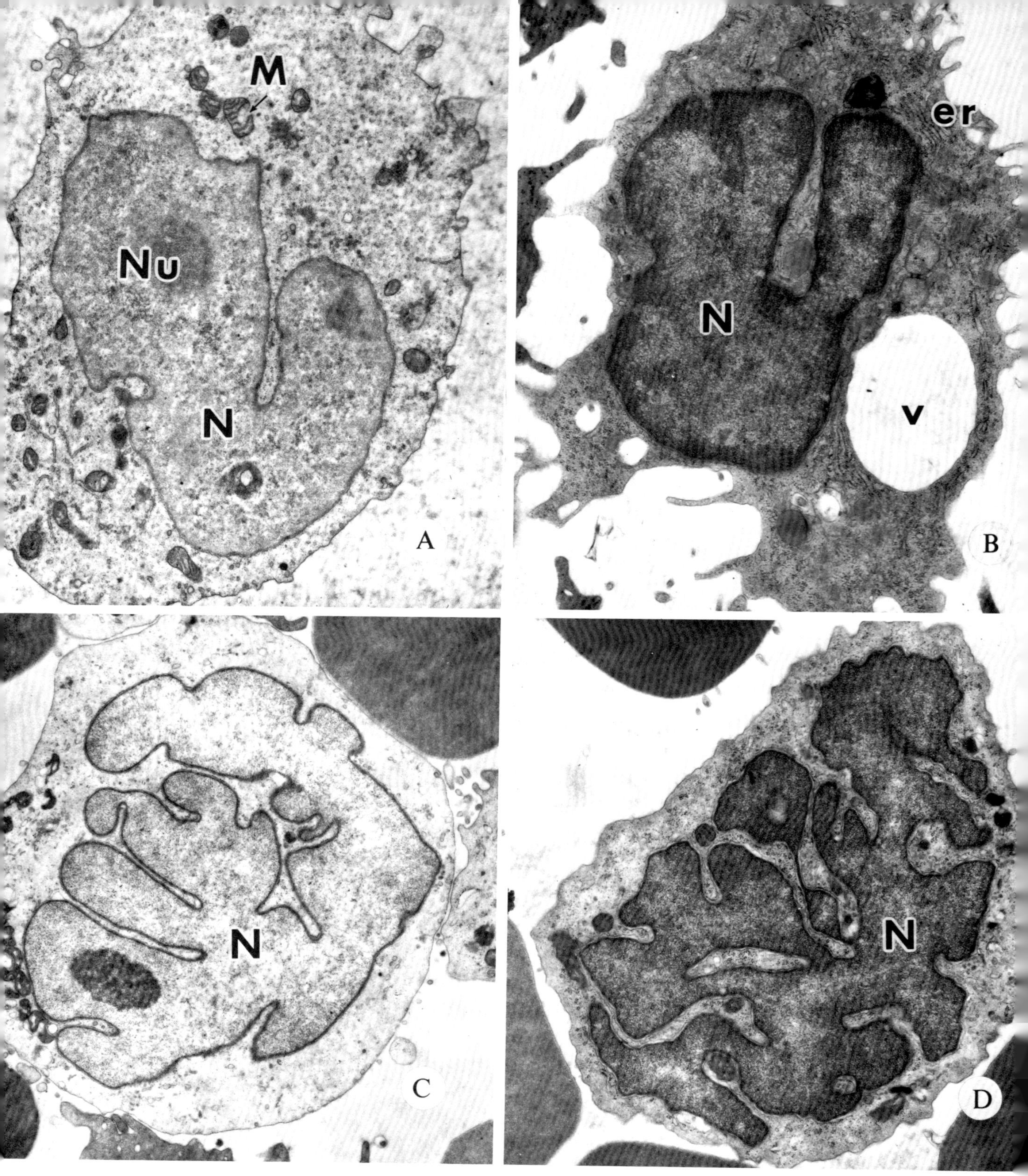
M
Nu
N
A
er
N
v
B
N
C
N
D

FIGURE 5-27. Range of abnormal cells in Sézary's syndrome.
A. Atypical lymphoid cell has indented nucleus (*N*) and pale nucleolus (*Nu*), small mitochondria (*M*), and limited other cytoplasmic organelles. *Fixation: Osmium. × 9,500.*
B. More like a histiocyte, this cell has developed endoplasmic reticulum (*er*), polyribosomes, a very large vacuole (*v*), a very irregular cytoplasmic surface, and a deeply invaginated nucleus (*N*). *× 9,500.*
C, D. Cytoplasm is similar to that of cells in Figure 5-27 **A** and **B**, respectively, but nuclei (*N*) are highly indented and irregular. The cells more nearly resemble mononuclear cells in subcutaneous tissues in cases of mycosis fungoides (Fig. 5-30). *× 7,800.*

Figures 5-28 and 5-29 appear on the following pages ⇨

FIGURE 5-28. Cytoplasm of lymphoid cells in Sézary's syndrome.
A. Cluster of glycogen (*gy*) granules. *Fixation: Osmium. × 58,000.*
B. Fine scatter of fibrils and highly irregular mitochondria (*M*) near immature nucleus (*N*). *× 58,000.*

FIGURE 5-29. Cytoplasm of lymphoid cells in Sézary's syndrome.
A. Cytoplasm of cell similar to cell in Figure 5-27**B** has a dense background, with scattered ribosomes, Golgi apparatus (*G*), round mitochondria (*M*), and dense lamellar structures (*arrow*). *× 58,000.*
B. Cytoplasm of cell similar to that in Figure 5-27**C** is pale, with numerous branched rough endoplasmic reticulum (*er*) and many ribosomes. *× 58,000.*

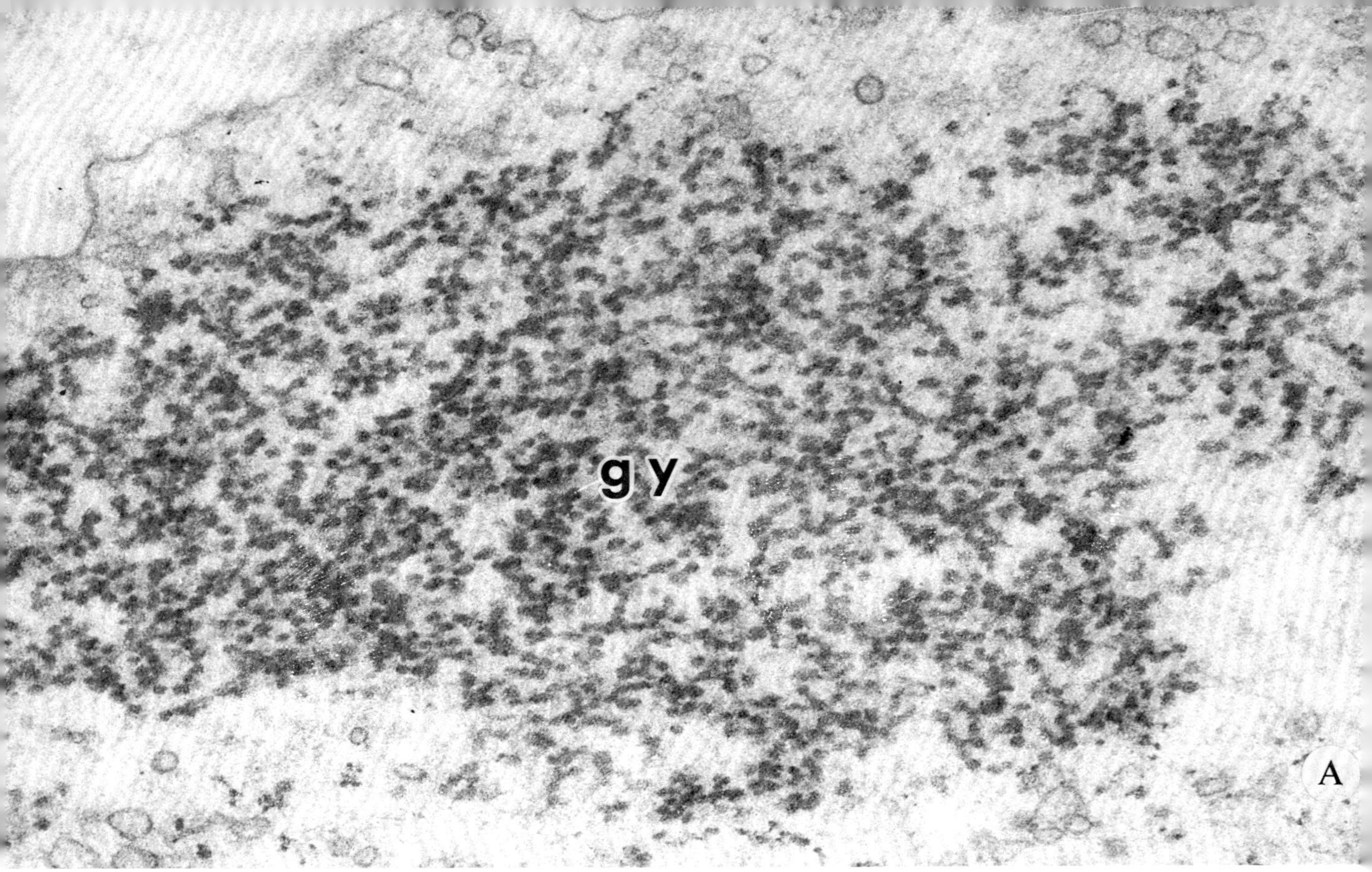
gy
A

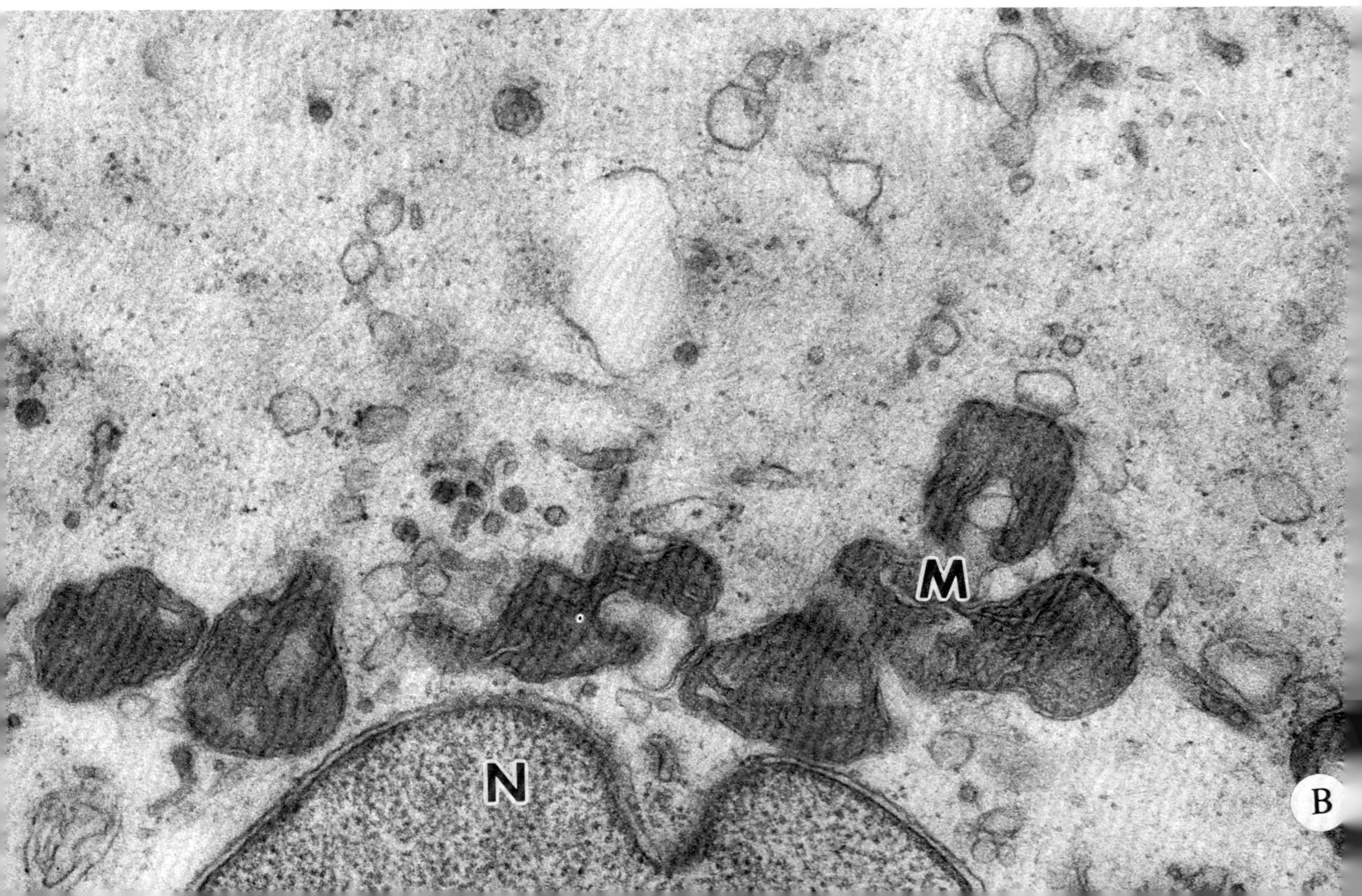
M
N
B

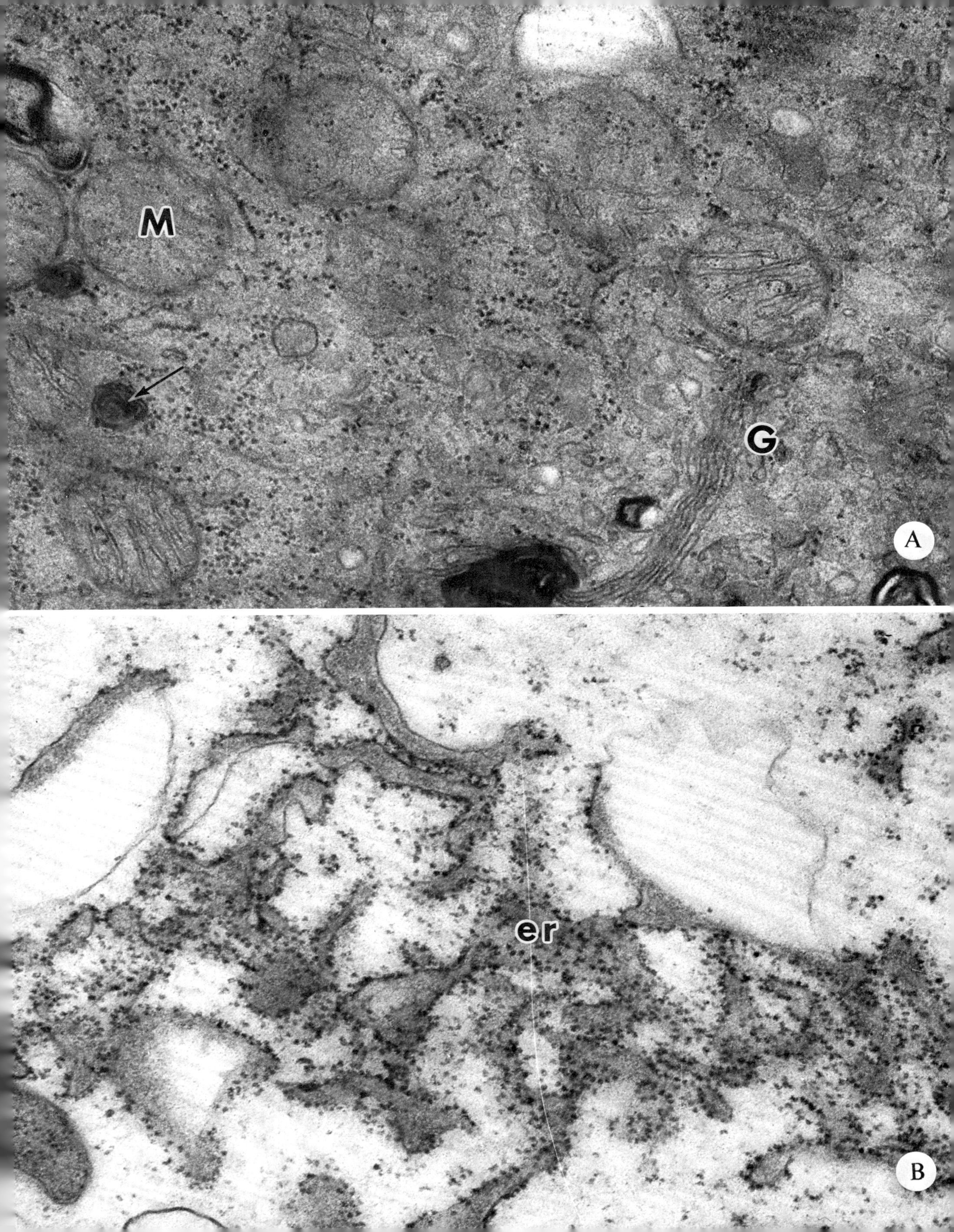
M
G
A
er
B

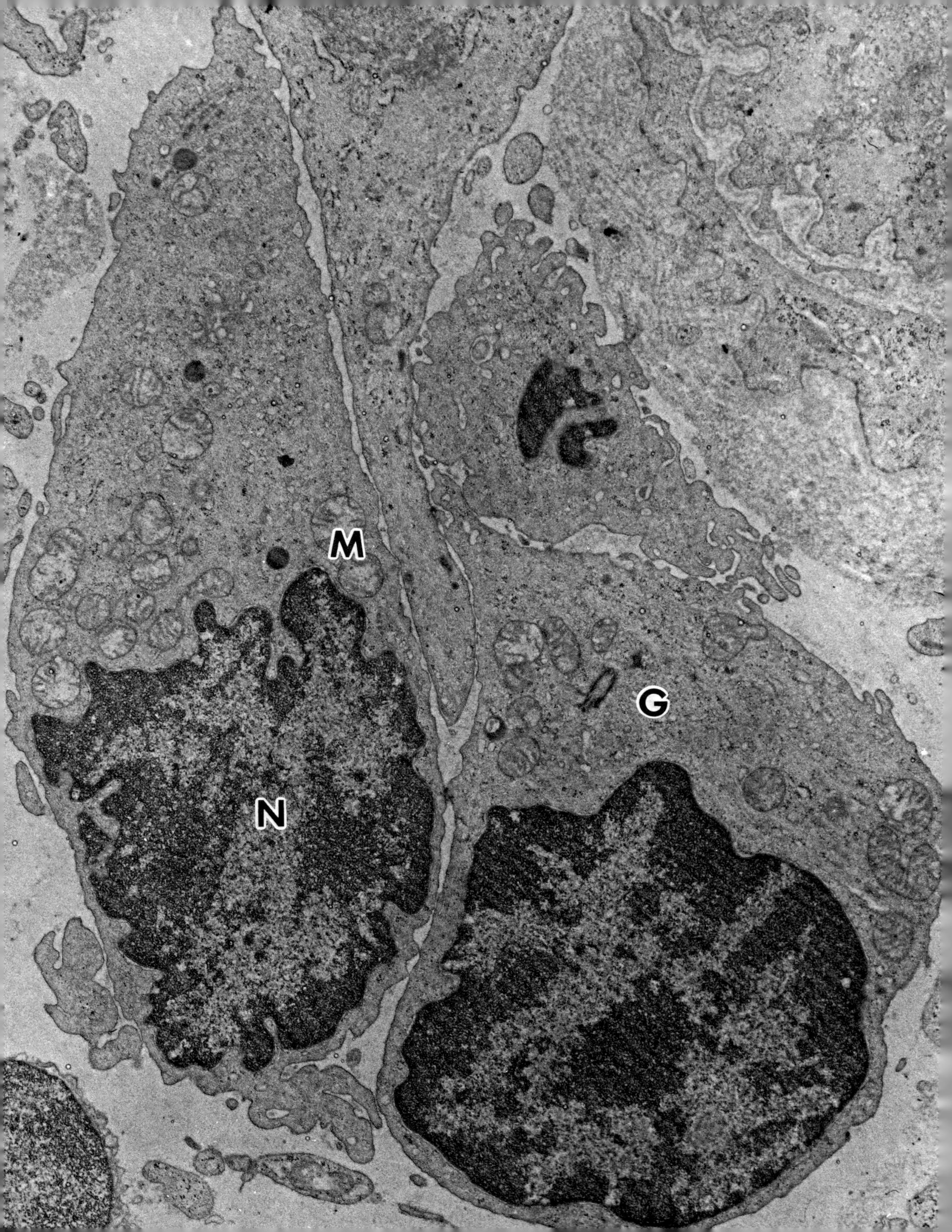
M
G
N

Sézary cells range in size from small lymphocytes to 25μ in diameter and show morphological variation between lymphocytes and histiomonocytes (Fig. 5-26). Their most characteristic feature is the presence of unusual indentation or lobulation of the nucleus; these cells are called "monstrous cells." Glycogen granules are frequent in the cytoplasm (Clendenning *et al.,* 1964). Taswell and Winkelmann (1961) described saliva-digestion-resistant, PAS-positive material in the cytoplasm of both circulating and skin cells and regarded this element as characteristic of Sézary cells, but this has not been confirmed by others (Clendenning *et al.,* 1964). Ultrastructural characteristics of these cells have been described by Lutzner and Jordan (1968), who claimed that the presence of a highly indented nucleus was pathognomonic of Sézary cells. In our experience, variation of Sézary cells from lymphoid (Fig. 5-27*A,C*) to histiocytic (Fig. 5-27*B,D*) is considerable in any given case, and no single type can possibly represent the malignant cells of this disorder. The variation in these cells may also be observed during the clinical course. Thus, we do not think that the type of cells described by Lutzner and Jordan (1968) are necessarily typical forms. Examples of heterogeneity of Sézary cells and their cytoplasmic characteristics are presented together with atypical lymphoid cells observed in skin (Figs. 5-28 through 5-31).

Viral Particles. There has been a search for viral particles in leukemic cells, based on the assumption that human leukemia may be caused by viruses, a concept which has been established in murine leukemia and various transplantable malignancies in animals. Searches for virus particles, as well as for structures resembling virus in size and shape, were undertaken in thin sections and in serum of leukemic patients (Dmochowski *et al.,* 1959, 1967; Braunsteiner *et al.,* 1960; Arnoult and Haguenau, 1966). Inoculation of material from suspected cases into animals and tissue culture were used frequently (Epstein *et al.,* 1965b) and considerable information has been accumulated. However, no conclusive evidence has yet been presented to prove the viral origin of human leukemia, though particles resembling virus have been seen and reported in malignant cells of blood-forming organs. Recently, Seman and Seman (1968) summarized their observations on 149 cases of leukemia and malignancy of blood-forming organs, and described both immature murine leukemia type A and mature type C particles. They claimed that there is a high incidence (50 per cent) of particle-positive cases in biopsy specimens, and a less effective (15 per cent) value of negative staining for viral particles in plasma. The significance of these particles is not known, and this prevalence of virus-like particles has not been reported by others.

FIGURE 5-30. Atypical lymphoid cells in Sézary's syndrome.
Atypical lymphoid cells in perivascular space of skin from case of Sézary's syndrome (mycosis fungoides). Some characteristics resemble those of mononuclear cells (Fig. 5-27**C, D**); however, the nucleus (*N*) is not nearly so indented. There are a number of mitochondria (*M*), and the Golgi complex (*G*) is apparent in cell at right. × *35,000.*

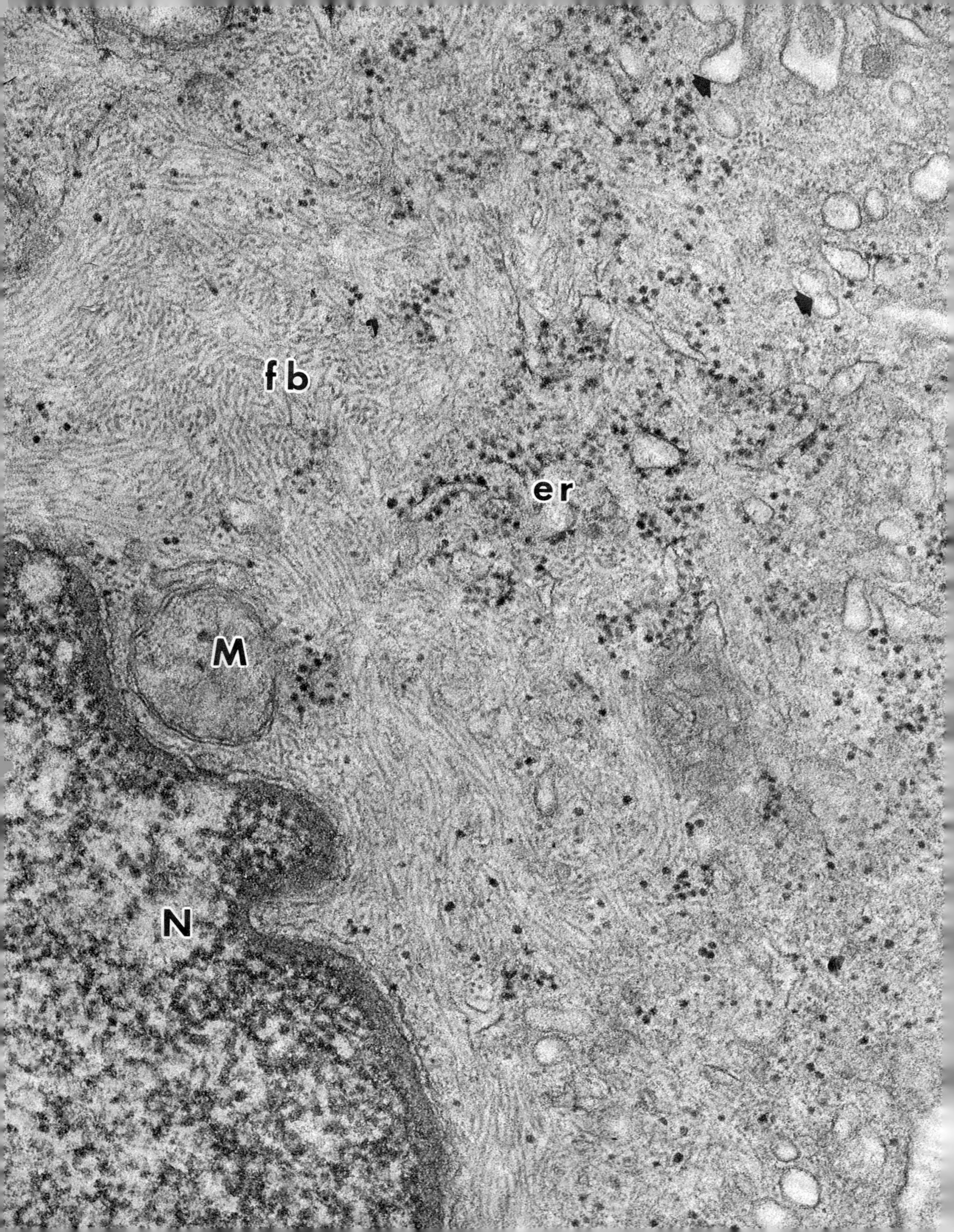

fb
er
M
N

FIGURE 5-31. Proliferating cell in Sézary's syndrome.
Cytoplasm shows extensive fibrillar formation (*fb*). Note number of pinocytotic vesicles (*arrows*), some endoplastic reticulum (*er*), a mitochondrion (*M*), and edge of the nucleus (*N*). × *72,000.*

REFERENCES

Able, M. E., Lee, J. C., and Rosenau, W. Lymphocyte-target cell interaction in vitro. *Amer J Path 60*:421, 1970.

Amano, S., Unno, G., and Hanaoka, M. Studies on the differentiation of lymphocytes and plasma cells. An advocation of "lymphogonia" theory. *Acta Haemat Jap 14*:108, 1951.

André-Schwartz, J. The morphologic responses of the lymphoid system to homografts. III. Electron microscopy study. *Blood 24*:113, 1964.

Arnason, B. G., Janković, B. D., Waksman, B. H., and Wennersten, C. Role of the thymus in immune reactions in rats. II. Suppressive effect of thymectomy at birth on reactions of delayed (cellular) hypersensitivity and the circulating small lymphocyte. *J Exp Med 116*:177, 1962.

Arnoult, J., and Haguenau, F. Problems raised by the search for virus particles in human leukemia. A study with the electron microscope of blood plasma, cerebrospinal, and megakaryocytes from bone marrow. *J Nat Cancer Inst 36*: 1089, 1966.

Awrorow, P. P., and Timofejewsky, A. D. Kultiverungsversuche von leukämischen Blute. *Virchow Arch Path Anat 216*:184, 1914.

Bach, F., and Hirschhorn, K. Lymphocyte interaction: A potential histocompatibility test *in vitro. Science 143*:813, 1964.

Bain, B., Vas, M. R., and Lowenstein, L. The development of large immature mononuclear cell in mixed leukocyte cultures. *Blood 23*:108, 1964.

Becker, A. J., McCulloch, E. A., and Till, J. E. Cytological demonstration of the clonal nature of spleen colonies derived from transplanted mouse marrow cells. *Nature* (*London*) *197*:452, 1963.

Benda, C. Uber den Bau der blutbildenden Organe und die Regeneration der Blutelemente beim Menschen. *Arch Anat Physiol* (*Physiol Abtl*), p. 347, 1896.

Bennett, J. M., and Dutcher, T. F. The cytochemistry of acute leukemia: Observations on glycogen and neutral fat in bone marrow aspirates. *Blood 33*:341, 1969.

Bernard, J., Bessis, M., Soulier, J. P., and Thiéry, J. P. Étude au microscope électronique d'une leucémie lymphoide avec cristaux intra-cytoplasmiques. *Rev Hemat 14*:227, 1959.

Bernhard, M., and Leplus, R. *Fine Structure of the Normal and Malignant Human Lymph Node.* Macmillan, New York, 1964.

Bernier, G. M., and Cebra, J. J. Frequency distribution of α, γ, K and λ polypeptide chains in human lymphoid tissues. *J Immun 95*:246, 1965.

Bessis, M. *Cytology of the Blood and Blood-forming Organs* (Ponder, E., transl.). Grune & Stratton, New York, 1956.

Binet, J. L., and Mathé, G. Étude en microscopie optique et électronique des "cellules immunologiquement compétentes" au cours des réactions de greffe. *C R Acad Sci 253*:1852, 1961.

Bluefarb, S. M. Is mycosis fungoides an entity? *Arch Derm* (*Chicago*) *71*:293, 1955.

Bloom, W., and Fawcett, D. W. *Textbook of Histology* (9th ed.). W. B. Saunders, Philadelphia, 1968.

Bosman, C., Feldman, J. D., and Pick, E. Heterogeneity of antibody-forming cells—an electron micrographic analysis. *J Exp Med 129*:1029, 1969.

Braunsteiner, H., Fellinger, K., and Pakesch, F. Electron microscopic investigation on sections from lymph nodes and bone marrow in malignant blood diseases. *Blood 12*:278, 1957.

Braunsteiner, H., Fellinger, K., and Pakesch, F. On the occurrence of virus-like bodies in human leukemia. *Blood 15*:476, 1960.

Bryant, B. J. Reutilization of lymphocyte DNA by cells of intestinal crypts and regenerating liver. *J Cell Biol 18*:515, 1963.

Caffrey, R. W., Rieke, W. O., and Everett, N. B. Radioautographic studies of small lymphocytes in the thoracic duct of the rat. *Acta Haemat 28*:145, 1962.

Cebra, J. J., Colberg, J. E., and Dray, S. Rabbit lymphoid cells differentiated with respect to α, γ and μ heavy polypeptide chains and to allotypic markers A_{A1} and A_{A2}. *J Exp Med 123*:547, 1966.

Chase, M. W. The cellular transfer of cutaneous hypersensitivity to tuberculin. *Proc Soc Exp Biol Med 59*:134, 1945.

Chessin, L. W., Börjeson, J., Welsh, P. D., Douglas, S. D., and Cooper, H. L. Studies on human peripheral blood lymphocytes *in vitro.* II. Morphological and biochemical studies on the transformation of lymphocytes by pokeweed mitogen. *J Exp Med 124*:873, 1966.

Clawson, C. C., Cooper, M. D., and Good, R. A. Lymphocyte fine structure in the bursa of Fabricius, the thymus and the germinal centers. *Lab Invest 16*:407, 1967.

Clendenning, W. E., Brecher, G., and Van Scott, E. J. Mycosis fungoides. *Arch Derm (Chicago) 89*:785, 1964.

Cooper, M. D., Perey, D. Y., McKneally, M. F., Gabrielsen, A. E., Sutherland, D. E. R., and Good, R. A. A mammalian equivalent of the avian bursa of Fabricius. *Lancet 1*:1388, 1966.

Cowling, D. C., and Quaglino, D. Effect of antigen mixtures on blastic transformation in leucocyte cultures. *Lancet 1*:117, 1964.

Cronkite, E. P., Jansen, C. R., Mather, G. C., Nielsen, N. O., Usenik, E. A., Adamik, E. R., and Sipe, C. R. Studies on lymphocytes. I. Lymphopenia produced by prolonged extracorporeal irradiation of circulating blood. *Blood 20*:203, 1962.

Cronkite, E. P., Jansen, C. R., Cottier, H., Rai, K., and Sipe, C. R. Lymphocyte production measured by extracorporeal irradiation, cannulation, and labeling techniques. *Ann NY Acad Sci 113*:566, 1964.

Curry, J. L., Trentin, J. J., and Cheng, V. Hemopoietic spleen colony studies. III. Hemopoietic nature of spleen colonies induced by lymph node or thymus cells, with or without phytohemagglutinin. *J Immun 99*:907, 1967.

Dameshek, W. "Immunoblasts" and "immunocytes." An attempt at a functional nomenclature. *Blood 21*:243, 1963.

Dameshek, W., and Gunz, G. *Leukemia* (2nd ed.). Grune & Stratton, New York, 1964.

de Man, J. C. H., and Meiner, W. B. H. Crystals of protein nature in the cytoplasm of lymphatic cells in a case of lymphoreticular malignancy. *Blood 20*:492, 1962.

de Petris, S., and Karlsbad, G. Localization of antibodies by electron microscopy in developing antibody-producing cells. *J Cell Biol 26*:759, 1965.

Dmochowski, L., Grey, C. E., Skyes, J. A., Shullenberger, C. C., and Howe, C. D. Studies on human leukemia. *Proc Soc Exp Biol Med 101*:686, 1959.

Dmochowski, L., Yumoto, T., Grey, C. E., Hales, R. L., Langford, P. L., Tayer, H. G., Freireich, E. J., Shullenberger, C. C., Shively, J. A., and Howe, C. D. Electron microscopy study of human leukemia and lymphoma. *Cancer 20*: 760, 1967.

Douglas, S. D., Hoffman, P. F., Börjeson, J., and Chessin, L. N. Studies on human peripheral blood lymphocytes *in vitro.* III. Fine structural features of lymphocyte transformation by pokeweed mitogen. *J Immun 98*:17, 1967.

Douglas, S. D., Fudenberg, H. H., Glade, P. R., Chessin, L. N., and Moses, H. L. Fine structure of leukocytes in infectious mononucleosis: *In vivo* and *in vitro* studies. *Blood 34*:42, 1969.

Downey, H., and McKinlay, C. A. Acute lymphadenosis compared with acute lymphatic leukemia. *Arch Intern Med 32*:82; 95, 1923.

Ehrlich, P. *Farbenanalytische Untersuchungen zur Histologie und Klinik des Blutes.* Hirchward, Berlin, 1891.

Epstein, M. A., and Achong, B. G. Fine structural organization of human lymphoblasts of a tissue culture strain (EB_1) from Burkitt's lymphoma. *J Nat Cancer Inst 34*:241, 1965a.

Epstein, M. A., Henle, G., Achong, B. G., and Barr, Y. M. Morphological and biological studies on a virus in cultured lymphoblasts from Burkitt's lymphoma. *J Exp Med 121*:761, 1965b.

Everett, N. B., Reinhardt, W. O., and Yoffey, J. M. The appearance of labelled cells in the thoracic duct lymph of the guinea pig after the administration of tritiated thymidine. *Blood 15*:82, 1960.

Everett, N. B., Caffrey, R. W., and Reike, W. D. Recirculation of lymphocytes. *Ann NY Acad Sci 113*:887, 1964.

Fagraeus, A. Antibody production in relation to the development of plasma cells. *In vivo* and *in vitro* experiments. *Acta Med Scand* (Suppl 204):1, 1948.

Feldman, J. D., and Nordquist, R. E. Immunologic competence of thoracic duct cells. II. Ultrastructure. *Lab Invest 16*:564, 1967.

Flemming, W. Studien über Regeneration des Gewebes. I. Zellvermehrung in den Lymphodrüsen und verwandten Organen und ihr Einfuss auf deren Bau. *Arch Mikr Anat. 24*:50; 338, 1885.

Fliedner, T. M., Kesse, M., Cronkite, E. P., and Robertson, J. S. Cell proliferation in germinal centers of the rat spleen. *Ann NY Acad Sci 113*: 578, 1964.

Foa, R., Foa, C., and Muratore, R. Aspect ultrastructural particular du réticulum endoplasmique dans un cas de leucémie lymphoide chronique. *Nouv Rev Franc Hemat 9*:795, 1969.

Frajola, W. J., Greider, M. H., and Bouroncle, B. A. Cytology of the Sternberg-Reed cell as revealed by the electron microscope. *Ann NY Acad Sci 73*:221, 1958.

Galbraith, P., Mitus, W. J., Gollerkeri, M., and Dameshek, W. The "infectious mononucleosis cell." A cytochemical study. *Blood 22*:630, 1963.

Gesner, B. M., and Gowans, J. L. The fate of lethally irradiated mice given isologous and heterologous thoracic duct lymphocytes. *Brit J Exp Path 43*:431, 1962.

Good, R. A., Gabrielsen, A. E., Peterson, R. D. A., and Cooper, M. D. The central lymphoid tissue in developmental immunobiology. *Trans Coll Physicians Phila 33*:180, 1966.

Govaerts, A. Cellular antibodies in kidney homotransplantation. *J. Immun 85*:516, 1960.

Gowans, J. L. The recirculation of lymphocytes from blood to lymph in the rat. *J Physiol 146*: 54, 1959.

Gowans, J. L., and Uhr, J. W. The carriage of immunological memory by small lymphocytes in the rat. *J Exp Med 124*:1017, 1966.

Grundmann, E. Die Bildung der Lymphocyten und Plasmazellen in lymphatischen Gewebe der Ratte. *Beitr Path Anat 119*:217, 1958.

Hall, J. G., Morris, B., Moreno, G. D., and Bessis, M. C. The ultrastructure and function of the cells in lymph following antigenic stimulation. *J Exp Med 125*:91, 1967.

Harris, T. N., Hummeler, K., and Harris, S. Electron microscopic observations on antibody-producing lymph node cells. *J Exp Med 123*:161, 1966.

Heilmeyer, L., and Begemann, H. *Atlas der Klinischen Haematologie und Cytologie.* Springer, Berlin, 1955.

Heiniger, H. J., Reidwyl, H., Giger, H., Sordat, B., and Cottier, H. Ultrastructural differences between thymic and lymph node small lymphycytes of mice. Nucleolar size and cytoplasmic volume. *Blood 30*:288, 1967.

Hellman, T. Lymphgefässe, Lymphknötchen und Lymphknoten. *Handbuch der Mikroskopischen Anatomie des Menschen,* Springer, Berlin, 1930, vol. 6 (part 1), p. 223.

Hodgkin, T. On some morbid appearances of the absorbent glands and spleen. *Med Chir Trans (London) 14*:58, 1832.

Hovig, T., Jeremic, M., and Stavem, P. A new type of inclusion bodies in lymphocytes. *Scand J Haemat 5*:81, 1968.

Hummeler, K., Harris, T. N., Tomassini, N., Hechtel, M., and Farber, M. B. Electron microscopic observations on antibody-producing cell in lymph blood. *J Exp Med 124*:255, 1966.

Hungerford, D. A., Donnelly, A. J., Nowell, P. C., and Beck, S. The chromosome constitution of human phenotypic intersex. *Amer J Human Genet 11*:215, 1959.

Kundrat, M. Ueber Lymph-Sarkomatoses. *Klin Wschr 6*:211, 1893.

Lawrence, H. S. The cellular transfer of cutaneous hypersensitivity to tuberculin in man. *Proc Soc Exp Biol Med 71*:516, 1949.

Lennert, K. Cytologie des ruhenden, aktivierten und entzündeten Lymphknotens. Lymphknoten, Diagnostik und Cytologie. *Handbuch der Speziellen pathologischen Anatomie und Histologie,* Bd 113. Springer, Berlin, 1961.

Lutzner, M. A., and Jordan, H. W. The ultrastructure of an abnormal cell in Sézary's syndrome. *Blood 31*:719, 1968.

Little, J. R., Brecher, G., Bradley, T. R., and Rose, S. Determination of lymphocyte turnover by continuous infusion of H^3 thymidine. *Blood 19*:236, 1962.

MacKinney, A. A., Jr., Stohlman, F., Jr., and Brecher, G. The kinetics of cell proliferation in cultures of human peripheral blood. *Blood 19*: 349, 1962.

MacKinney, A. A., Jr. Studies of plasma protein synthesis by peripheral cells from normal persons and patients with infectious mononucleosis. *Blood 32*:217, 1968.

Malpighi, M. *De Viscerum Structura.* Bonn, 1666. Cited from Garrison, F. H. *An Introduction to the History of Medicine* (4th ed.). Saunders, Philadelphia, 1960.

Marchesi, V. T., and Gowans, J. L. The migration of lymphocytes through the endothelium of venules in lymph nodes, an electron microscope study. *Proc Roy Soc [Biol] 159*:283, 1964.

Martinez, C., Dalmasso, A. P., and Good, R. A. Effect of thymectomy on development of immunological competence in mice. *Ann NY Acad Sci 113*:933, 1964.

Maruyama, K., and Masuda, T. Electron microscope observation on germinal center of the lymph node in guinea pigs sensitized with sheep erythrocytes. *Ann Rep Inst Virus Res Kyoto Univ 7*:149, 1964.

Maximow, A. A. Bindegewebe und blutbildende Gewebe. Die Gewebe. *Handbuch Mikr Anat Mensch 2*:232, 1927a.

Maximow, A. A. Development of non-granular leukocytes (lymphocytes and monocytes) into polyblasts (macrophages) and fibroblasts *in vitro. Proc Soc Exp Biol Med 24*:570, 1927b.

Mellors, R. C., and Korngold, L. The cellular origin of human immunoglobulins (γ_2, γ_{1M}, γ_1A). *J Exp Med 118*:387, 1963.

Mekori, T., Chieco-Bianci, L., and Feldman, M. Production of colonies of lymphoid cell populations. *Nature (London) 206*:367, 1965.

Merchant, B., and Brahmi, Z. Duplicate plating of immune cell products. Analyses of globulin class secretion by single cells. *Science 167*:69, 1970.

Meuwissen, H. J., Stutman, O., and Good, R. A. Functions of lymphocytes. *Seminars Hemat 6*: 28, 1969.

Michalowski, A., Bartoszewicz, W., and Kozubowski, J. Blastic transformation in leucocyte cultures. *Lancet 2*:1130, 1966.

Mori, Y., and Lennert, K. *Electron Microscopic Atlas of Lymph Node Cytology and Pathology* (Kirchemann, K., transl.). Springer, Berlin, 1969.

Morse, S. I., and Reister, S. K. Studies on the leukocytosis and lymphocytosis induced by Bordetella pertussis. II. The effect of pertussis vaccine on the thoracic duct lymph and lymphocytes of mice. *J Exp Med 125*:619, 1967.

Moses, H. L., Glade, P. R., Kasel, J. A., Rosenthal, A. S., Hirschaut, Y., and Chessin, L. N. Infectious mononucleosis: Detection of herpes like virus and reticular aggregates of small cytoplasmic particles in continuous lymphoid cell lines derived from peripheral blood. *Proc Nat Acad Sci 60*:489, 1968.

Murray, R. G., and Woods, P. A. Studies on the fate of lymphocytes. III. The migration and metamorphosis of *in situ* labeled thymic lymphocytes. *Anat Rec 150*:113, 1964.

Niederman, J. C., McCollum, R. W., Henle, G., and Henle, W. Infectious mononucleosis. Clinical manifestation in relation to EB virus antibodies. *JAMA 203*:205, 1968.

Nossal, G. J. V., Szenberg, A., Ada, G. L., and Austin, C. M. Single cell studies on 19S antibody production. *J Exp Med 119*:485, 1964.

Ogawa, K. Electronenoptische Untershehungen bei einem Fall von sog. Hodgkin-sarkom. *Frankfurt ztschr Path 71*:677, 1962.

Owen, J. J. T., and Ritter, M. A. Tissue interaction in the development of thymus lymphocytes. *J Exp Med 129*:431, 1969.

Paegle, R. D. Electron microscopic study of leukocytes in infectious mononucleosis. *Blood 17*: 687, 1961.

Papermaster, B. W., Condie, R. M., Finstad, J., and Good, R. A. Evolution of the immune response. I. The phylogenetic development of adaptive immunologic responsiveness in vetebrates. *J Exp Med 119*:105, 1964.

Paul, J. R., and Bunnell, W. W. The presence of heterophile antibodies in infectious mononucleosis. *Amer J Med Sci 183*:90, 1932.

Pearmain, G., Lycette, R. R., and Fitzgerald, P. H. Tuberculin-induced mitosis in peripheral blood leucocytes. *Lancet 1*:627, 1963.

Perry, S., Craddock, C. G., Paul, G., and Lawrence, J. S. Lymphocyte production and turnover. *Arch Intern Med 103*:224, 1959.

Pfeiffer, E. Drüsenfieber. *Jahrbuch Kinderheilk 29*: 257, 1889.

Policard, A. *Physiologie et Pathologie du Système lymphöid.* Masson, Paris, 1963.

Quaglino, D., and Hayhoe, F. G. Observations on the periodic acid-Schiff reaction in lymphoproliferative diseases. *J Path Bact 78*:521, 1959.

Rappaport, H. Tumors of the Hemopoietic System. In *Atlas of Tumor Pathology, Section III Fascicle 8.* Armed Forces Institute of Pathology, Washington, 1966.

Reinhardt, W. O., and Yoffey, J. M. Lymphocyte content of lymph from the thoracic and cervical ducts in guinea pig. *J Physiol 136*:227, 1957.

Robbins, J. H. Tissue culture studies of the human lymphocyte. *Science 146*:1648, 1964.

Robinson, S. H., Brecher, G., Lourie, I. S., and Haley, J. E. Leukocyte labeling in rats during and after continuous infusion of tritiated thymidine: Implications for lymphocyte longevity and DNA reutilization. *Blood 26*:281, 1965.

Rosenau, W., and Moon, H. D. Lysis of homologous cells by sensitized lymphocytes in tissue culture. *J Nat Cancer Inst 27*:471, 1961.

Schöpf, E., Schulz, K. H., and Gromm, M. Transformationen und Mitosen von Lymphocyten *in vitro* durch Quecksilber (II) Chlorid. *Naturwissenschaften 54*:568, 1967.

Schumacher, H. R., McFeely, A. E., and Maugel, T. K. The mononucleosis cell. III. Electron microscopy. *Blood 33*:833, 1969.

Seman, G., and Seman, C. Electron microscopic search for virus particles in patients with leukemia and lymphoma. *Cancer 22*:1033, 1968.

Sézary, A., and Bouvrain, Y. Erythrodermie avec présence de cellules monstreuse dans le derm et dans le sang circulant. *Bull Soc Franc Derm Syph 45*:254, 1938.

Sézary, A. Une nouvelle reticulose cutanée la reticulose maligne leucémique A. Histomonocytes monatreux et à forme d'érythrodermie vedemateuse et pigmentée. *Ann Derm Syph (Paris) 9*:5, 1949.

Sjövall, H. *Experimentelle Untersuchungen über das Blut und die blutbildenden Organe besonders das lymphatische gewebe des Kanichens bei wiederholten Aderlassen Hakan Ohlssons Boktrycken.* Lund, 1936. Cited by Yoffey and Courtice (1956).

Spriggs, A. I., and Jerrome, D. W. Electron-microscopy of Türk cells. *Brit J Haemat 13*:764, 1967.

Sprunt, T. P., and Evans, F. A. Mononuclear leucocytosis in reaction to acute infections ("infectious mononucleosis"). *Bull Hopkins Hosp 31*: 410, 1920.

St. Pierre, R. L. The thymus as a lymphoid organ. *Anat Rec 165*:113, 1969.

Stefani, S. S., and Tonaki, H. Fibrillar bundles in the nucleus of blood lymphocytes from leukemic and non-leukemic patients. *Blood 35*: 243, 1970.

Sundberg, R. D. Lymphocytes and plasma cells. *Ann NY Acad Sci 59*:671, 1955.

Svehag, S. E., and Mandel, B. The formation and properties of poliovirus-neutralizing antibody. I. 19S and 7S antibody formation: Differences in kinetics and antigen dose requirement for induction. *J Exp Med 119*:1, 1964a.

Svehag, S. E., and Mandel, B. The formation and properties of poliovirus-neutralizing antibody. II. 19S and 7S antibody formation: Difference in antigen dose requirement for sustained synthesis, anamnesis, and sensitivity to x-irradiation. *J Exp Med 119*:21, 1964b.

Symmers, D. The relationship of the toxic lymphoid hyperplasia to lymphosarcoma and allied diseases. *Arch Intern Med 21*:237, 1918.

Takeda, A., Takeda, Y., Huang, C. C., and Ambrus, J. L. Biphasic pattern of thymus regeneration after whole body irradiation. *J Exp Med 129*: 445, 1969.

Tanaka, H. Electron microscopic studies on the lymphatic cells in the lymph node and thymus, with special reference to lymphogonia. *Acta Haemat Jap 20*:237, 1957.

Tanaka, Y., Epstein, L. B., Brecher, G., and Stohlman, F., Jr. Transformation of lymphocytes in culture of human peripheral blood. *Blood 22*: 614, 1963.

Tanaka, Y. Fibrillar structures in the cells of blood-forming organs. *J Nat Cancer Inst 33*:467, 1964.

Tanaka, Y., and Liddy, T. J. Lipids and acid phosphatase in cultured lymphocytes of peripheral blood. A histochemical and electron microscopic study. *Lab Invest 15*:455, 1966.

Tanaka, Y., Bell, W. R., and Brindley, D. Pseudoviral inclusion bodies in acute leukemia. A report of two cases. *J Nat Cancer Inst 38*:629, 1967.

Taswell, H. F., and Winkelmann, R. K., Jr. Sézary's syndrome. A malignant reticulemic erythrodermia. *JAMA 177*:465, 1961.

Till, J. E., and McCulloch, E. A. A direct measurement of the radiation sensitivity of normal mouse bone marrow cells. *Radiat Res 14*:213, 1961.

Türk, W. Ein System der Lymphomatosen. *Klin Wschr 16*:1073, 1903.

Uhr, J. W., and Finkelstein, M. S. Antibody formation. IV. Formation of rapidly and slowly sedimenting antibodies and immunological memory to bacteriophage ΦX 174. *J Exp Med 117*:457, 1963.

van Furth, R., Schuit, H. R. E., and Hijmans, W. The formation of immunoglobulins by human tissues *in vitro.* IV. Circulating lymphocytes in normal and pathological conditions. *Immunology 11*:29, 1966.

Wakefield, J. D., and Thorbecke, G. J. Relationship of germinal centers in lymphoid tissue to immunological memory. I. Evidence for the formation of small lymphocytes upon transfer of primed splenic white pulp to syngeneic mice. *J Exp Med 128*:153, 1968.

Waksman, B. H., Arnason, B. G., and Jankovic, B. D. Role of the thymus in immune reactions in rats. III. Changes in the lymphoid organs of thymectomized rats. *J Exp Med 116*:187, 1962.

Weber, A. F., and Joel, D. Tabular and ultrastructural studies of agranulocytes of the thoracic duct of calves. *Blood 28*:266, 1966.

Weiss, L. Interactions of sensitized lymphoid cells and homologous target cells in tissue culture and in graphs: An electron microscopic and immunofluorescent study. *J Immun 101*:1346, 1968.

Weissman, J. L. Thymus cell migration. *J Exp Med 126*:291, 1967.

Wesslen, T. Passive transfer of tuberculin hypersensitivity by viable lymphocytes from the thoracic duct lymphocytes of mice. *Acta Tuberc Scand 26*:38, 1952.

Wiener, J., Spiro, D., and Russell, P. S. An electron microscopic study of the homograft rejection. *Amer J Path 44*:319, 1964.

Wivel, N. A., Mandel, M. A., and Asofsky, R. M. Ultrastructural study of thoracic duct lymphocyte of mice. *Amer J Anat 128*:57, 1970.

Yoffey, J. M., and Courtice, F. C. *Lymphatics, Lymph and Lymphoid Tissue.* Arnold, London, 1956.

Yoffey, J. M. *Quantitative Cellular Haematology.* Thomas, Springfield, Ill., 1960.

Yoffey, J. M., Winter, G. C. G., Osmond, D. G., and Meek, E. S. Morphological studies in the culture of human lymphocytes with phytohaemagglutinin. *Brit J Haemat 11*:488, 1965.

Zucker-Franklin, D. The ultrastructure of cells in human thoracic duct lymph. *J Ultrastruct Res 9*:325, 1963a.

Zucker-Franklin, D. Virus-like particles in the lymphocytes of a patient with chronic lymphocytic leukemia. *Blood 21*:509, 1963b.

Zucker-Franklin, D. The ultrastructure of lymphocytes. *Seminars Hemat 6*:4, 1969.

Zuelzer, W. W., and Flatz, G. Acute childhood leukemia, a ten year study. *Amer J Dis Child 100*: 886, 1960.

chapter 6
PLASMA CELLS

The term "Plasmazellen" (plasma cell) was introduced by Waldeyer (1875) for cells with abundant cytoplasm which contained many granules and which were found in many tissues. However, this was not the type of cell we know today as the plasma cell. Ramón y Cajal (1890) first described the plasma cell, which he found in subcutaneous tissues of patients suffering from syphilitic condylomas, and characterized it as the "cyanophil cell" because the cytoplasm stained a deep blue with basic dyes. Independent of this, Unna (1891) found the same type of cell in the skin of patients with lupus and described it as a "plasma cell." Plasma cells were distinguished from lymphocytes by the extensive investigations of Unna, Marschalkó, and Pappenheim around the beginning of the twentieth century (reviewed by Michels, 1931). The next important development came in the late 1940's with the development of the concept of its role in antibody formation (summarized by Ehrlich, 1956).

The more recent revelations of the cytoplasmic ultrastructure in plasma cells have been a significant contribution of electron microscopy to the field of hematology and represent an outstanding example of the correlation of ultrastructural morphology to cellular function. The functional significance of these cytoplasmic structures, the extensive endoplasmic reticulum, was suggested in the first electron micrographic descriptions of Braunsteiner *et al.* (1953, 1955). They described plasma cells rich in endoplasmic reticulum in normal human bone marrow and in three cases of multiple myeloma. The highly developed cytoplasmic cisternae with attached ribosomes were thought to be the important organelle for protein synthesis. Similar structures had been seen in cells of various secretory glands involved in protein excretion. This unique morphology, the prominence of a highly developed rough-surfaced endoplasmic

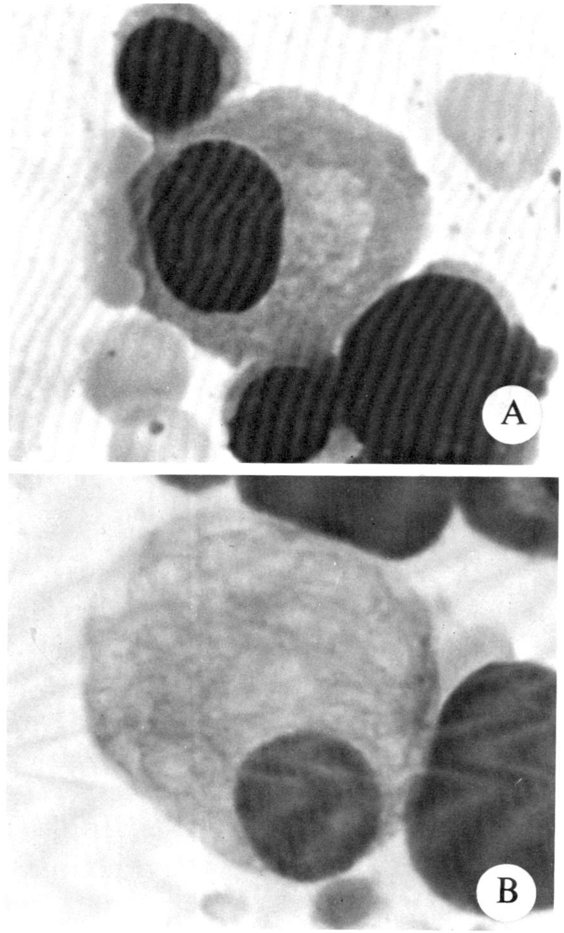

FIGURE 6-1. Two mature plasma cells from human bone marrow.
A. Typical cell has a clear zone in the abundant cytoplasm and eccentric nucleus. *Giemsa stain. × 2,000.*
B. Mature cell has extended cytoplasm of a vesicular appearance. *Giemsa stain. × 2,000.*

FIGURE 6-2. Normal mature plasma cells from bone marrow.
The large cell with an eccentrically located nucleus (*N*) has extensive areas of endoplasmic reticulum (*er*), a large Golgi (*G*) zone, several mitochondria (*M*), and multivesicular structure (*arrow*). Variable-sized vesicles contain material of differing density in the Golgi area, some of which may correspond to the azurophilic granules seen by light microscopy. This is clearly seen in the top cell. The nucleus has some chromatin concentrated around its periphery, a characteristic of the maturing cell. Electron-dense particles and part of a macrophage (*Ma*) are in the right upper corner, as well as a blood vessel (left upper corner). *× 15,000.*

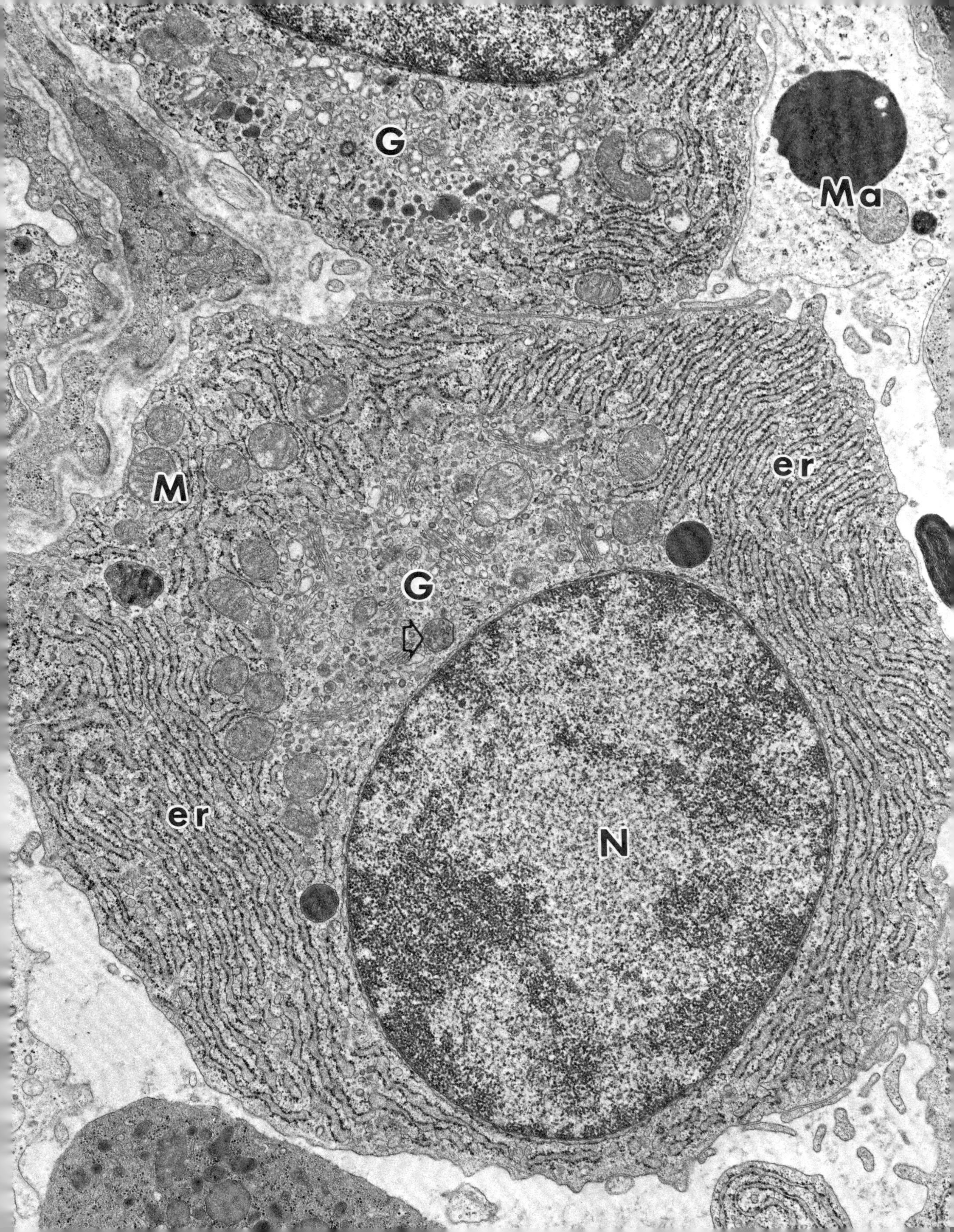
G
Ma
er
M
G
er
N

reticulum, is now generally accepted as the identifiable characteristic of plasma cells.

MORPHOLOGY

The typical plasma cell is a normal component of human bone marrow. The physiological response to some antigenic stimuli includes an increase in the number of normal plasma cells while other pathological entities involve abnormalities of the plasma cell per se. The reactive or stimulatory conditions, such as chronic inflammation, involve increased numbers of these cells grouped around capillaries or sinuses in the bone marrow. The plasma cell is more commonly noted in such lymphoreticular tissues as lymph nodes and spleen, where the numbers are also increased in the presence of a chronic inflammatory or reactive process. They are rarely seen in clusters like those of erythroblasts, although this has been described (Thiéry, 1962).

By light microscopy, the Giemsa stain of the mature plasma cell shows a large spherical or ovoid cell with abundant deep blue cytoplasm (Fig. 6-1*A*). The nucleus is round, eccentrically placed, and contains dense masses of chromatin, frequently arranged in wheel-spoke fashion. Nucleoli are seen only in immature forms. A large, well-defined, pale area near the paranuclear area contains the Golgi complex (Fig. 6-1*A*). In reactive or stimulated conditions, intracytoplasmic inclusions are common. Some of these are called Russell bodies (Dubreuil and Favre, 1920–1921; Apitz, 1937; Pease, 1949) and may appear as refractile areas in phase microscopy (Thiéry, 1958). In stained preparations they are often gray-blue and may take PAS stain, which indicates the presence of mucopolysaccharide (Welsh, 1962). An extensive accumulation of material containing protein and carbohydrate causes gross distention of the cisternae (Fig. 6-1*B*), which has led to their description in this state as "flame cells" (Undritz, 1952; Maldonado *et al.,* 1965), "Mott cells" or "grape cells" (Zlotnick, 1956).

By electron microscopy, the distinctive feature of the normal mature plasma cells is the well-packed, rough-surfaced endoplasmic reticulum (Figs. 6-2 through 6-4). When this endoplasmic reticulum is distended, it can also be discerned by phase microscopy (Thiéry, 1955, 1958). The rough-surfaced membranes (Fig. 6-5) have ribosomes on one surface which are RNA-containing particles (150 to 250 Å in diameter) and are responsible for the deep blue color of the cytoplasm when stained with basic dyes. These ribosomes are usually regularly spaced, with about 200 to 300 Å between particles. An occasional tangential cut of the endoplasmic reticulum suggests a spatial arrangement in rosettes or whorls about 1,000 to 1,500 Å in diameter, made up of eight to 16 ribosomes connected by a thin filament and arranged as in Figure 6-5*B*. Similar struc-

(*text continues on page 284*)

FIGURE 6-3. Mature plasma cell.
One plasma cell and parts of three others from marginal site of a metastatic focus of squamous cell carcinoma of the brain. The central plasma cell is highly differentiated and shows distended endoplasmic reticulum (*er*). Mitochondria (*M*) are distributed around a wide Golgi (*G*) area, and nucleus (*N*) is eccentrically located. Note small cytoplasmic blebs along upper and lower margins of cell membrane (*arrows*). Plasma cells at right and left upper corner have abundant flattened endoplasmic reticulum. × *15,000.*

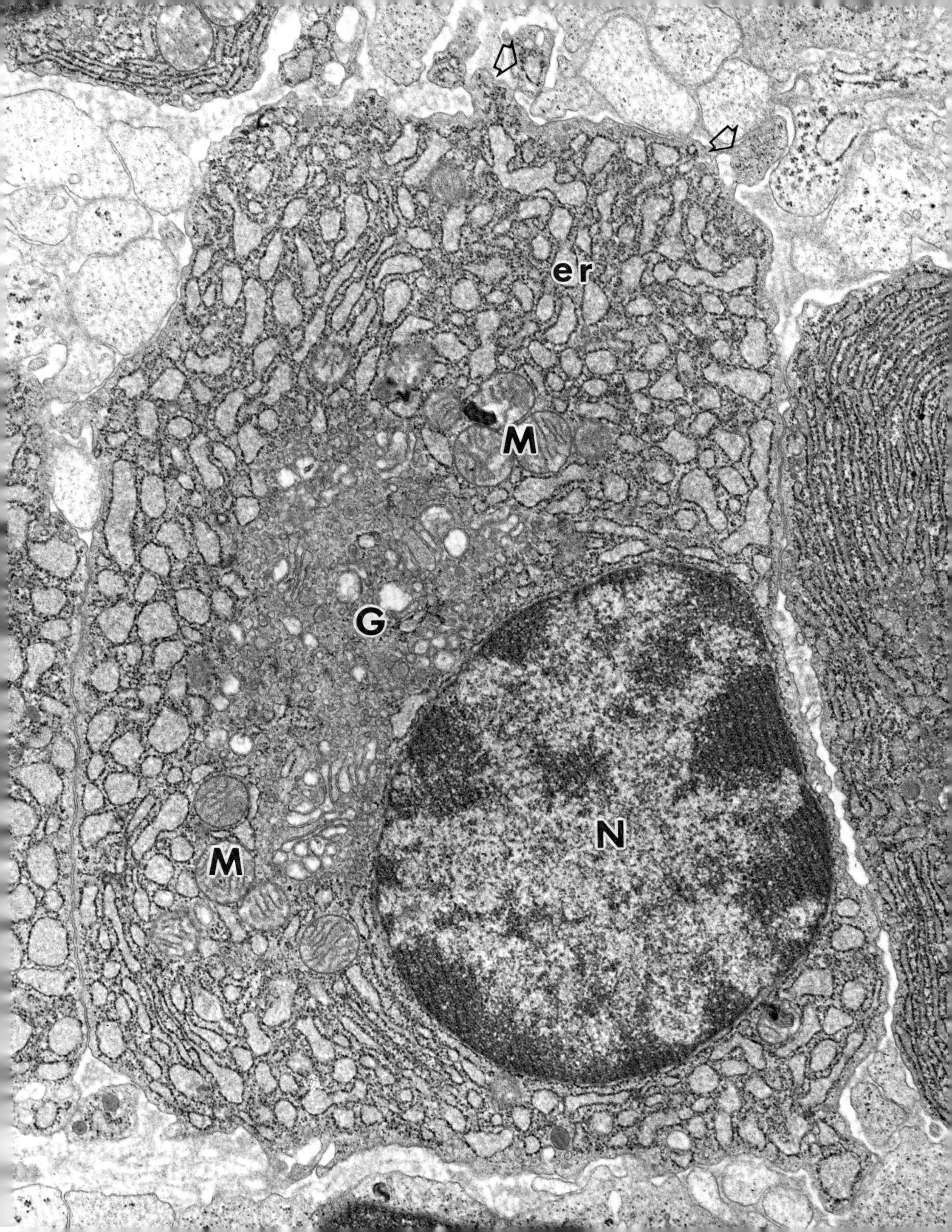
er
M
G
M
N

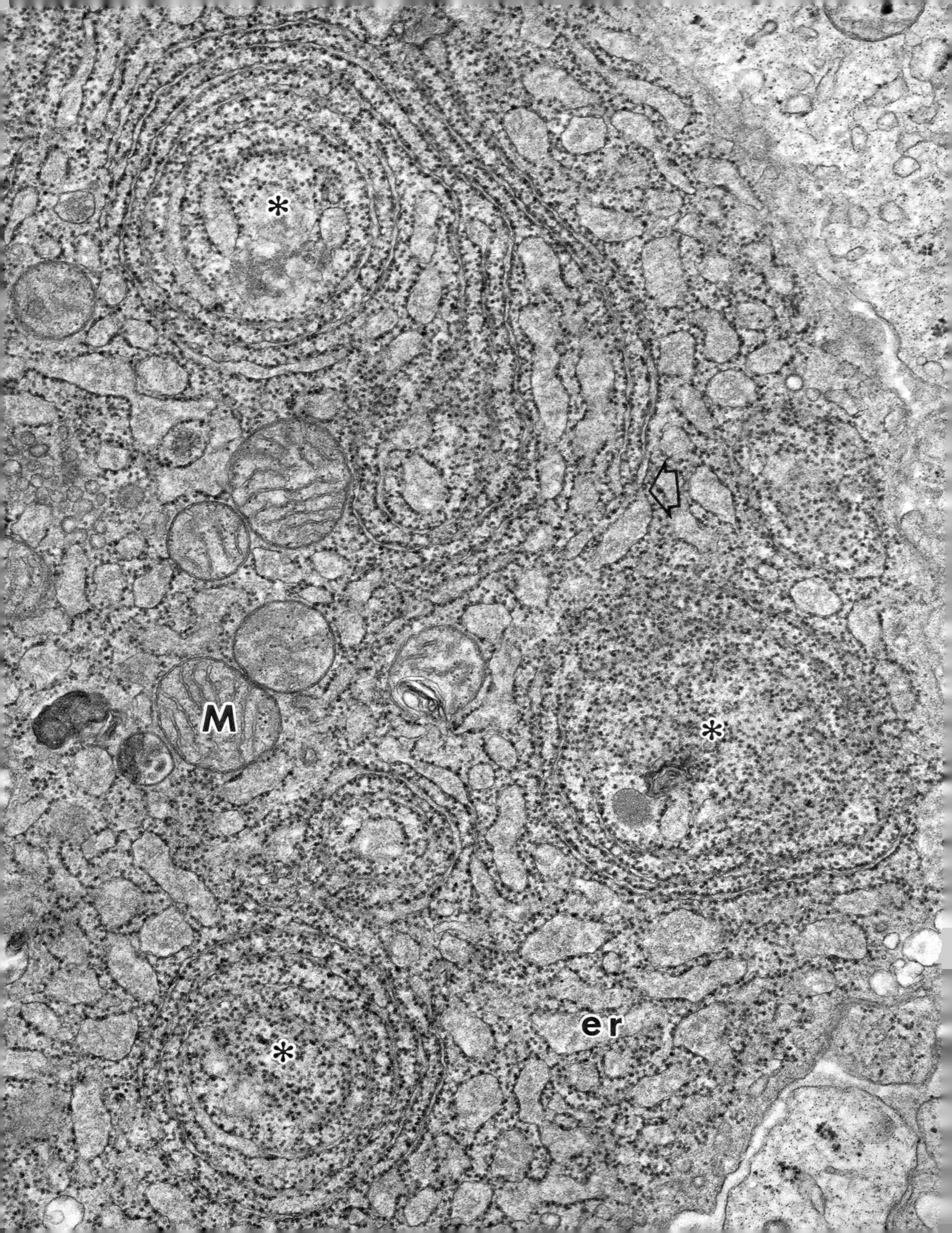
*
M
*
*
er

FIGURE 6-4. Mature plasma cell.
Cytoplasm has peculiar whorls (*asterisks*) of flattened endoplasmic reticulum (*er*) within distended endoplasmic reticulum. Communication of flattened with distended type (*arrow*) is an unusual phenomenon and suggests the whorl arrangement of flattened endoplasmic reticulum at more than one center. Large mitochondria (*M*) are seen at edge of Golgi area. × *32,300.*

Figures 6-5 and 6-6 appear on the following pages

FIGURE 6-5. Mature plasma cells.
A. This portion shows lamellar arrangement of endoplasmic reticulum (*er*). The ribosomes (*r*) are only on the outside of the membrane pair, and a small amount of protein material is present in cisternae. Particles dispersed in cytoplasm are ferritin granules. × *87,000.*
B. Distended endoplasmic reticulum (*er*) contains amorphous material, presumably globulin produced by this structure. The orderly lamellar structure seen in Figure 6-5**A** is disrupted as cisternae enlarge. The plane of section cut some endoplasmic membranes perpendicular to their surface; they appear as sharp lines with dots of ribosomal (*r*) RNA on one surface, while the angle of cut in other aeas is tangential. Membranes cut at an angle of less than 30° are generally not visualized by electron microscopy. These latter locations show the rosette arrangement (*arrows*) of ribosomal RNA particles on the membrane surface. × *98,000.*

FIGURE 6-6. Golgi apparatus in mature plasma cell.
This Golgi area of a mature plasma cell has a tangentially cut centriole (*Ce*). There are many small and larger vesicles (*v*) which contain amorphous material (*asterisk*). A portion of the flattened sacs (*s*) or vesicles typical of Golgi structures are also seen. A mitochondrion (*M*) is located near outer edges of Golgi zone. Some Golgi vesicles near rough-surfaced endoplasmic reticulum (*er*) appear to be connected to membranes with scattered ribosomal particles. × *65,000.*

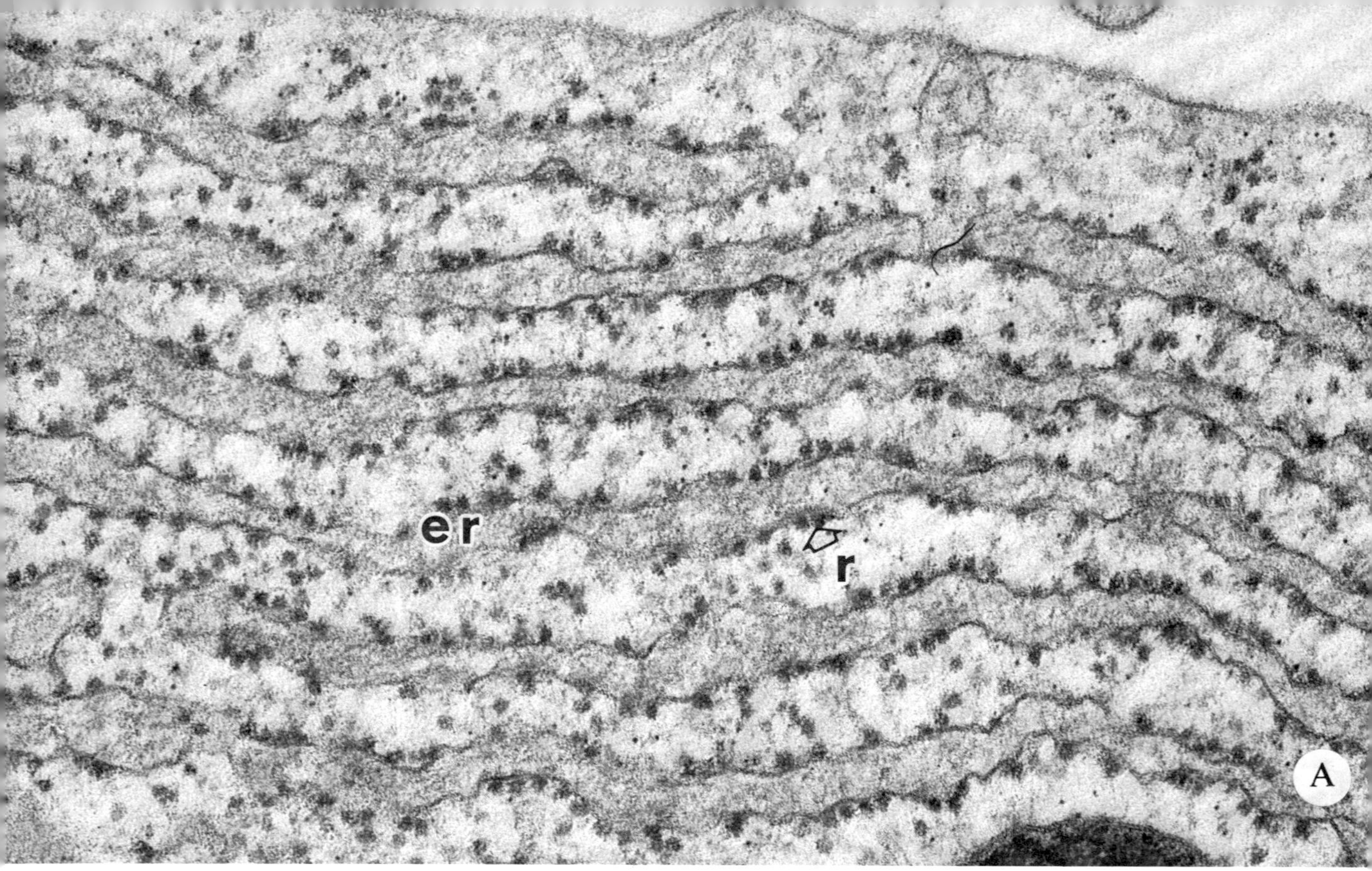
er
r
A

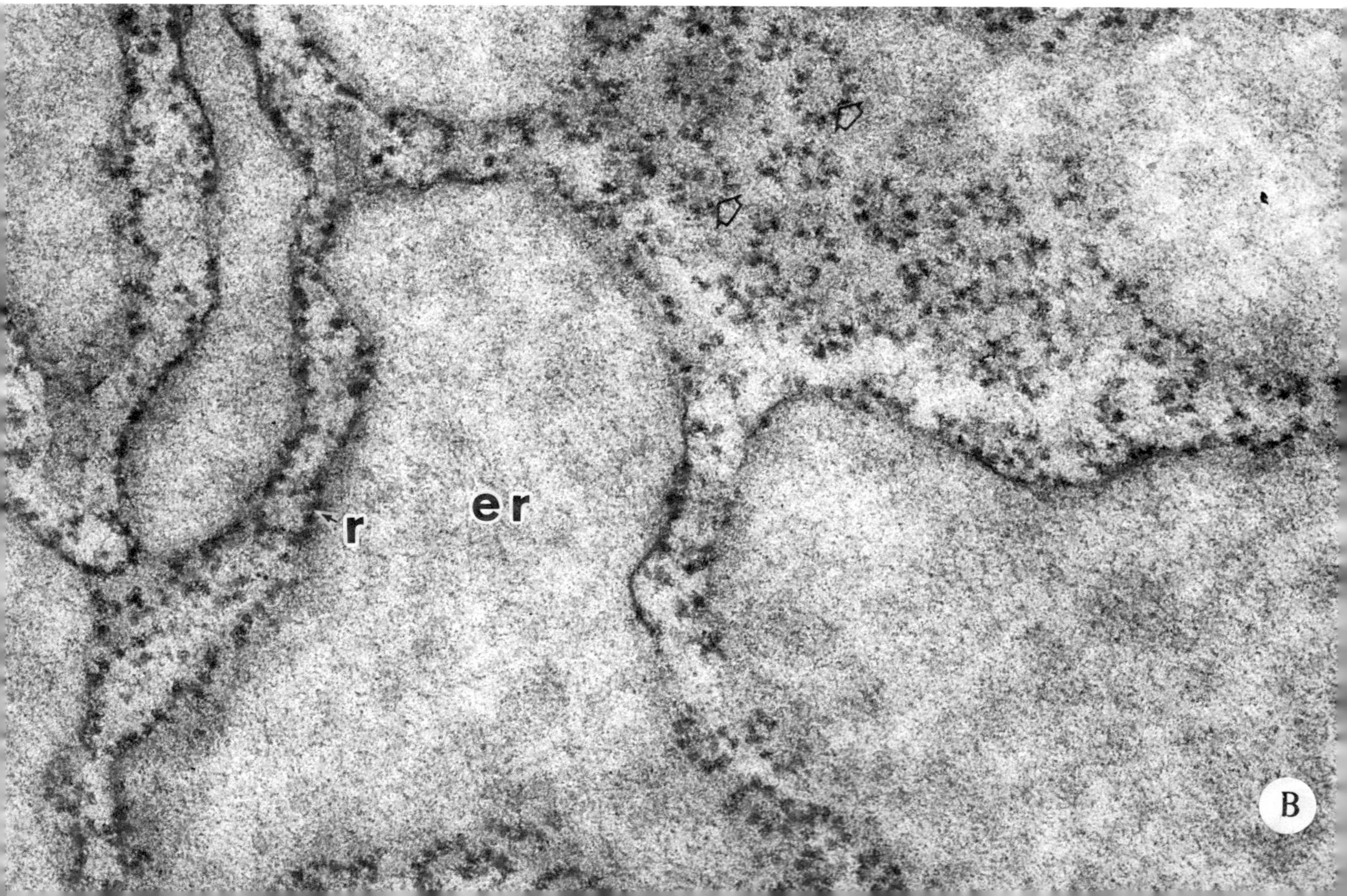
r
er
B

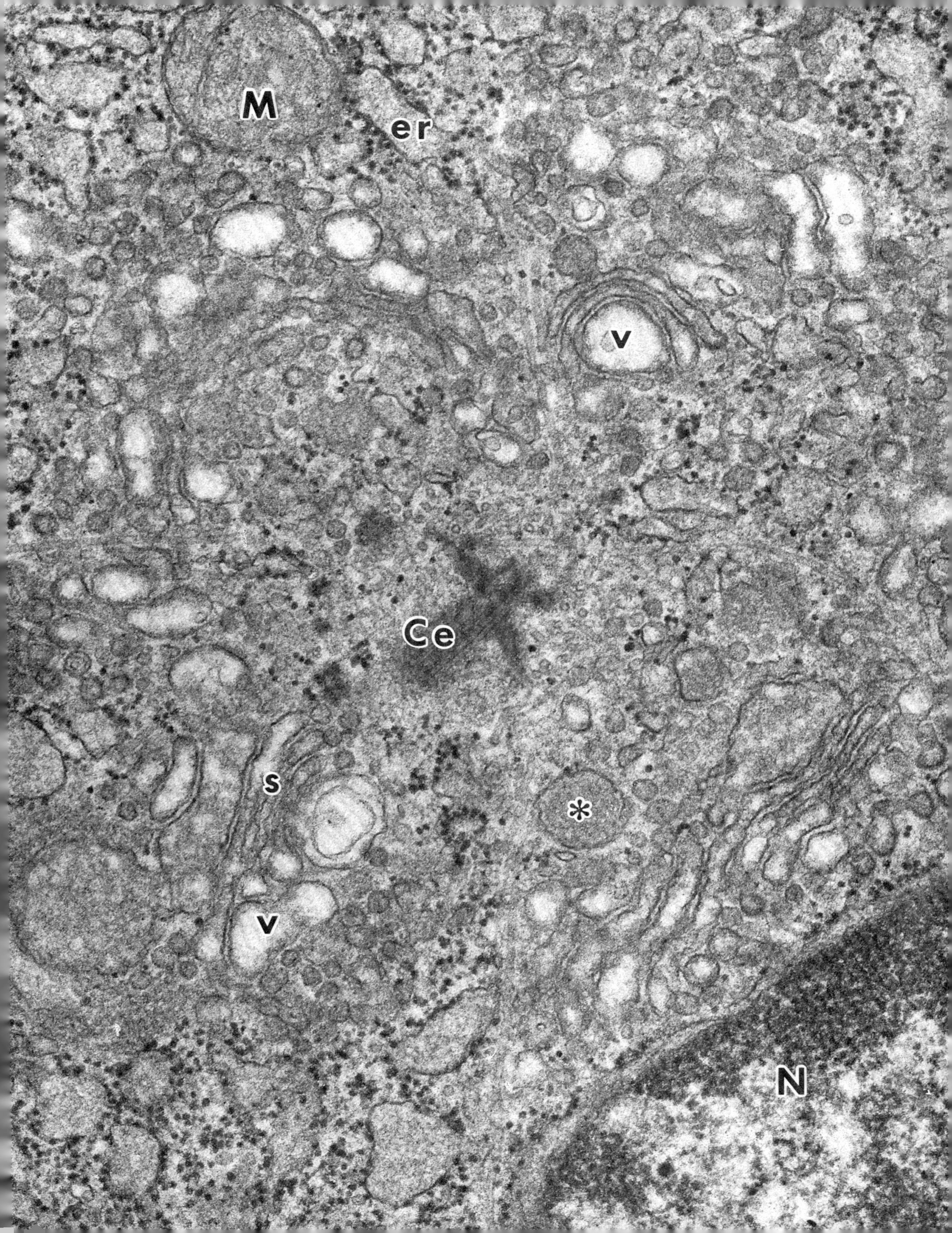
M
er
v
Ce
s
*
v
N

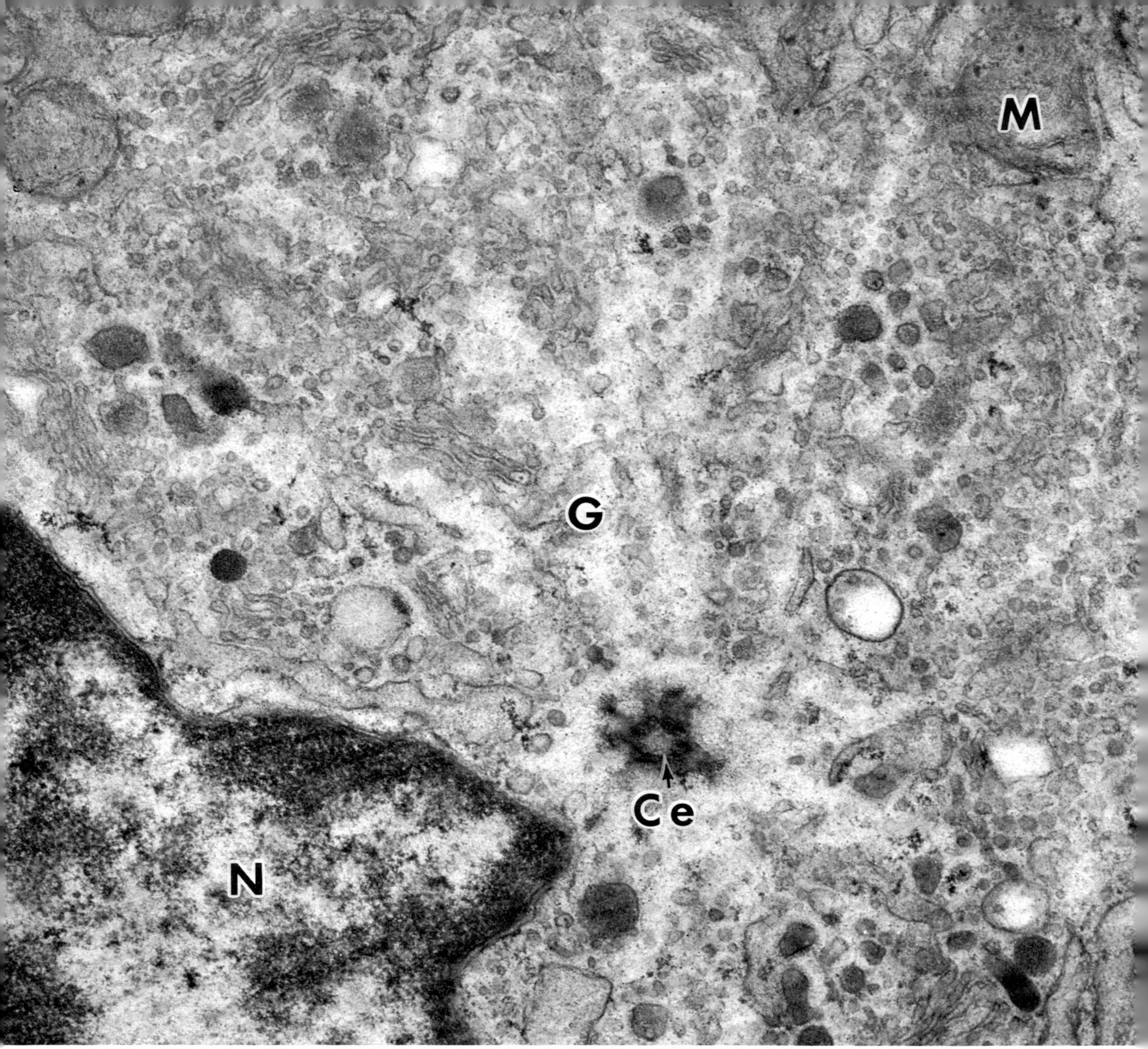

FIGURE 6-7. An unusual Golgi apparatus in plasma cell.
Plasma cell from a patient with refractory sideroblastic anemia contains a prominent centriole (*Ce*) in the Golgi (*G*) area with a radiant array of lighter streaks emanating from the centriole through the vesicular portion of the Golgi zone. This structural characteristic was seen in several sections of this cell. The nucleus (*N*) has a heavy concentration of chromatin along the nuclear envelope, and mitochondria (*M*) are present on the edge of the Golgi zone. *Fixation: Osmium. Plastic: Maraglas.* × *42,000.*

FIGURE 6-8. Russell bodies in plasma cell.
Cell from marrow of patient with refractory normoblastic anemia exhibits spheroid structures interpreted as Russell bodies (*Ru*). Dense inclusions vary in size (up to 4μ diameter) and may show some variation in density. Angular inclusions with less dense material (*asterisks*) are also seen in the cytoplasm. The nucleus (*N*) shows two nuclear inclusions. The Golgi zone (*G*) with a centriole (*Ce*) is apparent, along with a few mitochondria (*M*). The endoplasmic reticulum is primarily a vesicular structure. *Fixation: Osmium in s-collidine buffer. Plastic: Maraglas.* × *19,400.*

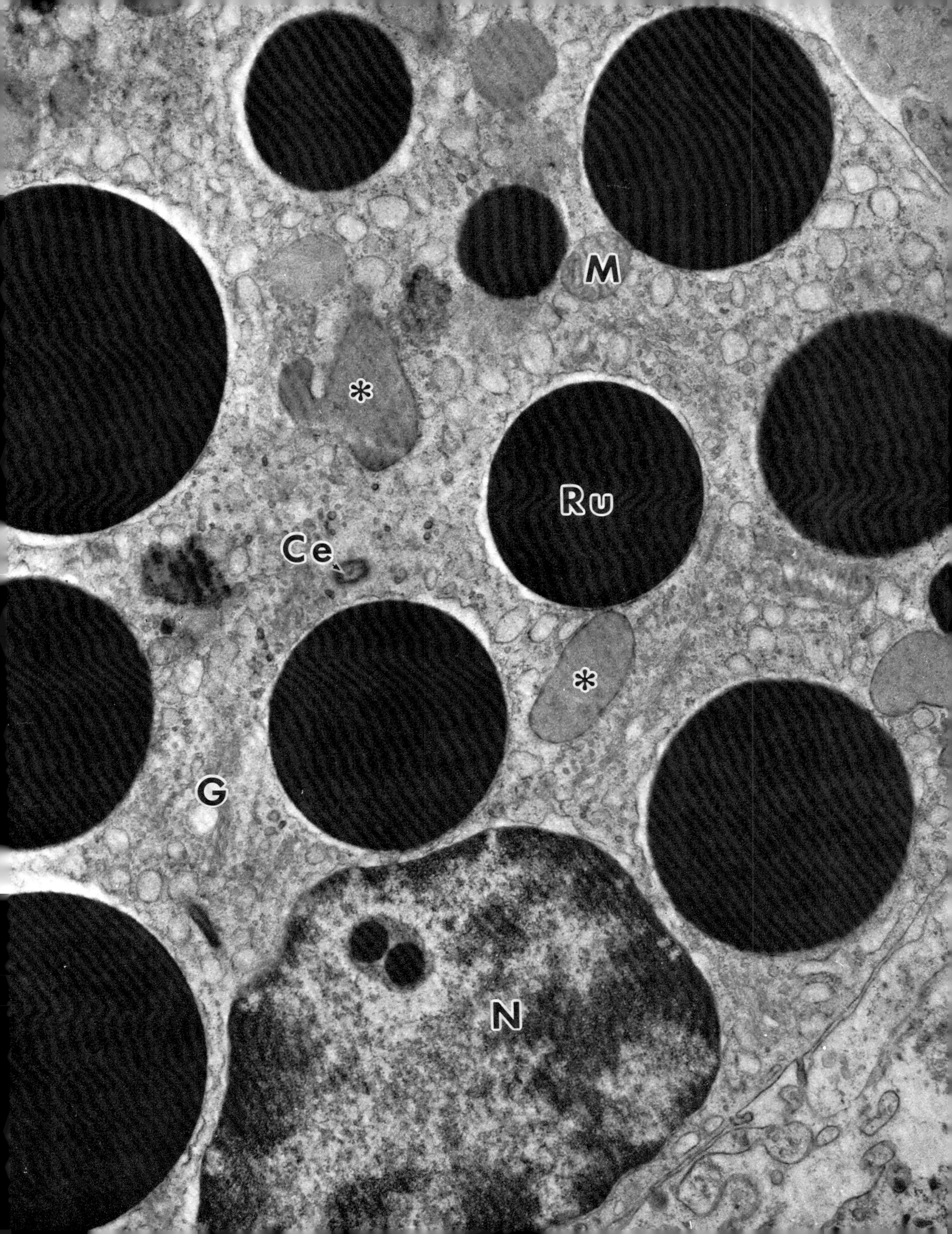
M
*
Ru
Ce
*
G
N

tures have also been described in hepatic cells and fibroblasts (Ross and Klebanoff, 1967). Ribosomes attached to the membranes are considered to be the site of protein synthesis.

The early functioning phase of the plasma cell with developed sheets of endoplasmic reticulum has flattened cisternae (Fig. 6-5*A*) which become dilated with synthesized protein as the cell reaches its more mature stage (Fig. 6-5*B*). The protein material in the cisternae of the endoplasmic reticulum varies from an amorphous to flocculent state. With specific labeling technics, these structures have been shown to produce immune gamma globulins (Rifkind *et al.*, 1962; de Petris *et al.*, 1963, 1965; Leduc *et al.*, 1968). The difference in appearance observed by electron microscopy may be related to variations in the chemical composition of synthesized immunoglobulin. These complex heterogeneous proteins—i.e., gamma globulins—may, depending on their class, contain relatively high amounts (10 per cent) of carbohydrate (Heremans *et al.*, 1959). Gamma globulins are known to vary in size, with sedimentation rates ranging from 7S to 19S in normal human serum and as high as 32S in some pathological states. A more complete description of these molecules can be found under Function.

The Golgi area (Figs. 6-6 and 6-7), with numerous vesicles and flattened sacs, is in the paranuclear clear zone of the plasma cell. It is one of the largest complexes of any bone marrow cell and serves as one of the prominent identifying characteristics of the plasma cell. A few granules in the Golgi apparatus increase in size and density to become large enough to be visualized by light microscopy, and may be the azurophilic granules of the Giemsa stain. The Golgi vesicles contain amorphous material which may be the carbohydrate that combines with the protein produced by the rough endoplasmic reticulum to form gamma globulin (Zagury *et al.*, 1970). Near the center of the Golgi area (Fig. 6-6) are centrioles, usually in pairs. When sections reveal both centrioles, their planes of orientation are always perpendicular to each other. Unusual Golgi (Fig. 6-7) are sometimes found in plasma cells.

During periods of activation, unusual structures are occasionally found within the endoplasmic reticulum and appear as electron-opaque spheroids (Fig. 6-8) or crystalloid shapes (Fig. 6-9). These structures, single or multiple, would be the condensed products of accumulated protein or protein complexes. Occasionally, the endoplasmic inclusions are less dense and very extensive (Fig. 6-10*A*). Cytochemically, typical Russell bodies (Fig. 6-8) are acid-fast, and in general react like protein. Also, crystalloid inclusions with internal periodicity up to 140 Å have been reported within the cisternae (Wellensiek, 1957; Thiéry, 1958; Movat and Fernando, 1962).

Crystalloid structures or crystals are rarely noted in granules of plasma cells. Ferritin or iron-staining material arranged in crystalloid form (Fig. 6-10*B*) is found only in severe, hypersiderotic conditions (Goodman and Hall, 1966). Other granules in plasma cells, which may be the azurophilic granules seen by light microscopy, occur less frequently and are the spheroid structures shown in Figure 6-11. They usually contain amorphous electron-dense material and may have an additional crescent-shaped body (Polli *et al.*, 1962) that is more electron-translucent. These structures may correspond to the vacuoles or blue vesicles noted in Giemsa-stained preparations.

The nucleus of the mature plasma cell, which is round or ovoid (Figs. 6-2 and

6-3), frequently has a characteristic wheel-spoke chromatin distribution, which can be seen by light microscopy but is not apparent by electron microscopy. The cut surface of a nucleus seldom shows the characteristic distribution pattern of the entire volume of the nucleus. A more uniform distribution of chromatin and the presence of nucleoli are considered to be indicative of a young or immature cell.

By phase microscopy the nuclei of plasma cells have been noted to have vacuoles, a phenomenon thought to represent nuclear elaboration of protein (Thiéry, 1957).

CYTOGENESIS

Recent progress in the study of cell origin has significantly altered the classic concept of cell generation in hemopoietic organs. As yet, there is no conclusive evidence that any single cytogenic origin applies to plasma cells. Two major hypotheses include their derivation from (1) lymphocytes, and/or (2) mesenchymal elements (cells of the reticuloendothelial system), either by direct transformation or through a committed blastic cell form known as a plasmoblast. However, a combination of both concepts may explain the phenomenon of plasmacytogenesis in different organs under various stimulations.

Maturation processes are studied by panoptical staining on smears and histologic preparations. Smear technics tend to destroy fragile cells and those adherent to structural elements during preparation so that cytological analyses are not satisfactory from histological preparations. Therefore, evaluations differ when different technics are employed. Morphological studies are generally based on intermediate forms arranged in progression from the mature plasma cell back to such well-known cell types as lymphocytes, histiocytes, and/or fixed mesenchymal elements called reticulum cells.

Lymphocytic origin of the plasma cell is the classic and, until recently, most widely accepted concept. Early investigators considered the lymphocyte or lymphoid cell as the more probable progenitor of the plasma cell (Maximow, 1928). Their primary concern was whether the parent cell was derived from circulating blood (hematogenous) or produced in loco (histogenous) (Downey, 1911; Maximow, 1928; Michels, 1931). The term "lymphoid cells" in older literature could include lymphocytes of the present morphology, histiocytes, and blastic cells of lymphoreticular tissues. Consequently, concepts based on a combination of these cell types would bias interpretations toward a lymphocytic origin of plasma cells. Originally, the lymphocytic origin theory was based on the simple morphological similarity between lymphocytes and plasma cells, particularly in their immature forms. Although there was no further evidence to support such a conclusion, this hypothesis has been preferred by many morphologists (Tompkins, 1960; Keuning *et al.,* 1963).

The role of lymphocytes in plasmacytogenesis is less well supported by more recent studies of reactive lymph nodes, and the formation of plasma cells, independent of the lymphocytic series, has been proposed (Miller, 1931; Sainte-Marie, 1964). The multiple origin of plasma cells has been hypothesized in similar experiments (McMillan and Engelbert, 1963). Although, at the present time, the lymphocytic theory is widely held, it should be reevaluated. Recent experiments have shown that circulating lymphocytes can transform themselves with proper stimulation (MacKinney *et al.,* 1962) into large blastic forms resembling hemocytoblasts

(text continues on page 290)

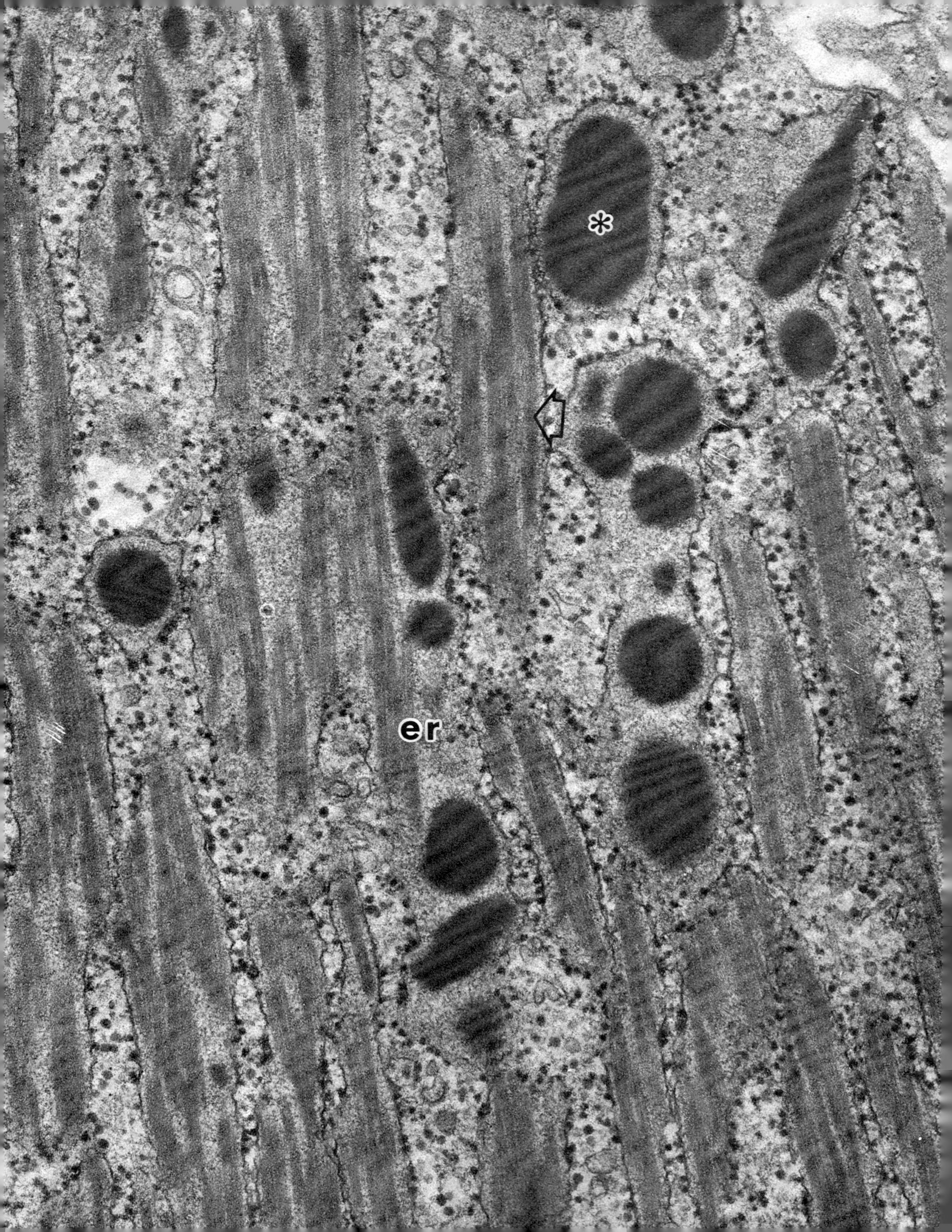
*
er

FIGURE 6-9. Crystalloid structures in plasma cell.
Occasional crystalloid structures (*arrow*) in cisternae of endoplasmic reticulum (*er*) may be polymerized protein (globulin) and are essentially similar to the Russell bodies in Figure 6-8. Amorphous dense spheres (*asterisk*) are also noted within the same endoplasmic reticulum. × *60,000.*

Figures 6-10 and 6-11 appear on the following pages ⇨

FIGURE 6-10. Cytoplasmic structures in plasma cell.
A. A very large amorphous mass lies within the endoplasmic reticulum (*er*) of this plasma cell from the bone marrow of a patient with refractory sideroblastic anemia. A portion of the nucleus (*N*) shows some clumping of finely granular chromatin; there are a few mitochondria but no Golgi apparatus. *Fixation: Osmium, s-collidine buffer. Plastic: Maraglas.* × *24,000.*
B. Inclusion in cytoplasm contains a large number of ferritin particles that are sometimes in rows, with a spacing of 100 to 110 Å. Subunits of ferritin particles are not clearly shown in this micrograph. × *193,000.*

FIGURE 6-11. Cytoplasmic structures in plasma cell.
A. This portion contains four different cytoplasmic inclusions that are not within the cisternae of endoplasmic reticulum: (1) homogeneous material enclosed with a single membrane; (2) structure with a crescent-shaped attachment; (3) structure with similar density but with a periodicity or crystalline form; (4) like the first, enclosed in a single membrane, but more dense and containing two very dense granules. Portion of nucleus (*N*), mitochondrion, and Golgi complex (*G*) are also seen. × *60,000.*
B. Two granules (*g*) with material of different density within a single membrane are near edge of Golgi zone. They are not within cisternae of endoplasmic reticulum but are equal in size to azurophilic granules seen with light microscopy. × *87,500.*
C. Occasional areas of increased density contain material arranged in platelike or crystalline manner. The lower granule (*g*) has a very dense large inner mass similar to smaller masses in granules seen in Figure 6-9**A**. *Fixation: Osmium.* × *87,500.*

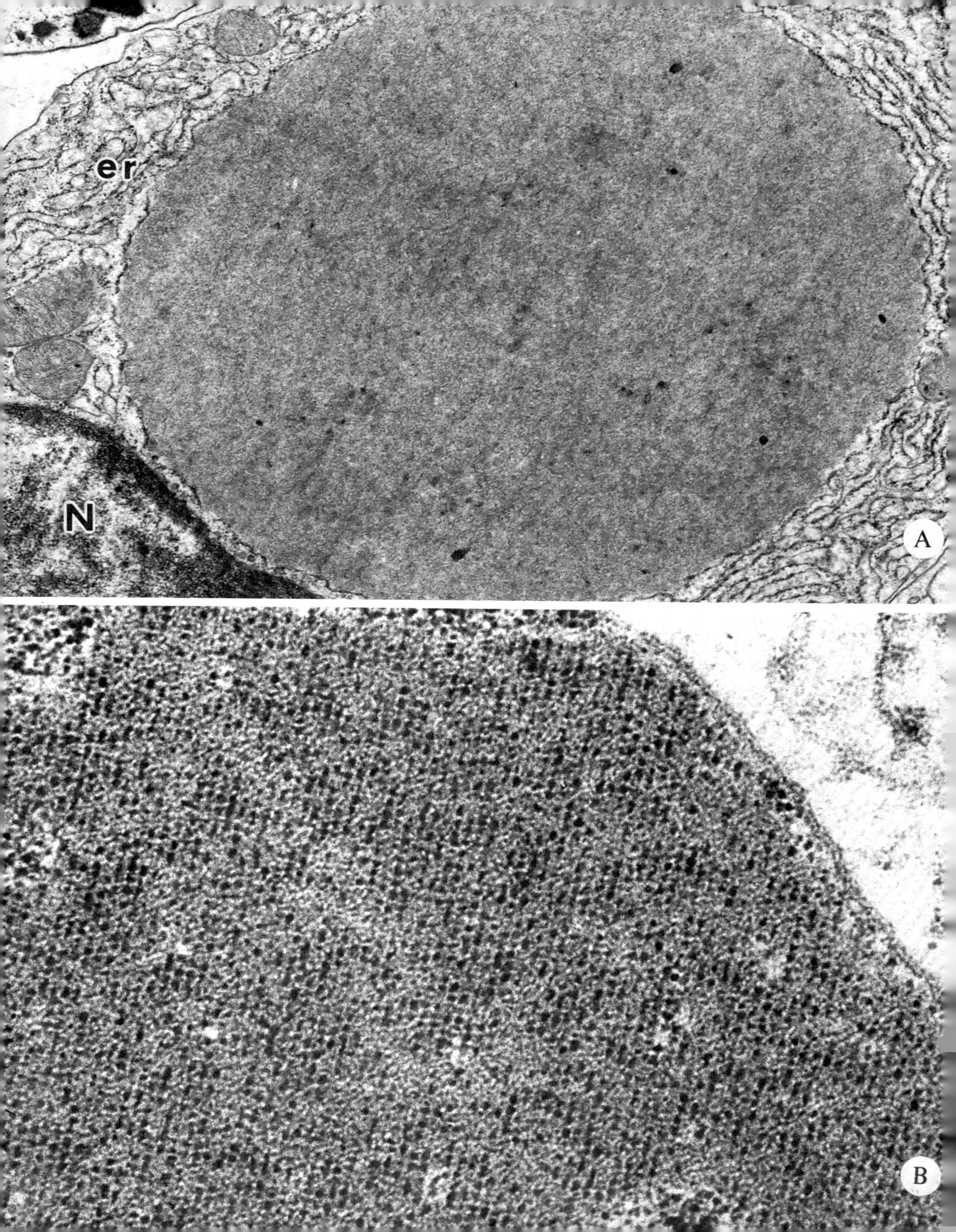
er
N
A
B

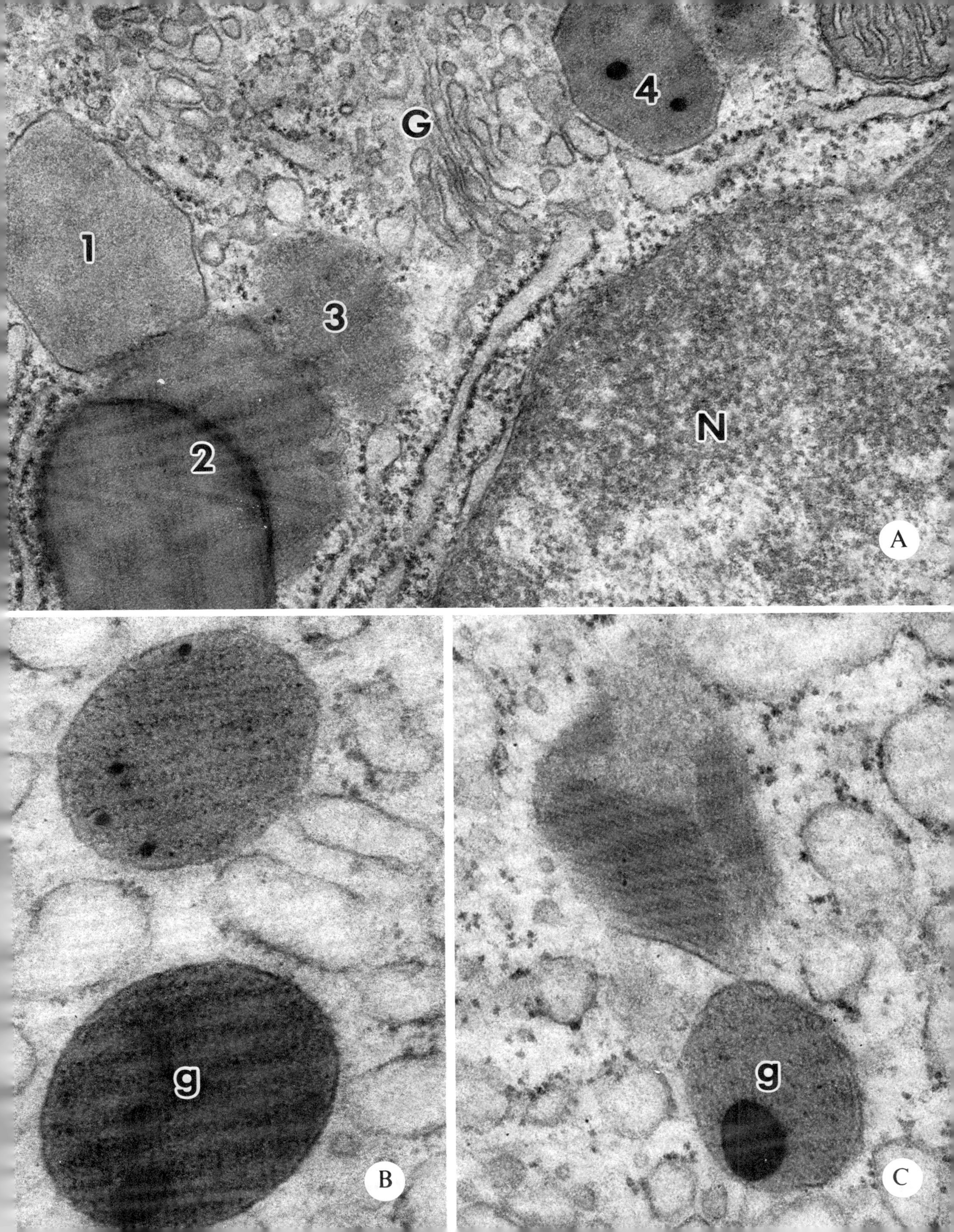
1
2
3
4
G
N
A
g
B
g
C

(Bernhard and Leplus, 1964). This suggests that lymphocytes could be the source of the "transitional cells" (Fagraeus, 1948) of active lymph nodes, though no evidence has been produced to demonstrate that the cultured blastic lymphocytic cells continue to develop into mature plasma cells. Recently Douglas and Fudenberg (1969) observed plasma cell development in lymphocyte cultures following use of a stimulant isolated from pokeweed.

Another concept which is receiving more support involves the transition from heterogeneous interstitial elements (known as undifferentiated mesenchymal cells) or immature cells of the reticuloendothelial system into plasma cells. The possible role of the undifferentiated mesenchymal cell was suggested by Ramón y Cajal (1890) in skin lesions and extended by many (including Downey, 1911, and Kingsley, 1924) to other organs, including lymph nodes (Kingsley, 1924; Miller, 1931; Parsons, 1943; Moe, 1964; Movat and Fernando, 1965), spleen (Fagraeus, 1948; Hanna *et al.,* 1966), and bone marrow (Rohr, 1936; Kolouch, 1938). Maturation progresses either by direct transformation (Bernhard and Leplus, 1964; Moe, 1964) of undifferentiated cells or develops from plasmablasts. The latter process has been well documented in lymph nodes and spleen in experimental animals following an initial antigenic stimulus (Movat and Fernando, 1965; Hanna *et al.,* 1966). After a second antigenic challenge, a proliferation of large basophilic cells with the large nucleus containing distinct nucleoli is noted near the reaction center of lymph nodes and in the red pulp near the follicles of the spleen (Fagraeus, 1948; Hanna *et al.,* 1966). This development in the lymph node is followed by a dominance of mature plasma cells around the reaction centers and along the medullar cords near the small vessels (Miller, 1931; Sainte-Marie, 1964) in spleen. Plasmacytosis is usually noted in red pulp (Fagraeus, 1948; Hanna *et al.,* 1966). These immature large basophilic cells, called "transitional cells" (Fagraeus, 1948), may become mature plasma cells. Morphologically, these immature cells are indistinguishable from the undifferentiated mesenchymal elements known as germinocytes, hemocytoblasts, lymphoid reticulum cells, lymphogonia, etc., (Lennert, 1961) and, therefore, can be regarded as the same cell.

The committed blastic form for plasmacytogenesis—i.e., plasmablast—may originate from transitional cells independent of the lymphocytic line. Because precursors of the plasmablasts are indistinguishable from the progenitor of the lymphoblast, Dameshek (1963) proposed the term "immunoblasts" to describe cells which showed these characteristics. Earlier, Osgood and Hunter (1934), on the basis of their study of myeloma cytology, proposed a specific blastic form as the origin of the plasma cell, a hypothesis which would not conflict with current concepts.

The nature of the difficulty is demonstrated by the atypical lymphocytes with strong basophilic cytoplasm which are seen frequently in peripheral blood of viral infected patients. These cells, known as Türk cells by light microscopists, have been classed as plasma cells by electron microscopy (Sprigg and Jerrome, 1967). Examples of atypical lymphocytes, shown in Figures 6-12 and 6-13, are from the peripheral blood of a patient with extensive dermatitis. It is very difficult to determine morphological differences between developing plasma cells and immature or atypical lymphocytes by light microscopy. However, the distinction is easier with the electron microscope—immature plasma cells (Figs. 6-13*A, B,* and 6-14) and atypical

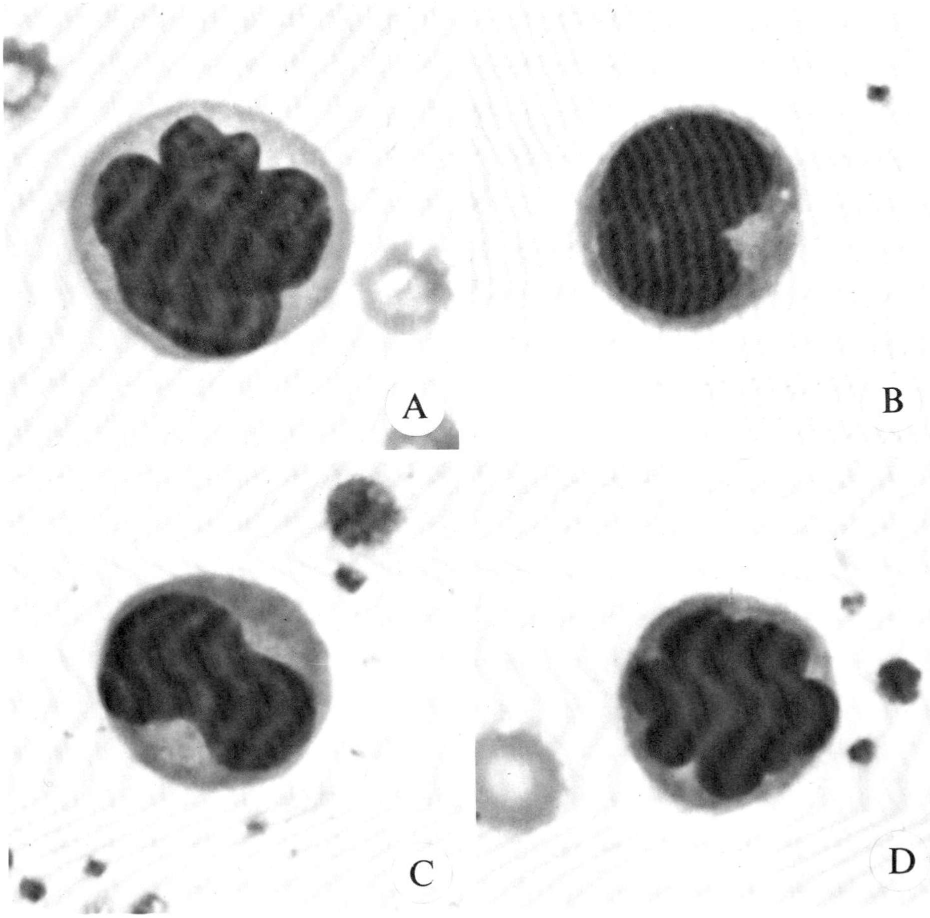

FIGURE 6-12. Atypical plasma cells.
A–D. Atypical peripheral ''lymphocytes'' from a patient with chronic dermatitis. Cells vary in size, with lobulated nuclei (**A**,**D**) and strong basophilic cytoplasm. × *2,000.*

plasma cells (Fig. 6-13*C, D*). The immature lymphocytes (Chap. 5) have considerably less endoplasmic reticulum.

Plasmacytogenesis by histiocytes and macrophages has also been postulated, but these hypotheses are less attractive, since macrophages or histiocytes are considered to be differentiated cells, which are unlikely to change into other cell types. In the study of plasma cell formation in various organs, the significance of perivascular mesenchymal cells (known as pericytes or adventitial cells) has been postulated. The concept of perivascular mesenchymal cells as a basis for plasmacytogenesis is not new. The phenomenon was observed by Hayamizu (1911) in experimental plasmacytosis in rabbit brain. The terms "adventitial cells" or "Marchand's leukocytoid cells" were used to describe these perivascular elements. Similar observations were made by others in various tissues (Miller, 1931; Amano *et al.,* 1944, 1951; Klein and Block, 1953; Hirata-Hibi, 1967). Some investigators tend to disregard the probability that immature lymphoid cells are the source of the plasma cell (Amano *et al.,* 1951). Sainte-Marie (1966) proposed that the plasma cell may originate from the endothelium of postcapillary venules in nodes. However, this concept has its limitations, since active lymphocyte migration is known to occur in this specific area (Gowans and Knight, 1964).

There is nothing intrinsic in any one of these concepts to completely exclude others. The problem of cells in antibody formation was also discussed in Chapter 5.

FUNCTION

Once the plasma cell was recognized, morphologists began to consider its function. According to Michels' excellent review (1931), these functional concepts included local absorption of chromatin material, transport of nutritive materials, or a physiologic condition of stimulated lymphocytes. The plasma cell was also regarded as a secretory corpuscle originating from lymphocytes. Other speculations more closely approximated current concepts that plasma cells are elements which are capable of elaborating a defense substance (antitoxin) important for the local immunization process, and that they are tissue elements produced by local metabolic changes. A close correla-

FIGURE 6-13. Atypical plasma cells.
Unusual cells are from peripheral blood of same patient with chronic dermatitis. In smears, most of these abnormal cells were interpreted as atypical lymphocytes (Fig. 6-12).
A. Medium-sized cell with highly indented nucleus (*N*) is comparable to hemocytoblasts or "transitional cells"; both are precursors of antibody-forming cells. There are many polyribosomes, a few profiles of tubular endoplasmic reticulum near the Golgi apparatus (*G*) and large mitochondria (*M*). × *11,400.*
B. Immature plasma cell with lamellar endoplasmic reticulum, several mitochondria (*M*), and a slightly eccentric position of the nucleus with rudimentary nucleolus (*Nu*). Many free polyribosomes and immature nuclear appearance help to define its immaturity. All characteristics of this cell suggest an intermediate state. × *11,400.*
C. Small mononuclear cell with large amount of distended endoplasmic reticulum is classified as a small lymphocyte by light microscopy. × *11,400.*
D. Though lymphoid in appearance, this cell's tubular endoplasmic reticulum suggests it is more like a developing plasma cell. It is uncertain whether this cell should be classified as lymphocyte or plasma cell. A platelet (*P*) is adjacent. × *11,400.*

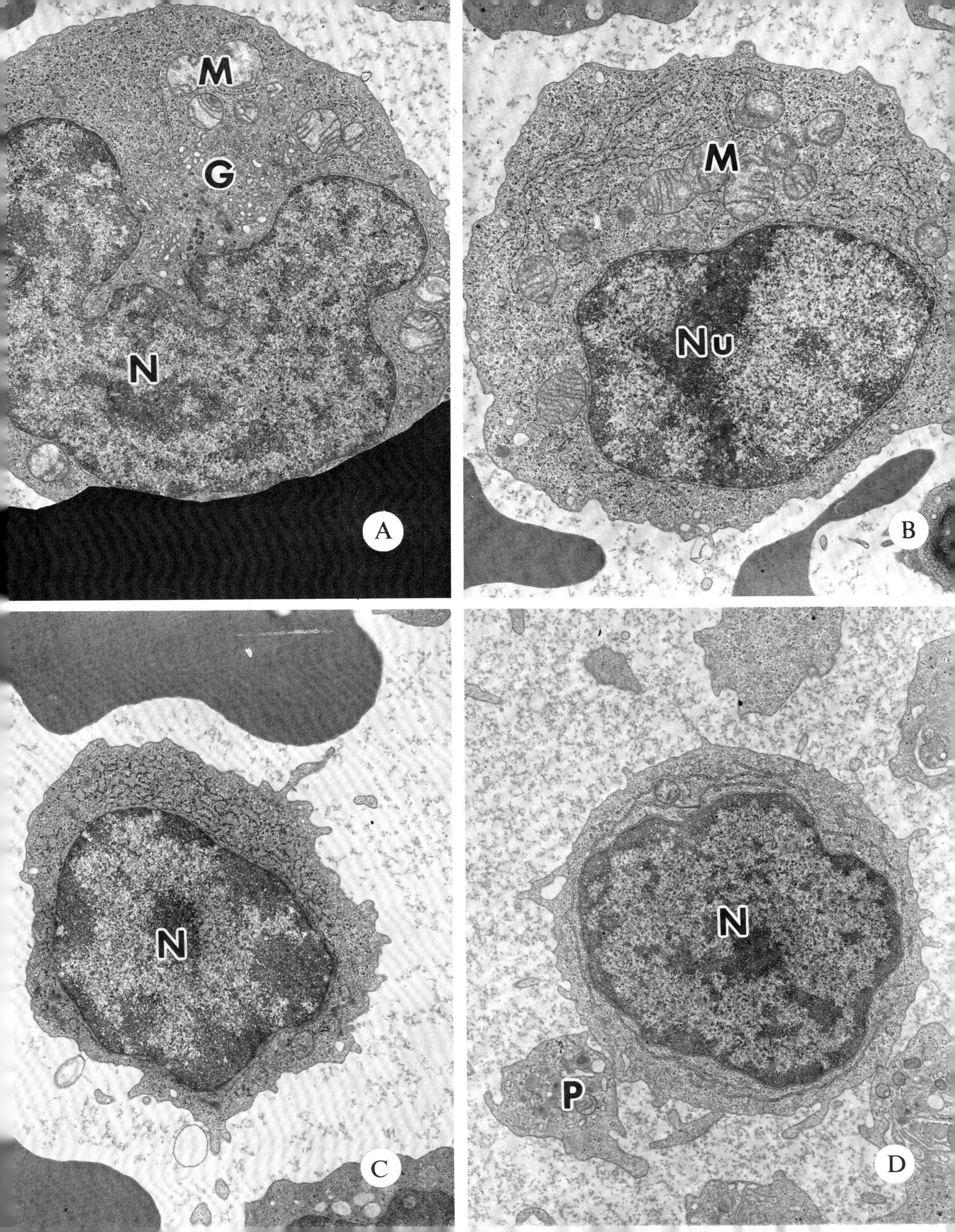
M
G
N
A
M
Nu
B
N
C
N
P
D

tion between the local development of plasma cells in lymph nodes and circulating antibodies, following injection of *Streptococcus viridans,* was described by Björneboe and Gormsen (1943). They produced hypergammaglobulinemia in rabbits and related the increase in circulating antibodies to the plasmacytosis that had developed. Similar observations, relating plasma cell production to hypergammaglobulinemia in man and animals, were made by Bing (1940). Direct evidence for the cellular site of production of human globulins in cells of lymphatic tissue was demonstrated by a two-stage fluorescent antibody method by Coons *et al.* (1955). Ortega and Mellors (1957) confirmed this and found three types of cells which reacted positively to the fluorescent stain; two were plasma cells.

IMMUNOGLOBULINS (Ig)

The plasma cell is a primary source of antibodies found in circulating blood—i.e., gamma globulins. The production of these proteins starts in the early plasma cell and continues in the mature plasma cell. Gamma globulins were first designated as a distinctive group of serum proteins by Tiselius (1937) using electrophoresis for their separation; later, serum antibodies were identified within this protein fraction (Tiselius and Kabat, 1938). Various physicochemical and biological methods have elucidated the molecular structure of these antibodies (Putnam, 1969; Milstein and Pink, 1970).

All immunoglobulin molecules consist of a basic unit of 4 polypeptide chains: one pair of heavy chains (molecular weight 50,000 to 70,000) and one pair of light chains (molecular weight about 20,000) linked by interchain disulfide bonds. Both heavy and light chains are further classified by their antigenic and structural properties. Five classes of heavy chains (gamma, alpha, mu, delta, and epsilon) and two types of light chains (kappa and lambda) have been distinguished. Each class of immunoglobulins is characterized by properties of its heavy chain. Both kappa and lambda light chains can associate with the heavy chains of all classes. A hypothetical model of the heavy polypeptide chains of an immunoglobulin is presented in Figure 6-15.

The predominant type of immunoglobulin is IgG, which constitutes about 80 per cent of the total circulating antibody in human adults. Its molecular weight is estimated as 140,000, with a sedimentation constant of 6.6 to 7S. The heavy chains, which determine the specificity of the molecule, are called the gamma chains and contain about 2.5 per cent carbohydrate by weight. Four subclasses, IgG1, IgG2, IgG3, and IgG4, have been identified.

IgA is the next most prevalent immunoglobulin, corresponding to about 10 per cent of circulating antibodies in the human adult (150 to 250 mg/100 ml). The

FIGURE 6-14. Two immature plasma cells from metastatic focus of squamous cell carcinoma of brain.
A. Large mononuclear cell with irregularly extended tubular endoplasmic reticulum. The nucleus (*N*) has limited chromatin margination and a rudimentary nucleolus (*Nu*). The cytoplasm still contains polyribosomes with a random distribution of mitochondria. Part of the Golgi apparatus (*G*) is seen. This cell could be classed as a "transitional cell." × *13,300.*
B. An uncommon lymphoid cell from the same specimen exhibits a reticular chromatin pattern in the nucleus (*N*), only a few layers of flattened endoplasmic reticulum (*er*), an aggregation of mitochondria (*M*), and part of the Golgi complex (*G*). × *13,300.*

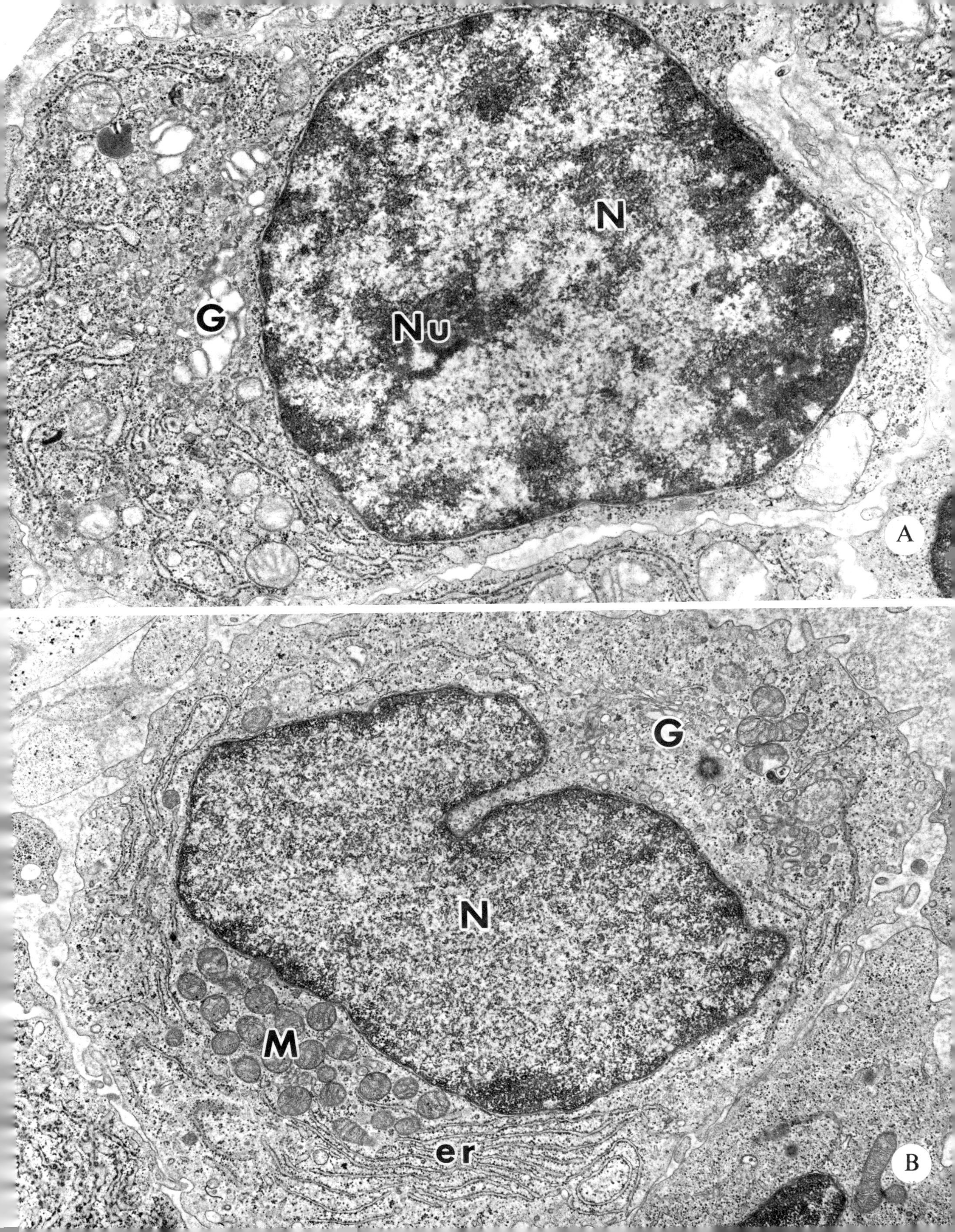
N
Nu
G
A
G
N
M
er
B

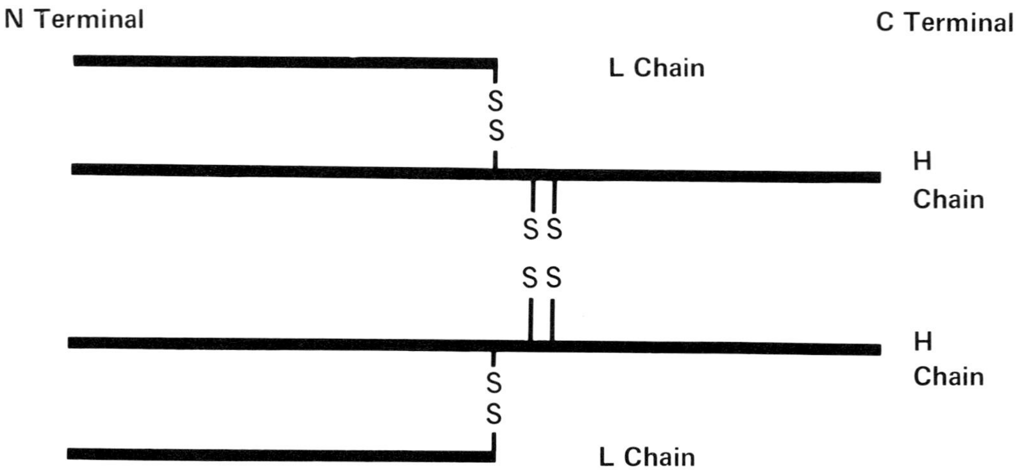

FIGURE 6-15. Schematic representation of molecular structure of IgG. The disulfide interchain bonds are always near the end of the light chain, but may vary in their attachment to the heavy chain. The IgM molecules are formed by the combination of five of these basic units. A spatial arrangement of these units has been proposed by Milstein and Pink (1970).

specific heavy chain of this protein is an alpha chain, and two subclasses have been identified. This molecule contains about 10 per cent carbohydrate by weight. Though the bulk of serum IgA has a molecular weight of 160,000 and a sedimentation rate of 7S (Heremans *et al.*, 1959), IgA also exists as polymers associated with a secretory piece (Cebra and Small, 1967) and sediments with the 11S fractions (Tomasi *et al.*, 1965).

The largest immunoglobulin molecule (molecular weight about 900,000 and sedimentation constant of 19S) is IgM, which represents about 5 to 10 per cent of the total serum antibodies in human adult (60 to 170 mg/ml). The specific heavy chain is called M chain. This IgM molecule contains five basic subunits. Like IgA, IgM contains about 10 per cent carbohydrate by weight.

Normal adult serum also has very small amounts of IgD (Rowe and Fahey, 1965) and IgE (Ishizaka *et al.*, 1966), which contain delta and epsilon heavy chains, respectively. Whole immunoglobulin molecules, particularly the larger classes, can be visualized by electron microscopy with the use of negative-staining methods (Svehag *et al.*, 1967; Chesebro *et al.*, 1968).

Antibody formation in the plasma cell follows the same basic principle of the protein biosynthesis illustrated in hemoglobin synthesis (Chap. 2). However, little is known clearly about the biosynthetic pathway of the antibody. Excess production of both heavy and light chains in myeloma cells suggests that heavy and light chains may be synthesized at different loci prior to assembly of the four peptides to form the complete molecule, in or near the ribosomes of endoplasmic reticulum. Conjugation of carbohydrate may occur just prior to secretion or near the Golgi apparatus after the whole peptide assembly has been completed (Zagury *et al.,* 1970).

The question of how and when the plasma cell is programmed to produce the mRNA which results in the synthesis of a specific antibody is not yet answered. The favored possibility is the proposal of Burnet (1959), that the antigen-sensitive cell is restricted to the synthesis of antibody molecules of only one specificity. An antigen stimulates its specific cell to proliferate and produce a specific antibody. Another possibility is the transfer of an informational molecule from the macrophage to lymphocytes, which are therefore multipotential. This will be discussed in Chapter 7, under Macrophages and Precursors.

The duration of immunity exceeds the life span of a single plasma cell, an observation leading to the hypothesis that either the antigen remains in the host as a stimulant for long periods or protein synthesis information is introduced into a stem cell or "immunoblast," which transmits the message to the maturing plasma cells for a number of cell generations. The capacity to make a protein that is specific for a given antigen relates to the question of the cell's origin and transformations, because the cell needs to have or receive the specific antigenic information to produce the specific antibody (gamma globulin). How and when the information for synthesis of specific antibody is given to the cell may be explained by knowing more about the cell's antecedents.

There has been little evidence that the mature plasma cell has the capacity to phagocytize; so the antigen does not appear to enter as a particle during the plasmacyte stage. A soluble or particulate antigen might be taken in by pinocytosis, but no significant action similar to erythroblastic pinocytosis has been observed by electron microscopy in mature plasma cells (Thiéry, 1962). Moreover, experiments with isotope-labeled antigen have shown that the antibody synthesizing cell contains no isotope label (Nossal *et al.,* 1968a,b). It has been suggested that plasma cell islands about a central macrophage could permit information to be transferred from the macrophage to the differentiating plasma cell (Thiéry, 1962). However, juxtaposition of these two cells is not common, and so far, there are limited data to support this theory (Thiéry, 1962; Nossal *et al.,* 1968a,b). Isotope-labeling experiments (Schooley, 1961) suggest that protein synthesis occurs in the proplasmacytic or early growth period. Consequently, the information which is germane to the specific character of the synthesized protein would need to be in the cell during the early transformation or transition of cell development. The transformation from reticulum cell or macrophage would account readily for programming of protein synthesis via pinocytosis or phagocytosis which might have taken place before transition into plasma cells. On the other hand, the more easily visualized transition from primitive lymphoid or reticulum cells and the location of many mature plasma cells in lymph nodes makes this idea attractive, although the antigenic access in this sequence is still not clear.

Recent but somewhat controversial work (Fishman *et al.,* 1963; Fishman and Adler, 1967) has suggested that the macrophage may process an antigen, which has been phagocytized, and then transfer immunogenic RNA to lymph node cells, stimulating them to produce antibodies. In this manner a stimulated reticulum cell or lymphoid type cell could become the antibody-producing plasma cell.

The synthesized protein that accumulates within the cisternae is released from

(text continues on page 302)

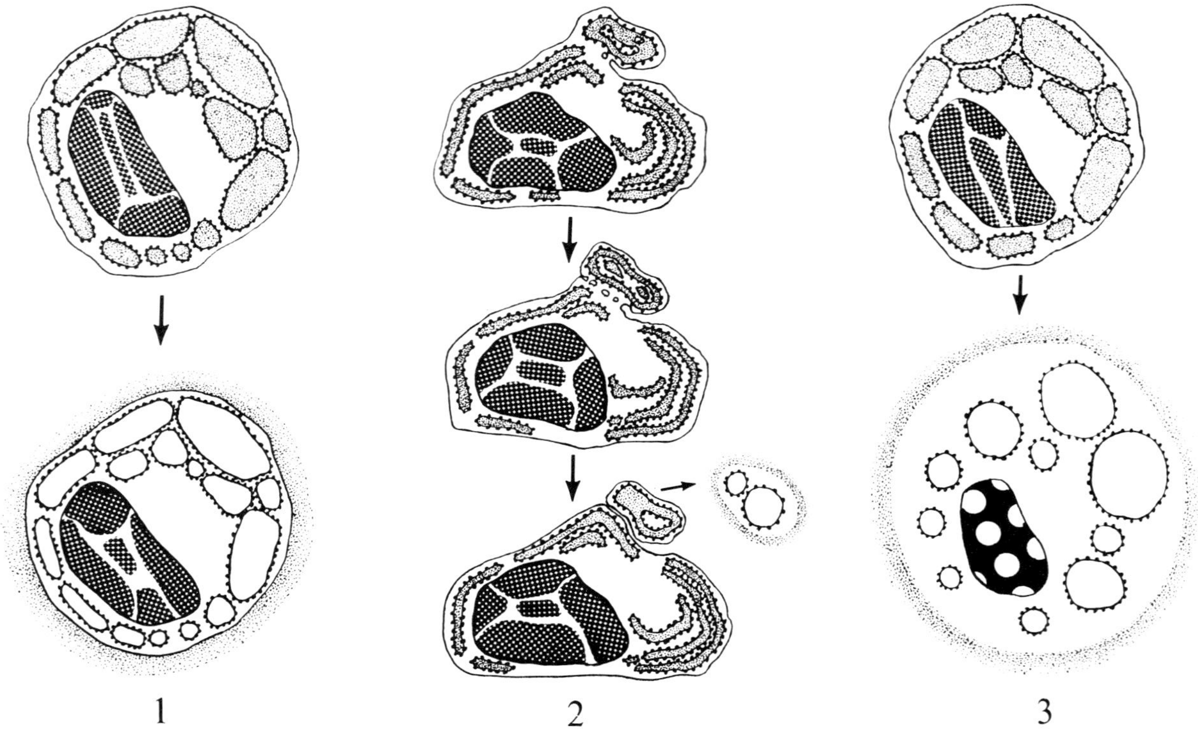

A

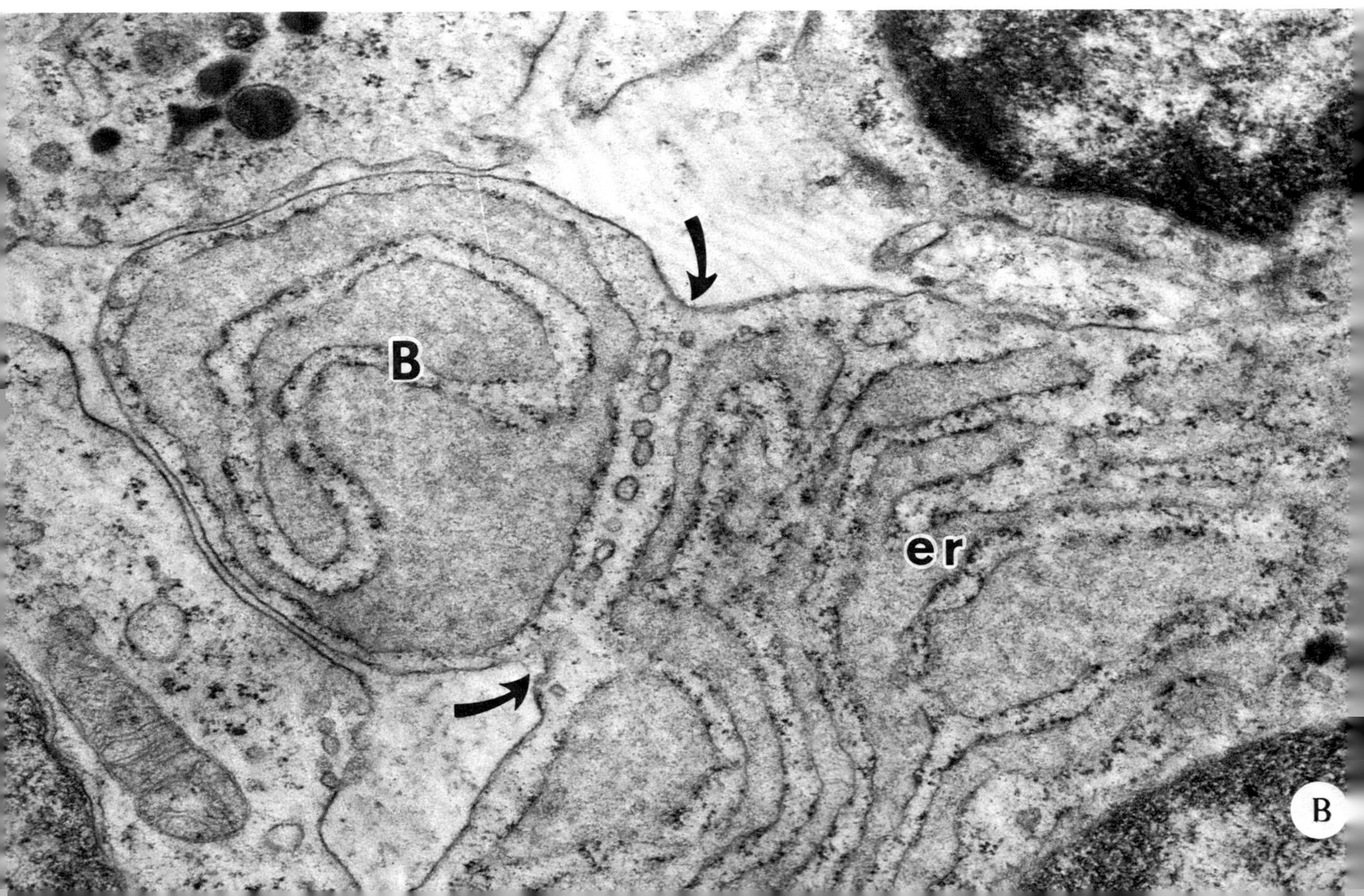

FIGURE 6-16. Mechanisms of antibody release from mature plasma cells.
A. Schematic representation of (1) diffusion through plasma membrane or direct communication of endoplasmic reticulum to outside; (2) blebbing off of part of cytoplasm; (3) lysis of whole plasma cell.
B. Portion of plasma cell from marrow of patient with refractory normoblastic anemia is forming a bleb (*B*) which contains rough endoplasmic reticulum (*er*) with protein in its cisternae. Series of small vesicles at the base of the bleb (*arrows*) will coalesce and sever it from the cytoplasm. Different stages of this process have been seen in various marrows and demonstrate one of the mechanisms of gamma globulin release from the cell. *Fixation: Osmium in s-collidine buffer. Plastic: Maraglas. × 39,000.*
Reprinted with permission from Goodman, J. R., and Hall, S. G. *Blood 28:*83, 1966.

Figures 6-17 and 6-18 appear on the following pages

FIGURE 6-17. Plasma cells in dysgammaglobulinemia.
Lymph node in dysgammaglobulinemia can have a proliferation of both normal-looking and atypical plasma cells. These large plasma cells have a near normal appearance. Chromatin concentration along the margin of the nucleus (N) is not sharply delineated. However, the endoplasmic reticulum (*er*) is well developed and encircles large Golgi complexes (*G*). There are a number of mitochondria (*M*) and a few dense granules (*g*). The cisternae of the endoplasmic reticulum have a moderate amount of amorphous material and several examples of cytoplasmic blebs (*arrow*) are present on cell peripheries. *× 12,000.*

FIGURE 6-18. Plasma cells in dysgammaglobulinemia.
These three atypical plasma cells are from same case as those in Figure 6-17. One with two nuclei (*N*) has distinct nucleoli (*Nu*), which are not commonly noted in typical plasma cells, and differentiated endoplasmic reticulum (er). Nucleoli in cells with developed endoplasmic reticulum suggest a dissociation of nuclear and cytoplasmic differentiation, characteristic in some plasma cells of lymph nodes in this disease. The cytoplasm of all these cells has typical endoplasmic reticulum, mitochondria (*M*), and Golgi complexes (*G*). One normal appearing plasma cell is present. × 12,000.

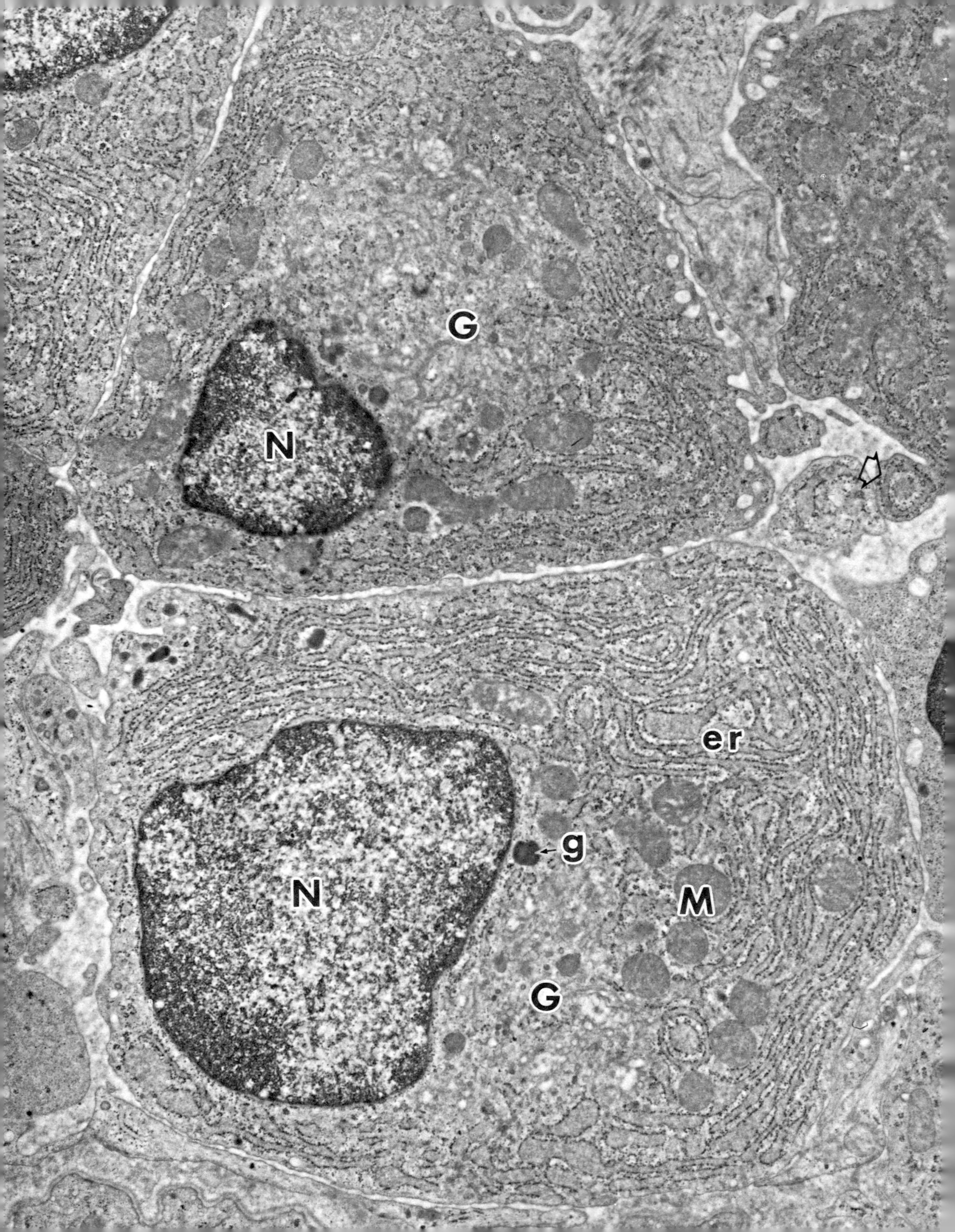
G
N
er
g
N
M
G

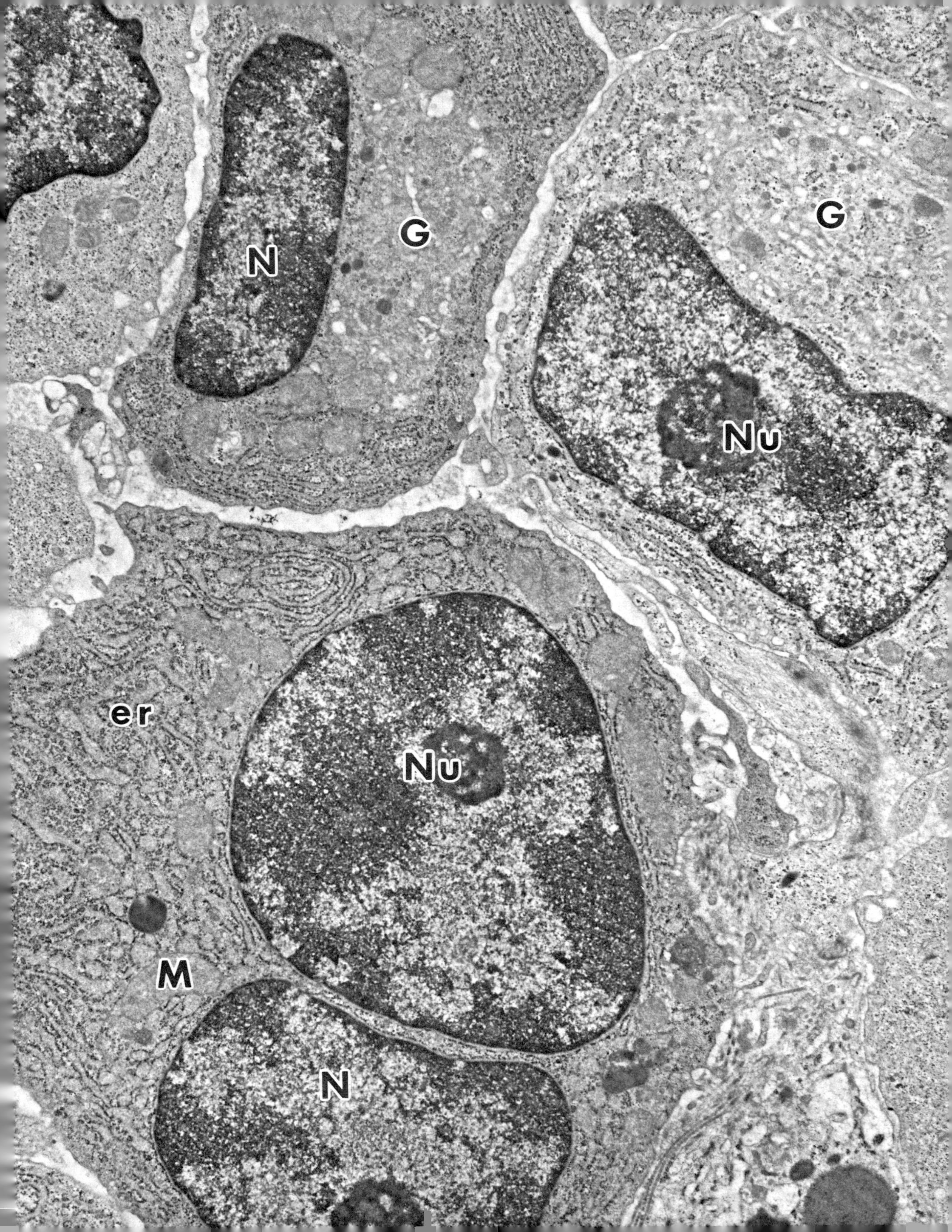
N
G
G
Nu
er
Nu
M
N

the cell to the circulating blood. The mechanism of protein release (Fig. 6-16*A*) could be accomplished by: (1) excretion through an opening of an endoplasmic reticulum cisterna into the extracellular fluid; (2) detachment or blebbing of portions of the cytoplasm containing endoplasmic reticulum filled with protein products that are released when the separated cytoplasmic fragments disintegrate; or (3) by the degradation of the whole cell. The first of these mechanisms has not yet been reported by electron microscopists. A rapid opening and closing of a cisterna lumen could be missed or masked by fixation of the cell. Studies by Harris *et al.* (1966), using the hemolytic plaque method, have shown that both lymphocytes and plasma cells release specific hemolytic antibodies in amounts sufficient to cause a plaque (clean area immediately surrounding the cell). This antibody may be released either by diffusion or from ruptured cytoplasmic blebs. A number of micrographs in the mechanism of bleb formation on plasma cells have been made (Thiéry, 1960; Goodman and Hall, 1966; Han *et al.,* 1966) (Fig. 6-16*B*). Repeated and excessive action of this type would, in effect, result in complete cell fragmentation. Thiéry (1960) reported this type of phenomenon in plasma cells incubated on microscopic slides. Schooley (1961) suggested a life span of only 3 days for plasma cells in lymph nodes, supporting the theory of a fairly rapid loss of the cell cytoplasm, if not the entire cell.

PATHOLOGY

DYSGAMMAGLOBULINEMIA (NONMALIGNANT)

Pathological syndromes that can be related to the plasma cell system include hypogammaglobulinemia (Gitlin *et al.,* 1959) or dysgammaglobulinemia (Rosen *et al.,* 1961, 1966). In these syndromes the failure to produce antibody is usually partial (Gilbert and Hong, 1964; Barth *et al.,* 1965), and rarely total (Gitlin *et al.,* 1959), although nearly complete absence of these circulating proteins has been found in men and animals. The individual with severe hypogammaglobulinemia suffers from repeated infections and repeated immune response to antigenic stimulation which frequently leads to early death. Failure of antibody production may be associated with (1) a defect or decrease in production of plasma cells (Good, 1954; Rosen and Janeway, 1966); (2) defects in the ability of immunologically competent cells to receive or transmit the required antigenic message for gamma globulin production (Rosen and Janeway, 1966); or (3) atypical plasma cells which are incapable of producing all types of immunoglobulins.

Of particular interest to morphologists is whether the absence of a particular immunoglobulin is directly related to the failure of plasma cell production, or whether the failure to produce a particular immunoglobulin can be associated with abnormalities in the plasma cell. We examined material from a patient with dysgammaglobulinemia whose serum proteins had been studied extensively (Barth *et al.,* 1965). The main protein abnormality was the markedly diminished 7S fraction and an elevation of 19S fraction. The morphology of plasma cells from the lymph nodes and bone marrow showed no essential cytoplasmic difference from that of typical plasma cells observed in normal specimens. The cells had a round-to-ovoid nucleus located eccentrically in the cytoplasm (Fig. 6-17), a wide Golgi area, and well-developed endoplasmic reticulum. The chromatin in the nucleus was somewhat coarser than that of typical plasma cells; however, chromatin clumping, similar to that in normal plasma cells, was also seen. Occasional nucleoli were observed (Fig. 6-18), a finding seen in immature normal cells, and also in an occasional binucleated cell. The endoplasmic reticulum cisternae were frequently dilated and contained homogeneous material of moderate opacity. Though this is found in normal plasma cells (Fig. 6-4), it seemed to be more prominent in this case (Fig. 6-19). These observations suggest that the circulating macroglobulin in this case may have been produced by the proliferating plasma cells, which differ little morphologically from those observed in physiological conditions. The Golgi area (Fig. 6-20) has all its normal components. The presence of many microtubules is not abnormal and is not thought to be related to the pathology. Some immature cells with a spare endoplasmic reticulum and abundant polyribosomes (Fig. 6-21*A*) were discovered, and others with more evidence of differentiation (Fig. 6-21*B*) suggest a clonal origin of cells similar to those observed in stimulated normal marrows and lymph nodes.

One striking abnormality was the presence of intranuclear inclusions (Fig. 6-21*C,D*) which were homogeneous and contained neither spheroid nor crystalloid structures. These are surrounded by a single membrane, usually near the middle of the nucleus, and vary from about 1μ to larger ones which occupy almost the entire nucleus. The cell containing the inclusions showed no morphological alteration to suggest cellular degeneration, and the significance of the inclusions is unknown. Similar nuclear inclusions have also been found in macroglobulinemia, which is known to have increased serum proteins of 19S and some as large as 32S.

MULTIPLE MYELOMA

Multiple myeloma is a malignant disorder which affects the bone marrow primarily and is associated with hypergammaglobulinemia and plasma cell proliferation. This condition may be defined as a malignancy of the plasma cell or of its precursor (Fig. 6-22). The disease may be extramedullary (Jackson *et al.,* 1931; Ewing and Foote, 1952) or in a leukemic form (Gluzinski and Reinchenstein, 1906; Newman *et al.,* 1952).

This disease was first described in three different reports: by Dalyrymple (1846), Bence-Jones (1847), and MacIntyre (1850). The lesion was defined as multiple myeloma by Rustizky (1873), and the syndrome was summarized as one disease by Kähler (1889) at a time when the plasma cell itself had not yet been defined. The plasma cell proliferation in this disease was first pointed out by Wright in 1900 and confirmed by Christian (1907). At first, it was implied that multiple myeloma was a tumorous condition which could involve any myeloid tissue, as morphological heterogeneity or proliferating cells was claimed. However, such interpretations prior to 1930 reflect the inadequate methodology in cytological diagnosis of proliferating cells (Snapper and Kahn, 1964). More recent publications report some variations in the type of proliferating cell (Gunn and Mahle, 1937; Herbut and Erf, 1946; Taylor, 1947), but the cytological classification may have been misinterpreted.

The cells in multiple myeloma are called myeloma or malignant plasma cells and differ from typical plasma cells in that they are usually larger and may have inclusions. There is an apparent discrepancy between the state of maturation of the nucleus and cytoplasm (Snapper and Kahn, 1964). Mitosis or multinucleated giant cells are observed frequently and

(text continues on page 312)

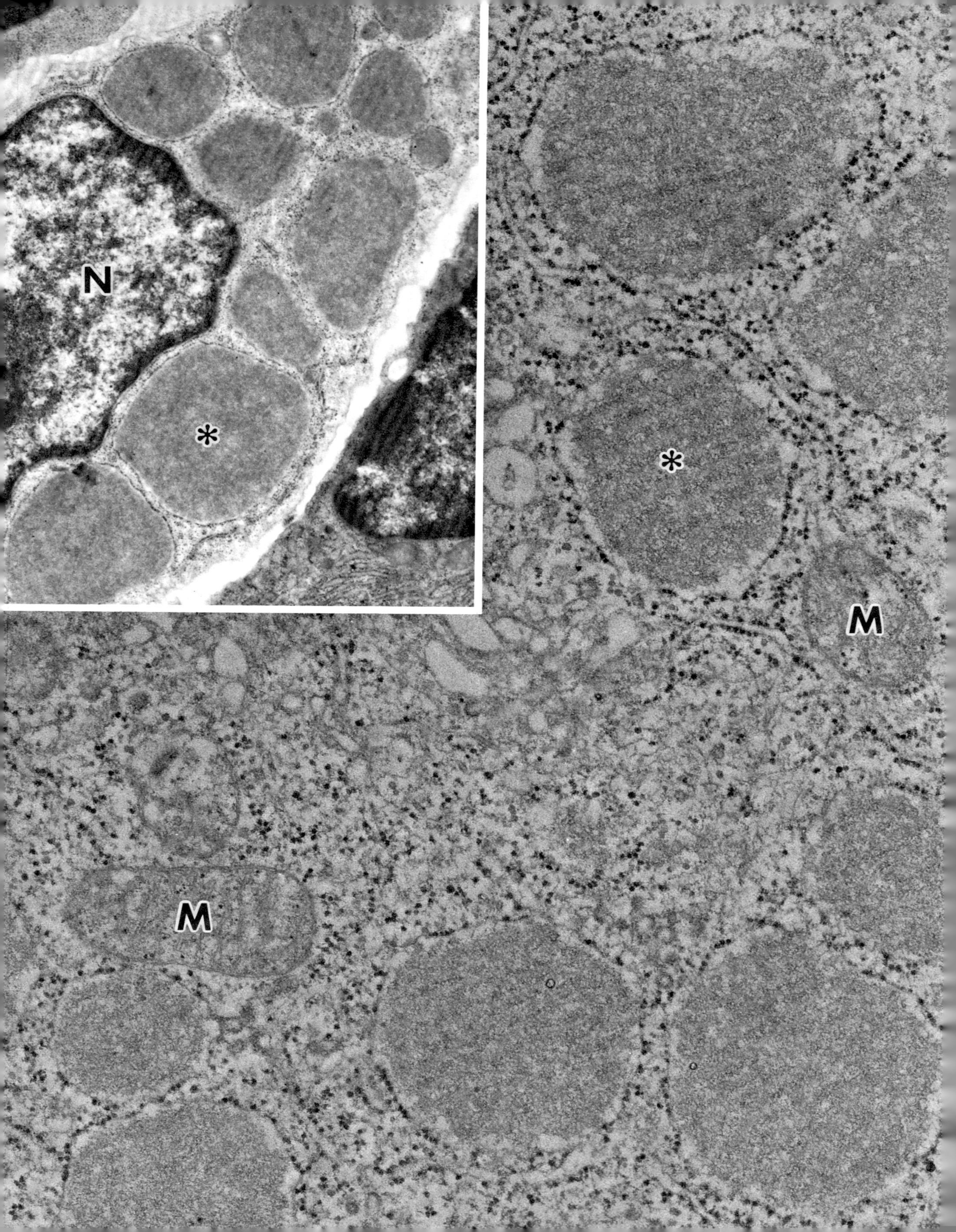
N
*
*
M
M

FIGURE 6-19. Plasma cells in dysgammaglobulinemia.
Cells with inclusions or masses of material within endoplasmic reticulum are commonly noted in dysgammaglobulinemia. Large masses of amorphous material (*asterisks*) occupy most of cytoplasmic area and stain PAS-positive. Cells showing these inclusions are considered to be plasma cells, with material distending the cisternae of endoplasmic reticulum. Low magnification (*inset,* × *15,000*) shows part of nucleus (*N*). Larger micrograph illustrates part of similar cell with two mitochondria (*M*). × *49,000.*

Figures 6-20 and 6-21 appear on the following pages ⇨

FIGURE 6-20. Plasma cell in dysgammaglobulinemia.
Golgi area of plasma cell contains centriole (*Ce*), with typical nine triads around a central core, many microtubules (*mt*), and small vesicles (*v*). A number of the vesicles contain some dense amorphous material. Some Golgi saccules (*s*) are dilated and electron-translucent. A sprinkling of ribosomes within the Golgi region appear to be unattached; others are present on membranes or in whorls. A mitochondrion (*M*) and the edge of the nucleus (*N*) are present. × *48,000.*

FIGURE 6-21. Immature plasma cells in dysgammaglobulinemia.
A. Large immature cell shows general structure similar to that of a hemocytoblast except for some increase in endoplasmic reticulum (*er*) and aggregation of mitochondria (*M*). Nucleus (*N*) is slightly eccentric. This could be early form of plasma cell in stage of transformation. × *11,000.*
B. Except for moderately developed endoplasmic reticulum (*er*), this is a characteristic plasma cell, with mitochondria (*M*), nucleus (*N*), and wide Golgi (*G*) area. × *10,000.*
C. Large plasma cell has an intranuclear inclusion (*in*) composed of amorphous material of moderate electron opacity. Mitochondria (*M*) are adjacent to nucleus (*N*). × *15,000.*
D. Atypical plasma cell has an intranuclear inclusion (*in*) similar to that in cells found in macroglobulinemia. The inclusion is amorphous and coarser than that in Figure 6-21**C.** Chromatin in the nucleus (*N*) is dense, and the Golgi area (*G*) is wide. × *15,000.*

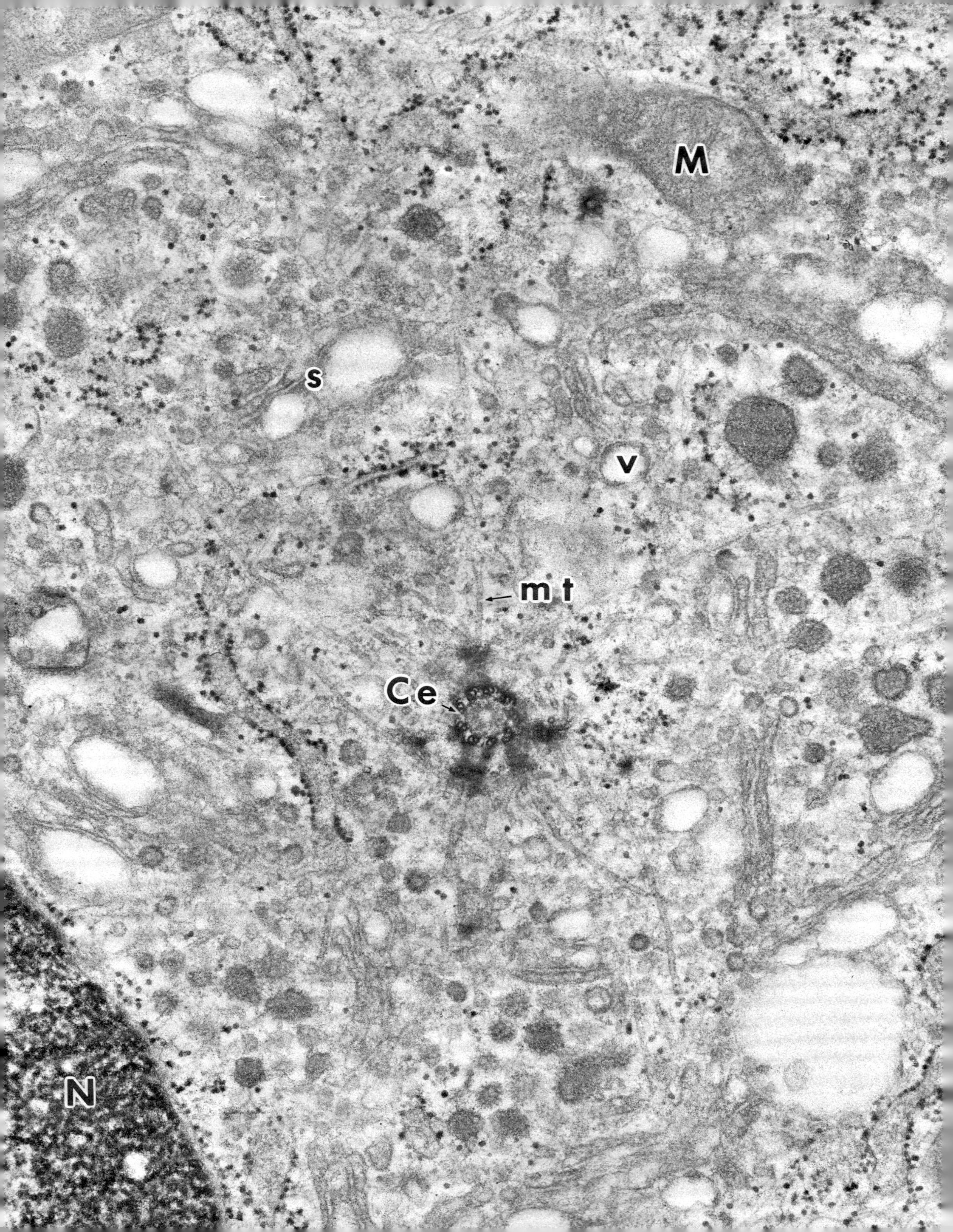
M
s
v
mt
Ce
N

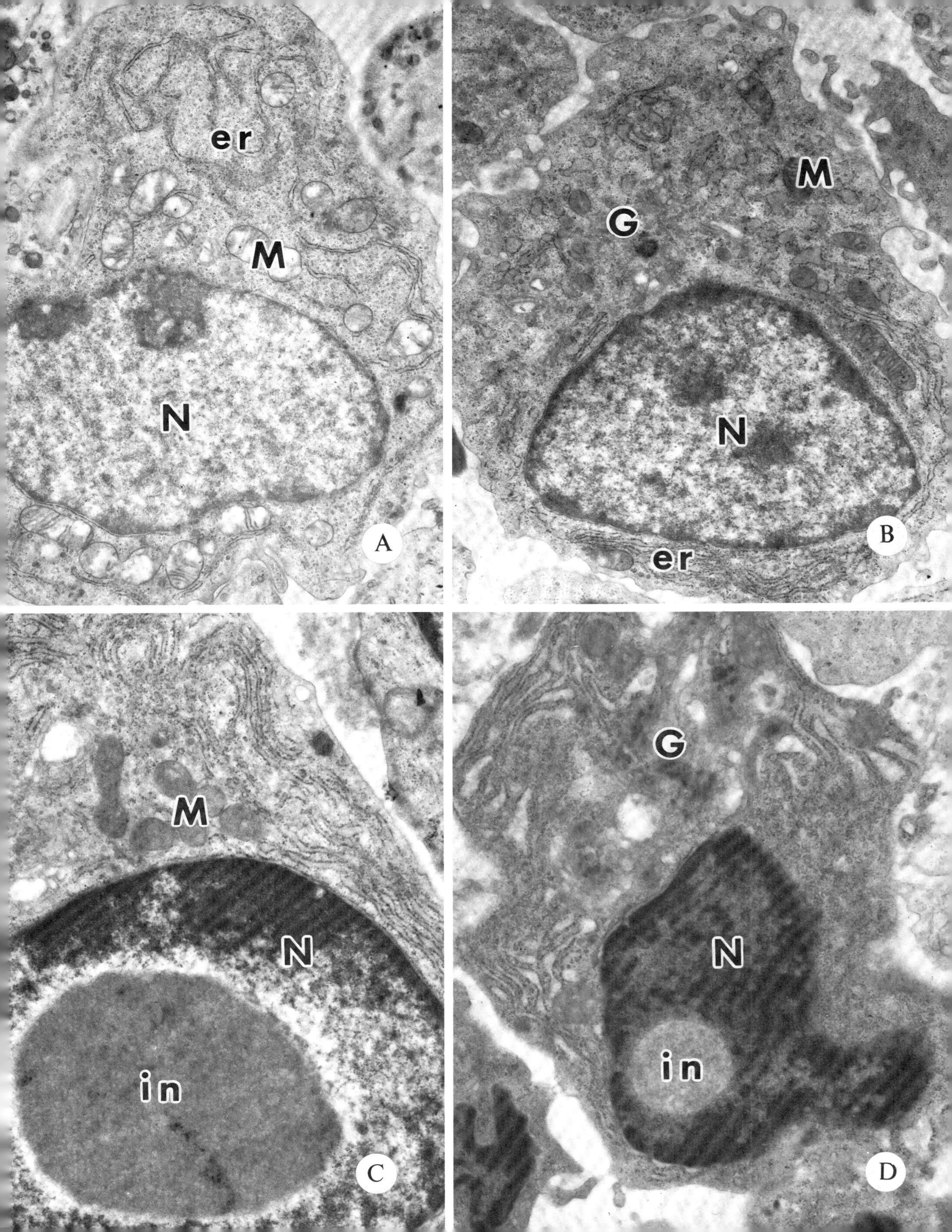
er
M
N
A
G
M
N
B
er
M
N
in
C
G
N
in
D

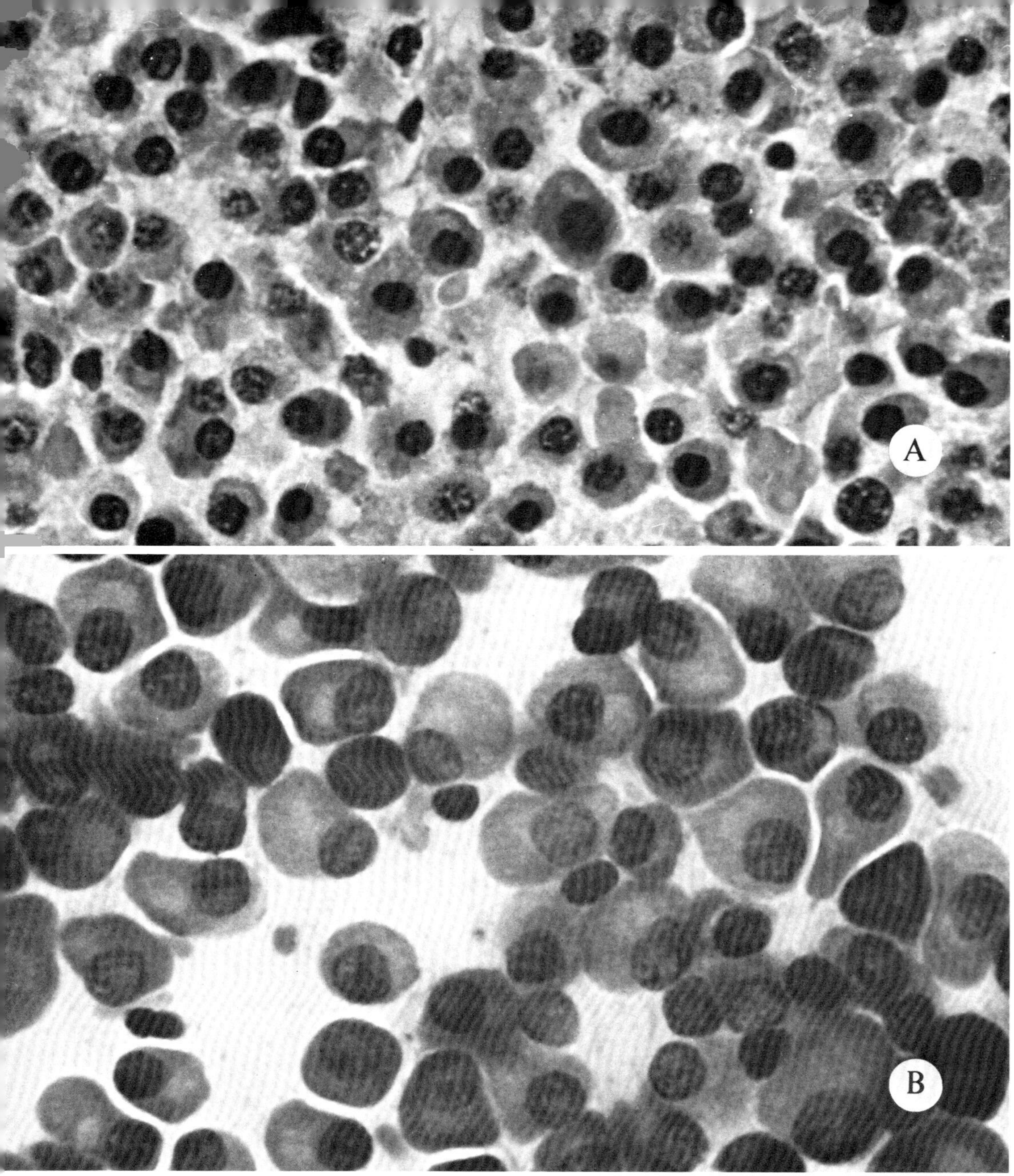

FIGURE 6-22. Myeloma cells in bone marrow.
A. Histological section of marrow fragment, formalin-fixed, paraffin-embedded, and stained with hemotoxylin and eosin. There is essentially complete replacement of normal cells by myeloma cells. × *1,000.*
B. Stained smear from same marrow. The cytological characteristics are similar to those of plasma cells. *Wright stain.* × *1,000.*

FIGURE 6-23. General appearance of myeloma cells.
Malignant cell from bone marrow of patient with myeloma. The nucleus (N) has uniform distribution of chromatin and a large distinct nucleolus (*Nu*). There are more mitochondria (*M*) than usual, one of which is very long (*arrow*). The edge of the Golgi zone has only a few typical elongated vessels or saccules. Several dense granules (g), and lighter-staining cytoplasmic inclusions (*asterisk*) are present, some of which have dense bodies within the single limiting membrane. The moderate amount of lamellar endoplasmic reticulum (*er*) appears normal. *Fixation: Osmium.* × 22,000.

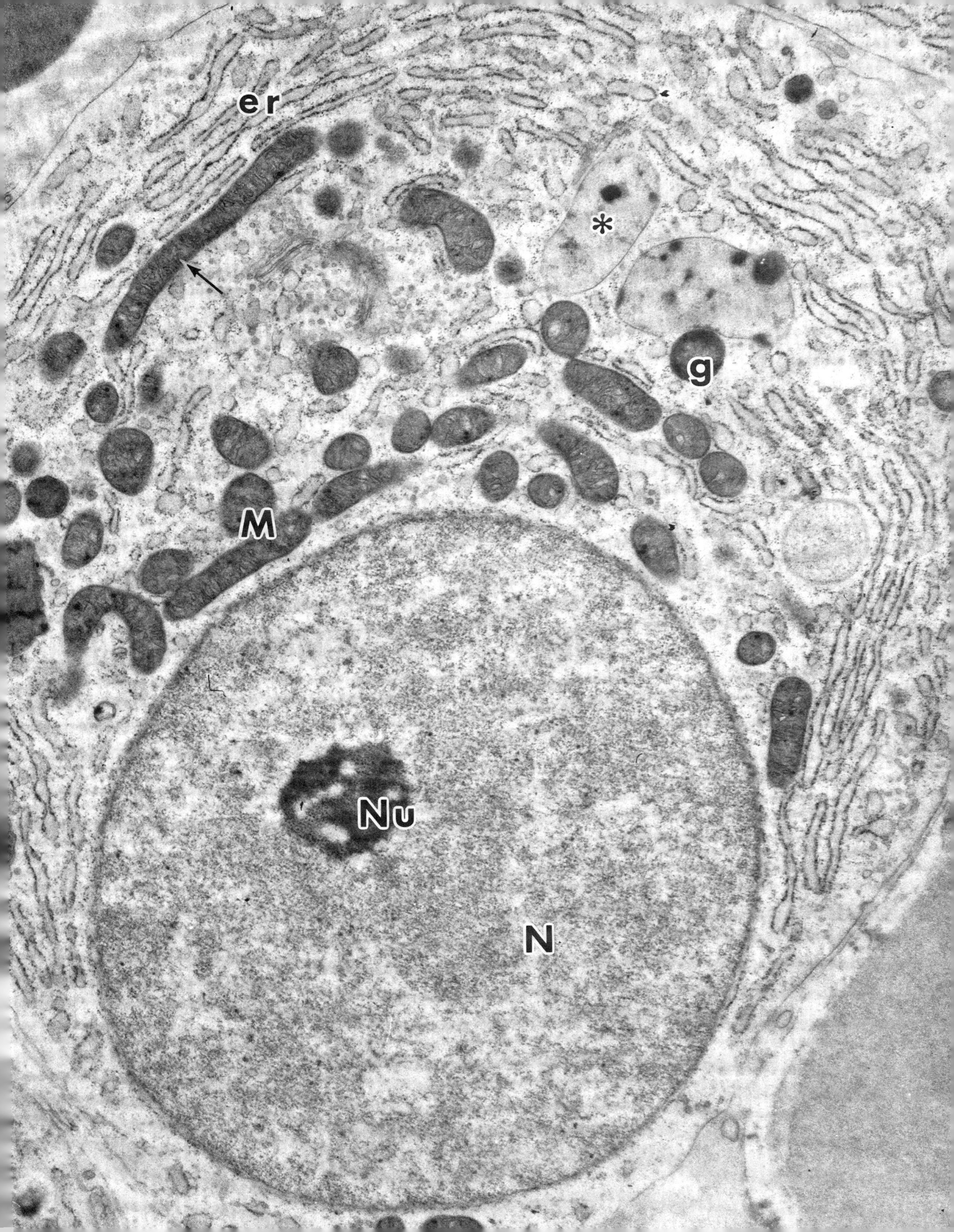
er
*
g
M
Nu
N

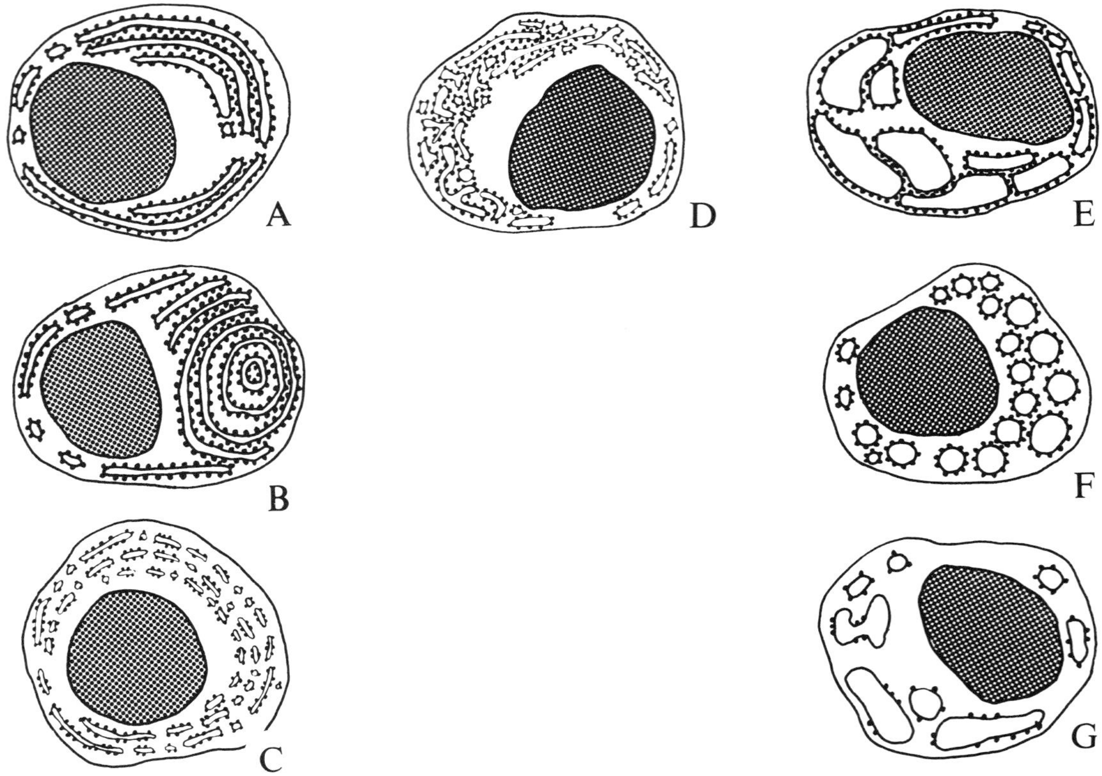

FIGURE 6-24. Endoplasmic reticulum in myeloma cells.
Various patterns of endoplasmic reticulum in myeloma cells can be classified as follows:
A–D, flattened type; **E–G,** distended type. The pattern in **E** could be formed by the distention of **A–D.** Pattern **F** could be formed by the distention of **C.** Pattern **G** is possibly related to the immaturity of the cell.
A. Lamellar, tubular
B. Concentrically lamellar, tubular
C. Concentrically lamellar, vesicular
D. Irregular or reticular, tubular
E. Intact but grossly distended
F. Vesicularly distended
G. Irregularly distended

FIGURE 6-25. Endoplasmic reticulum in myeloma cell.
A. This rough-surfaced endoplasmic reticulum (*er*) has a normal lamellar pattern. Ribosomal (*r*) particles appear smaller than normal (Fig. 6-5**A**) while cisternae contain homogeneous material of moderate density. × *43,000.*
B. Endoplasmic reticulum (*er*) of this cell is grossly distended with very electron-translucent material. The cytoplasmic space between cisternae is reduced to thin layers (*arrow*). Two mitochondria are tightly held in these thin strips of cytoplasm bound by endoplasmic reticulum. × *54,000.*

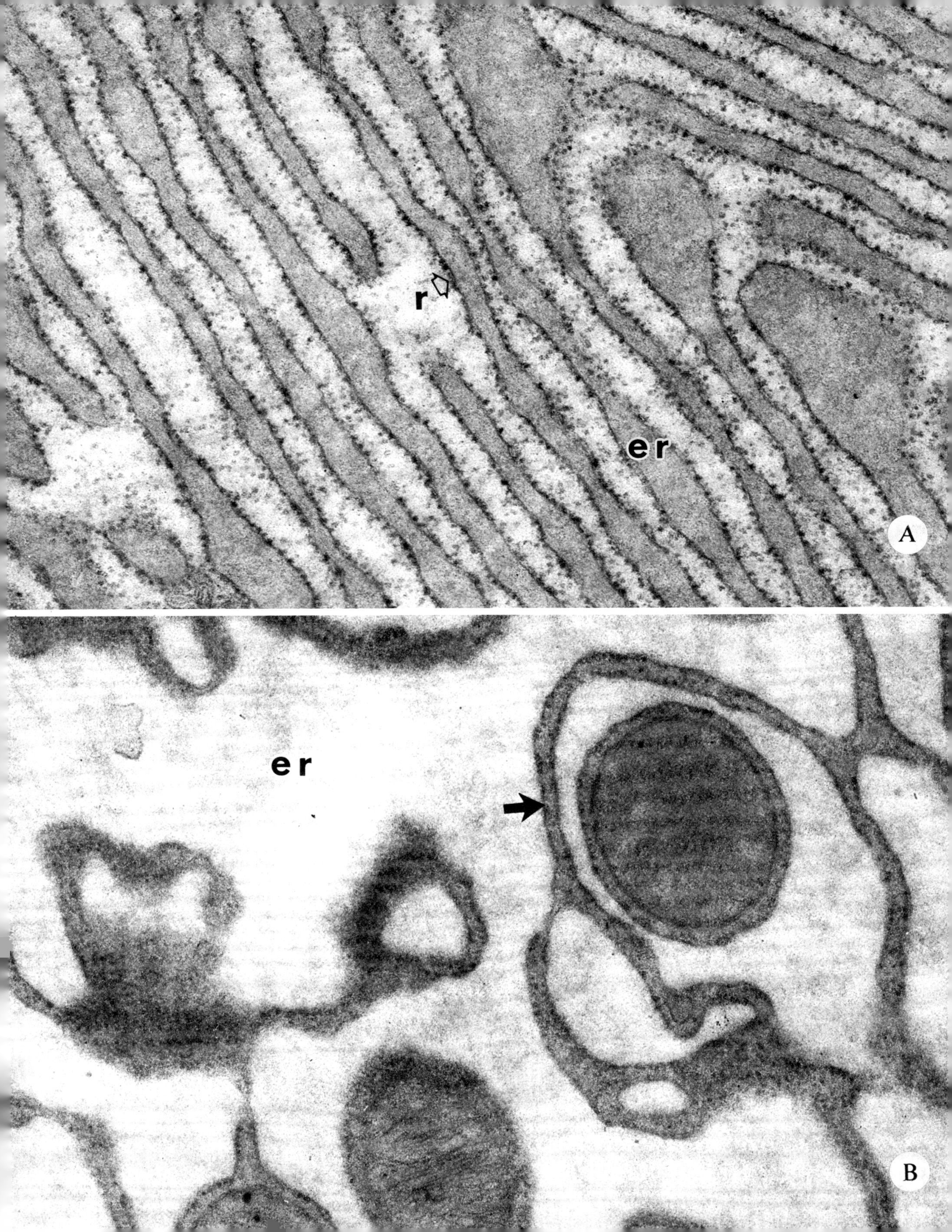
r
er
A
er
B

the most immature forms are often called "paraplasmablasts." The cellular morphology varies from one case to another, and ranges from typical plasma cells to the lymphoid cells frequently observed in Waldenström's macroglobulinemia. An abnormal protein in the serum is a common finding, with the serum electrophoretic pattern usually showing a single sharp peak (Osserman and Takatsuki, 1963; Snapper and Kahn, 1964). This abnormal protein is a globulin but almost invariably lacks antibody activity and is usually relatively homogeneous. The abnormal myeloma grobulins have been identified by immunochemical and ultracentrifugal technics as classes of IgG, IgD (Rowe and Fahey, 1965), IgM, IgA, and IgE globulins. The serum and urine frequently contain an abnormal polypeptide called the Bence-Jones protein. In malignant conditions, asynchronous production of peptides may occur, with an excess of one of the peptides. The excess production of the light chain is excreted as the Bence-Jones protein (Williams *et al.,* 1966). Excess amounts of the heavy chain, which has different solubility characteristics, have only recently been recognized (Osserman and Takatsuki, 1963; Franklin and Lowenstein, 1964). The relative homogeneity of an abnormal myeloma protein would result from a single clone which produces a single protein in successive cellular generations (Waldenström, 1962). Experimental plasma cell tumor in mice has demonstrated that the protein in this tumor maintains its antigenic property throughout repeated transplantations (Potter *et al.,* 1964).

The ultrastructure of the myeloma cell varies from well-differentiated, nearly normal plasma cell forms (Fig. 6-23) to quite atypical plasma cell forms. Most of the malignant cells are of medium size, with well-developed endoplasmic reticulum of various patterns which are quite characteristic (Fig. 6-24). The plasma border is sometimes irregular and suggests highly active movement in vivo. Cellular size may vary from giant cells (30μ in diameter, sometimes with multiple nuclei) to normal. The electron opacity of the cytoplasm is generally lighter when compared with a normal plasma cell, probably because of a decrease of cytoplasmic ribosomes—either free or attached to the membrane of endoplasmic reticulum (Zucker-Franklin, 1964). The nucleus is large, with occasional identation, and located in a slightly eccentric position in the cytoplasm. The chromatin is always coarse, often with a significantly large and pleomorphic nucleolus. The Golgi area of these malignant cells is large and relatively well defined, with a large number of vesicular elements.

Well-developed endoplasmic reticulum, with morphological characteristics of the normal plasma cell, is also noted (Fig. 6-25). The arrangement may be classified into: (1) lamellar, including circular lamellae; (2) concentric; and (3) reticular or vesicular (Fig. 6-24). The patterns seem to be preserved during the maturation process and are fairly uniform in any single

FIGURE 6-26. Mitochondria in myeloma cells.
A. Myeloma cells occasionally have mitochondria (*M*) with very dilated cristae filled with amorphous material. The sectioned organelle has a botryoidal appearance. The vesicular type of endoplasmic reticulum (er) is distended with amorphous material (*asterisk*) of moderate density. *× 55,000.*
B. Many normal-appearing mitochondria (*M*) show possible increase in the number of dense granules (*arrow*). There is one large dense cytoplasmic granule, probably azurophilic (*g*). Endoplasmic reticulum (*er*) has smaller and irregularly placed ribosomes. *Fixation: Osmium. × 40,000.*

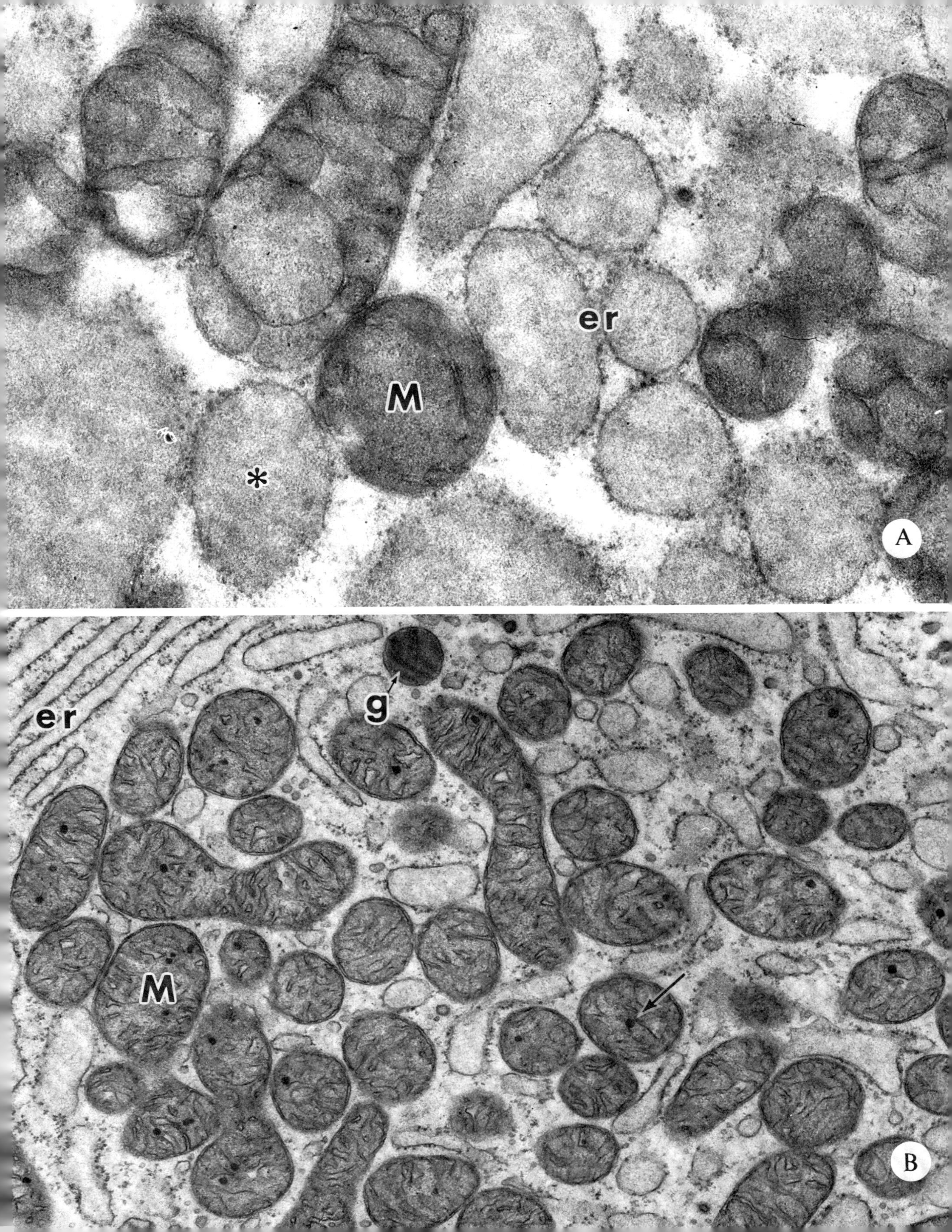
er
M
*
A
er
g
M
B

case. The distribution of ribosomes on the membrane is usually uniform, and the rosette formation is frequently seen in cells with well-differentiated endoplasmic reticulum. At times, however, the distribution can be quite irregular and the particles diminished in size. In extreme conditions, the membrane may have RNA granules far smaller than the normal—about 30 Å (Zucker-Franklin, 1964), probably reflecting the distorted activity of protein production. The endoplasmic reticulum may be distended and contain amorphous fine filamentous or flocculated substances. According to Bessis *et al.* (1963), cells with distended endoplasmic reticulum are most commonly seen in cases with IgA myeloma. However, we have observed this disgree of distended endoplasmic reticulum to be common in almost any type of hypergammaglobulinemia. The electron opacity of the accumulated material varies from almost none to moderate; a regular periodicity of about 100 Å has been reported in material condensed in the cisternae (Sorenson, 1964). Comparative cytological studies suggest that the material in the endoplasmic reticulum is closely related to the abnormal proteins in serum. Immunocytological use of ferritin-conjugated antimyeloma globulin in mice has disclosed the presence of myeloma protein in these cells (Rifkind *et al.,* 1962). When the endoplasmic reticulum is excessively distended, the cells become enlarged and are then recognized as foamy cells (Zlotnick, 1956). These cells (Schamezellen—morular cells), sometimes show diffuse PAS-positive cytoplasm and are then called flaming cells (Maldonado *et al.,* 1965). The mitochondria of myeloma cells are usually large, with fairly regular or occasionally irregular cristae (Fig. 6-26*A*) and are rarely doughnut-shaped organelles. Large numbers of mitochondria are sometimes found (Fig. 6-26*B*) and intramitochondrial granules with high electron density are frequent. Cytoplasmic inclusions (Fig. 6-27*A*) range from electron-translucent to those with dense areas within limiting membrane. Some cells have many small dense bodies concentrated mainly near the Golgi area (Fig. 6-27).

The distended endoplasmic reticulum may contain spheroids of various sizes (Fig. 6-28*A*), Russell bodies, or crystals (Liévre *et al.,* 1961), which may correspond to structures reported by light microscopy (Glaus, 1917; Apitz, 1937). Inclusions are reported as PAS-positive or negative, probably depending on the amount of hexose in the accumulated proteins. In general, a Russell body is considered to be the structure formed by

(text continues on page 320)

FIGURE 6-27. Cytoplasmic inclusions in myeloma cells.
Cytoplasmic inclusions (rarely observed in normal plasma cells) are not within the cisternae of the endoplasmic reticulum (where Russell bodies are usually found).

A. These large pale inclusions have single membranes. One (*asterisk*) contains several dense areas and has a more fibrous appearance. An edge of the nucleus (*N*), a few mitochondria (*M*), and some endoplasmic reticulum (*er*) are also present. These inclusions may appear as crystalloid structures under the phase microscope with a negative PAS-reaction. *Fixation: Osmium.* × *48,000.*

B. This myeloma cell has many small electron dense inclusions (*asterisk*), most of which appear homogeneous although a few are lighter, with small areas of increased density. They extend outward from the Golgi area (*G*), generally increasing in size with distance from the center. This suggests their origin from the Golgi apparatus and several may coalesce as they move from the center. Some endoplasmic reticulum (*er*) and mitochondria (*M*) are also present. × *20,000.*

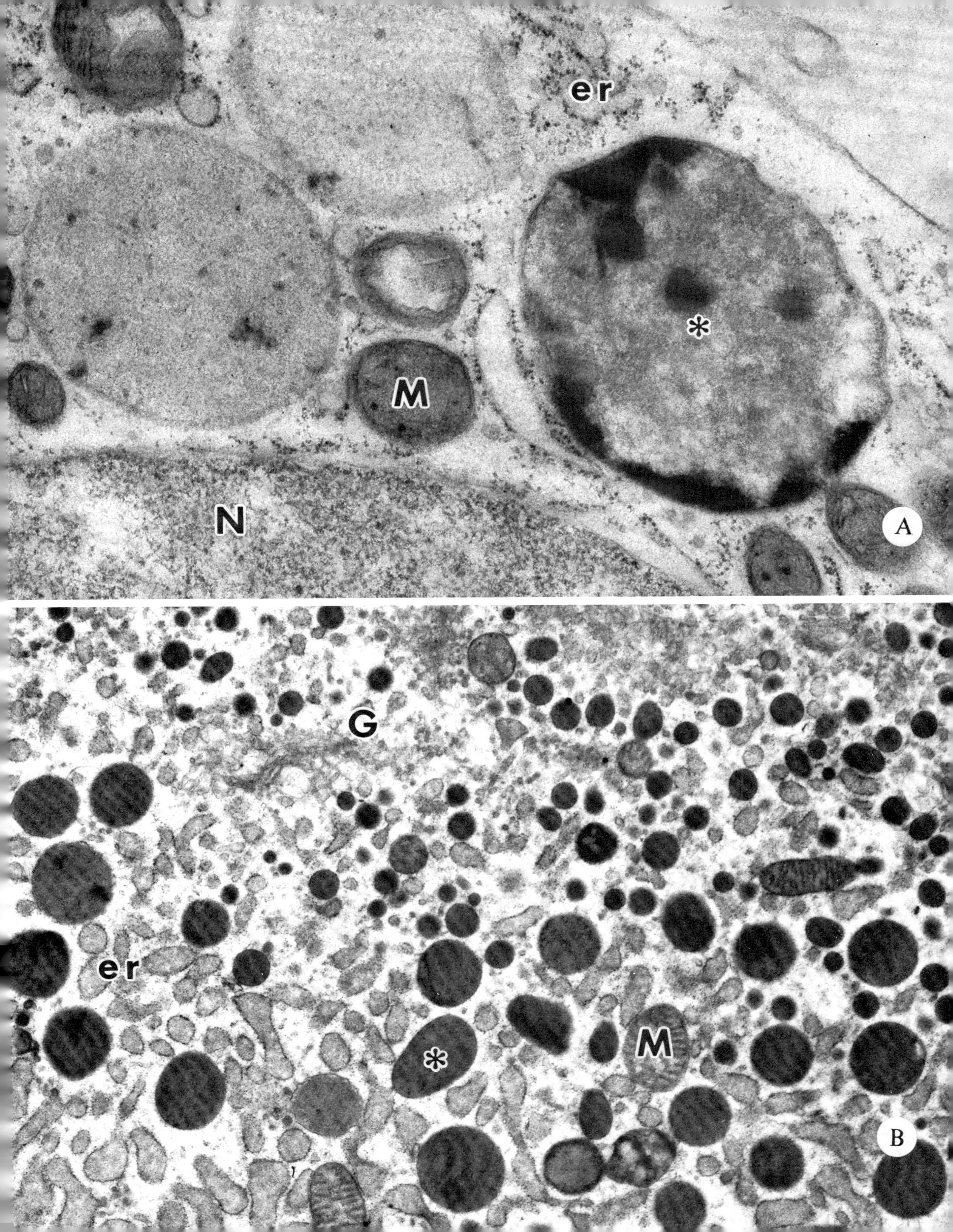
er
*
M
N
A
G
er
*
M
B

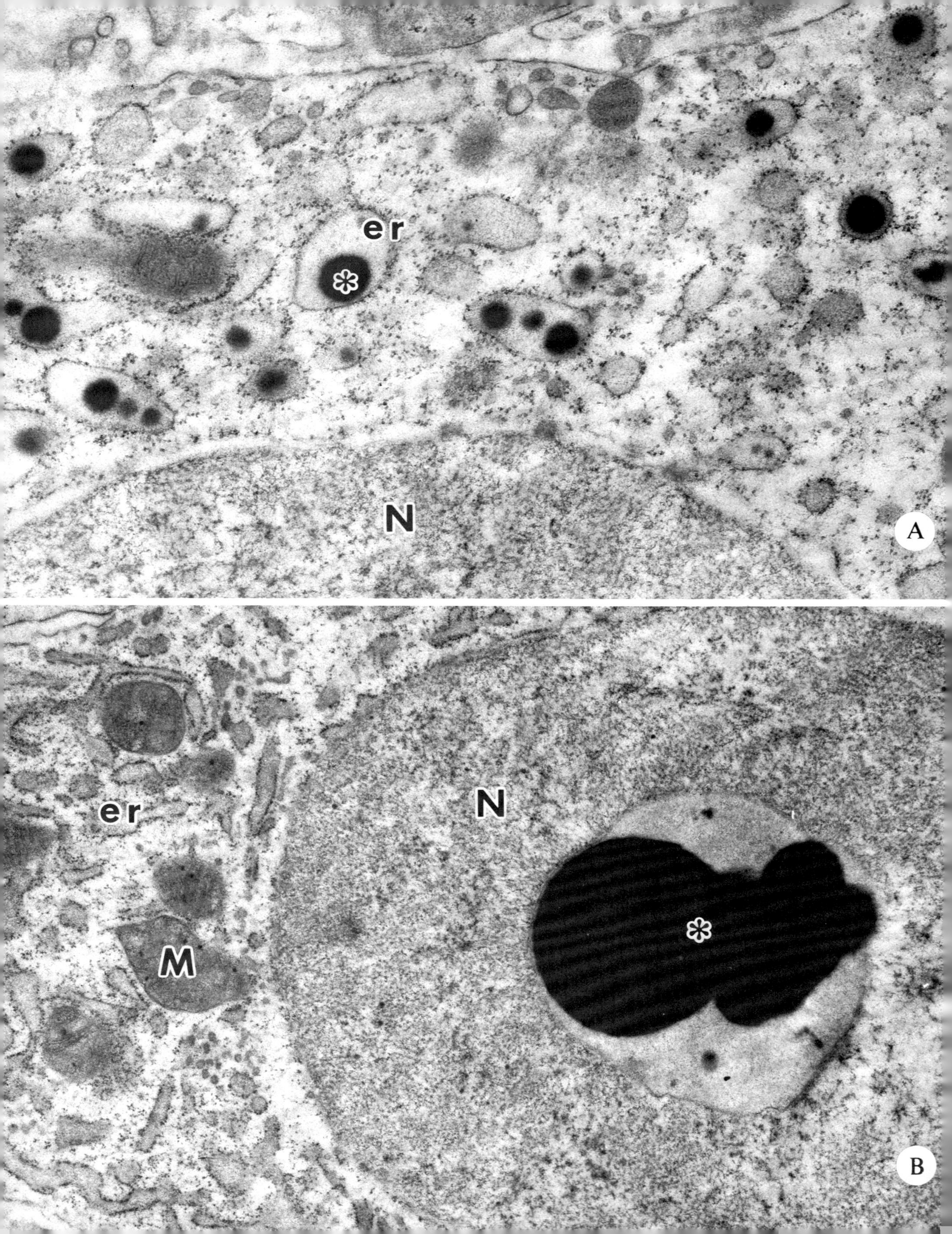
er
N
A
er
N
M
B

FIGURE 6-28. Inclusion bodies in myeloma.
A. Inclusions (*asterisk*) within cisternae of endoplasmic reticulum (*er*) contrast with cytoplasmic inclusions shown in Figure 6-27**B.** The electron-opaque spheres differ from Russell bodies (Fig. 6-8) only in their size. Many are too small to be visible by light microscopy. *Fixation: Osmium.* × *34,000.*
B. About 25 per cent of the myeloma cells of this case have electron-opaque spheroids of amorphous material within the nucleus. The single membrane which separates the inclusions (*asterisk*) from the nucleus (*N*) also contains diffuse, more translucent granular material. The endoplasmic reticulum (*er*) is vesicular and has several irregular, branched structures. Several mitochondria (*M*) are present. *Fixation: Osmium.* × *27,000.*

Figures 6-29 and 6-30 appear on the following pages ⇨

FIGURE 6-29. Double population of myeloma cells.
Two distinctive types (shown in parts **A** and **B**, and **C** and **D**) of proliferating cells, with irregular and distended translucent material, were found in a single specimen from marrow in a case of myeloma.
A. Immature cell resembles mesenchymal cell, with a large nucleolus (*Nu*) in the nucleus. × *10,000.*
B. More mature cell with developed endoplasmic reticulum has a larger Golgi apparatus (*G*) and more mitochondria (*M*). × *10,000.*
C. In immature cell with lymphoid appearance and no endoplasmic reticulum, a wide Golgi area (*G*), small mitochondria (*M*), and many free ribosomes are primary constituents. × *10,000.*
D. Cell with large distinct nucleolus (*Nu*) in a rounded, eccentrically located nucleus, has well-developed endoplasmic reticulum (*er*), mitochondria (*M*), and typical Golgi area. × *10,000.*

FIGURE 6-30. Myeloma cell variations.
A. Cell has distended endoplasmic reticulum (*er*) containing electron-lucent material, a Golgi complex (*G*), several mitochondria (*M*), and a large nucleus. The nucleus has a very large nucleolus (*Nu*) and uniform distribution of chromatin, suggesting that this is an immature cell, although the cytoplasm has characteristics more consistent with a mature cell. × *10,000.*
B. Another cell from same marrow has unusual arrangement of endoplasmic reticulum (*er*) containing some material of moderate density, but the cytoplasm is quite clear and almost devoid of ribosomes. The nucleus and nucleolus (*Nu*) suggest that this is an immature cell. × *10,000.*
C. Marrow cell with lymphoid appearance was diagnosed by light microscopy as lymphosarcoma; however, by electron microscopy it was found to be myeloma. This cell has developed a moderate amount of endoplasmic reticulum, a Golgi complex, and several mitochondria (*M*). The nucleus (*N*) contains a nucleolus, and the cell appears to be relatively immature. *Fixation: Osmium.* × *14,000.*
D. Cell from another case shows cellular proliferation classed as "plasmocytic reticulum cell sarcoma." There are a large number of mitochondria (*M*), a large Golgi (*G*), and well-developed endoplasmic reticulum. The nucleus is large and irregular and contains a large distinct nucleolus (*Nu*). × *10,000.*

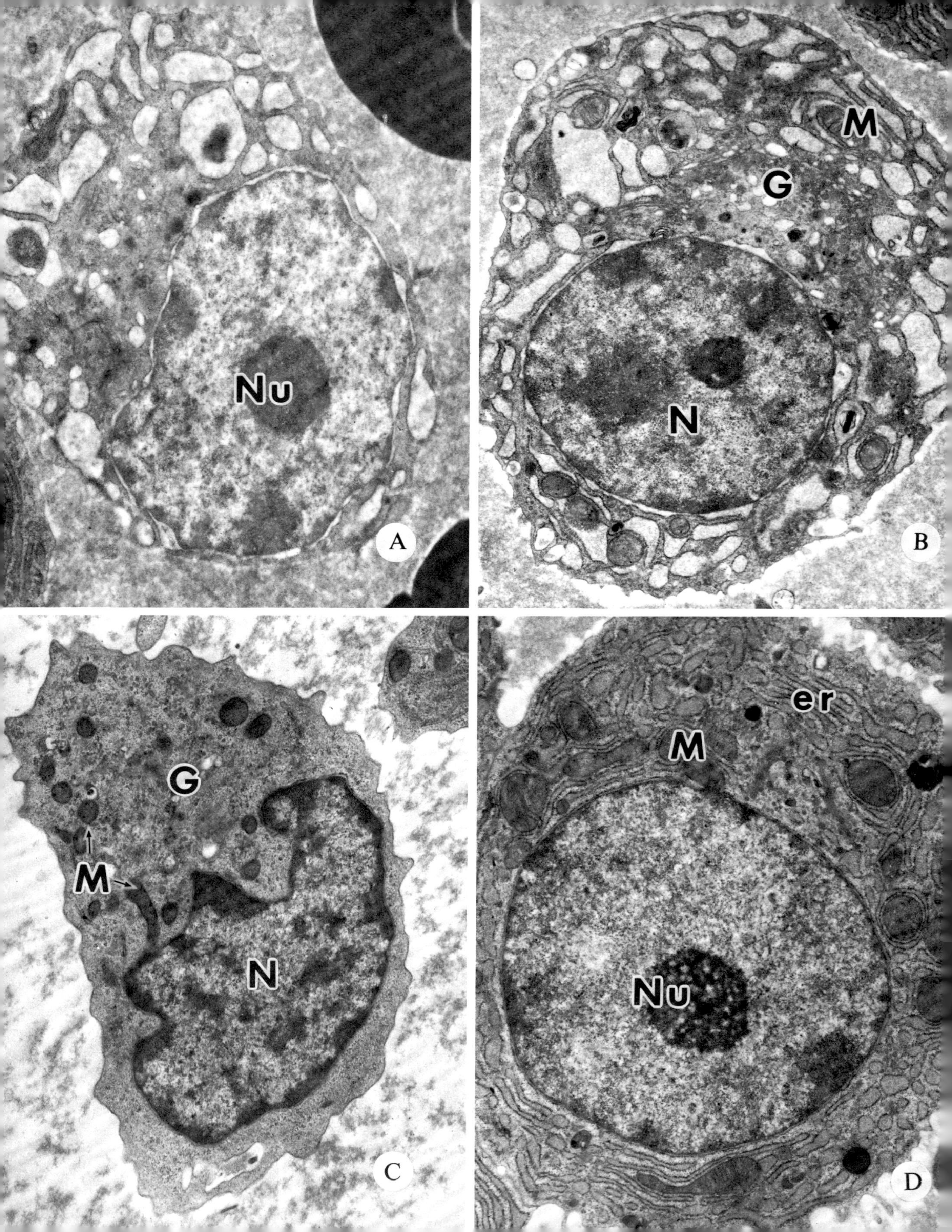
Nu
A
M
G
N
B
G
M
N
C
er
M
Nu
D

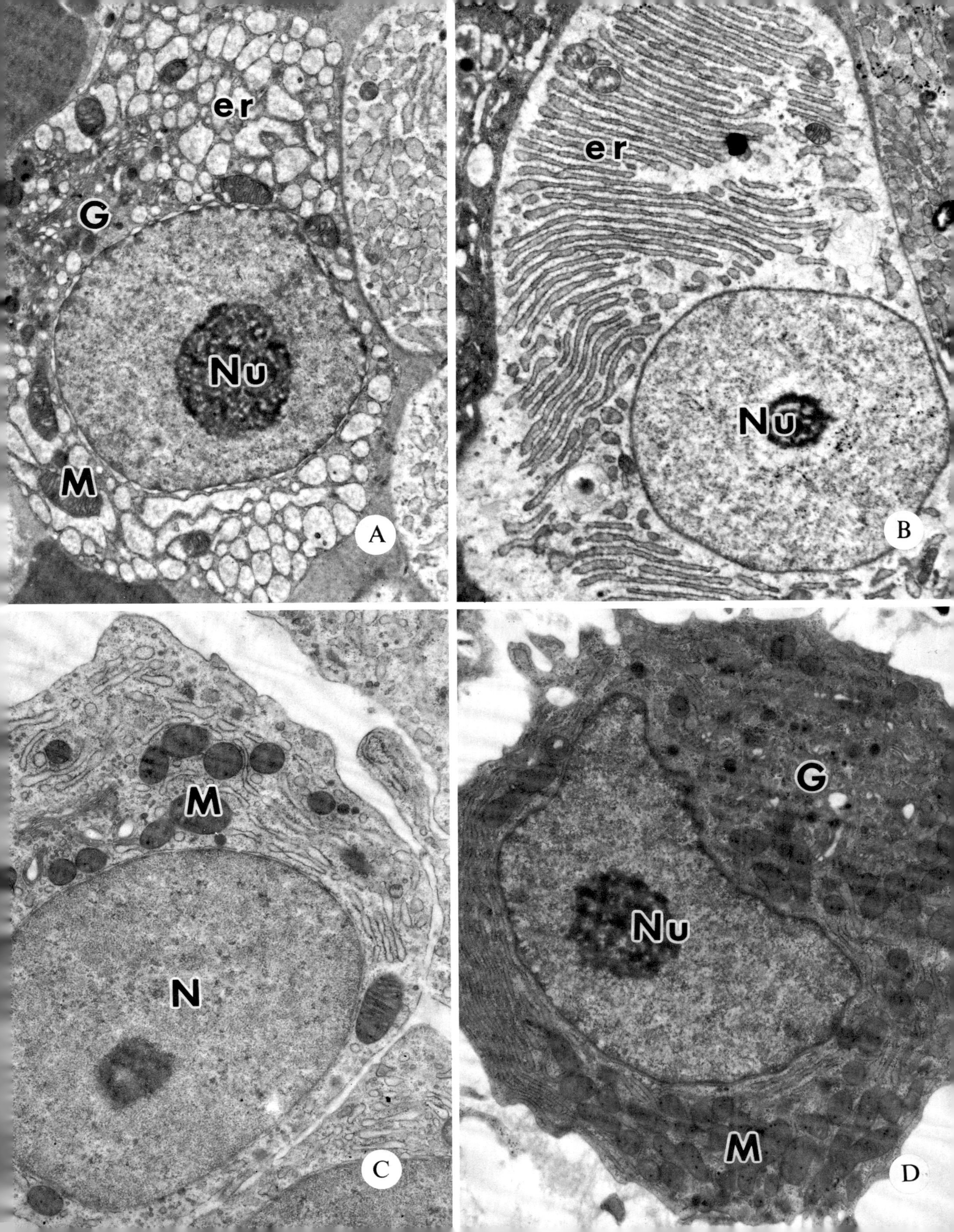
er
G
Nu
M
A
er
Nu
B
M
N
C
G
Nu
M
D

coacervation of produced protein. No periodicity has been reported in these electron-opaque structures.

The synthesized material in the endoplasmic reticulum may be discharged to the environment by the mechanism described for normal cells. In myeloma cells, drastic excretion mechanisms, such as clasmatosis or whole cell lysis, are probably more common than in normal cells and may reflect an increased fragility of the malignant cell.

On rare occasions, intranuclear inclusions composed of amorphous material have been observed (Fig. 6-28*B*), including spheroids of various sizes (Apitz, 1937; Fruhling and Porte, 1958; Brittin *et al.,* 1963). These were first described by Apitz (1937), who used Weigert fibrin stain and reported round structures consisting of two portions: a central bluish hyaline spheroid(s) and a thin peripheral rim of dark-staining material. The smallest were colorless or only faintly blue. Inclusions were sometimes single, although some had several in a single nucleus. Electron microscopic examination of many intranuclear inclusions suggests development from a fine granular substance to larger, coarser particles, probably by the coacervation of accumulated proteins (Brittin *et al.,* 1963). They were usually noted in the middle of the nucleus, bordered by a single membrane. The communication of the inclusion to the nuclear envelope has been seen frequently (Fruhling and Porte, 1958), but no internal crystalline structures have been identified in the spheroid. Inclusions may be formed in the nucleus (Brittin *et al.,* 1963) or by the engulfment of cytoplasmic materials in an invagination of the nuclear envelope (Fruhling and Porte, 1958).

Various technics, including ordinary light microscopy (Franklin and Lowenstein, 1964; Brecher *et al.,* 1964), immunofluorescence microscopy (Solomon *et al.,* 1963), and electron microscopy (Brecher *et al.,* 1964), have failed to correlate cytological aspects, biochemical changes, and the clinical course of multiple myeloma. This is due mainly to the wide morphologic variation of myeloma cells in a single case, which is as wide as the difference in cellular morphology among different cases (Figs. 6-29 and 6-30). However, several morphologic characteristics have been suggested in association with myeloma protein: (1) frequently observed proliferation of immature myeloma cells in cases with significant Bence-Jones protein in blood and urine (Williams *et al.,* 1966); (2) flaming plasma cells, intranuclear PAS-positive inclusions and thesaurocytes noted particularly in IgA myeloma (Paraskevas *et al.,* 1961; Drivsholm and Clausen, 1964; Maldonado *et al.,* 1965); (3) proliferation of lymphoid plasma cells; and (4) intranuclear inclusion of PAS-positive material in some cases of Waldenström's macroglobulinemia (Dutcher and Fahey, 1959). These correlations between morphology and biochemical quality of serum proteins are not consistent enough for diagnostic use.

In examination of myeloma cells by light and electron microscopy, many intermediate forms between undifferentiated and differentiated plasma cells are noted (Maldonado *et al.,* 1966). On occasion, several different types of myeloma cells have been distinguished in the same specimens (Fig. 6-29) (Brecher *et al.,* 1964; Maldonado *et al.,* 1966). Some appear to be derived from lymphoid precursors while others have a more irregular form of endoplasmic reticulum and may be of reticulum cell derivation. In one case of plasma cell sarcoma (Bessis, 1956; Okano *et al.,* 1966), the proliferating cells showed significantly developed endoplasmic reticulum arranged in lamellar pattern (Fig. 6-30*D*). However, from the whole structure of the cell, it could have been described as an atypical plasma cell rather than as a reticulum cell.

MACROGLOBULINEMIA

Macroglobulinemia, or an increased level of serum IgM, occurs in several pathologic states, including infections (Ritzman *et al.,* 1960; Rosen, 1962). This is classed as secondary macroglobulinemia while the term "primary macrobulinemia" refers to conditions in which the primary stimulus producing the increased macroglobulin is unknown but is associated with a proliferation of IgM-synthesizing cells (Ritzman *et al.,* 1960).

Waldenström (1944) first described a lymphoproliferative disorder associated with macroglobulinemia and a severe hemorrhagic tendency. This disease is now classed as a malignancy of the lymphoreticular cells or cells of reticuloendothelial origin capable of producing macroglobulin (Dutcher and Fahey, 1959; Ritzman *et al.,* 1960). It is relatively rare and has about the same incidence as multiple myeloma (Rosen, 1962). High molecular weight substances far exceed physiological levels and may contribute to the clinical signs, such as bleeding tendency or central nervous symptoms unique for this disorder. Conditions associated with the latter symptom include deafness, drowsiness, and coma, a combination known as Bing-Neel's syndrome (Ritzman *et al.,* 1960; Rosen, 1962). These symptoms are thought to be due to disturbance of intracranial circulation and cellular infiltration (Ritzman *et al.,* 1960; Rosen, 1962).

Since the proliferating cells in macroglobulinemia are often pleomorphic, resembling lymphocytes and plasma cells, the term "lymphoid plasma cell" is frequently used (Dutcher and Fahey, 1959). A study of the literature on macroglobulinemia suggests that conditions reported as primary macroglobulinemia could be categorized within one disorder typified by proliferation of plasma-reticulum cells. Cellular infiltrates of heterogeneous morphology usually have a dominant cell type that resembles either a lymphocyte or a mature plasma cell. This infiltrate may vary in each case as to its site or stage of disease (Schaub, 1952). This could account for the variation in diagnoses—i.e., macroglobulinemia with lymphoma (sarcoma) or macroglobulinemia with myeloma (Dutcher and Fahey, 1959). The dominant cell type in a given case may distinguish three subtypes—a lymphocytic, plasmacytic, and an intermediate form (lymphoid-plasma cell).

In our electron microscopic investigation on 13 cases of primary microglobulinemia, cells proliferating in 11 cases showed the general appearance of myeloma or atypical plasma cells (Brecher *et al.,* 1964). In three cases, most of the proliferating cells were hardly distinguishable from myeloma cells (Fig. 6-31). In 8 other cases, infiltrates had more pleomorphic elements but resembled myeloma cells (Fig. 6-32). The two abnormal cases had bizarre proliferating cells, one with two or three layers of endoplasmic reticulum in a narrow rim of cytoplasm (Fig. 6-33*A*). In general appearance the cells resembled those described by Zucker-Franklin (1964). In the other case, the predominant cells were round with a spherical nucleus, the cytoplasm had only scattered endoplasmic reticulum (Fig. 6-33*B*) and only a few plasma cells.

These 13 cases of macroglobulinemia, together with other reports on this disorder (Braunsteiner *et al,* 1956; Fruhling *et al.,* 1960; Stockringer, 1962; Bessis *et al.,* 1963; Zucker-Franklin, 1964; Kuhn, 1967), are the basis for describing the ultrastructural characteristics of proliferating elements in this disease. The malignant cells are mixtures of cells with more or less dominant endoplasmic reticulum. The latter category may fit the description of lymphocytes in smear technics, whereas cells with dominant endoplasmic reticulum frequently distended with amorphous material of moderate density, resemble myeloma cells. By light microscopy, the cells with endoplasmic reticulum have all the characteristics of plasma cells, such as well-developed, basic-staining cytoplasm and an eccentrically located nucleus adjacent to the well-developed Golgi apparatus. Cells with only a little endoplasmic reticulum of a vesicular nature commonly have a lymphoid appearance, which suggests a possible variance from a lymphocytic series.

It is not unusual to find bizarre multinuclear cells in macroglobulinemia. The nuclear margin is usually smooth, as in the plasma cell, with chromatin clumping; frequently, indentation, lobulation, and multiplication of the nucleus are seen in the pleomorphic cells (Fig. 6-32*B, C, D*). The Golgi apparatus is well organized into lamellar, vacuolar, and vesicular components, with moderately opaque material within the vacuoles. Mitochondria do not appear to differ from those seen in myeloma cells, although swollen or degraded structures are frequently seen in the pleomorphic cell type. The rough-surfaced endoplasmic reticulum arrangement may be irregular and distended, with disrupted or distorted ribosomal distribution in the bizarre cells. Material accumulated in the cisternae varies from homogeneous to coarsely flocculated, probably reflecting biochemical differences (Fig. 6-34). Although high molecular weight protein is synthesized, spheroid or crystalloid structures are less frequently seen than in myeloma cells, particularly in IgA myeloma.

The cytoplasm of the malignant cell has granules similar to those seen in myeloma cells and usually less than 1μ in diameter. Vacuoles with double compartments may be seen.

Intranuclear PAS-positive inclusions are one of the more significant structures in macroglobulinemia (Dutcher and Fahey, 1959; Stockinger, 1962; Brittin *et al.,* 1963; Kuhn, 1967). Histochemically, they are positive with the Millon, PAS and diatase-PAS reaction; not metachromatic with toluidine blue; and negative with alcian blue and Sudan black B (Dutcher and Fahey, 1959; Brittin *et al.,* 1963). The material contains neither DNA with Feulgen reaction nor RNA with pyronine stain. A developing sequence has been suggested for these inclusions in cells from a case of macroglobulinemia (Dutcher and Fahey, 1959). The inclusion is usually homogeneous, as seen by electron microscopy (Fig. 6-35*A*), although crystalline or spherical structures similar to those seen in myeloma cells (Fig. 6-35*B*) have been reported (Stockinger, 1962; Brittin *et al.,* 1963; Kuhn, 1967). Immunofluorescent studies reveal a positive reaction for 19S macroglobulin, corresponding to this intranuclear material (Dutcher and Fahey, 1960).

(text continues on page 328)

FIGURE 6-31. Cells in macroglobulinemia.
The darker cell (bottom) is more mature, with distended cisternae in endoplasmic reticulum (*er*), normal-appearing mitochondria (*M*), a Golgi complex, and several dense myelin laminar bodies (*arrow*). The upper cell is less dense and possibly less mature, with a very large Golgi apparatus (*G*), moderately distended cisternae, mitochondria (*M*), many free ribosomes in the cytoplasm, and a small laminar inclusion (*arrow*). Nucleus (*N*) shows some clumping of chromatin. $\times$ *16,000.*

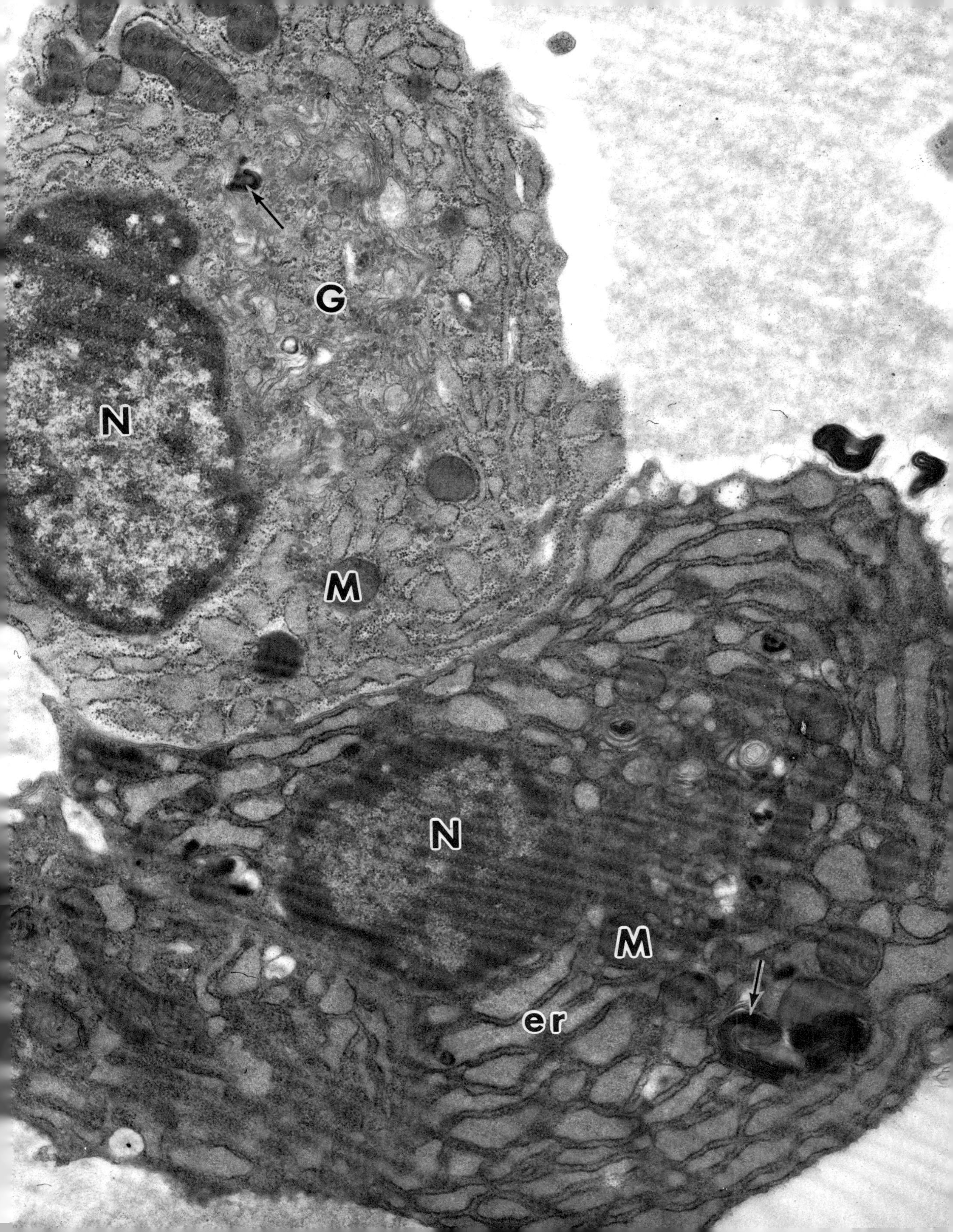
G
N
M
N
M
er

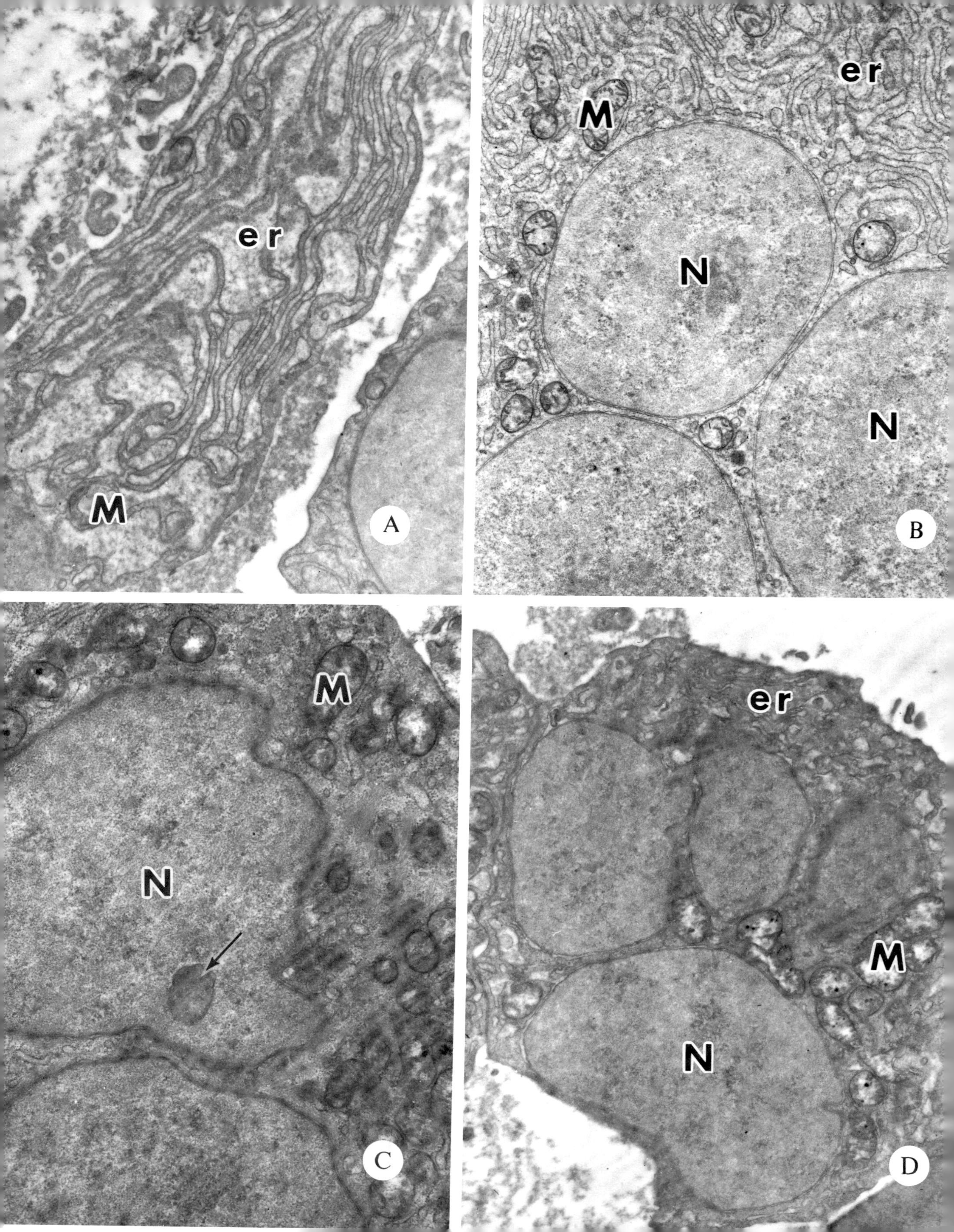
er
M
A
er
M
N
N
B
M
N
C
er
M
N
D

FIGURE 6-32. Cells in macroglobulinemia.
The cells in parts **A** through **D** are all from the same patient.
A. This cell is similar to typical plasma cell with distended endoplasmic reticulum (*er*), small mitochondria (*M*), and part of a nucleus. *Fixation: Osmium.* × *11,300.*
B. Cell has three nuclei (*N*) with fine granular chromatin, small distinct mitochondria (*M*), and well-developed endoplasmic reticulum (*er*). *Fixation: Osmium.* × *11,300.*
C. In a binucleated cell there is a small inclusion (*arrow*) in one nucleus (*N*), an irregular nuclear outline, many mitochondria (*M*) and some fine fibrillar structures. *Fixation: Osmium.* × *17,500.*
D. Cell with four nuclei (*N*) has an irregular profile, endoplasmic reticulum (*er*), and pale areas in mitochondria (*M*). In general, it lacks the appearance of a typical plasma myeloma cell. *Fixation: Osmium.* × *11,300.*

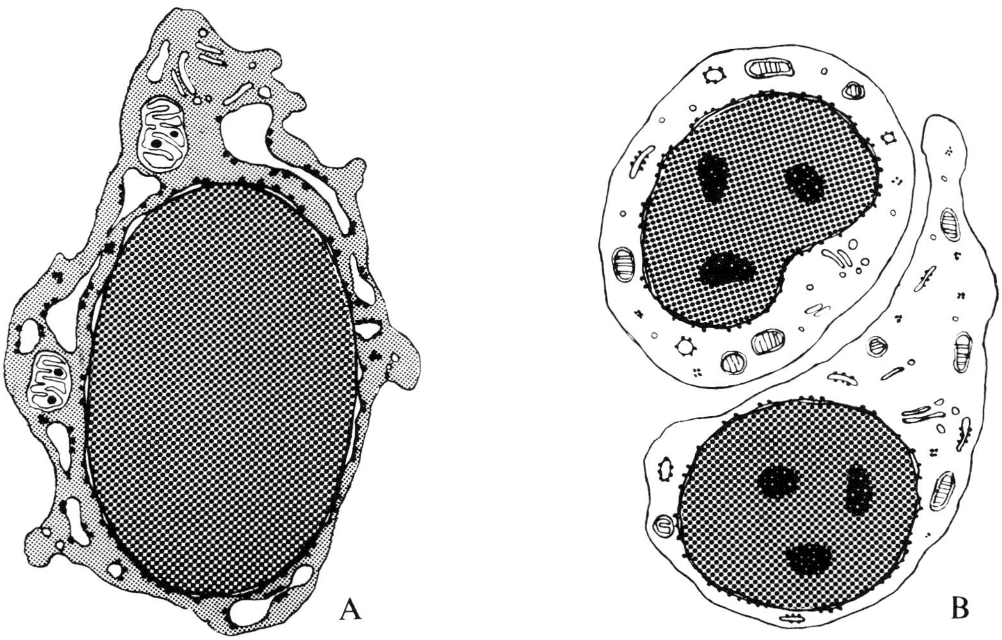

FIGURE 6-33. Uncommon types of proliferative cells in macroglobulinemia.
A. Small cell has dense background material and small amount of endoplasmic reticulum.
B. Mononuclear cells with distictive nucleoli and scattered vesicular or tubular endoplasmic reticulum. Cells similar to plasma cells are also observed with these proliferating cells.

Figures 6-34 and 6-35 appear on the following pages

FIGURE 6-34. Cytoplasm of proliferating cells in macroglobulinemia.
Endoplasmic reticulum from a case of macroglobulinemia with "myeloma cell" proliferation shows nature of content in cisternae.
A. Cytoplasm has vesicular type of endoplasmic reticulum (*er*), several mitochondria (*M*), and abundance of ribosomes, many of which appear to be free; a few are arranged in whorls (*arrow*) or are attached to membranes of the cisternae. × *43,000.*
B. Distended cisternae in endoplasmic reticulum (*er*) contains flocculated material, which appears to have a fine fibrillar structure. Several mitochondria (*M*) and the edge of the nucleus (*N*) are present. *Fixation: Osmium.* × *43,000.*

FIGURE 6-35. Intranuclear inclusions in macroglobulinemia.
A. Amorphous material (*asterisk*) is contained in a single membrane. The nucleus (*N*) has uniform distribution of chromatin. Part of the Golgi complex (*G*) is present in the cytoplasm. *Fixation: Osmium.* × *40,000.*
B. Many spheroids in an amorphous matrix are in this intranuclear inclusion (*asterisk*), which has a single membrane. The nucleus (*N*) has uniform distribution of chromatin, and the cytoplasm shows a portion of the Golgi apparatus (*G*), a tangentially cut centriole (*Ce*) and part of a mitochondrion (*M*). *Fixation: Osmium.* × *32,000.*

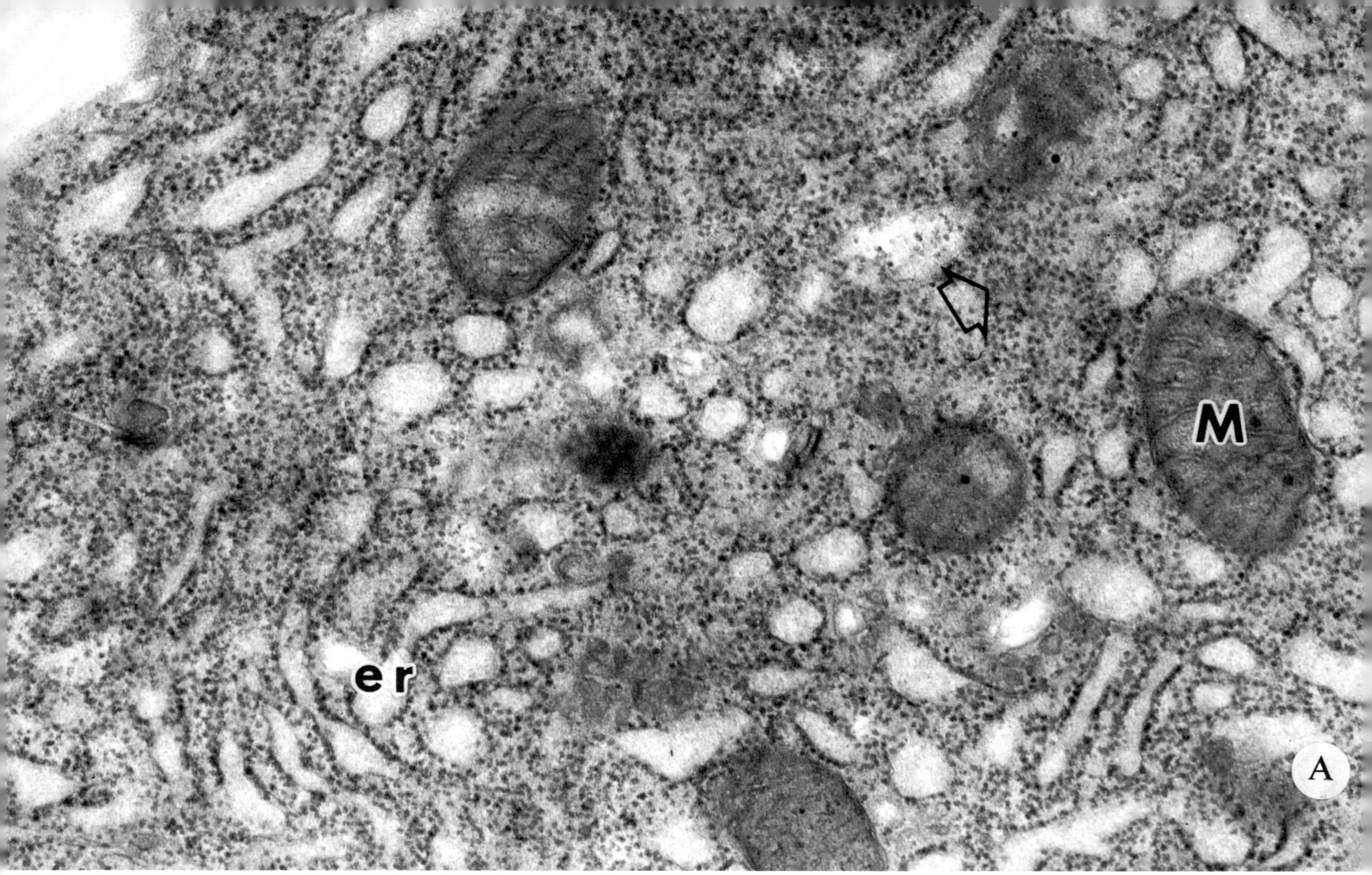
M
er
A

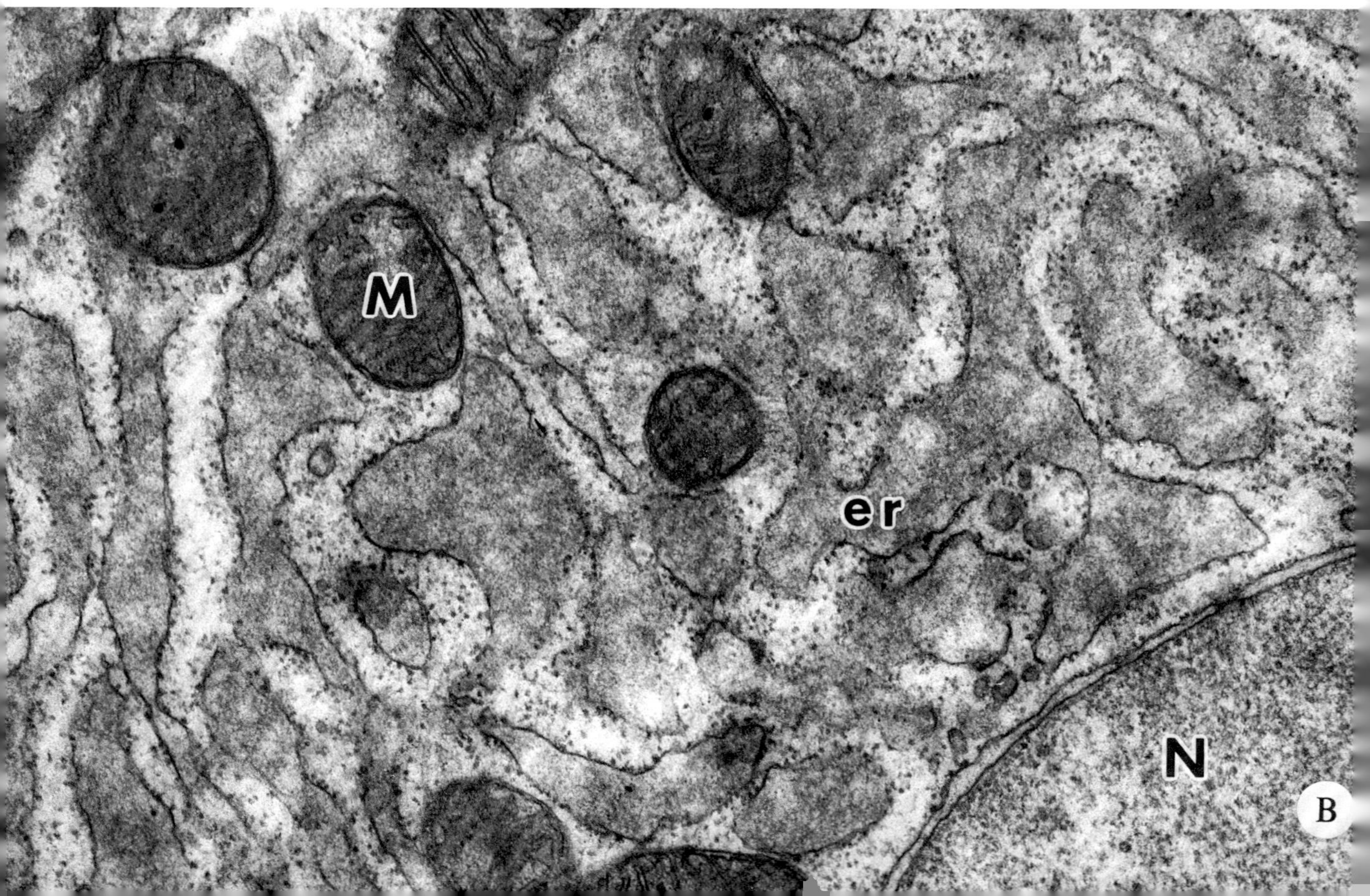
M
er
N
B

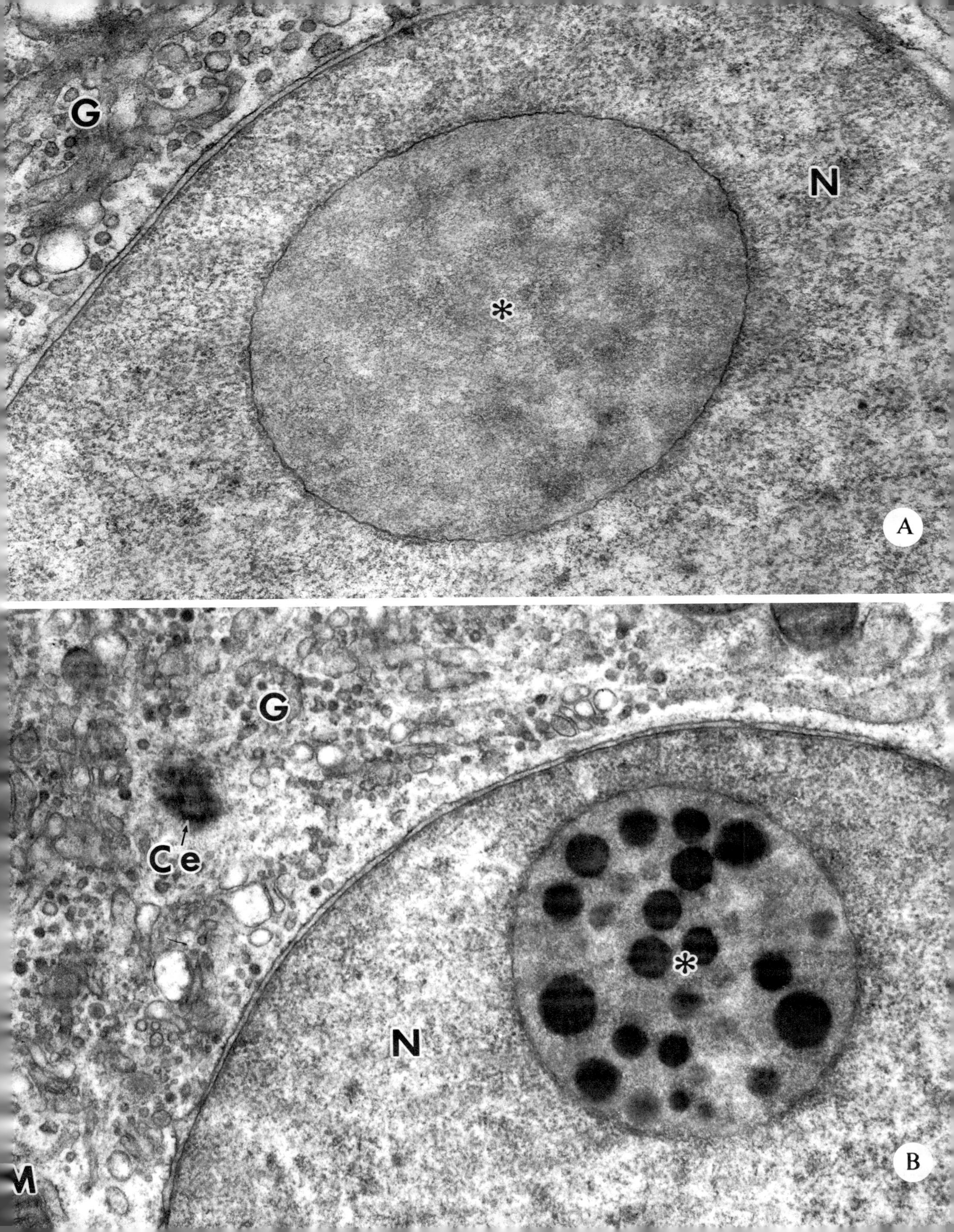
G
N
*
A
G
Ce
N
*
B
M

The inclusion may relate to the abnormal elaboration of an intracellular protein in these disorders (Brittin *et al.,* 1963).

Electron microscopic examination of the cytoplasm of the malignant cell shows fibrillar structures, particularly in cells of atypical appearance (Tanaka, 1964), with filaments about 50 to 100 Å in thickness that occasionally have a beaded appearance similar to that observed in various cells of the reticuloendothelial system.

Mastocytosis is frequently observed in Waldeström's macrolobulinemia (Dutcher and Fahey, 1959). The proliferation of mast cells possibly reflects the stimulated state of the reticuloendothelial system; however, its significance for clinical manifestations is not understood.

REFERENCES

Amano, S., Hirata, M., and Fuji, S. Studies on inflammatory cells. IV. Adventitial cells. (In Japanese) *Trans Soc Path Jap 34*:26, 1944.

Amano, S., Unno, G., and Hanaoka, M. Studies on the differentiation of lymphocytes and plasma cells. An advocation of "lymphogonia" theory. *Acta Haemat Jap 14*:108, 1951.

Apitz, K. Ueber die Bildung Russellscher Körperchen in den Plasmazellen multipler Myelome. 2. Beitrag zur Pathologie des Zellkernes. *Virchow Arch Path Anat 300*:113, 1937.

Barth, W. F., Asofsky, R., Liddy, T. J., Tanaka, Y., Rowe, D. S., and Fahey, J. L. An antibody deficiency syndrome. Selective immunoglobin deficiency with reduced synthesis of γ and α immunoglobin polypeptide chains. *Amer J Med 39*:319, 1965.

Bence-Jones, H. On a new substance occurring in the urine of a patient with "mollities ossium." *Trans Roy Soc London 5*:673, 1847.

Bernhard, W., and Leplus, R. *Fine Structure of the Human Lymph Nodes, Normal and Malignant.* Pergamon, New York, 1964.

Bessis, M. *Cytology of the Blood and Blood Forming Organs* (Ponder, E., transl.). Grune & Stratton, New York, 1956.

Bessis, M., Breton-Gorius, J., and Binet, J. L. Étude comparée du plasmocytome et du syndrome de Waldenström. Examen au microscope électronique. *Nouv Rev Franc Hemat 3*:159, 1963.

Bing, J. Further investigations on hyperglobulinemia. II. Is serum-globulin formed from plasma cells and reticulo-endothelial cells? *Acta Med Scand 103*:564, 1940.

Björneboe, M., and Gormsen, H. Experimental studies on the role of plasma cells as antibody producers. *Acta Path Microbiol Scand 20*:649, 1943.

Braunsteiner, H., Fellinger, K., and Pakesch, F. Demonstration of a cytoplasmic structure in plasma cells. *Blood 8*:916, 1953.

Braunsteiner, H., and Pakesch, F. Electron microscopy and the functional significance of a new cellular structure in plasmocytes: A review. *Blood 10*:650, 1955.

Braunsteiner, H., Oswald, E., Pakesch, F., and Reimer, E. Lymphoretikulosen mit Makroglobulinamie. *Wien Z Inn Med 37*:349, 1956.

Brecher, G., Tanaka, Y., Malmgren, R. A., and Fahey, J. F. Morphology and protein synthesis in multiple myeloma and macroglobulinemia. *Ann NY Acad Sci 113*:642, 1964.

Brittin, G. M., Tanaka, Y., and Brecher, G. Intranuclear inclusions in multiple myeloma and macroglobulinemia. *Blood 21*:335, 1963.

Burnet, F. H. *Clonal Selection Theory of Acquired Immunity.* Cambridge Univ. Press, London, 1959.

Cebra, J. J., and Small, P. A. Polypeptide chain structure of rabbit immunoglobulins. III. Secretory A-immunoglobin from colostrum. *Biochemistry 6*:503, 1967.

Chesebro, B., Bloth, B., and Svehag, S. E. The ultrastructure of normal and pathological IgM immunoglobulins. *J Exp Med 127*:399, 1968.

Christian, H. A. Multiple myeloma: A histological comparison of six cases. *J Exp Med 9*:325, 1907.

Coons, A. H., Leduc, E. H., and Connolly, J. M. Studies on antibody production. I. A method for the histochemical demonstration of specific antibody and its application to a study of the hyperimmune rabbit. *J Exp Med 102*:49, 1955.

Dalyrymple, J. On the microscopical character of mollities ossium. *Dublin Quar J Med Sci 2*:85, 1846.

Dameshek, W. "Immunoblasts" and "immunocytes." An attempt at a functional nomenclature. *Blood 21*:243, 1963.

de Petris, S., Karlsbad, G., and Pernis, B. Localization of antibodies in plasma cells by electron microscopy. *J Exp Med 117*:849, 1963.

de Petris, S., and Karlsbad, G. Localization of antibodies by electron microscopy in developing antibody-producing cells. *J Cell Biol 26*:759, 1965.

Douglas, S. D., and Fudenberg, H. H. In vitro development of plasma cells from lymphocytes following pokeweed mitogen stimulation. A fine structural study. *Exp Cell Res 54*:277, 1969.

Downey, H. The origin and structure of the plasma cells of normal vetebrates, especially of the cold blood vetebrates and the eosinophils of the lung of amblystoma. *Folia Haemat 11*:275, 1911.

Drivsholm, A. A., and Clausen, J. The relationship between the cytology and immuno-electrophoretic pattern in 105 cases of myelomatosis. *Acta Med Scand 175*:609, 1964.

Dubreuil, G., and Favre, M. Cellules plasmatique, plasma d' granulations specifique cellules à corps Russell. *Arch Anat Micr 17*:302, 1920–21.

Dutcher, T. F., and Fahey, J. L. The histopathology of the macroglobulinemia of Waldenström. *J Nat Cancer Inst 22*:887, 1959.

Dutcher, T. F., and Fahey, J. L. Immunocytochemical demonstration of intranuclear localization of 18S gamma macroglobulin in macroglobulinemia of Waldenström, *Proc Soc Exp Biol Med 103*:452, 1960.

Ehrlich, W. E. Identität der Plasmazellen. Entzündung und Immunität Reaktionen. *Handbuch Allg Path 7*(1):163, 1956.

Ewing, M. R., and Foote, F. W. Plasma cell tumors of the mouth and upper air passages. *Cancer 5*:499, 1952.

Fagraeus, A. The plasma cellular reaction and its relation to the formation of antibodies in vitro. *J Immun 58*:1, 1948.

Fishman, M., Hammerstrom, R. A., and Bond, V. P. In vitro transfer of macrophage RNA to lymph node cells. *Nature* (*London*) *198*:549, 1963.

Fishman, M., and Adler, F. L. The role of macrophage RNA in the immune response. *Sympos Quant Biol 22*:343, 1967.

Franklin, E. C., and Lowenstein, J. Protein abnormalities associated with proliferative disorders of plasma cells and lymphocytes. *Seminars Hemat 1*:144, 1964.

Fruhling, L., and Porte, A. Contribution de la microscopie électronique à létude d'un sarcome plasmocytaire. *Ann Anat Path 3*:538, 1958.

Fruhling, L., Porte, A. and Roger, S. La maladie de Waldenström. Étude d'un case en microscopies optique et electronique. *Ann Anat Path 5*:508, 1960.

Gilbert, C., and Hong, R. Qualitative and quantitative immunoglobulin deficiency. *Amer J Med 37*:602, 1964.

Gitlin, D., Gross, P. A. M., and Janeway, C. A. The gamma globulins and their clinical significance. II. Hypogammaglobulinemia. *New Eng J Med 260*:72, 1959.

Glaus, A. Über multiples Myelozytom mit eigenartigen zum Teil kristallähnlichen Zelleinlargerungen kombiniert mit Elastolyse und ausgedehnter Amyloidose und Verkalkung. *Virchow Arch Path Anat 223*:301, 1917.

Gluzinski, A., and Reinchenstein, M. Myeloma und leukemi lymphatica plasmocellularis. *Wien Klin Wschr 19*:336, 1906.

Good, R. A. Agammaglobulinemia: an experimental study. *Amer J Dis Child 88*:625, 1954.

Goodman, J. R., and Hall, S. G. Plasma cells containing iron: An electron micrographic study. *Blood 28*:83, 1966.

Gowans, J. L., and Knight, E. J. The route of re-circulation of lymphocytes in the rats. *Proc Roy Soc [Biol] 159*:257, 1964.

Gunn, F. D., and Mahle, A. E. Megakaryoblastic myeloma with crystalline protein in the renal tubules. *Trans Chicago Path Soc 15*:23, 1937.

Han, S. S., Han, I. H., and Johnson, A. G. Antibody response in the rat. II. Microclasmatosis, a possible mode of antibody release. *Proc Soc Exp Biol Med 121*:782, 1966.

Hanna, M. G., Jr., Swartzendruber, D. C., and Congdon, C. C. Morphologic changes in spleen lymphatic tissue during antibody production. *Exp Molec Path Suppl 3*:75, 1966.

Harris, T. N., Hammeler, K., and Harris, S. Electron microscopic observations on antibody-producing lymph node cells. *J Exp Med 123*:161, 1966.

Hayamizu, T. Studies on the origin of plasma cells. (In Japanese), *Trans Soc Path Jap 1*:215, 1911.

Herbut, P. A., and Erf, L. A. Lipoblastic and megakaryocytoid multiple myeloma. *Amer J Clin Path 6*:13, 1946.

Heremans, J. F., Heremans, M-Th., and Schultze, H. E. Isolation and description of a few properties of β-2A globulins of human serum. *Clin Chim Acta 4*:96, 1959.

Hirata-Hibi, M. Evidence for the origin of plasma cells from adventitial cells. I. Sensitized subcutaneous connective tissue examined by light microscopy. *Blood 29*:41, 1967.

Ishizaka, K., Ishizaka, T., and Hornbrook, M. M. Physiochemical properties of reaginic antibody. *J Immun 97*:840, 1966.

Jackson, H., Jr., Parker, F., Jr., and Bethea, J. M. Studies of diseases of the lymphoid and myeloid tissues. II. Plasmocytomata and their relation to multiple myelomata. *Amer J Med Sci 181*:169, 1931.

Kähler, O. Zur Symptomatologie des multiplen Myeloms: Beobachtung von Albumosurine. *Prag Med Wschr 14*:33, 1889.

Keuning, F. J., Van der Meer, J., Nieuwenhuis, P., and Oudendjik, P. The histiophysiology of the antibody response. II. Antibody responses and splenic plasma cell reactions in sublethally x-irradiated rabbits. *Lab Invest 12*:156, 1963.

Kingsley, D. W. Regressive structures and the lymphocyte: The plasma cell, its origin and development: A study of the mammalian nictitating membrane. *Anat Rec 29*:1, 1924.

Klein, H., and Block, M. Bone marrow plasmacytosis. A review of sixty cases. *Blood 8*:1034, 1953.

Kolouch, F., Jr. Origin of bone marrow plasma cells associated with allergic and immune states in the rabbits. *Proc Soc Exp Biol Med 39*:147, 1938.

Kuhn, C. Nuclear bodies and intranuclear globulin inclusions in Waldenström's macroglobulinemia. *Lab Invest 17*:404, 1967.

Leduc, E. H., Avrameas, S., and Bouteille, M. Ultrastructural localization of antibody in differentiating plasma cells. *J Exp Med 127*:109, 1968.

Lennert, K. Cytologie des ruhenden, aktivierten und entzündeten Lymphoknotens. *Lymphknote, Diagnostik und Cytologie. Hand buch der Speziellen Pathologischen Anatomie und Histologie,* vol. 3, no. 3. Springer, Berlin, 1961.

Liévre, J. A., Camus, J. P., Lévy, R., Badin, J., Bessis, M., and Tessier, F. Myelome à globuline cristallisable. Étude physico-chimique et microscopie électronique. *Nouv Rev Franc Hemat 1*: 23, 1961.

MacIntyre, W. A case of mollities and fragilities ossium, accompanied with urine strongly changed with animal matter. *Med Chir Trans London 33*:211, 1850.

MacKinney, A. A., Jr., Stohlman, F., Jr., and Brecher, G. The kinetics of cell proliferation in cultures of human peripheral blood. *Blood 19*: 349, 1962.

Maldonado, J. E., Bayrd, E. D., and Brown, A. L., Jr. The flaming cell in multiple myeloma. A light and electron microscopy study. *Amer J Clin Path 44*:605, 1965.

Maldonado, J. E., Kyle, R. A., Brown, A. L., Jr., and Bayrd, E. D. "Intermediate" cell types and mixed cell proliferation in multiple myeloma: Electron microscopic observations. *Blood 27*: 212, 1966.

Maximow, A. The Lymphocyte and Plasma Cell. In *Special Cytology* (Cowdry, E. V., ed.). Hoeber, Inc., New York, 1928, Vol. 1, p. 353.

McMillan, D. B., and Engelbert, V. E. The developmental history of the plasmacyte. *Amer J Path 42*:315, 1963.

Michels, N. A. The plasma cell. *Arch Path 11*:775, 1931.

Miller, F. R. The induced development and histogenesis of plasma cells. *J Exp Med 54*:333, 1931.

Milstein, C. and Pink, J. R. L. Structure and evolution of immunoglobulins. *Progr Biophys 21*:209, 1970.

Moe, R. E. Electron microscopic appearance of the parenchyma of lymph nodes. *Amer J Anat 114*: 341, 1964.

Movat, H. Z., and Fernando, N. V. P. The fine structure of connective tissue. II. The plasma cell. *Exp Molec Path 1*:535, 1962.

Movat, H. Z., and Fernando, N. V. P. The fine structure of the lymphoid tissue during antibody formation. *Exp Molec Path 4*:155, 1965.

Newman, W., Diefenbach, W. C. L., Quinn, M., and Meyer, L. M. A case of acute plasma cell leukemia supporting the concept of unity of plasmacellular neoplasia. *Cancer 5*:514, 1952.

Nossal, G. J. V., Abbot, A., and Mitchel, J. Antigens in immunity. XIV. Electron microscopic radioautographic studies of antigen capture in lymph node medulla. *J Exp Med 127*:263, 1968a.

Nossal, G. J. V., Abbot, A., Mitchel, J. and Lummus, Z. Antigens in immunity. XV. Ultrastructural features of antigen capture in primary and secondary lymphoid follicles. *J Exp Med 127*: 277, 1968b.

Okano, H., Azar, H. A., and Osserman, E. F. Plasmacyte reticulum cells sarcoma. Case report with electron microscope studies. *Amer J Clin Path 46*:546, 1966.

Ortega, L. G., and Mellors, R. C. Cellular sites of formation of gamma globulin. *J Exp Med 106*: 627, 1957.

Osgood, E. E., and Hunter, W. C. Plasma cell leukemia. *Folia Haemat 52*:369, 1934.

Osserman, E., and Takatsuki, K. Plasma cell myeloma: gamma globulin synthesis and structure. *Medicine 42*:357, 1963.

Paraskevas, F., Heremans, J., and Waldenström, J. Cytology and electrophoretic pattern in IA (Beta 2A) myeloma. *Acta Med Scand 170*:575, 1961.

Parsons, L. D. Cellular changes in lymph nodes of experimental mice with special reference to plasma cell development. *J Path Bact 55*:397, 1943.

Pease, A. G. E. The nature of Russell bodies and Kurloff bodies: observations on cytochemistry of plasma cells and reticulum cells. *J Clin Path 2*: 81, 1949.

Polli, E. E., Lanzavecchia, G., and Bosision, M. Inclusion Bodies of Human Plasma Cells in Some Myeloproliferative Disorders. In *Proceedings of the 5th International Congress on Electron Microscopy* (Breese, S. S., ed.). Academic Press, New York, 1962, vol. 2, p. SS–170.

Potter, M., Dreyer, W. J., Kuff, E. L., and McIntire, K. R. Heritable variation in Bence-Jones protein structure in an inbred strain of mice. *J Mol Biol 8*:814, 1964.

Putnam, F. W. Immunoglobulin structure: variability and homology. *Science 163*:633, 1969.

Ramón, y Cajal, S. Estudios Histologicos sobre los Tumores Epitheliales. In *Manual de Anatomie Pathologica*. Barcelona, 1890. Cited by Michels (1931).

Rifkind, R. A., Osserman, E. F., Hsu, K. C., and Morgan, C. The intracellular distribution of gamma globulin in a mouse plasma cell tumor (x-5563) as revealed by fluorescence and electron microscopy. *J Exp Med 116*:423, 1962.

Ritzman, S. E., Thurm, R. H., Traux, W. E., and Levin, W. C. The syndrome of macroglobulinemia. *Arch Intern Med 105*:939, 1960.

Rohr, K. Blut und Knochenmarksmorphologie der Agranulozytosen. *Folia Haemat 55*:305, 1936.

Rosen, F. S., Kevy, S. V., Merler, E., Janeway, C. A., and Gitlin, D. Recurrent bacterial infections and dysgammaglobulinemia: Deficiency of 7S gamma-globulins in the presence of elevated 19S gamma-globulins. *Pediatrics 28*:182, 1961.

Rosen, F. S. The macroglobulins. *New Eng J Med 267*:491, 1962.

Rosen, F. S., and Janeway, C. A. The gamma globulins. III. The antibody deficiency syndromes. *New Eng J Med 275*:769, 1966.

Ross, R., and Klebanoff, S. J. Fine structural changes in uterine smooth muscle and fibroblasts in response to estrogen. *J Cell Biol 32*: 155, 1967.

Rowe, D. S., and Fahey, J. L. A new class of human immunoglobulins. I. A unique myeloma protein. *J Exp Med 121*:171, 1965.

Rustizky, Von J. Multiple myelome. *Deutsch Z Chir 3*:162, 1873.

Sainte-Marie, G. Study on plasmocytopoiesis. I. Description of plasmocytes and of their mitoses in the mediastinal lymph nodes of ten-week old rats. *Amer J Anat 114*:207, 1964.

Sainte-Marie, G. Cytokinetics of antibody formation. *J Cell Physiol 67* (Suppl. 1):109, 1966.

Schaub, F. Zum Krankheitsbild und zur Differentialdiagnose der Makroglobulinanamie Waldenström *Schweiz Med Wschr 82*:890, 1952.

Schooley, J. C. Autoradiographic observations of plasma cell formation. *J Immun 86*:331, 1961.

Snapper, I. and Kahn, A. I. Multiple myeloma. *Seminars Hemat 1*:87, 1964.

Solomon, A., Fahey, J. L., and Malmgren, R. A. Immunohistologic localization of gamma-1- macroglobulins, beta-2A-myeloma proteins, 6.6S gamma-myeloma proteins and Bence-Jones proteins. *Blood 21*:403, 1963.

Sorenson, G. D. Electron microscopic observations of bone marrow from patients with multiple myeloma. *Lab Invest 13*:196, 1964.

Sprigg, A. I., and Jerrome, D. W. Electron microscopy of Türk cells. *Brit J Haemat 13*:764, 1967.

Stockinger, L. Electronenoptiche Darstellung einer Macroglobulinretention in Plasmazellen des menschlichen Knockenmarks. *J Cell Biol 15*: 131, 1962.

Svehag, S. E., Chesebro, B., and Bloth, B. Ultrastructure of gamma M Immunoglobulin and alpha macroglobulin. Electron microscopic study. *Science 158*:933, 1967.

Tanaka, Y. Fibrillar structures in the cells of blood-forming organs. *J Nat Cancer Inst 33*:467, 1964.

Taylor, C. E. Erythroid multiple myeloma. *Amer J Clin Path 17*:222, 1947.

Thiéry, J. P. L'ergastoplasme des plasmocytes à l'état vivant. *Rev Hemat 10*:745, 1955.

Thiéry, J. P. Étude sur le plasmocyte à l'état vivant. II. Ecrettion de vacuoles d'origine nucléaire. *Rev Hemat 12*:211, 1957.

Thiéry, J. P. Étude sur le plasmocyte en contraste de phase et en microscopie électronique. III. Plasmocytes à corps de Russell et à cristaux. *Rev Hemat 13*:61, 1958.

Thiéry, J. P. Microcinematographic Contributions to the Study of Plasma Cells. In *Cellular Aspects of Immunity.* Ciba Foundation Symposium. Churchill, London, 1960, p. 59.

Thiéry, J. P. Étude au microscope électronique de l'îlot plasmocytaire. *J Micr 1*:275, 1962.

Tiselius, A. Electrophoresis of serum globulin. II. Electrophoretic analysis of normal and immune sera. *Biochem J 31*:1464, 1937.

Tiselius, A., and Kabat, E. A. Electrophoresis of immune serum. *Science 87*:416, 1938.

Tomasi, T. B., Tan, E. M., Solomon, A., and Prendergast, R. A. Characteristics of an immune system common to certain external secretions. *J Exp Med 121*:101, 1965.

Tompkins, E. H. The conversion of lymphocytes with "atypical nuclei" into plasma cells of the Marshalkó type. *Amer J Path 37*:175, 1960.

Undritz, E. *Atlas of Haematology.* Sandoz, Basel, 1952.

Unna, P. Ueber Plasmazellen insebesondere beim Lupus, *Mschr Prakt Derm 12*:296, 1891.

Waldenström, J. Incipient myelomatosis or "essential" hyperglobulinemia with fibrinogenopenia—a new syndrome? *Acta Med Scand 117*: 216, 1944.

Waldenström, J. Monoclonal and polyclonal gammopathies and the biological system of gamma globulins. *Progr Allerg 6*:320, 1962.

Waldeyer, W. Ueber Bindegewebszellen. *Arch Mikr Anat 11*:176, 1875.

Wellensiek, H. J. Zur submikroskopischen Morphologie von Plasmazellen mit Russellschen Körperchen und Eiweisskristallen. *Beitr Path Anat 118*:173, 1957.

Welsh, R. A. Light and electron microscopic correlation of the periodic acid-Schiff reaction in the human plasma cell. *Amer J Path 40*:285, 1962.

Williams, R. C., Jr., Brunning, R. D., and Wollheim, F. A. Light-chain disease: An abortive variant of multiple myeloma. *Ann Intern Med 65*:471, 1966.

Wright, J. H. A case of multiple myeloma. *Trans Ass Amer Physicians 15*:137, 1900.

Zagury, D., Uhr, J. W., Jamieson, J. D., and Palade, G. E. Immunoglobulin synthesis and secretion. II. Radioautographic studies of sites of addition of carbohydrate moieties and intracellular transport. *J Cell Biol 40*:52, 1970.

Zlotnick, A. The "morular cell" and the "grape cell" in bone marrow and peripheral blood. *Blood 11*:1140, 1956.

Zucker-Franklin, D. Structural features of cells associated with the paraproteinemias. *Seminars Hemat 1*:165, 1964.

chapter 7

BONE MARROW STRUCTURE

The generation of blood cells from bone marrow was discovered by Neumann (1868, 1882), who described both red and yellow marrows. The study of bone marrow structure was attempted by Rindfleisch in 1880, and later by Van der Stich in 1892. In 1900, Naegeli postulated the presence of the parental cell of all blood cells in the bone marrow and introduced the term "myeloblasts." The morphology and definition of Naegeli's myeloblasts were apparently different from cells currently defined by that term. The exploration of the immature compartment of bone marrow and the theories of the origin of the cells were the most popular subjects in hematology at that time. By the end of 1920, the role of basophilic, nongranulated components of the bone marrow was established as constituting the immature compartment for cell generation. Morphologically, these elements corresponded to the large lymphoid cells observed in yolk sacs called "hemocytoblasts" by Ferrata (1918, 1920). Cells of similar morphology were believed to be responsible for generation in postnatal bone marrow. The delicate tissues contained in the middle of various hard bone shells were regarded as one functional system and estimated to be larger in total cell mass than that of liver (Wetzel, 1920).

Alteration of bone marrow cells in various hematologic disorders was observed after technics of bone marrow aspiration were introduced. These methods are now routinely used to obtain specimens for the diagnosis of disease and evaluation of the therapeutic effects of drugs.

An interest in the relationship of the immature compartment or bone marrow structural cells to hematopoiesis has developed from the use of autologous marrow infusions to initiate hematopoiesis following acute radiation damage. These marrow infusions, coupled with the spleen-colony methods of Till and McCulloch (1961) have provided an additional approach to the study of stem cells. However, the structure of bone marrow and cytology of this immature compartment are the least explored of all marrow cells. The use of the electron microscope in conjunction with some of the recent experimental approaches may help to increase the understanding of problems on origin and cytogenic relationships of stem cells.

MORPHOLOGY

Structurally, the bone marrow is composed of a sponge-like framework of blood vessels (Figs. 7-1 through 7-4) and cellular reticulum (Fig. 7-4*B*). The cells which participate in the formation of this cellular matrix are called reticulum cells; large macrophages with elongated cytoplasm and fat cells are also included as part of this matrix. The reticulum cells are apparently connected to each other and form the fundamental architecture of bone marrow. Unlike other organs, fibrils (reticulin fibers) and other extracellular structures such as collagen are sparsely scattered in bone marrow. This suggests that the cellular framework is flexible and able to adapt rapidly to variations in number of marrow cells.

Bone marrow anatomy may be easily understood when the structure is analyzed by following the blood pathways. Detailed studies on the marrow vessels are available in femurs and other long bones of small animals (Doan, 1922; Drinker *et al.*, 1922; Bergmann, 1930; Fliedner *et al.*, 1956). An extensive and complete review on this topic was made recently by Brånemark (1968).

The distribution of blood vessels is best traced by using dye injection technics. The artery enters the marrow cavity of the femur near the proximal end of the long bone and divides into two major branches, ascending and descending. The ascending branches, which are relatively short, are further divided into arteries until they reach the epiphysis. Descending arteries run parallel along the bone axis in a significant twisting pattern (Fig. 7-1*B*), branching in only a few places. Consequently, arteries of fairly large size reach the epiphyseal region, where significant anastomosis of arteries and veins occurs. Anastomosis between two adjacent small arteries is rarely observed. In the diaphysis, several large arteries branch into smaller ones, which lead toward the periphery of the marrow. Here, near the subendosteum, they further divide into many small vessels (Fig. 7-1*B* and 7-3*A*) which connect to sinuses (Fig. 7-3*B*). Numerous arterial capillaries also penetrate to the bone cortices. The sinuses begin after the capillary connection; because of the complex connections, the initial part of the sinus is called sinus contori (Fliedner *et al.*, 1956). In the diaphsis, blood flows through the sinus recti into the central vein at the middle of the

(*text continues on page 346*)

FIGURE 7-1. Structure of femoral marrow in rat.
The marrow was fixed by glutaraldehyde perfusion and India ink was injected. These sections are a few millimeters in thickness and embedded in balsam.
A. In this cross section, dense structures (A) are small arteries containing large amount of India ink; bas relief of arrangement of sinuses (*S*) is apparent. × *130.*
B. Longitudinal section shows a twisted artery (*A*) and several arterioles (*asterisk*). Cross sections of sinusoids (*S*) are discernible. × *130.*

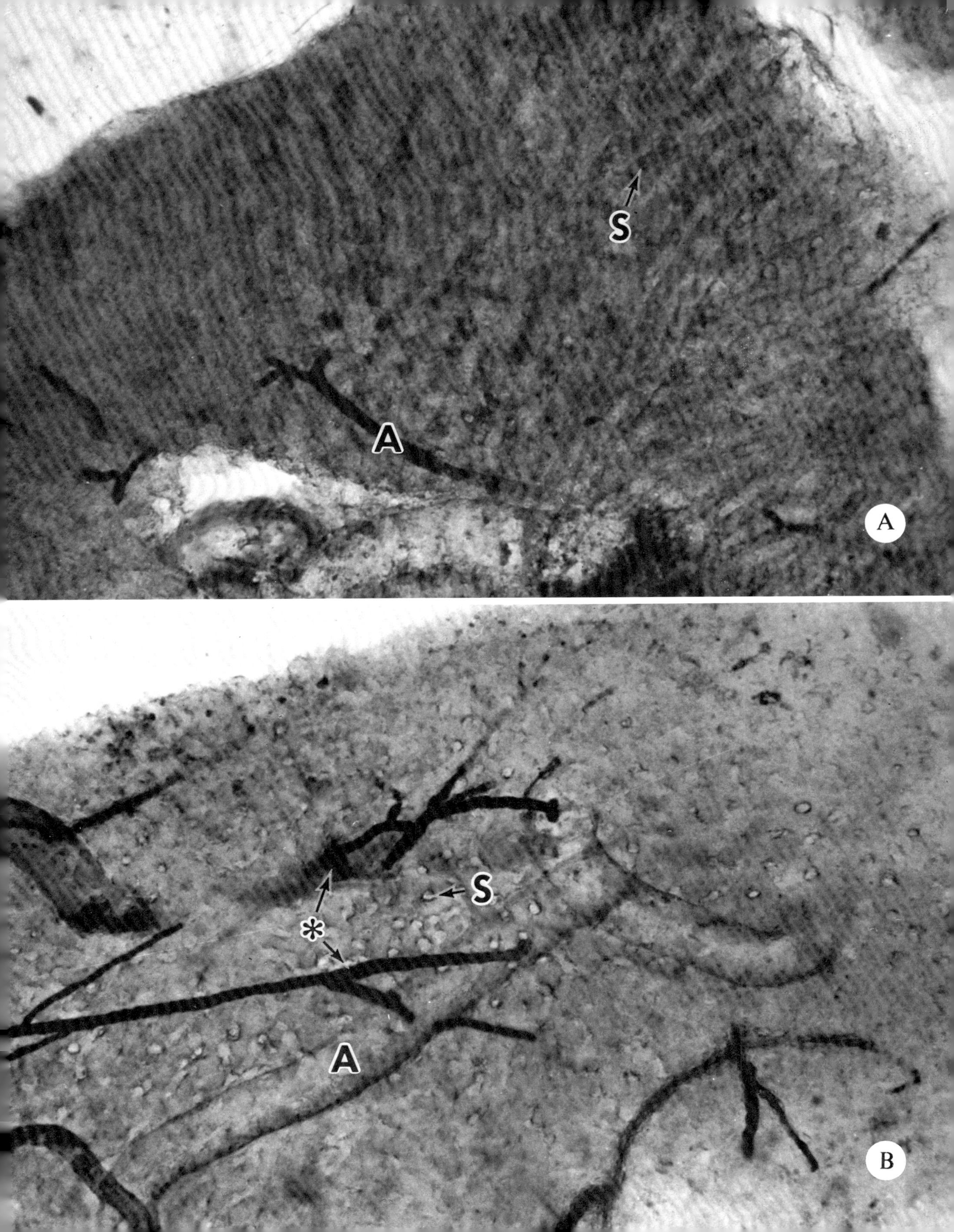
S
A
A
S
*
A
B

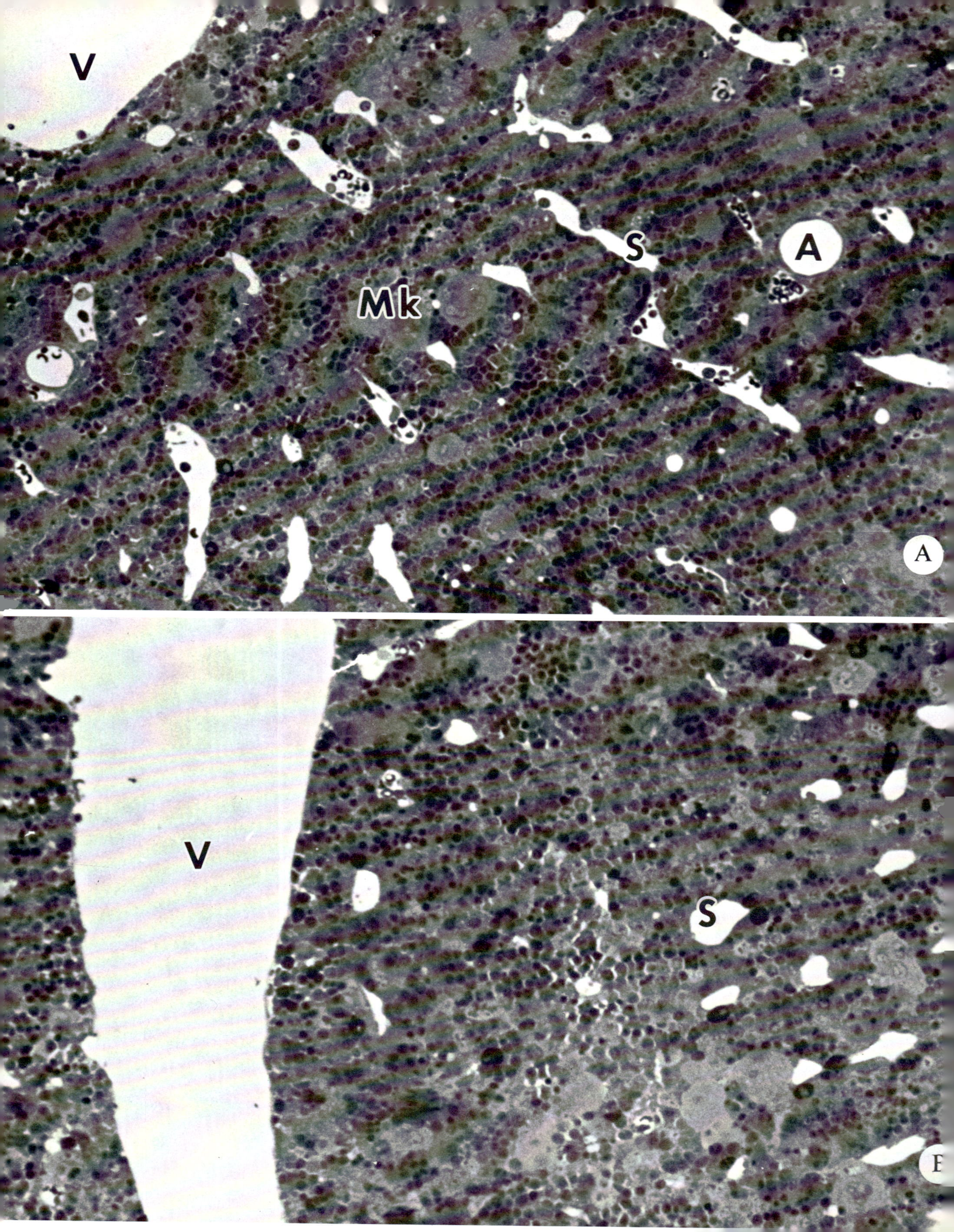
V
S
A
Mk
A
V
S
B

FIGURE 7-2. Structure of femoral marrow in rat.
Hyperplastic marrow from a phenylhydrazine hydrochloride-treated rat was cut from a block embedded for electron microscopy and stained by the Huber method.
A. Sinuses lead toward central vein (*V*). Noted dilated arteries (*A*) or arterioles, which are rounded structures. The array of sinusoids (*S*) is apparent. A proliferation of megakaryocytes (*Mk*) is easily identified. × *360.*
B. Section cut on a longitudinal plane shows central vein (*V*) and cross sections of sinus lumen (*S*). × *360.*

Figures 7-3 and 7-4 appear on the following pages

FIGURE 7-3. Plastic cast of rat marrow vessels.
Cast was prepared by plastic infiltration and polymerization, with subsequent removal of tissue by digestion.
A. Large artery (*A*) shows small branches toward periphery (*arrow*). Large dilated structures are apparently sinuses (*S*). × *150.*
B. Sinus (*S*) connects (*arrow*) to capillary vessel. × *230.*
C. Branches of sinus (*S*) are clearly demonstrated. × *230.*

FIGURE 7-4. Structure of marrow in rat.
A. Marrow was prepared in same manner as that for Figure 7-2. Note spatial relationships between free cells and interstitial structures (*arrow*) bewteen sinuses (*S*) and blood vessels. These interstitial cells can be seen, but not distictly. A megakaryocyte (*Mk*) is present. × *1,280.*
B. Schematic interpretation of relationship of bone marrow structure and free cells. Sinus with its endothelial lining cells (*middle*) is supported intermittently by interstitial cells and cytoplasm (*shaded cells*). Some of these structural cells are scattered throughout the intersinusoidal space and tend to support the two fat cells in opposite corners. The cells bounded by dotted lines represent immature elements (see text and Figs. 7-15 and 7-18).

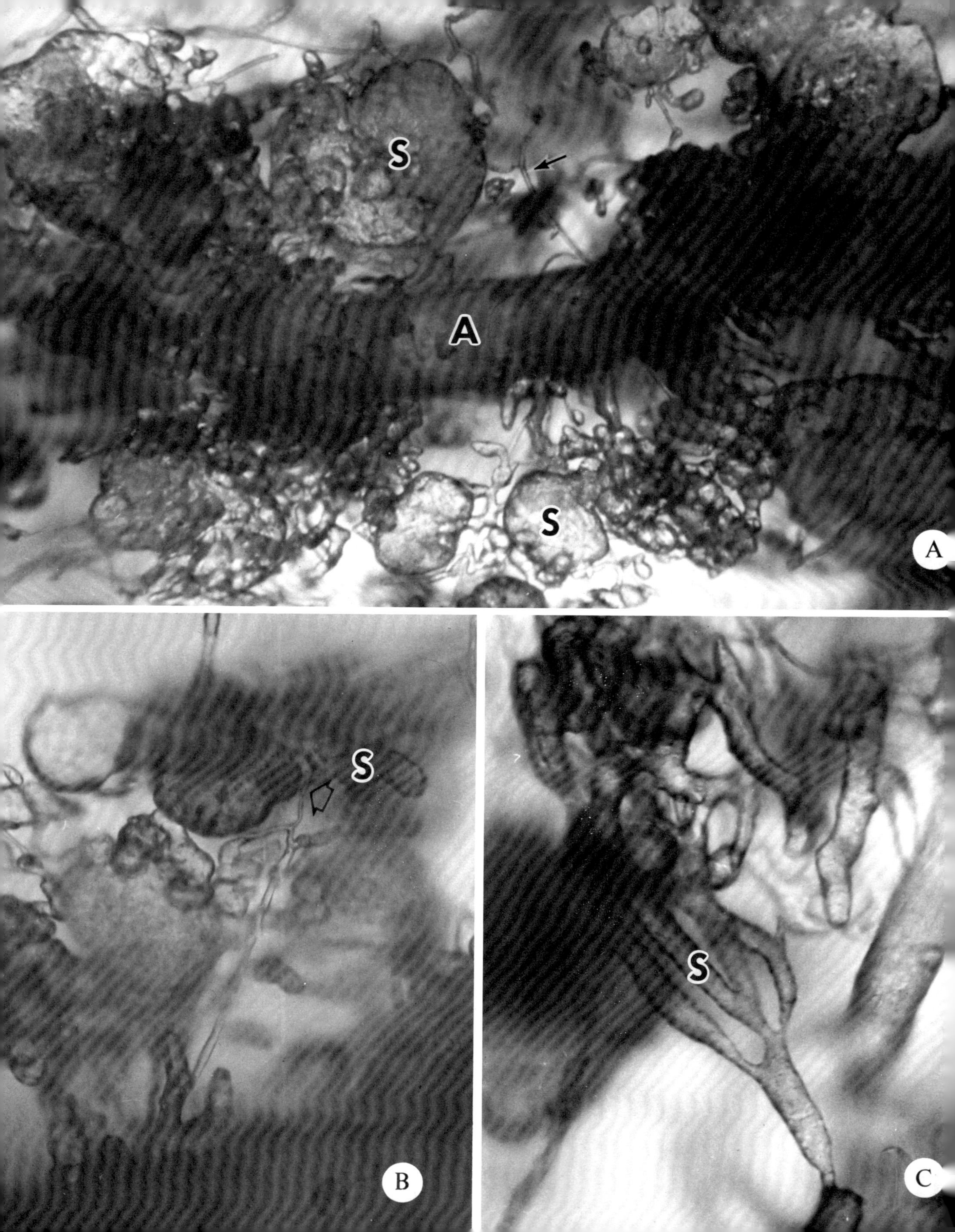
S
A
S
A
S
B
S
C

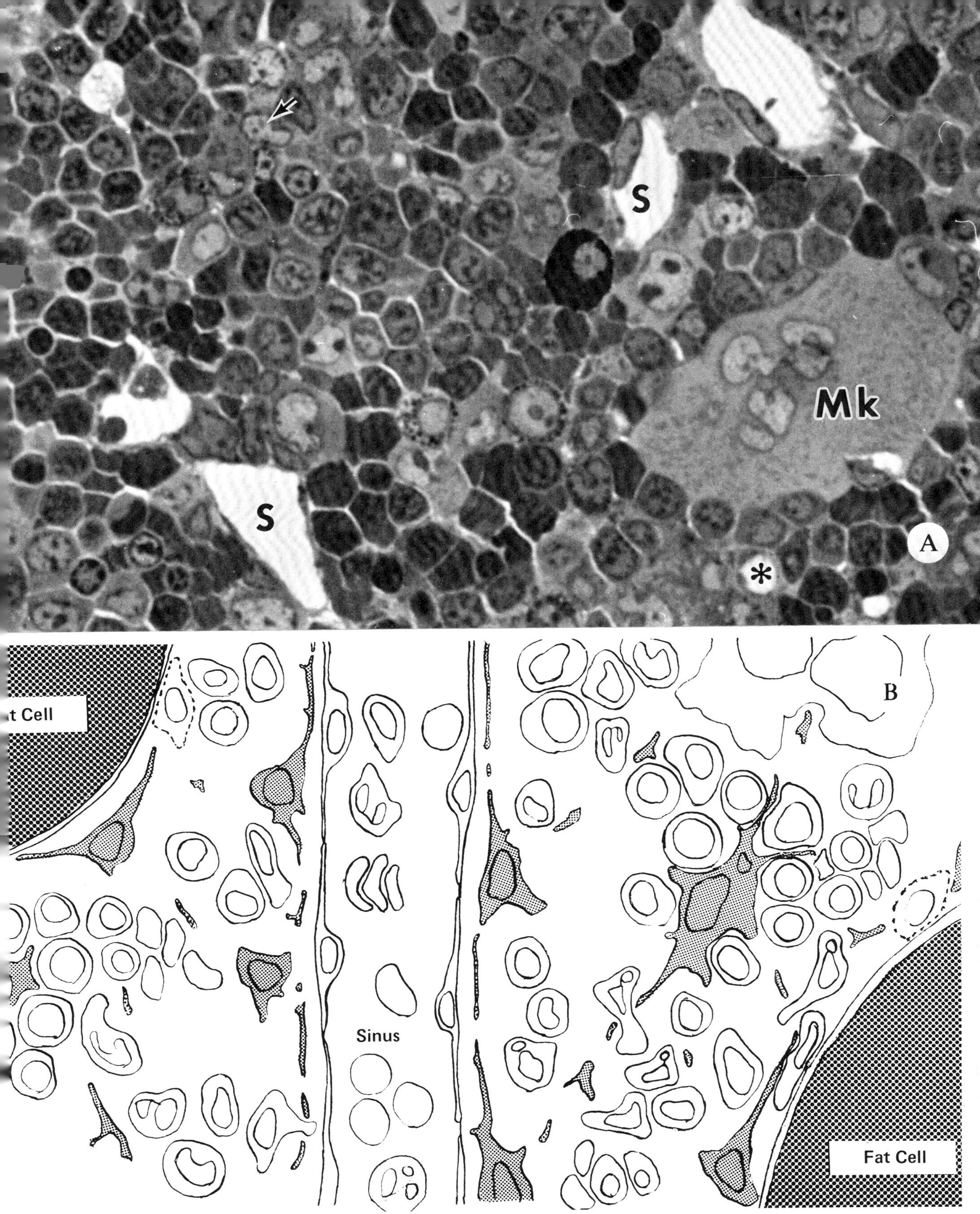
S
S
Mk
A
*
t Cell
B
Sinus
Fat Cell

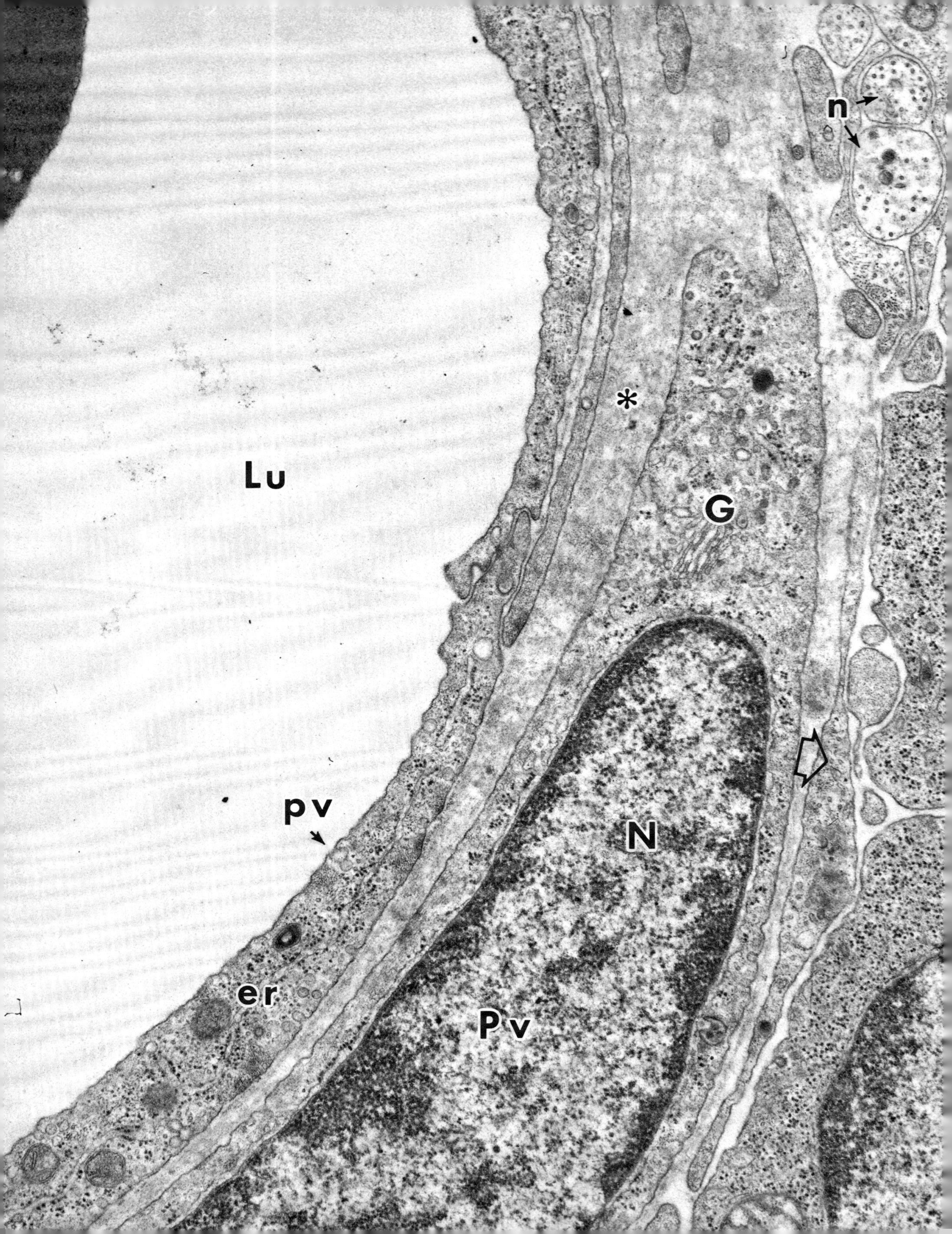

n
*
Lu
G
pv
N
er
Pv

FIGURE 7-5. Tissue surrounding small artery in rat bone marrow.
Section is from same block of tissue as that from which sections for Figures 7-2 and 7-4**A** were taken. Vessel lumen (*lu*) is distended as a result of the pressure of the glutaraldehyde perfusion. Inner vessel surface has elongated sheets of endothelial cell cytoplasm which contains some endoplasmic reticulum (*er*), ribosomes and numerous pinocytotic vessels (*pv*). The next layer of intercellular amorphous material (*asterisk*) is followed by a perivascular cell (*Pv*) with a portion of the nucleus (*N*) and the Golgi complex (*G*). The amorphous material in the perivascular space is separated from intersinusoidal spaces by projections of reticulum cytoplasm (*large arrow*). Structures in upper right corner (*n*) are unmyelinated nerve fibers. × *29,600.*

Figures 7-6 and 7-7 appear on the following pages

FIGURE 7-6. Ultrastructure of human marrow.
The lumen (*Lu*) of a small blood vessel is nearly closed. It is formed by portions of four endothelial cells (*En*) held together by tight junctions (*arrows*), with layer of amorphous material (*asterisk*) between endothelial cells and cytoplasm of perivascular cell (*Pv*). The Golgi apparatus (*G*) of one endothelial cell is prominent. × *13,200.*

FIGURE 7-7. Endothelium in marrow of rat.
Section, from same block of tissue as that used for Figures 7-2 and 7-4, shows relationship between sinus endothelial (*En*) and reticulum cells (*Rc*) in rat marrow. The sinusoidal space in the middle, with mononuclear cell (*asterisk*), is lined with tightly connected endothelial cells. There are no gaps between the adjacent vales of cytoplasm, although apparent fenestrations (*arrows*) are seen occasionally. Small amounts of amorphous material and fibrillar structures (*open arrow*) are seen between endothelial cells, thin strips of reticulum cell (*Rc*) cytoplasm and a mast cell (*Mc*). × *8,400.*

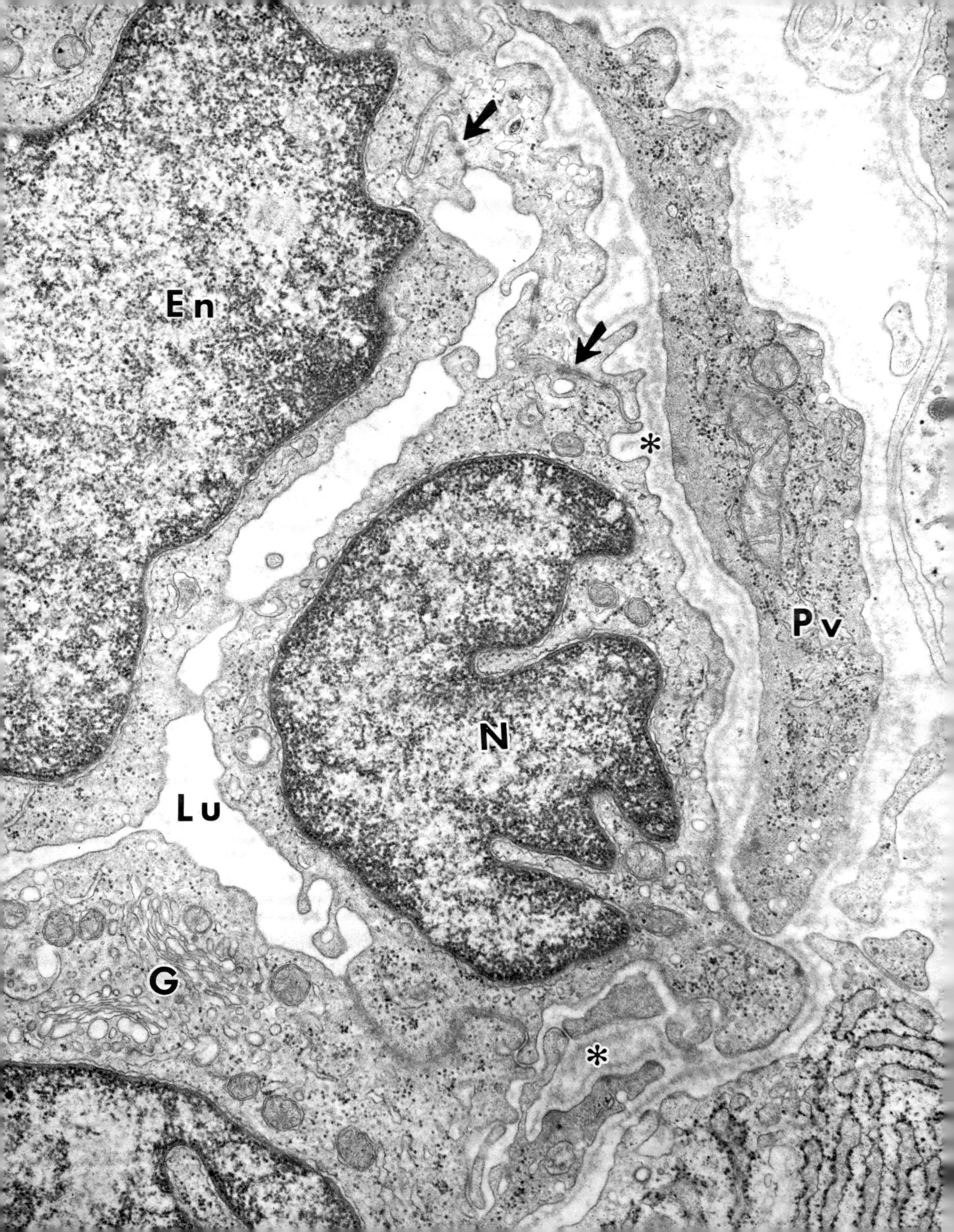
En
Pv
N
Lu
G
*
*

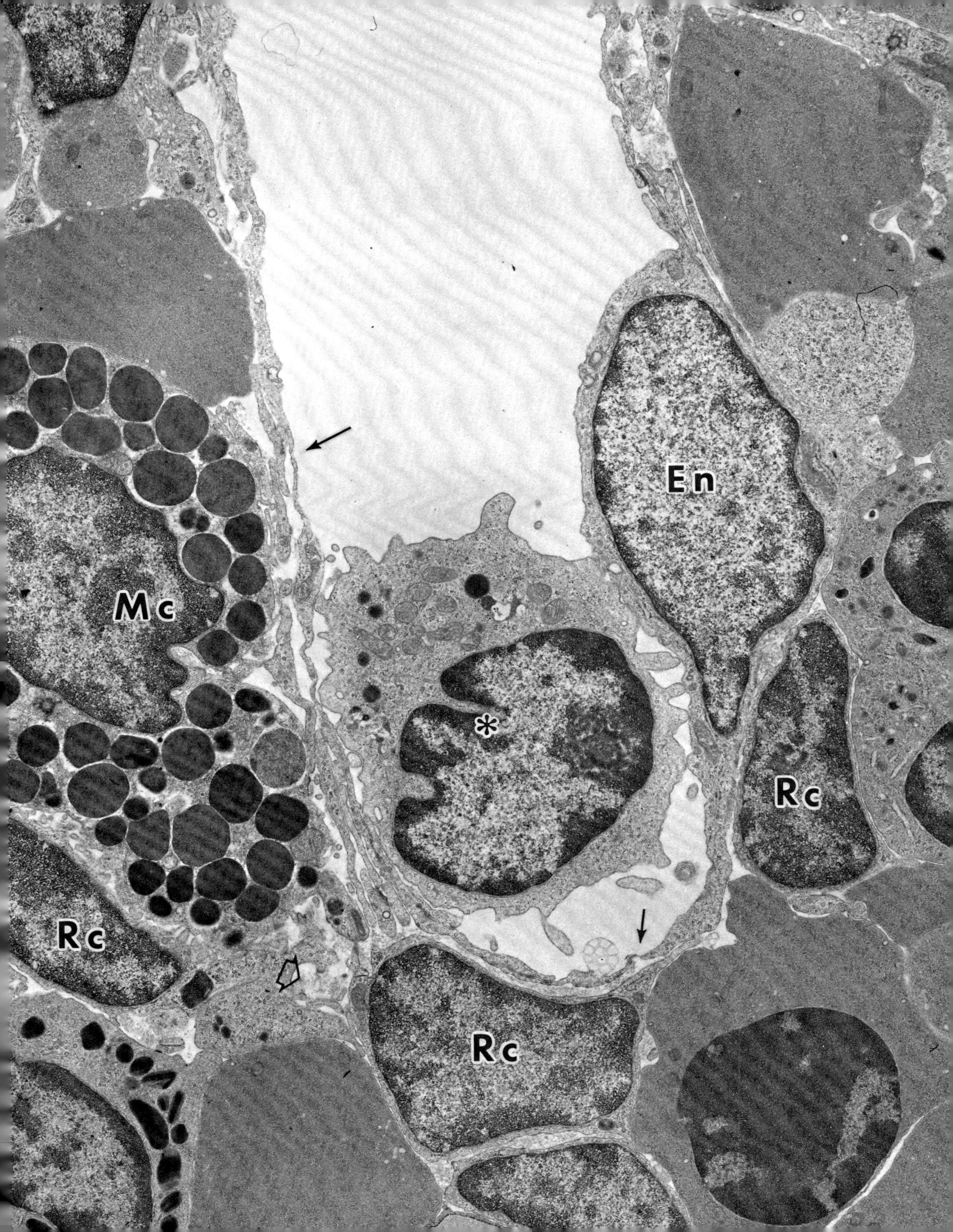
En
Mc
*
Rc
Rc
Rc

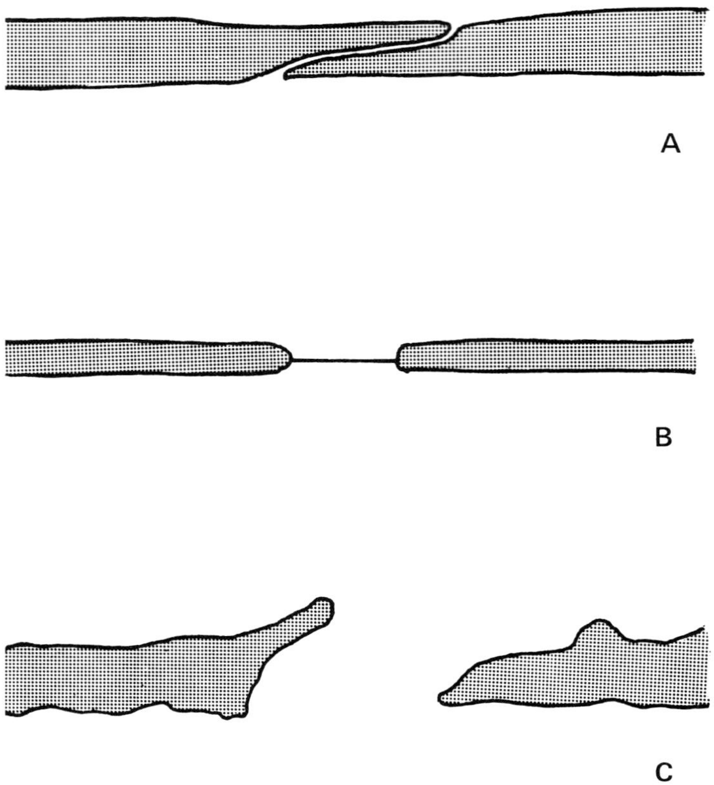

FIGURE 7-8. Types of endothelial cell contacts.
A. Overlapping junctions, frequently bound by desmosomes.
B. Fenestration in continuous cytoplasm.
C. Complete gap between two cells, which may be a transient state and, at another point in time, may close.

FIGURE 7-9. Cytoplasmic detail of rat endothelial cell.
Lumen is at left, and tip of nucleus (*N*) is at top. There are several pinocytotic vesicles (*pv*), inclusions (*in*), some endoplasmic reticulum (*er*), a band of extracellular fibers (*fb*) between the endothelial cell and portions of reticulum cells (*Rc*) containing some intracellular fibers (*asterisks*). × *45,000.*

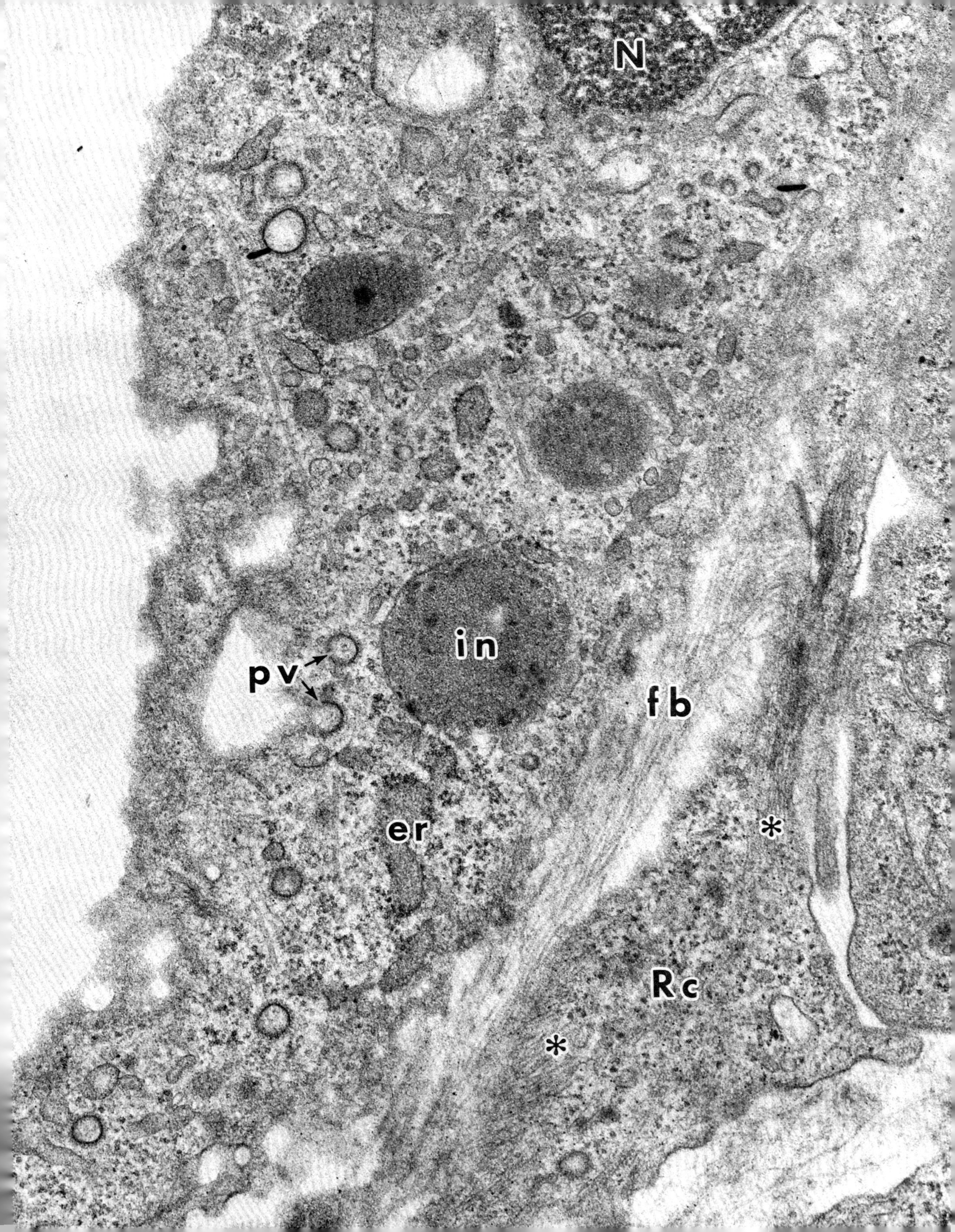
N
in
pv
fb
er
*
Rc
*

bone marrow. All blood is drained by veins which connect with the outside venous circulation.

Sinuses are completely covered by a layer of endothelium; however, the space between sinuses contains many free myeloid elements. Intersinusoidal spaces are formed mainly by the framework of interstitial elements, which include elongated macrophages. Extracellular fibrils are noted only around the large vessels, endothelial cells of sinuses, and the fat cells. These are the essential features of the anatomy of the bone marrow and appear to be highly similar in various animal species. Details of each cellular element will be described in the following sections.

VASCULATURE

Until recently, only a few publications were available on the ultrastructure of marrow vasculature (Figs. 7-5 through 7-10). It is difficult to obtain a topographic orientation of the vasculature in situ since marrow structures are concealed in the hard bone, and significant distortion of the delicate structures occurs during preparation for electron microscopy. No topographical orientation is possible on human specimens, since the aspirated or biopsied material consists only of tissue fragments. To obtain better understanding of the bone marrow, we examined rat bone marrows fixed in situ by perfusion technics. This method eliminates the distortion of the anatomy of marrow when it is removed before fixation. The large arteries of the bone marrow do not differ significantly from those observed in other organs. They seem to have a definite internal elastic membrane and outside muscle coating. The arterial wall of medium to small sized vessels consists of elongated cells intermingled with elastic fibrils. Elastic fibrils are observed in the walls of arterioles with luminal diameters of 20μ or less (Fig. 7-5). Arteries of larger size have a few layers of elongated cells. Both elastic fibrils and neighboring cells gradually disappear as the diameter decreases and the vessel becomes a capillary. Small vessels of similar characteristics may be seen in human bone marrows (Fig. 7-6). The ultrastructural anatomy of the junction between capillaries and sinuses is not clearly understood, because anastomosis occurs at the subendosteal regions of bone and the study of these particular areas is not easily made by routine approaches. The anastomosing sinuses form a highly complicated meshwork, with enlarging vessels, until they finally connect with the central vein. The major portion of blood sinuses are the sinus recti. Their relation to the central vein is illustrated in Figure 7-2.

Ultrastructurally, the endothelium of marrow sinuses consists of thin elongated cells which connect by direct cytoplasmic contact (Fig. 7-8*A*, *B*). Usually no gaps are seen between two adjacent cells except for cytoplasmic fenestration in the endothelial cells (Figs. 7-7 and 7-8*B*). There is no significant variation in morphology of endothelial cell connections, regardless of the location of the sinuses. This is also true for the morphology of the central vein

FIGURE 7-10. Lining cells of central vein of rat bone marrow.
Lumen has an endothelial cell (*En*) on its inner surface, followed by alternate layers of amorphous material (*asterisks*), perivascular cell (*Pv*) or other perivascular cell cytoplasm. There are many small bundles of fibrils (*arrow*). × *22,200.*

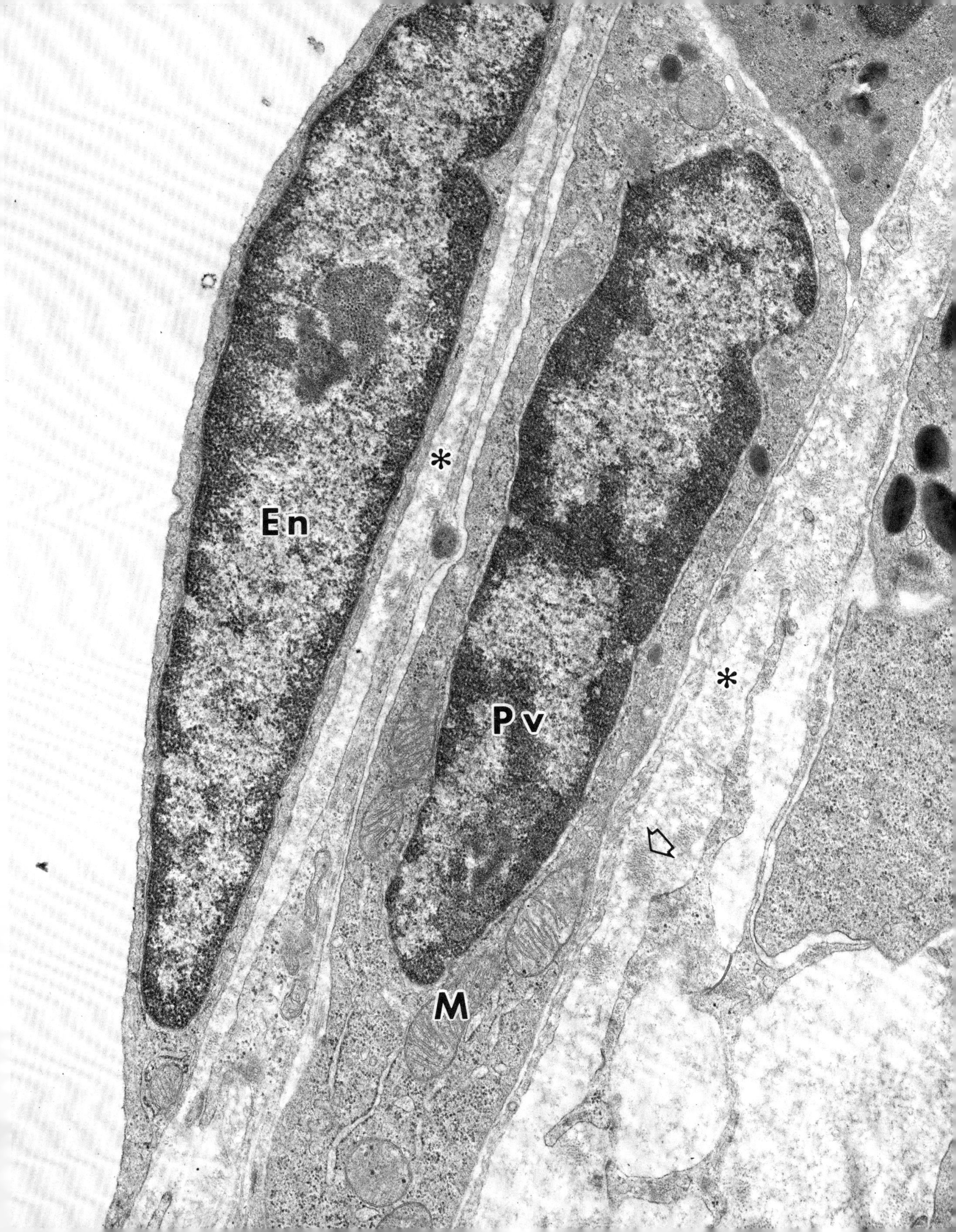

*
En
Pv
*
M

(Fig. 7-10), outside of which only a few extra cell layers are observed. This is a variation of the observation made on human bone marrow, in which dissociation of endothelial lining is reported to be common (Tanaka, 1969) (Fig. 7-8*C*). Endothelial lining cells are believed to remove foreign particles from the circulation, although the macrophages in the stromal spaces are much more active in phagocytosis of degenerating myeloid and erythroid cells.

Ultrastructural findings in marrow sinuses are somewhat controversial. Reports by Weiss (1961, 1965) claimed that no real endothelial cell was present on the sinus wall and that the cells covering sinuses were actually reticulum cells. This is in agreement with the conclusion of Fresen (1960, 1964) who also regarded sinus endothelium as consisting of reticulum cells. On the other hand, Zamboni and Pease (1961) considered the lining cells of the sinuses to be only endothelial cells with no reticulum cells present. Watanabe (1966) stated that the wall of the bone marrow sinuses consisted of a monolayer of endothelial cells supported by reticulum cells. This reaffirmed the classic view of bone marrow anatomy and our own observations (Tanaka, 1969).

Nerve tissues are observed rarely in bone marrow; however, nerves of both myelinated and unmyelinated types are distributed throughout the bone marrow along the blood vessels (Brånemark, 1968; Calvo, 1968). Small nerve fibers are seen near the arterial walls (Fig. 7-5), but it is not known how these fibrils are distributed or how they terminate.

RETICULUM CELLS

A sponge-like frame of cells in bone marrow is formed mainly by interstitial cells categorized vaguely as reticulum cells and constitutes the basic architecture of the marrow intersinuosoidal spaces in numerous species of animals. These interstitial elements may be classified into two major groups, phagocytic and nonphagocytic types (Tanaka, 1969), and have been recognized histologically for many years.

The morphology of the nonphagocytic cells has not been clearly defined, but the cells are generally considered to have an oval, vesicular nucleus and scant cytoplasm, with or without syncytial forms. These elements are regarded as immature compartments of bone marrow whose role is to generate blood cells (Maximow, 1927). Electron microscopically, cells of nonphagocytic type can be divided into two subtypes by their morphology: cells with intracytoplasmic fibrils, and cells with an immature appearance of both nucleus and cytoplasm (Tanaka, 1969). The first group conforms to the classic morphology of nonphagocytic reticulum cells described elsewhere.

Nonphagocytic cells with intracytoplasmic fibrils can be clearly distinguished from macrophages and immature cells in human bone marrow (Tanaka, 1969). They are often present around the sinus walls, as if they were a lining layer

(text continues on page 354)

FIGURE 7-11. Nonphagocytic reticulum cell with intracytoplasmic fibrils.
Nonphagocytic reticulum cell (*center*) has a large vesicular nucleus (*N*), a prominent nucleolus (*Nu*), many large mitochondria (*M*), and both smooth and rough endoplasmic reticulum. Golgi area (*G*) is just above the nucleus. There are very fine fibrils loosely scattered in cytoplasm, with concentrations near the cell surface (*arrows*). The lumen of the sinus (*S*) contains plasma protein with a thin sheet of endothelial cell (*En*) cytoplasm, followed by some amorphous material and part of a mast cell (*Mc*). × *9,300.*

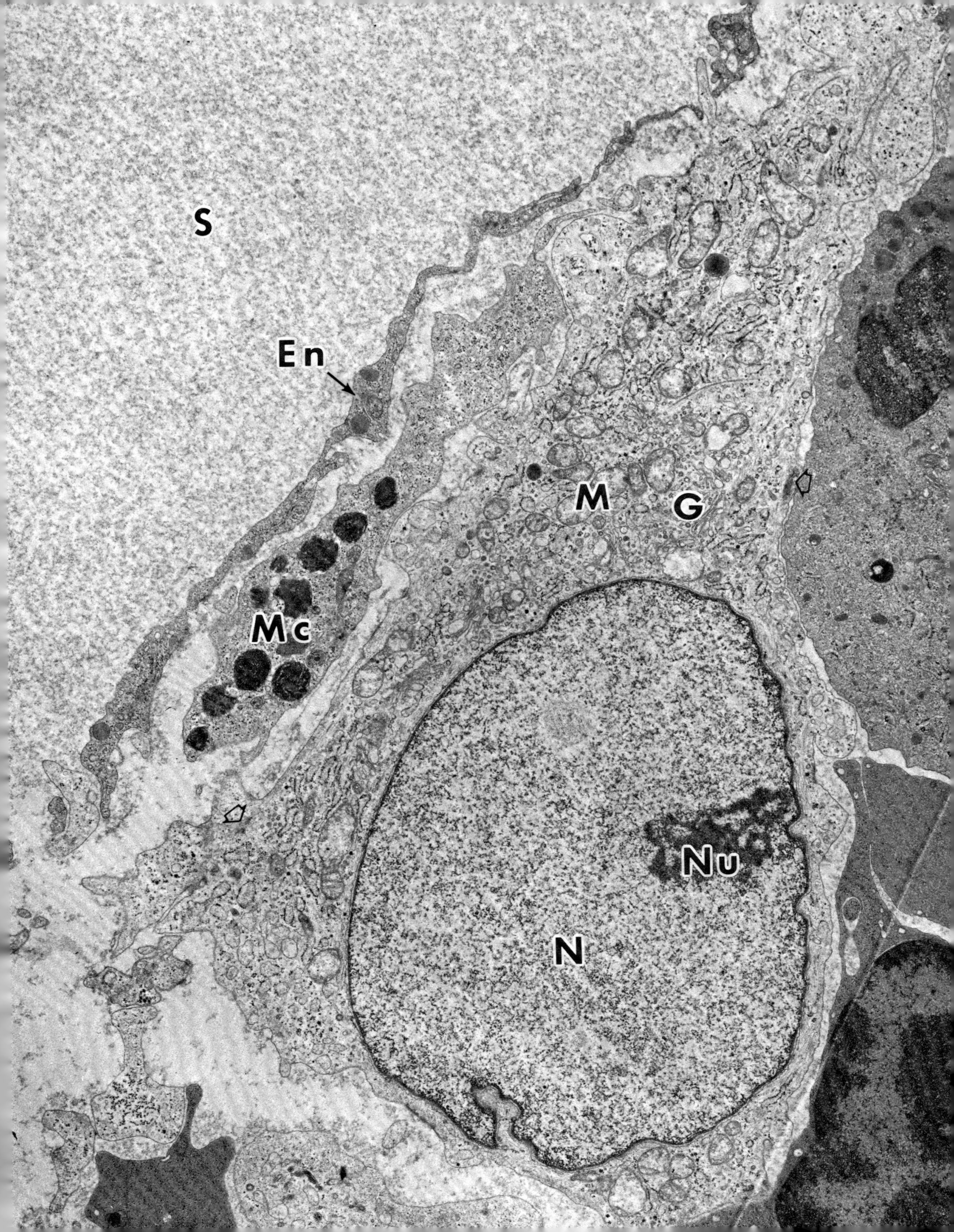
S
En
M
G
Mc
Nu
N

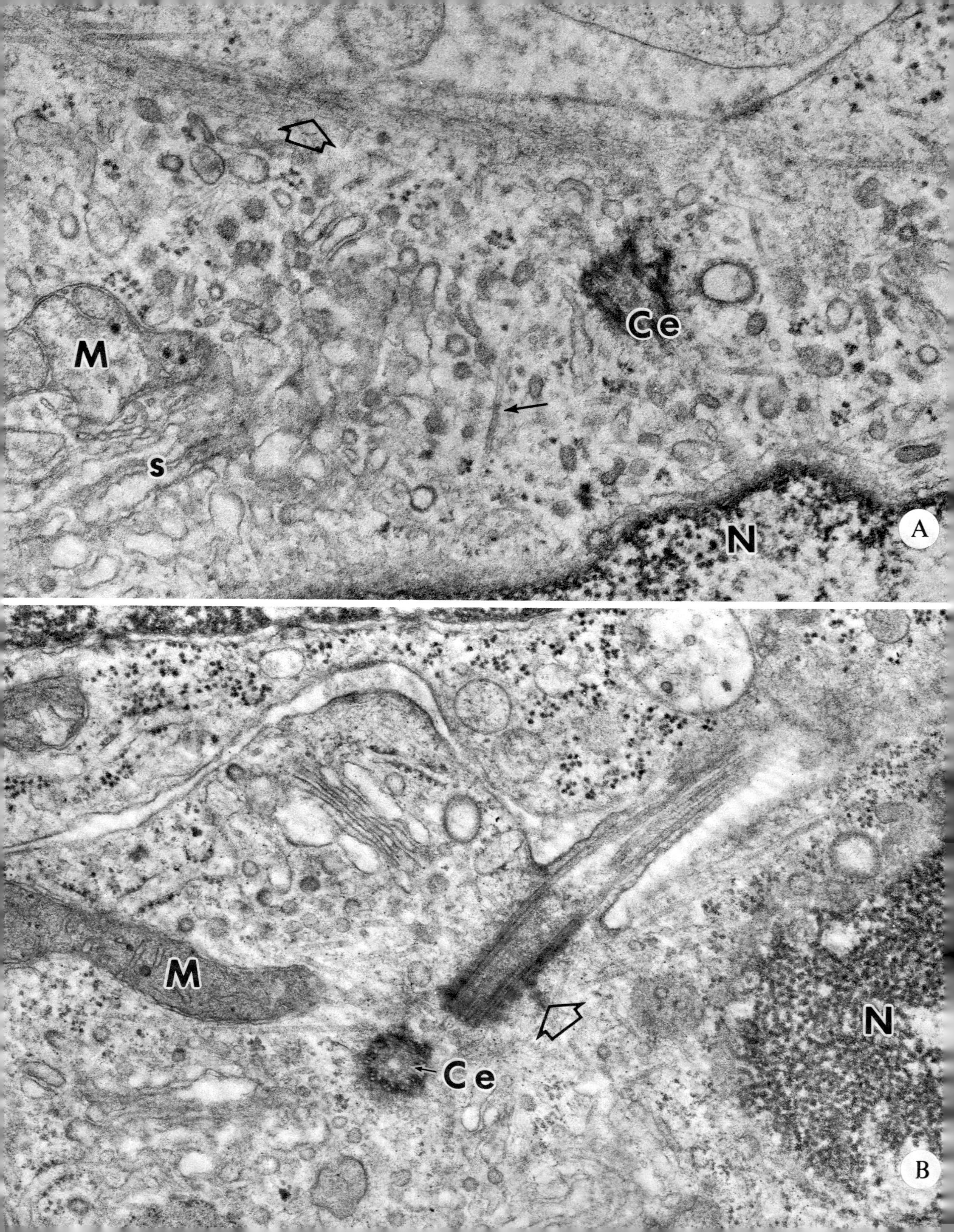
Ce
M
S
N
A
M
Ce
N
B

FIGURE 7-12. Nonphagocytic reticulum cell with intracytoplasmic fibrils.
A. Group of fine fibrils (*open arrow*), a few characteristic tubular filaments (*small arrow*), edge of the nucleus (*N*), saccules (*s*) of the Golgi complex and a centriole (*Ce*) are present. × *44,000.*
B. Bottom of cilia and its intracellular base structure (*arrow*). Note well-developed Golgi and centriole (*Ce*). An elongated mitochondrion (*M*) and a portion of the nucleus (*N*) are present. × *44,000.*

Figures 7-13 and 7-14 appear on the following pages

FIGURE 7-13. Nonphagocytic reticulum cell with intracytoplasmic fibrils.
Reticulum cell of the endothelial lining in human marrow shows fine fibrils (*open arrow*) near cell surface and scattered individual forms dispersed among endoplasmic reticulum (*er*) and mitochondria (*M*). Portion of the nucleus is at the bottom. × *60,000.*

FIGURE 7-14. Nonphagocytic reticulum cell of rat, with intracytoplasmic fibrils.
Reticulum cell (*Rc*) of rat marrow, directly beneath endothelial (*En*) cell, closely resembles the cell type in human marrow. There are a few fibrils (*open arrow*) in the intercellular space and in the cytoplasm (*arrow*). A few inclusions with ferritin particles (*f*) are also seen. × *19,000.*

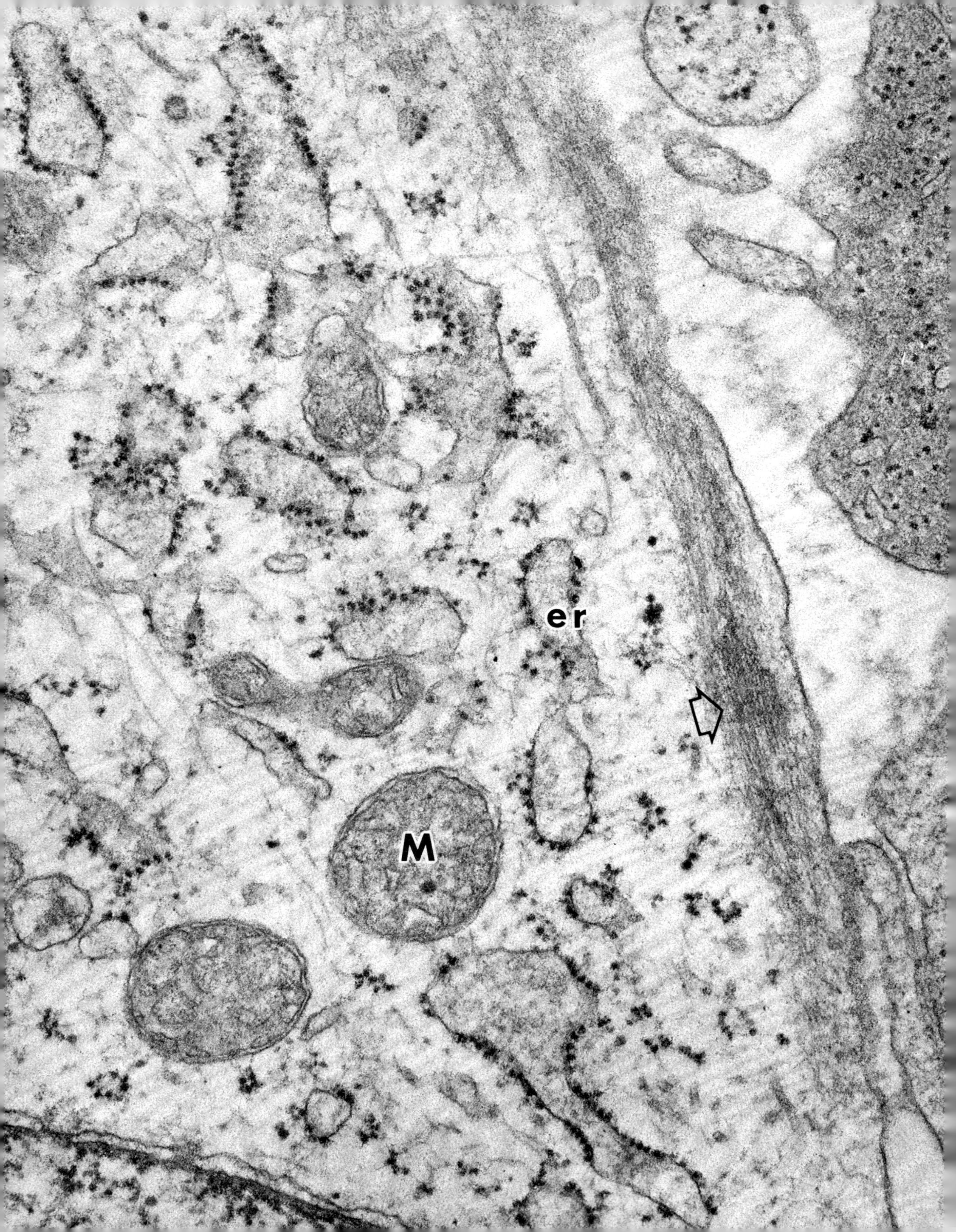

er
M

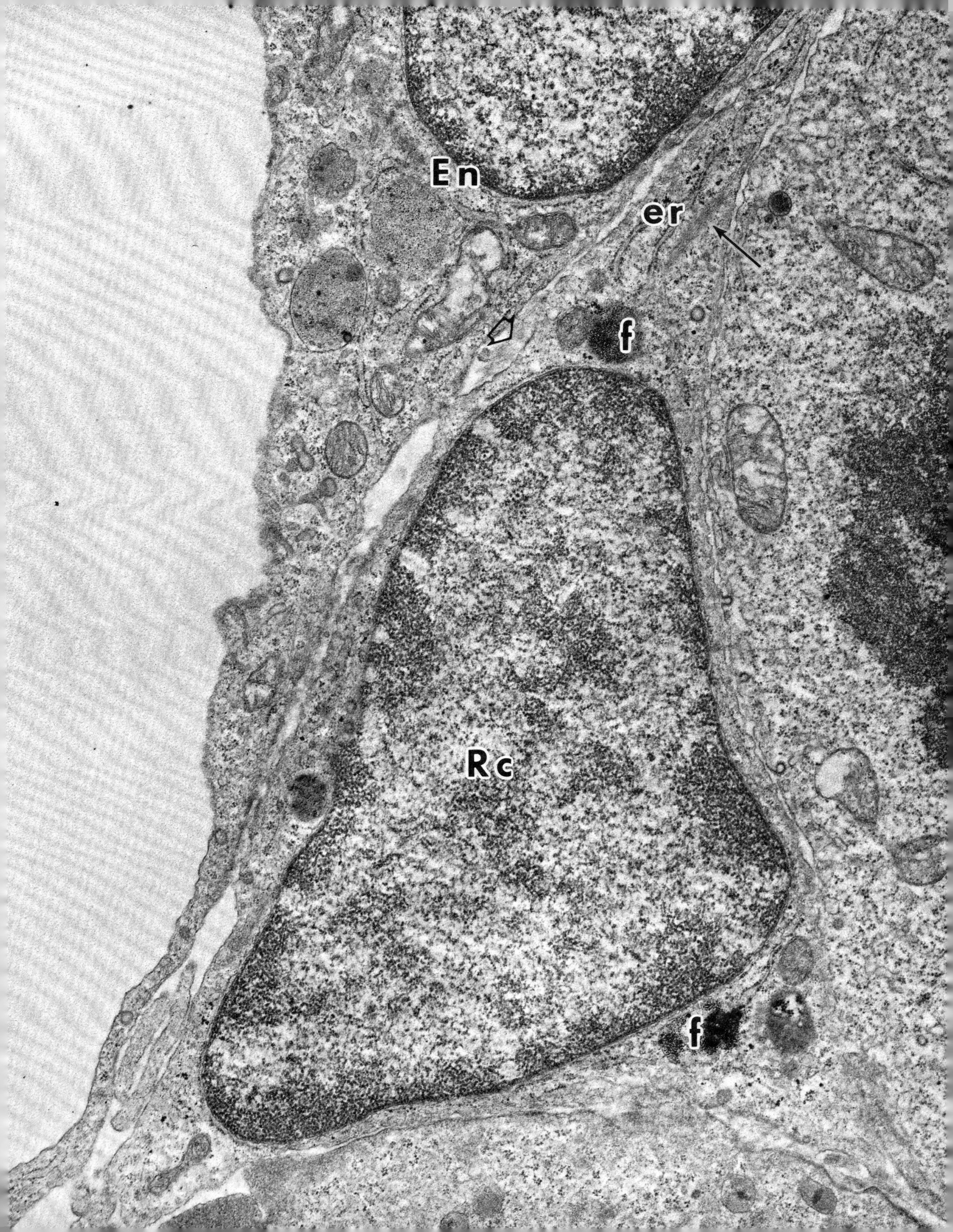
En
er
f
Rc
f

supporting the surface endothelial cells (Fig. 7-11), and they communicate with other interstitial elements, such as another nonphagocytic cell with intracytoplasmic fibrils, elongated macrophages, and fat cells, to form the structure of intersinusoidal spaces. An association of extracellular substances, fibrillar (Fig. 7-9) or afibrillar, may also be seen. These nonphagocytic cells possess a large nucleus with fine chromatin pattern which creates a vesicular appearance of the nucleus by light microscopy. A nucleolus is usually observed. The elongated cytoplasm contains many vesicular elements and moderate amounts of endoplasmic reticulum (Figs. 7-11, 7-12*A*, and 7-13). Filamentous structures, both fine fibrillar and tubular forms, are common (Figs. 7-11, 7-12*A*, and 7-13). Electron-opaque condensations of finer fibrils may be noted near the plasma membrane (Tanaka, 1964). There is no active phagocytosis, even in lipidoses, in which many phagocytic cells contain various forms of lipid granules. No syncytial forms are noted. In many studies of human marrows which show hyperplasia of free cells, the nonphagocytic cells appear to be unrelated to the hematopoietic activity. Because of the apparent unresponsive feature of these cells, we consider that they are probably important, as the structural architecture of the bone marrow and the presence of fibrils tend to support such an interpretation.

Similar endothelial lining cells have been observed in bone marrow of rats (Fig. 7-14), rabbits, and guinea pigs. Similar cells in rat bone marrow have been described by Ito (1965), who suggested that they may be the immature compartment of bone marrow.

The morphology of lining cells in animals differs slightly from that in humans; a more condensed chromatin pattern and phagocytic material is frequently seen in the former. However, the general characteristics, such as topography and the elongated shape of these cells, are retained in a manner similar to the cells observed in humans. Intracytoplasmic fibrils may be observed around or near the cell membrane and surface cilia (Fig. 7-12*B*) may be associated with either extracellular fibrils or amorphous material.

Immature Cells

Immature cells specific for blood-cell generation have been postulated for many years. However, no one has yet clearly demonstrated their actual morphology. Various experimental approaches have proved that the bone marrow contains a self-maintaining compartment and that migration of cells from other sources into the bone marrow is not required. The morphology of this compartment has been explored in many hematopoietic tissues of both humans and animals. It has been generally accepted that possible parental

FIGURE 7-15. Immature cells with ill-defined or indistinct cell surface seen occasionally in human bone marrow.

A. Nucleus (*N*) contains large nucleolus (*Nu*). No clear membrane is discernible where cytoplasm is in contact with erythroblast (*Eb*) and myelocyte (*My*). Cytoplasm has mitochondria (*M*) and scattered ribosomes. × *16,000.*

B. Reticulum cell with very irregular and partially indistinct surface, has moderate-sized Golgi complex (*G*), numerous small dense mitochondria (*M*), large vesicles (*v*) and practically no polyribosomes. × *12,200.*

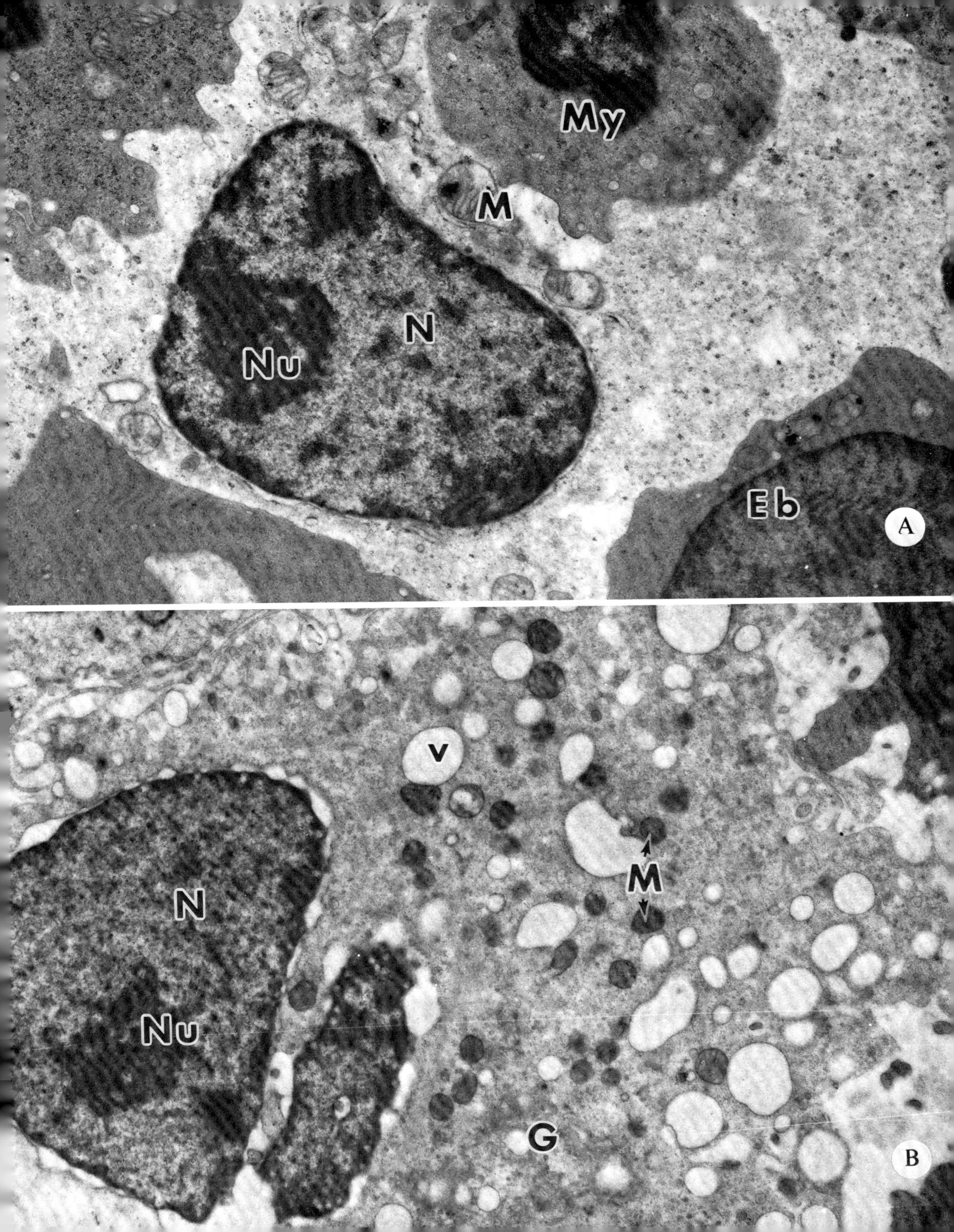
My
M
N
Nu
Eb
A
V
M
N
Nu
G
B

cells could be the elongated mesenchymal cells with nonphagocytic activity (primitive reticulum cells), large lymphoid cells called hemocytoblasts, and mononuclear cells resembling either small lymphocytes or monocytes. In postnatal human bone marrows, the cells of the first two categories are regarded as self-generating elements. Recent cytokinetic studies have led many investigators to favor the conclusion that cells of a free, unattached form may play an important role in marrow hematopoiesis, and the classic view, which stressed the significance of fixed immature elements, is now regarded as less important (Loutit, 1968). Studies of marrow regeneration in rabbits have demonstrated that whole marrow structure can be re-formed after the elimination of all free cells from the bone marrow either by curettage (Steinberg and Hufford, 1947; Mital and Cohen, 1966) or washing. Mechanically damaged rabbit bone marrow can restore structural and hematopoietic compartments from stem cells originally present in the bone marrow. No circulating hemic stem cells appear to be required (Maloney and Patt, 1969). This indicates that the immature cells of fixed type left in the bone marrow re-form and regenerate not only the original architecture of bone marrow but also restore hematopoiesis. These experiments suggest that fixed mesenchymal cells may be more important than free blastic forms for generation of cells in bone marrow. However, Crosby (1970) has reported interdependence of the fixed structural and free blastic cells following x-irradiation. For this reason, we favor the classic view that cytogenesis is dependent on fixed immature cells, until clearer evidence excludes either the fixed or migratory cell systems as the progenitors of bone marrow activity.

Light microscopical morphology of nonphagocytic *blastic mesenchymal* cells has been reported, but there has been no clear delineation on the distribution of the blastic cells or their morphology as they transform to committed blastic forms during differentiation. In a study of large numbers of pathological bone marrows, we noted interstitial cells with distinctive morphology which had not been described previously. On the basis of the pure morphological analysis, these cells might be the immature compartment of adult bone marrows (Tanaka *et al.,* 1966; Tanaka, 1967). Since such elements are not commonly noted in normal subjects, the illustrations used here are from hyperplastic marrows of nonmalignant diseases. The extremely immature forms (Fig. 7-15*A*) appear as cells of interstitial elements which proliferate between free cells. They do not show the clear outer cell membrane usually seen. The extent of the cytoplasm can only be suggested by the presence of polyribosomes in amorphous background material of moderate electron opacity. A lacking or defective cell membrane is unknown. However, this lack of a definitive cell

(*text continues on page 368*)

FIGURE 7-16. Interstitial cells in mitosis.
The cells have distinct cell boundary. Mitosis suggests they may be viable forms rather than degenerating remnants.

A. Chromosomes (*Ch*) are distinct; cytoplasm contains few mitochondria (*M*) or other organelles and few or no ribosomes. An erythroblast (*Eb*) is adjacent. × *17,500.*

B. Several mitotic spindle fibers (*arrows*) are near the chromosomes (Ch). The cell contains a few vesicles and very small dense granules. × *12,800.*

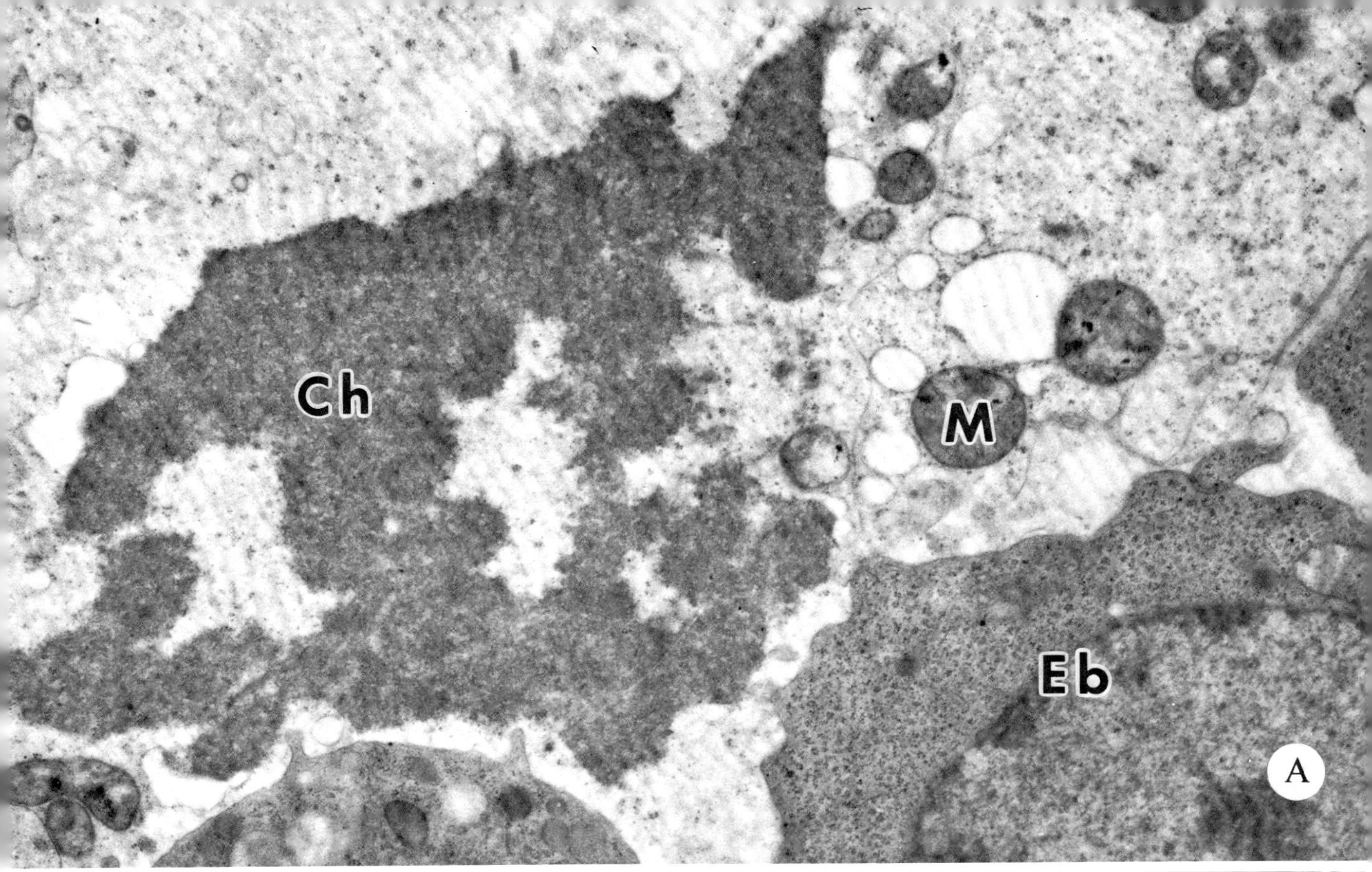
Ch
M
Eb
A

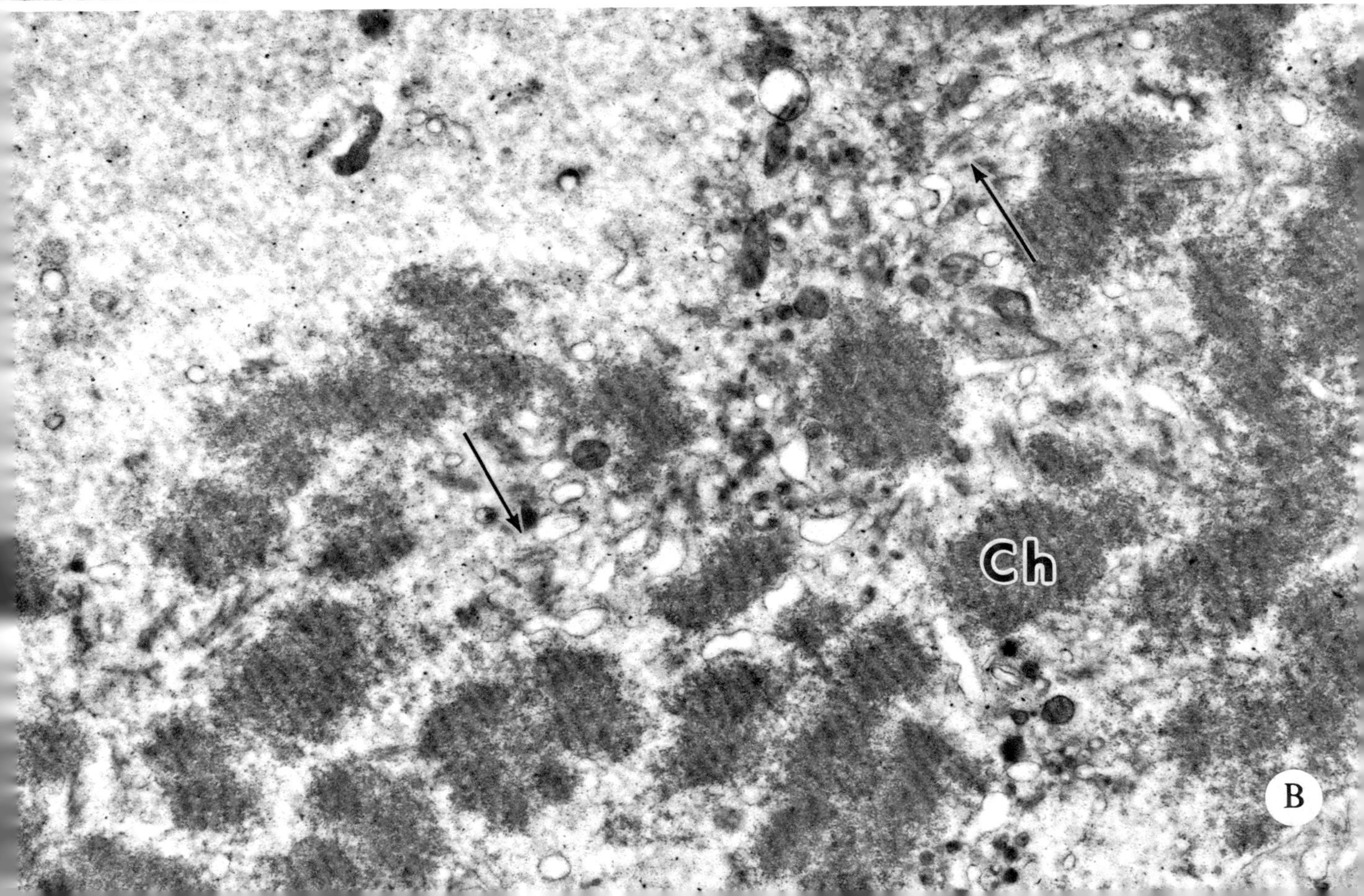
Ch
B

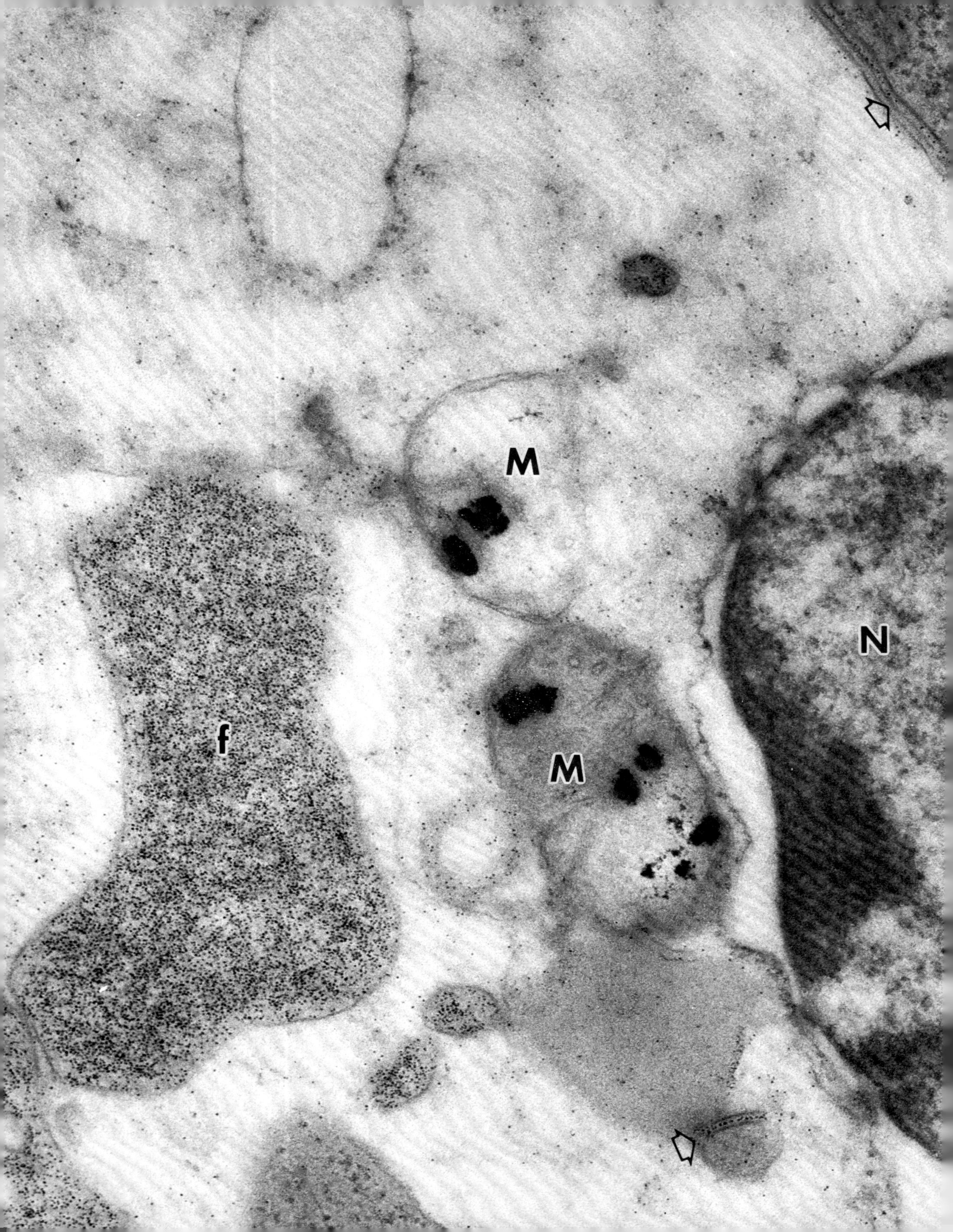
M
N
f
M

FIGURE 7-17. Interstitial cell from marrow of siderotic patient.
Interstitial cell, with indistinct boundary, has accumulation of iron in mitochondria (*M*), scattered in the cytoplasm, and in the intercellular spaces (*arrows*). The ferritin provides a marker for an apparent deep membrane fold. Lack of cytoplasmic ribosomes and the delicate nature of cytoplasmic surface are apparent adjacent to the nucleus (*N*). Part of an adjacent machophage is filled with ferritin (*f*). × *66,500.*

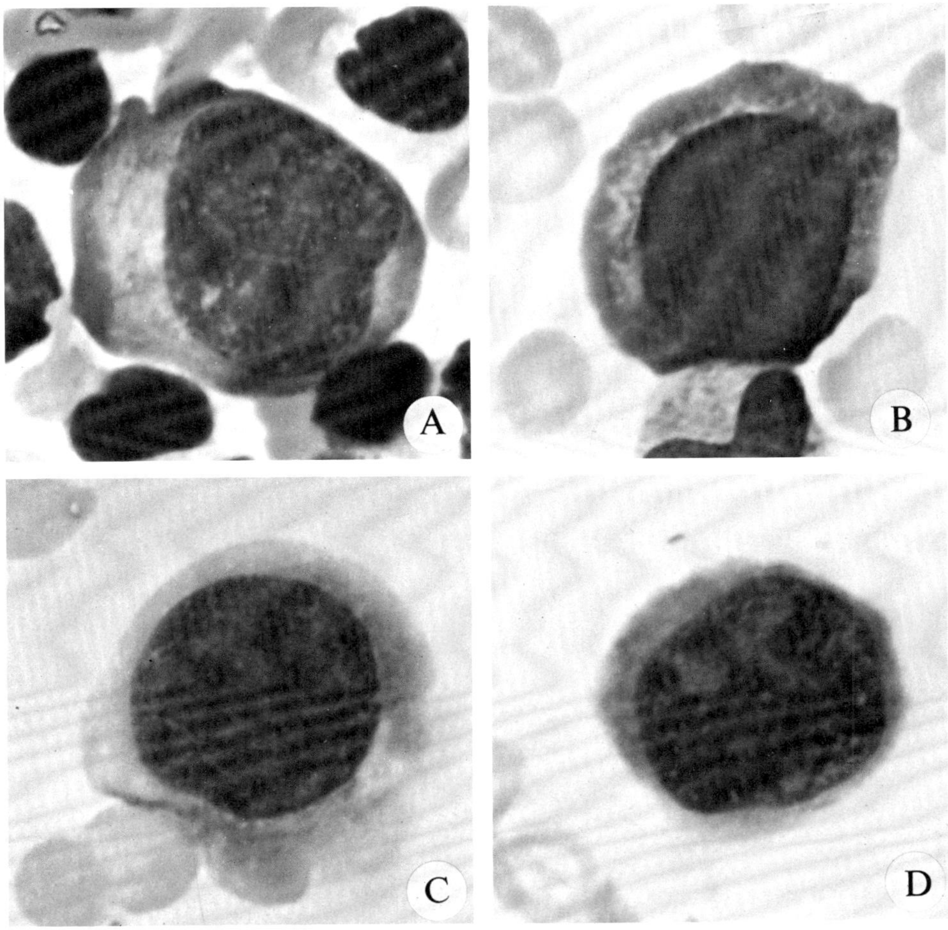

FIGURE 7-18. Immature round cells in human bone marrow.
These cells might be classified as immature forms of committed cell line—i.e., proerythroblast (**A,B**) or myeloblast (**C,D**). However, they may correspond to very immature cells which are uncommitted (see Figures 7-20 through 7-26). × *2,000.*

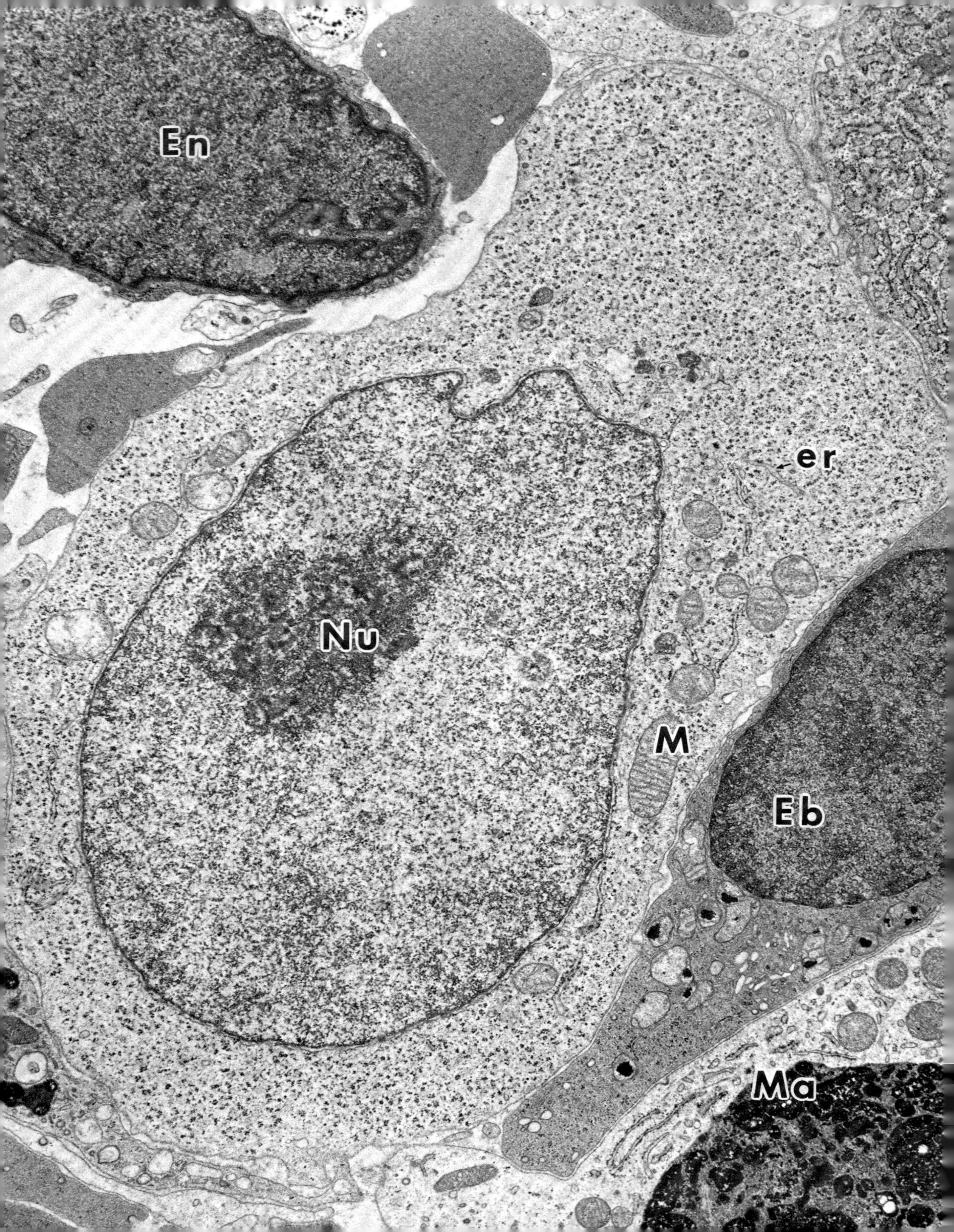
En
er
Nu
M
Eb
Ma

FIGURE 7-19. Immature cell from hyperplastic human bone marrow.
This immature cell has a distinct cell surface and abundant polyribosomes. It appears more immature than either a proerythroblast or myeloblast (Chaps. 2 and 3), as the nuclear chromatin is widely diffused and there is a large distinct nucleolus (*Nu*), a number of large mitochondria (*M*), a small amount of endoplasmic reticulum (*er*), and no apparent Golgi apparatus. This cell has the general appearance of lymph node hemocytoblasts. An erythroblast (*Eb*) with iron-containing mitochondria, a macrophage (*Ma*), and an endothelial cell (*En*) are also present. × *11,000.*

Figures 7-20 and 7-21 appear on the following pages ⇨

FIGURE 7-20. Immature cell from hyperplastic marrow.
This is the same cell as that in Figure 7-19, showing cytoplasmic details. There are many polyribosomes (*r*) and very little background material. The few vesicles near the nucleus (*N*) cannot be classified. × *48,000.*

FIGURE 7-21. Mononuclear cells with very immature characteristics.
A. Cell boundary (*arrow*) is delicate, cytoplasm has very few organelles, and nucleus contains scattered chromatin, numerous small dense aggregates, and a distinctive nucleolus (*Nu*). × *10,000.*
B. Cell boundary is more definite, and cytoplasm contains several mitochondria (*M*), Golgi vesicles (G) and granules. Nucleus has granular chromatin and large nucleolus (*Nu*). × *9,500.*
C. Mononuclear cell resembles that shown in Figure 7-19 but is smaller, with finely granular nucleus (*N*) and essentially only mitochondria (*M*) for cytoplasmic organelles. × *12,000.*
D. Narrow rim of fat cell (*Fc*) cytoplasm (*open arrow*) is adjacent to the fat body. There is only a small portion of thin cytoplasm of the immature mononuclear cell (*arrow*). × *14,000.*

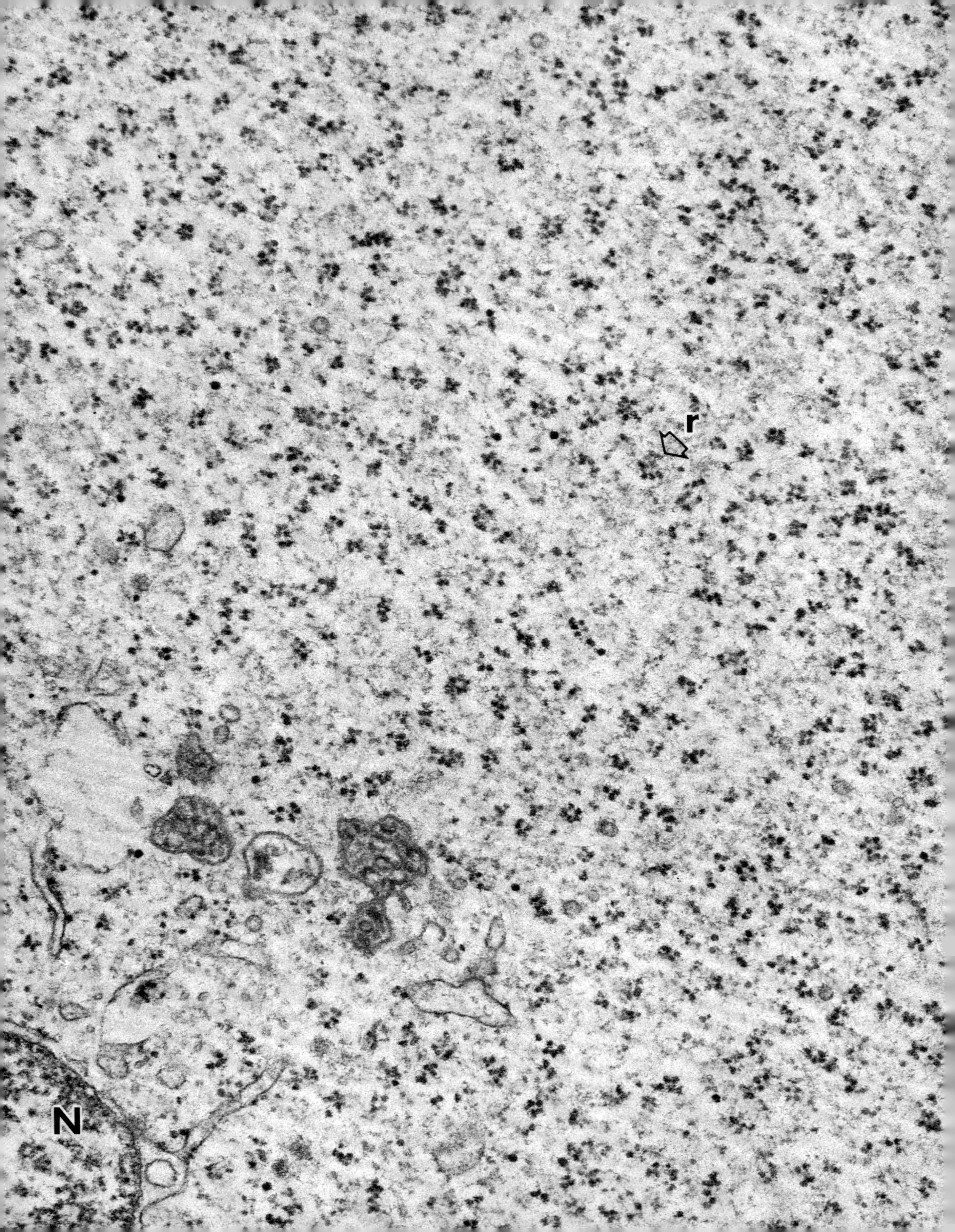
r
N

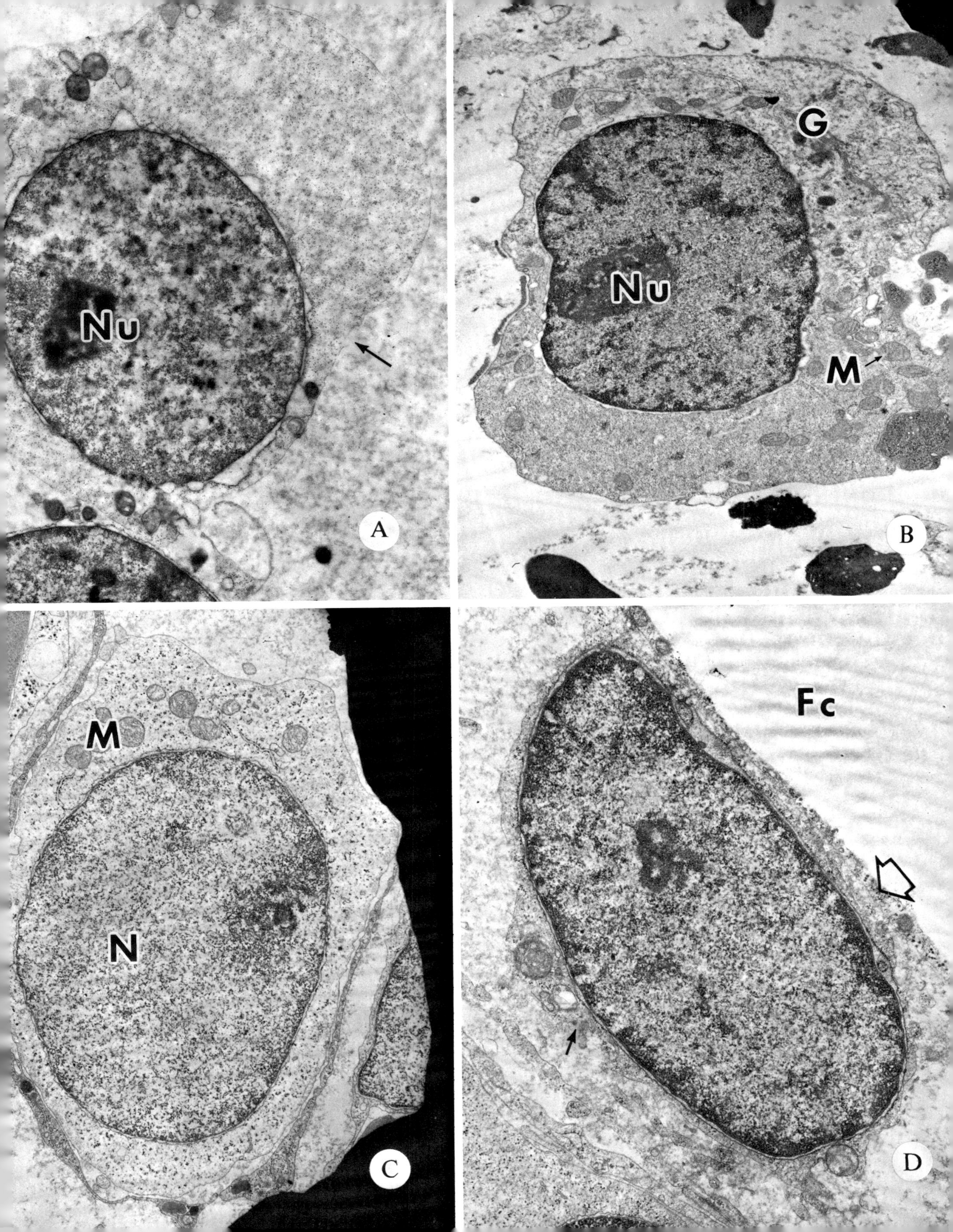
Nu
A
G
Nu
M
B
M
N
C
Fc
D

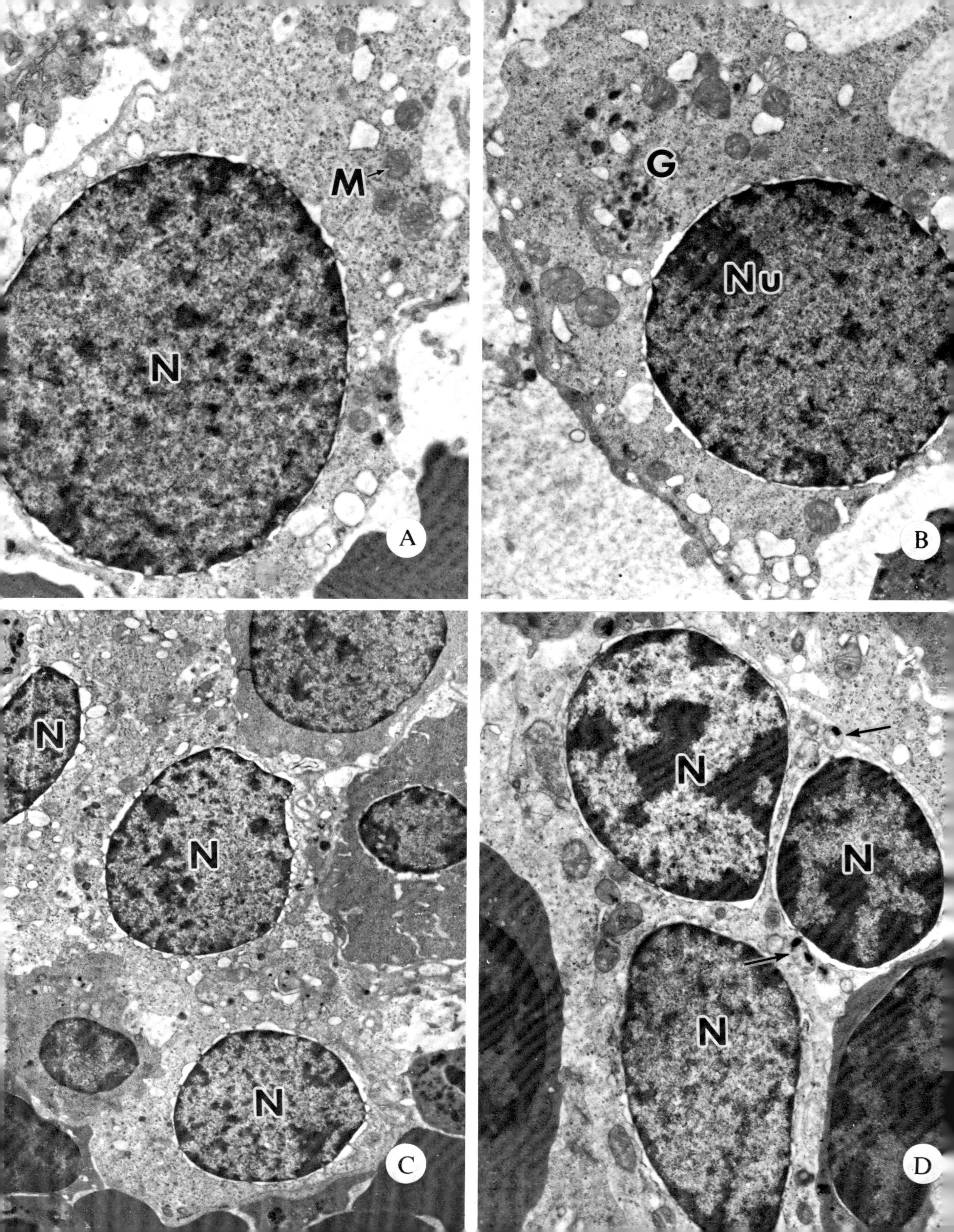
M
N
A
G
Nu
B
N
N
N
C
N
N
N
D

FIGURE 7-22. Immature cells, with many ribosomes and definite boundary, which may be erythroid precursors.

A. Chromatin in eccentrically located nucleus (*N*) has a reticular distribution. Cytoplasm contains a few large round mitochondria (M), vacuoles, and many polyribosomes. × *9,700.*

Reprinted with permission from Tanaka, Y., Brecher, G., and Bull, B. *Blood 28*: 758, 1966.

B. Cell similar to one in Figure 7-22**A** also has a nucleolus (*Nu*) and Golgi area (*G*) containing some granules. × *9,000.*

C. In marrow from patient with sideroblastic anemia, there is either one cell whose cytoplasm contains three nuclei (*N*) and appears to be continuous or there are three cells with indistinct boundaries. Bottom cell appears to be a very early erythroblast, but the cytoplasm is still apparently contiguous with that of the other cells. × *5,000.*

D. Three nuclei seem to share a common cytoplasm with immature characteristics. The cytoplasmic nuclear contact is loose, compared with that of two erythroblasts, and the chromatin in two nuclei has started to condense and marginate. The presence of iron in the mitochondria (*arrows*) suggests that these may be early erythroid cells. × *10,000.*

Figures 7-23 and 7-24 appear on the following pages ⇨

FIGURE 7-23. Immature cells from human marrow.
Rounded immature cells are adjacent to thin rim (*arrow*) of fat cell cytoplasm (*Fc*). Chromatin is finely dispersed in nuclei (*N*), one of which shows a nucleolus (*Nu*). Cytoplasm has many polyribosomes and numerous large mitochondria (*M*), many of which are on the opposite side of the cell from the Golgi apparatus (*G*) in the central cell. This cell might be precursor of either myeloid or erythroid cell lines. × *12,600.*

FIGURE 7-24. Immature cells from human marrow.
Two immature cells resemble hemocytoblasts of lymph nodes (similar to cells shown in Figure 7-23). Nucleus (*N*) contains finely dispersed chromatin in one; the other has a very prominent nucleolus (*Nu*). A portion of a plasma cell (*Pc*) is at bottom, and a macrophage (*Ma*) at upper right. × *9,000.*

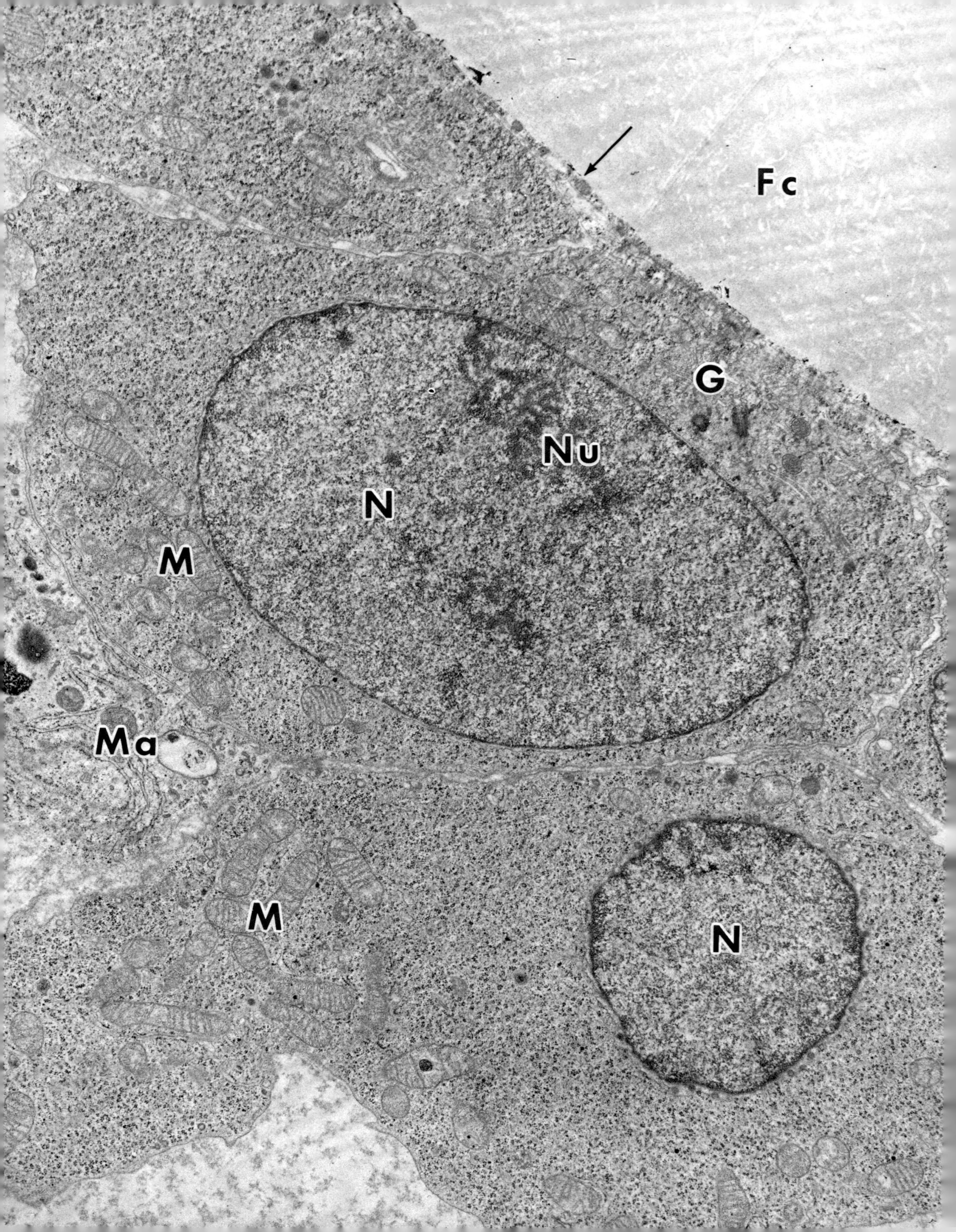
Fc
G
Nu
N
M
Ma
M
N

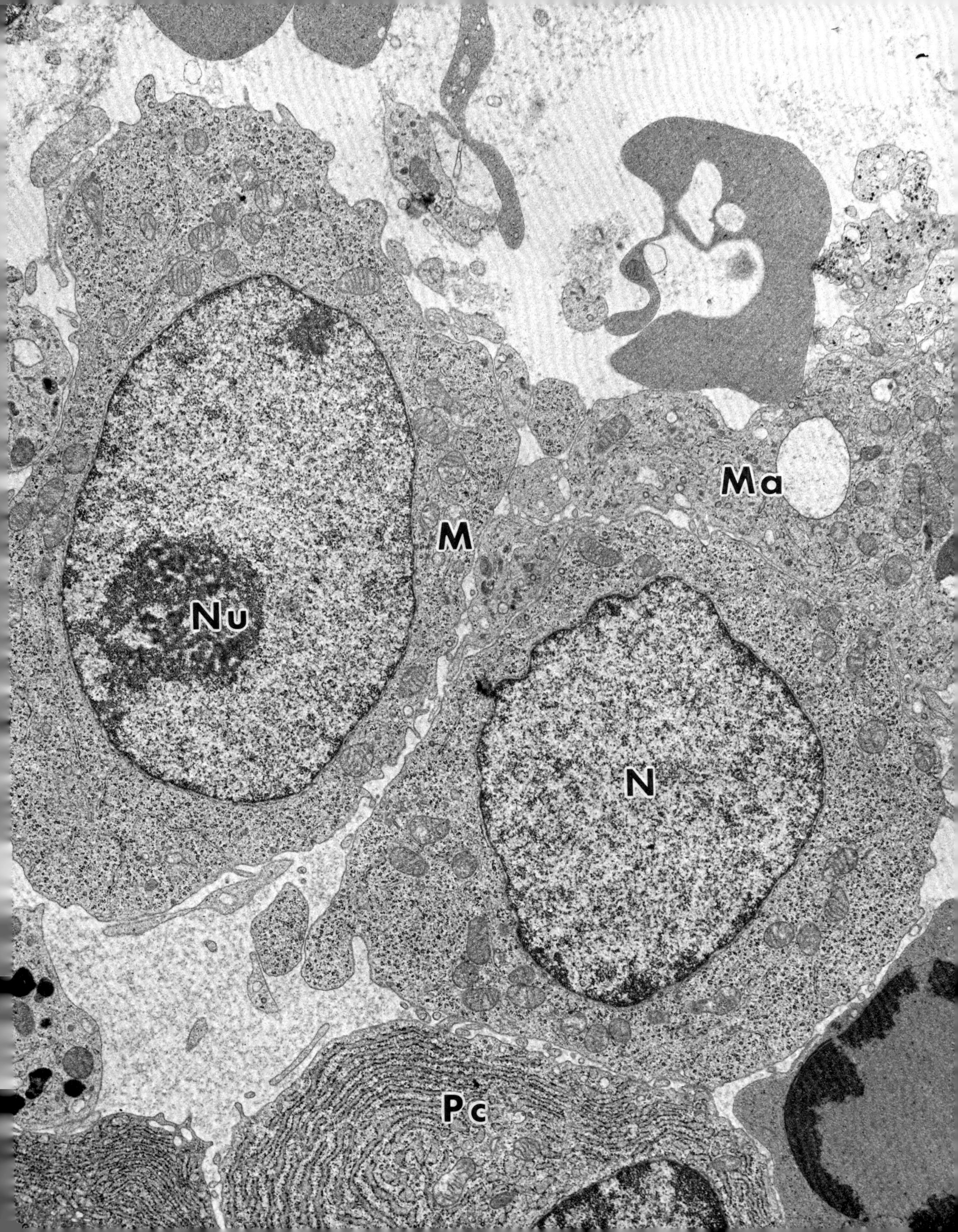
Ma
M
Nu
N
Pc

boundary is observed in various forms of mesenchymal elements, including reticulum cells of lymph nodes, fibroblasts, and osteochondroblasts of bone. Thus we speculate that this feature may be related to the specific nature of the plasma membrane of these cells (Tanaka, 1967). Mitoses of these cells can be seen (Fig. 7-16), where a few cytoplasmic organelles are noted around the nucleus. Also, iron deposition may be seen in hypersiderotic conditions within the mitochondria of these cells (Fig. 7-15*A*).

Cells with similar characteristics but with partially intact cell membrane have also been observed (Fig. 7-15*B*). These cells are usually large, have an oval nucleus, and are ameboid in general appearance. A nucleolus is present occasionally. They measure more than 20μ on their longest axis. The cell membrane, when present, is usually enfolded and highly irregular, and there may be more than one nucleus in the same cytoplasm (Fig. 7-22*D*). The mitochondria are distributed randomly and may contain iron (Fig. 7-17). This may also occur extracellularly, as in siderotic bone marrows. Search for similar cells with intact cell membranes reveals the presence of such cells in some bone marrows. Such elements have been found, as shown in Figures 7-18 through 7-24. These cells do not resemble any known committed blastic forms of either myeloid elements or small lymphocytes. A diffuse chromatin pattern in the nucleus is typical of these immature cells. All their cytoplasmic features are extremely immature and resemble those hemocytoblasts in lymph nodes. The rounded cells are seen in various conditions, in contrast to the extreme rarity of the diffusely extended type; they are associated with other supporting cells of the intersinusoidal spaces, particularly fat cells. Rarely, the cells with distinctive cell membranes are closely associated with the diffuse mesenchymal elements, a relationship suggesting that they are originating from them (Fig. 7-22*C*). However, the interpretation needs verification, with additional examples from human marrows.

Hyperplasia of immature cells achieved experimentally in animals by the administration of hemolytic agents, shows proliferation of large (up to 30μ) mononuclear cells with polyribosomes (Fig. 7-25). The size of these mononuclear cells and their lack of any cytoplasmic organelles other than mitochondria easily distinguish them from immature erythroblasts and myeloblasts. Search for various intermediate forms which resemble the committed blastic cells of each line reveals the presence of transitional cells for erythroblasts, myelocytes, and megakaryocytes, as well as lymphoid forms and immature interstitial elements. The significance of the latter two forms in cell-generation activity is far from conclusive. Experimentally induced hyperplastic animal marrows, fixed by perfusion, did not provide examples of the diffuse mesenchymal proliferation which appeared to be present in a few cases of hyperplastic erythroid human marrows.

Hyperplastic bone marrows of man have *interstitial cells* with cytoplasmic characteristics other than those previ-

(*text continues on page 374*)

FIGURE 7-25. Large immature cell from rat marrow.
This cell, adjacent to sinusoid (*S*), is comparable to human cell in Figure 7-19. A large nucleolus (*Nu*) is in the vesicular nucleus, with innumerable polyribosomes and large mitochondria (*M*). Note adjacent erythroid cells, endothelial cell (*En*), and neutrophil (*Ne*). × *14,000.*

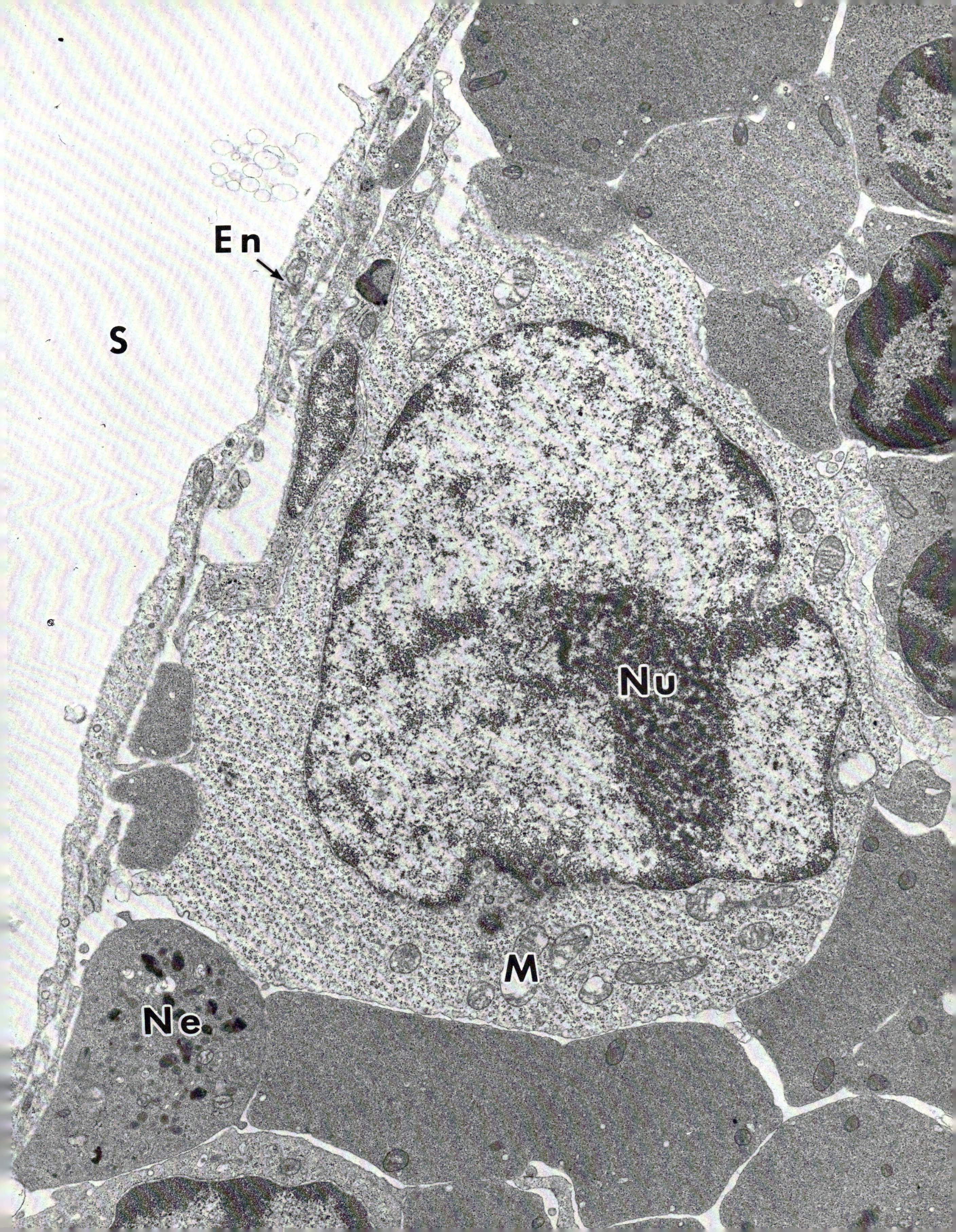

En
S
Nu
M
Ne

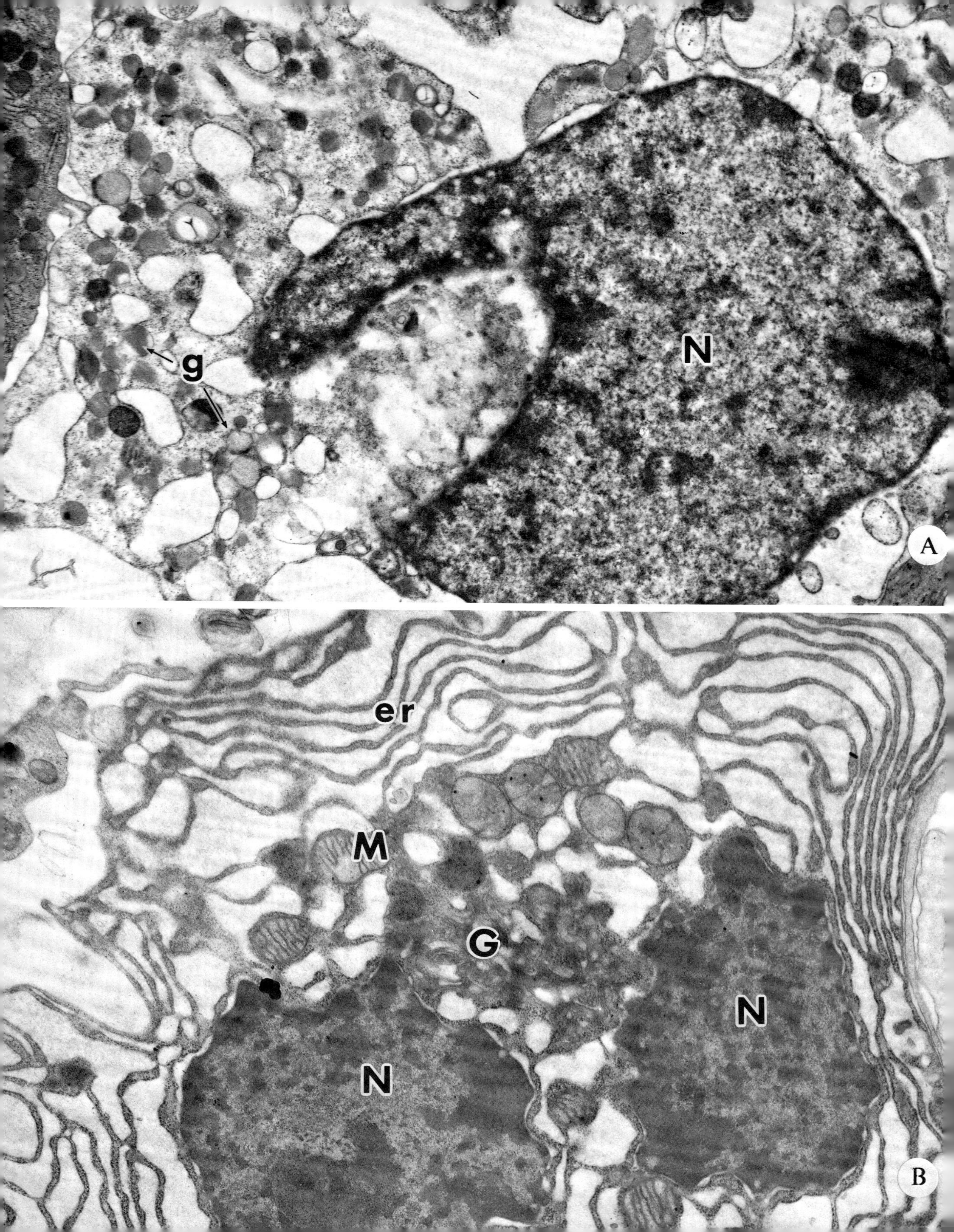
g
N
A
er
M
G
N
N
B

FIGURE 7-26. Nonphagocytic interstitial cells from human marrow.
A. Vacuolated cytoplasm contains numerous granules (*g*) and reticular distribution of chromatin in an irregularly shaped nucleus (*N*). × *15,500.*
B. Cell with two nuclei (*N*), Golgi complex (*G*), mitochondria (*M*), and distended endoplasmic reticulum (*er*) filled with light amorphous material is indistinguishable from atypical plasma cell except for its highly irregular cell boundary. × *13,200.*

Figures 7-27 and 7-28 appear on the following pages

FIGURE 7-27. Macrophage (phagocytic reticulum cell).
The cytoplasm has numerous digestive vesicles containing ingested material, large mitochondria (*M*) and scattered endoplasmic reticulum. A portion of the nucleus (*N*) is at lower left. × *28,000.*

FIGURE 7-28. Macrophages (phagocytic reticulum cells).
A. Macrophage from patient with hemolytic anemia has several ingested erythroid fragments (*asterisks*). × *15,000.*
B. Macrophage from patient with lipidosis contains at least two partly degraded ingested myelocytes (*My*). × *18,400.*

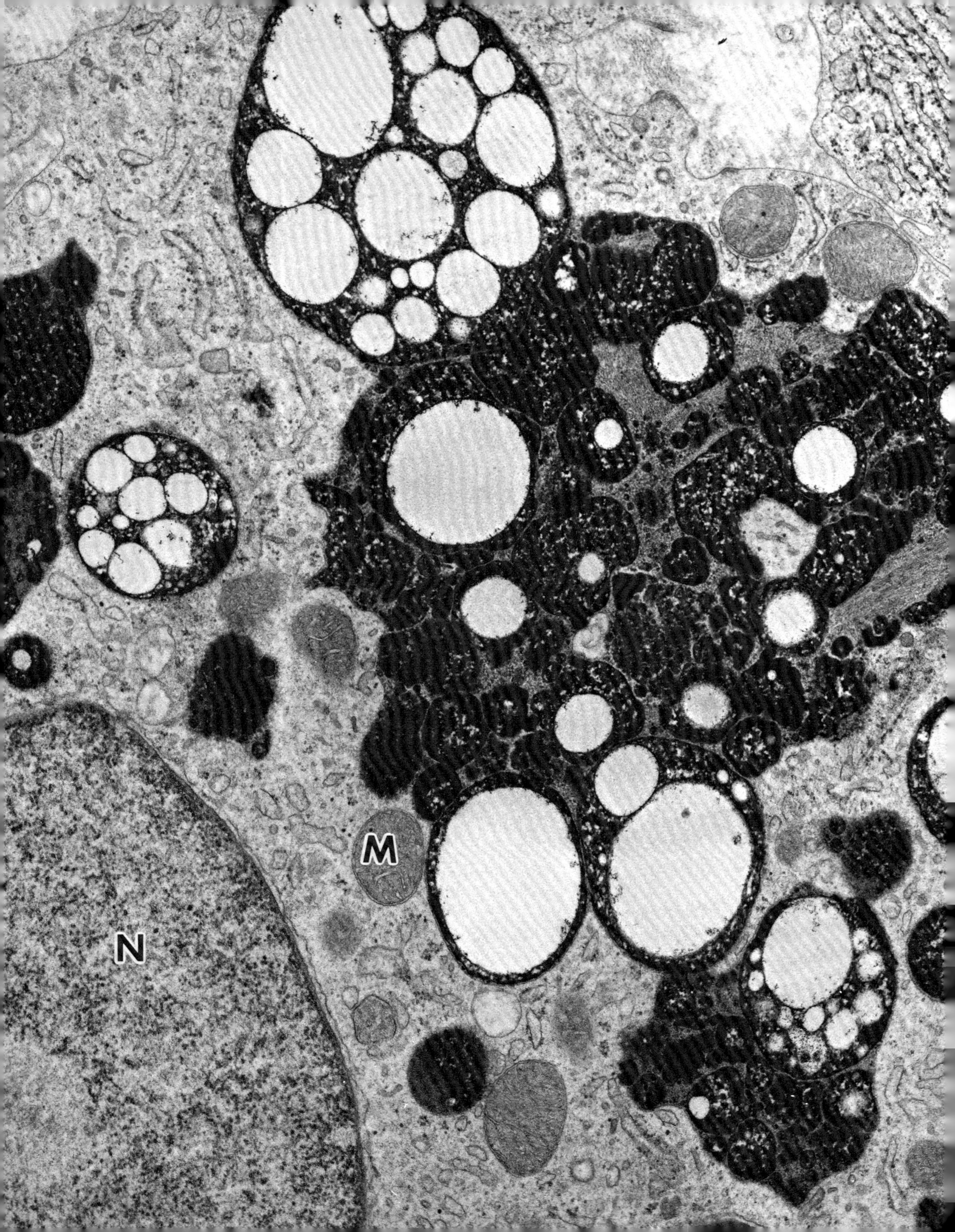
M
N

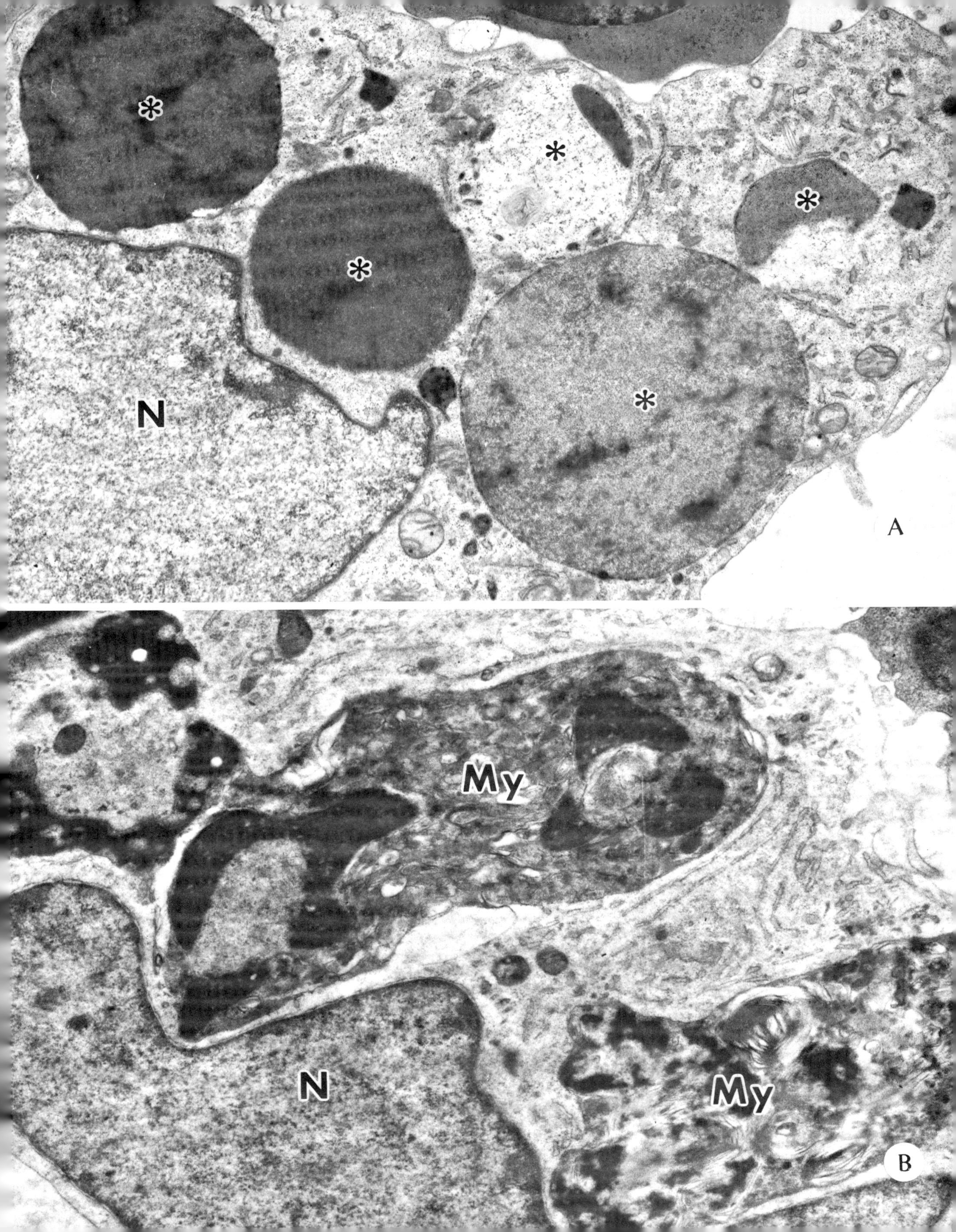
N
A
My
N
My
B

ously mentioned; one frequently seen is a cell with cytoplasmic granules. The presence of such granulated cells was reported (Franco and Ferrata, 1919; Ferrata, 1921), but their identity was not established, since cells with a similar appearance were found to contain artifacts produced during the preparation of smears (Ringeon, 1924, 1925; Lambin, 1927). We observed, with the electron microscope, interstitial cells with granulation in human bone marrows. These elements were distinguishable from granulated myelocytes and were not believed to be formed by artifacts (Fig. 7-26*A*). The significance of these cells is not known, nor has their contribution to the myelocyte generation been established.

One other common form is the cell with extensive endoplasmic reticulum (Fig. 7-26*B*). Sometimes differentiation of the endoplasmic reticulum is so developed in these cells that they are difficult to distinguish from plasma cells. Amano and Tanaka (1956) studied the concept of marrow perivascular mesenchyma as a progenitor of plasma cells, a role which has been accepted by many investigators for other tissues. Though the perivascular localization of the mature plasma cells may be seen in the bone marrow (see Chap. 6), such a relationship is not clearly established. The possibility that they contribute to plasmacytogenesis in human bone marrow has not been excluded (Rohr, 1960).

MACROPHANGES

Cells with signs of active phagocytosis are observed commonly in the interstitial space of bone marrow (Hudson and Yoffey, 1963, 1968), and can be identified easily by the variety of phagocytized material in the cytoplasm (Figs. 7-27 through 7-29). They are usually elongated and possess large amounts of cytoplasm which may have very extensive thin strips reaching between other cells (see Fig. 2-1). These cells are considered as fixed and are among the important members of the cellular reticulum. Macrophages contain many vesicular elements, and large amounts of phagocytized material (Fig. 7-27) originating from degenerated erythroid cells (Fig. 7-28*A*), granulocytes (Fig. 7-28*B*), and foreign substances. The condition of the patient determines the pleomorphic appearance of these cells and the grade of phagocytotic activity. A large amount of iron, either as ferritin (Fig. 7-29) or hemosiderin (Goodman *et al.,* 1968), is a common finding in these cells. Residues in phagocytes frequently appear as myelin figures (Fig. 7-29), which are apparently created by the crystalloid arrangement of lipid-containing material derived from degenerated cells. Many macrophages are noted in bone marrow, particularly in impaired cell generation in some anemias (Goodman *et al.,* 1968). This phenomenon is related to the elimination of degenerating or defective cells which fail to mature.

Hyperplastic bone marrow has interstitial cells of both ill-defined boundary and clear cytoplasmic border with a well-developed vesicular system. These cells occasionally show slight signs of phagocytosis and may be an early transitional form of immature interstitial cells (Fig. 7-30*A*). A free phagocytic cell, resembling neither a monocyte nor a lymphocyte, is

(text continues on page 380)

FIGURE 7-29. Macrophage.
Portion of macrophage shows two common residues of digestion: myelin figures (*arrows*) and dispersed ferritin particles (*circles*). × *244,000.*

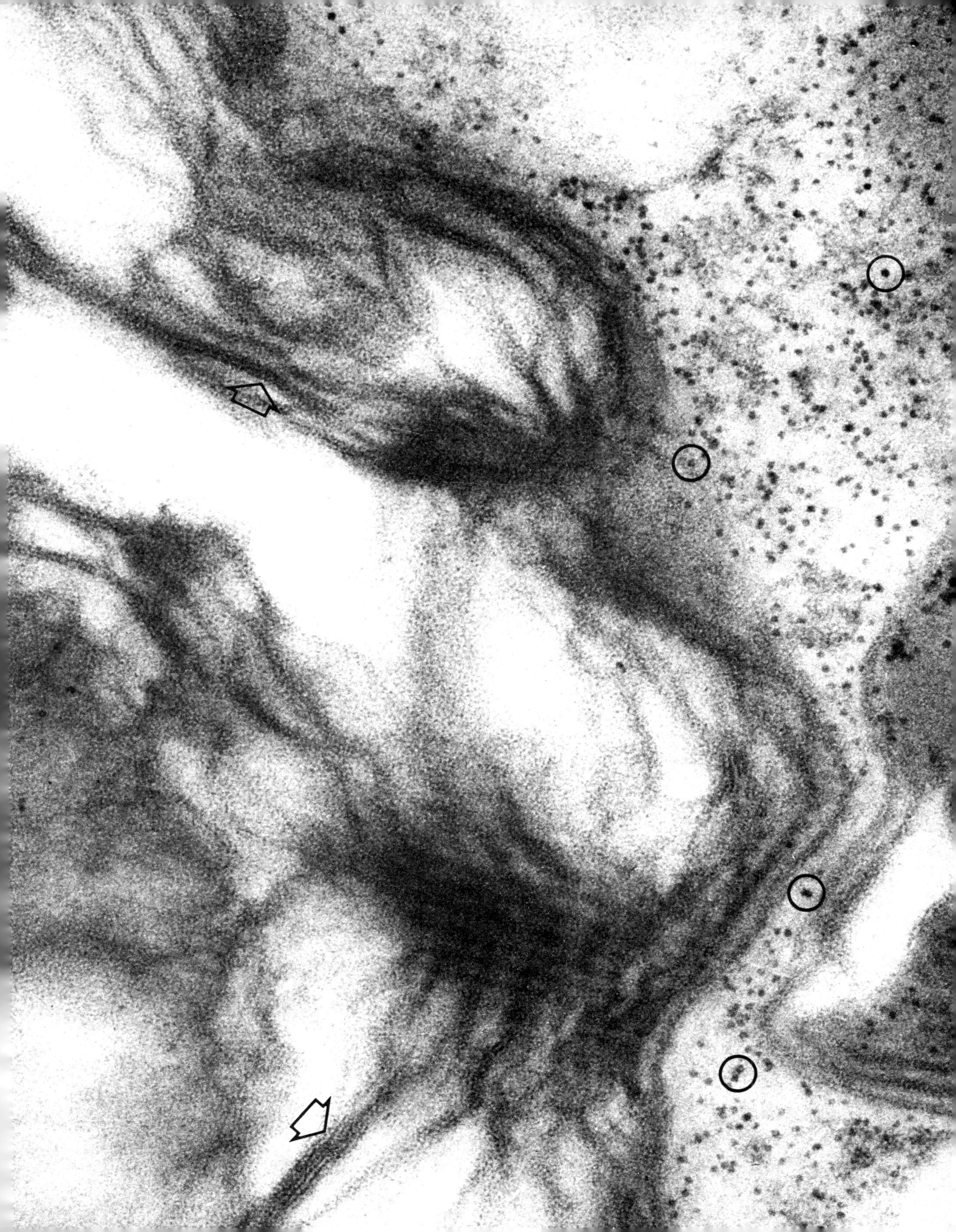

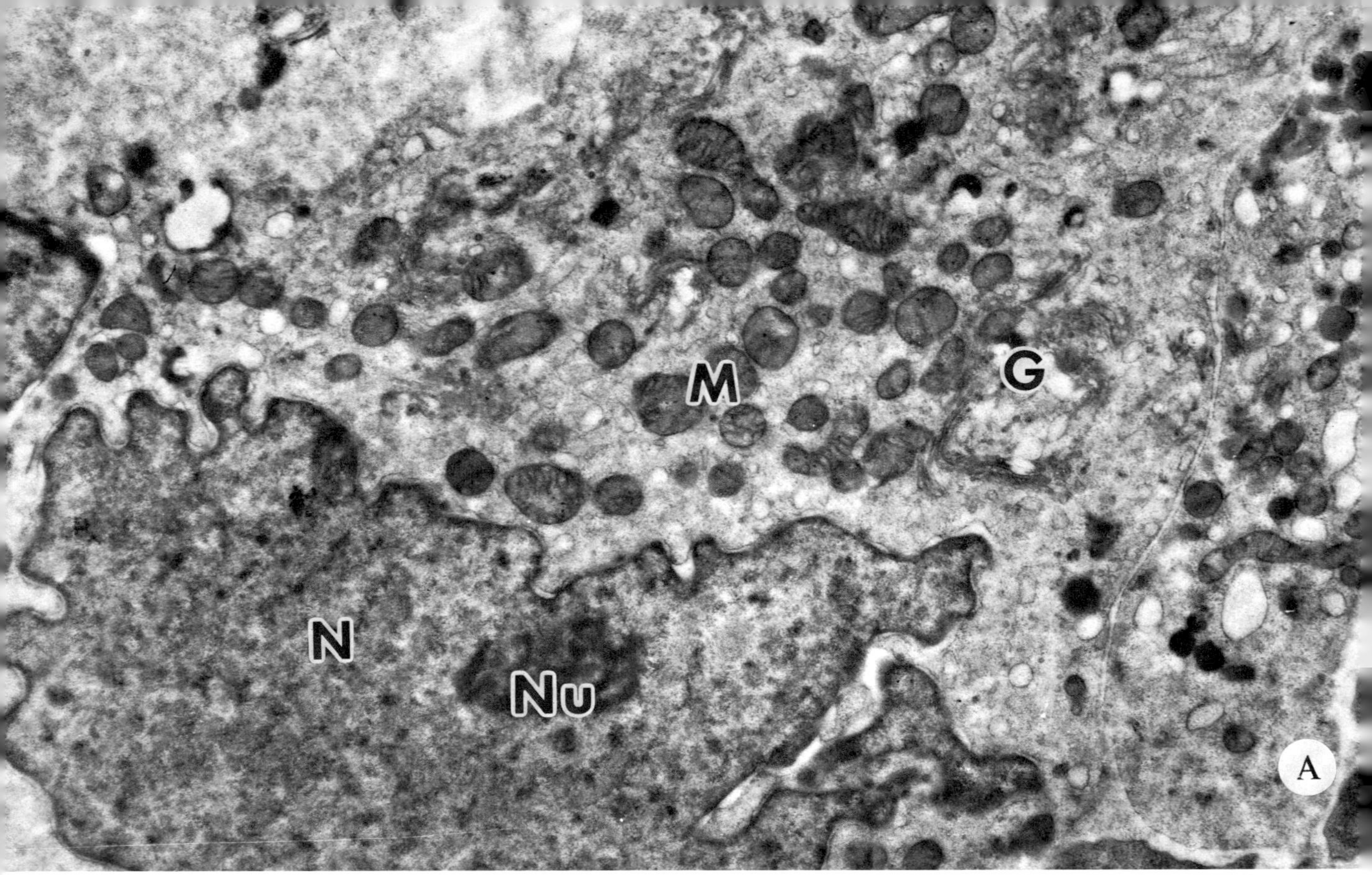
M
G
N
Nu
A

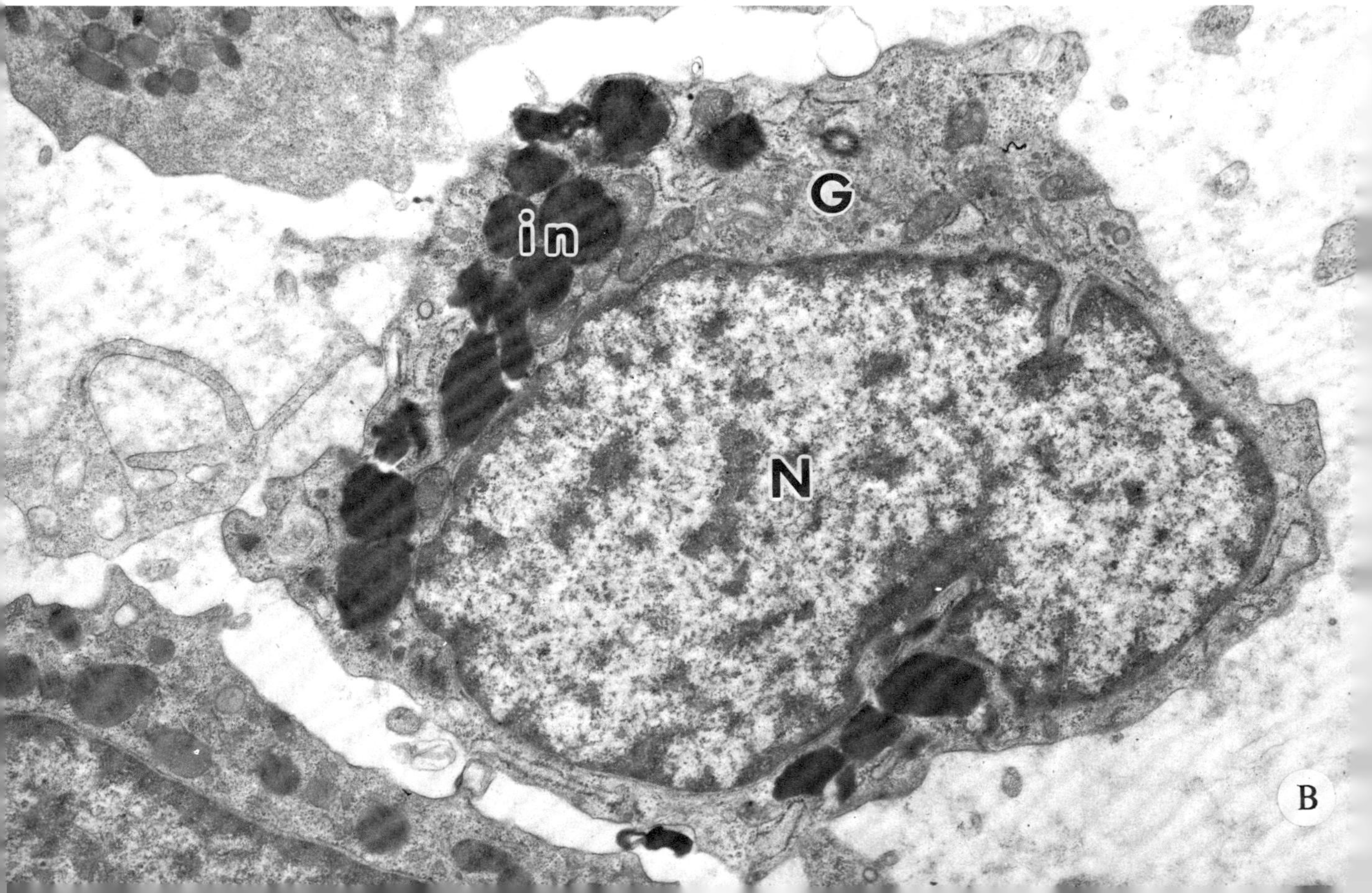
G
in
N
B

FIGURE 7-30. Phagocytic cells from hyperplastic marrow.
A. Interstitial cell with some ultrastructural characteristics of immature phagocyte and large number of mitochondria (*M*), a vesicular system, and large Golgi area (*G*) in the cytoplasm. The reticular nucleus (*N*) is very irregular in outline and has a distinct nucleolus (*Nu*). × *11,700.*
B. Mononuclear cell from patient with lipidosis contains ingested lipid (*in*). The vesicular appearance of the nucleus (*N*), lack of cytoplasmic granules, and presence of inclusions suggest that it is neither a lymphocyte nor monocyte but possibly histiocyte. Cell contains a Golgi area (*G*). × *15,500.*

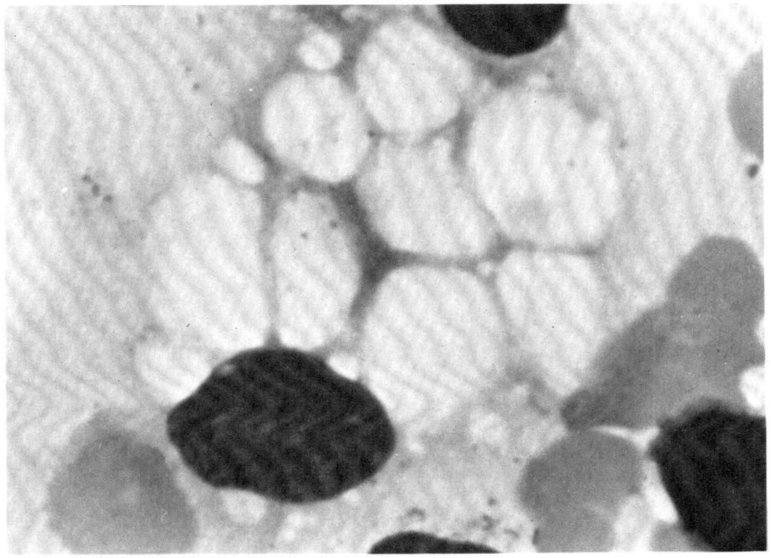

FIGURE 7-31. Fat cells in marrow.
Light micrograph of typical fat cells from human bone marrow smear. *Giemsa stain.* × *2,000.*

Figures 7-32 and 7-33 appear on the following pages

FIGURE 7-32. Fat cells and related structures.
Thin strips of fat cell cytoplasm (*open arrow*), including mitochondria (*M*), line the fat cells—small segment at upper right and larger portion (*Fc*). The large elliptical nucleus (*N*) is in reticulum cell (*Rc*) which has small amount of cytoplasm. Several long vales of reticulum cell cytoplasm (*solid arrows*) are present. Lumen of sinus (*S*) in the middle is flat and a myelocyte (*My*) is in the intersinusoidal space. An endothelial cell (*En*) is adjacent to sinus. × *19,000.*

FIGURE 7-33. Fat cell cytoplasm.
A portion of the cytoplasm of a fat cell near the nucleus (*N*) contains several small lipid vacuoles (*F*). Dense granular inclusions in lipid droplets are of unknown chemical composition and are seen only occasionally. Cytoplasm also contains numerous small mitochondria (*M*), many ribosomes, and some endoplasmic reticulum (*er*). A few fine intracellular fibrils can also be seen. × *34,000.*

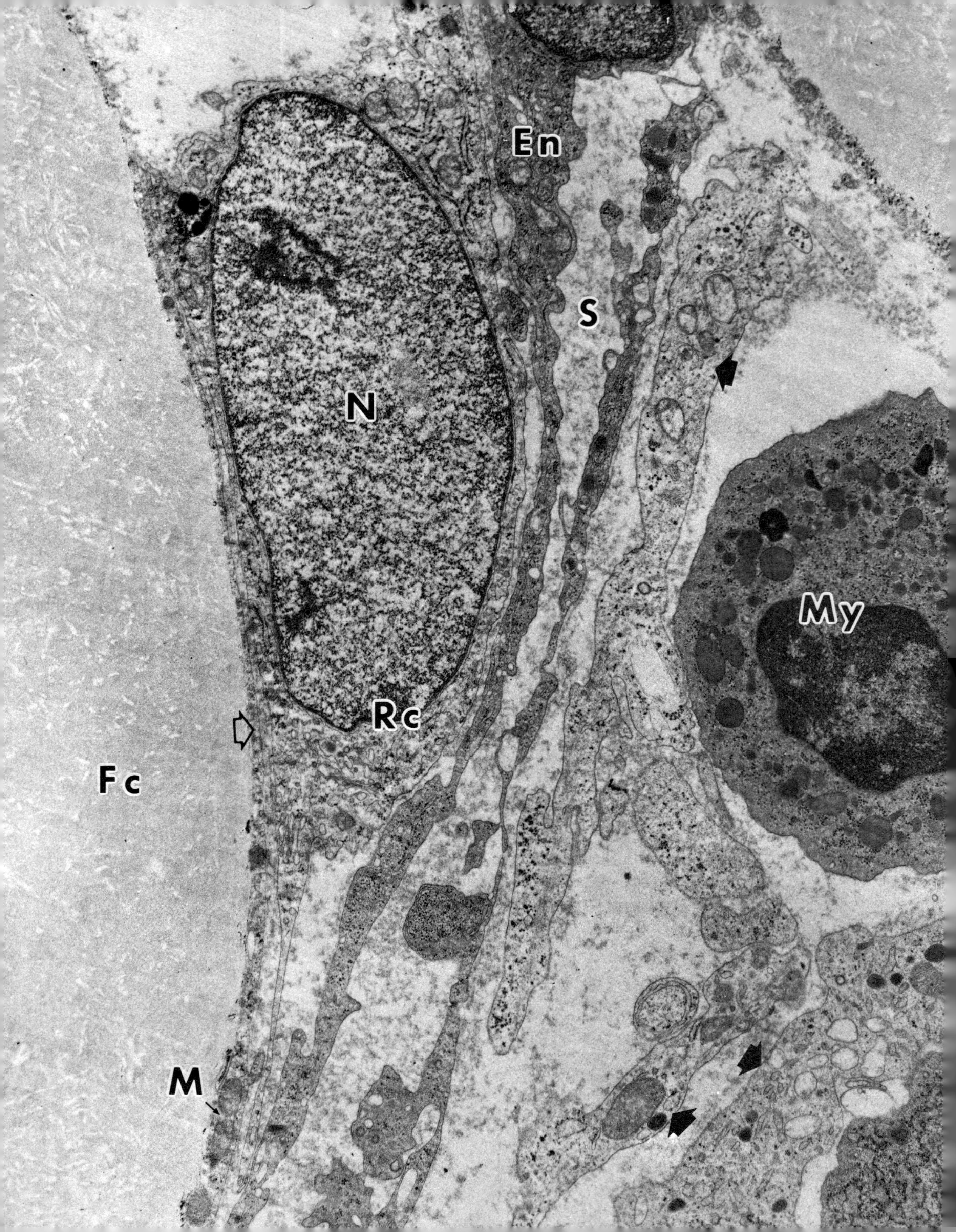
En
S
N
My
Rc
Fc
M

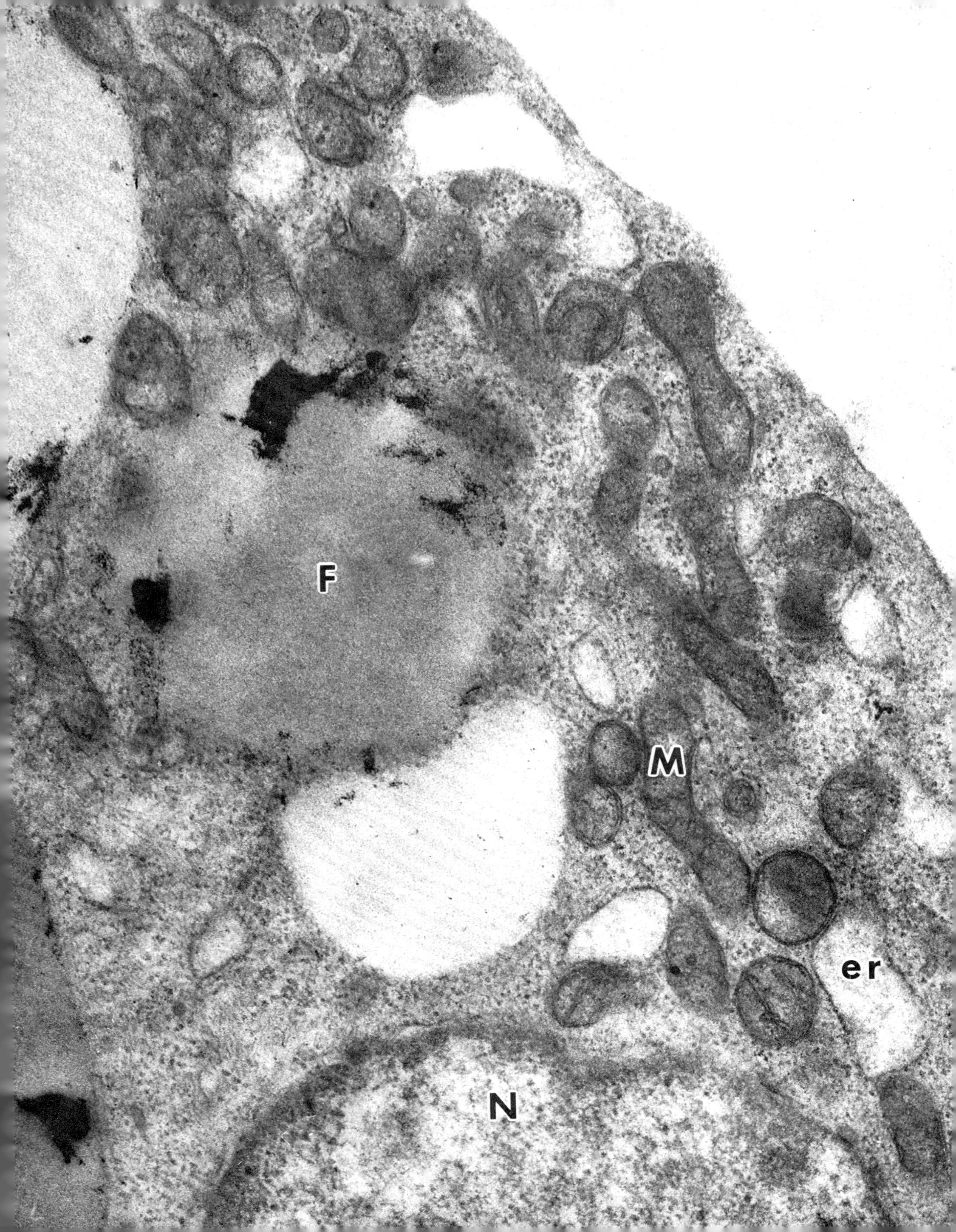
F
M
er
N

shown in Figure 7-30*B*. This cell could be called a histiocyte. Whether the bone marrow can generate free phagocytic elements other than monocytes is as yet unknown.

FAT CELLS

It is well known that large numbers of fat cells are present in postnatal bone marrow (Fig. 7-31). When yellow, the bone marrow consists almost entirely of fat cells, between which are marrow vessels, reticulum cells, and extracellular fibrils (Fig. 7-32). The number of fat cells varies widely according to the physiological state of the subject—e.g., their number increases with age. Myelopoiesis can be induced in fat marrow by appropriate stimuli though the origin of fat and how the cell collects or synthesizes fat are not well understood. Harris (1960) suggested that accumulated fat in the cells can be utilized during rapid regeneration of bone marrow cells.

It is difficult to fix bone marrows which are laden with many fat cells, and there is considerable difficulty in getting a uniform cut and smooth thin sections of such specimens. No extensive study has yet appeared on the ultrastructural study of marrow fat cells. Fragmentary observations show that their ultrastructure (Figs. 7-33 and 7-34) is different from reticulum cells of both phagocytic and nonphagocytic types (Tanaka, 1969). Regenerating bone marrow has small fat vacuoles in elongated reticulum cells (Ito, 1965) which could be the mother cells of the very large lipid-containing cells in the bone marrow (Shimamine, 1952; Ito, 1965; Watanabe, 1966).

CYTOGENESIS

BONE MARROW RETICULUM CELLS

Kinetic studies on bone marrow reticulum cells are rare. Caffrey *et al.* (1966) studied rat bone marrows by radioisotope methods and showed that reticulum cells, which form a part of the fixed reticular network, are probably a slowly proliferating compartment. These data on rate of reproduction tend to conflict with the hypothesis that hemocytoblasts are derived from cells of the fixed reticulum networks; on the other hand, they confirm that the hemocytoblast compartment could be the precursor of committed blastic forms. This is in good agreement with morphological data that nonphagocytic reticulum cells with classic reticulum cell appearance do not contribute to cell degeneration (Tanaka, 1969).

Fixed macrophages, blood monocytes, and sinus endothelial cells of bone marrow are regarded as cells of the reticuloendothelial system (RES) although this is confusing when RES is used to delineate cell function other than phagocytosis. Since this problem has not been discussed extensively, we will present a brief review of the cells of RES and their activity in hematopoiesis, based on a modification of Akazaki's view (1952, 1963).

FIGURE 7-34. Fat cell cytoplasm.
Cytoplasm of another fat cell contains numerous large mitochondria (*M*) with dense matrix and prominent intramitochondrial dense granules (*arrows*). Pale fat vacuoles (*asterisks*) appear to be moving to join the large fat droplet (*F*). Intracytoplasmic fibrils (*fb*) are present, and many pinocytotic vesicles (*pv*) are near the cell surface. × *44,500.*

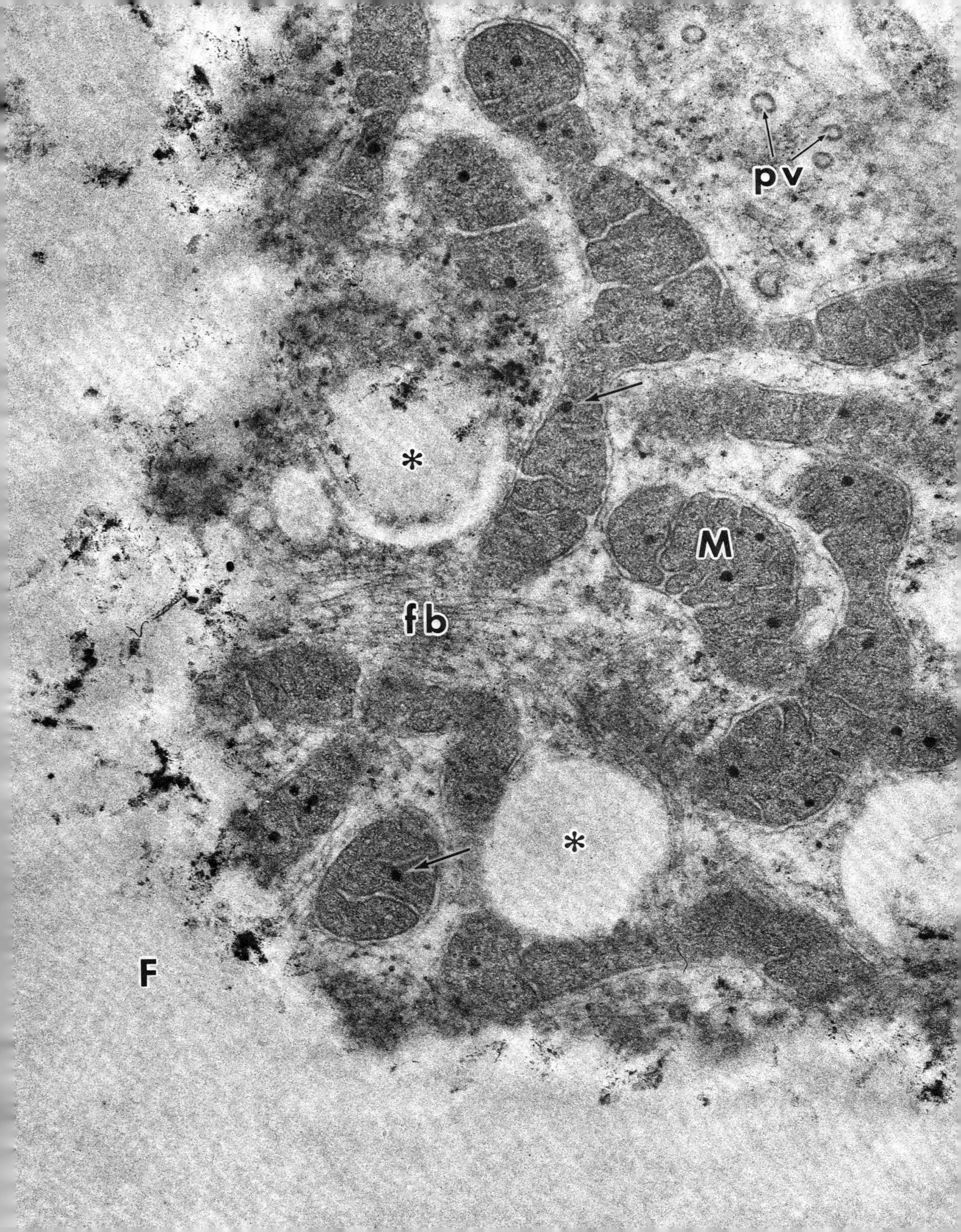
pv
*
M
fb
*
F

RETICULOENDOTHELIAL SYSTEM AND ITS RELATIONSHIP TO BLOOD-FORMING ACTIVITY

Cells of heterogeneous morphology, with a significant phagocytotic activity, may be detected when colloidal pigments are injected into animals. Using this technic, Aschoff (1924) introduced the term "reticuloendothelial system," derived from three points of similarity of the two major elements of this system: reticulum cells of lymphoreticular tissues and endothelial lining cells of sinusoids. Common properties of these two cells are phagocytic activity, association with reticulum fibers, and location—e.g., the inner surface of blood and lymph spaces. Aschoff's original concept also included the histiocyte and blood monocytes in this system. He knew that cells grouped in this system were involved in a variety of functions other than phagocytosis but thought their primary activity was phagocytosis. The concept was accepted by many others, who extended the classification beyond phagocytosis (Jaffe, 1927) and included fat cells (Wells, 1940). Doan (1940) proposed a family tree of cells. The most critical point of this concept is that cells with heterogeneous morphology and cytogenesis are grouped on the basis of one functional role. The identification of a specific group of cells as defined by their function in static histologic sections produces a dilemma for morphologists. An attempt to visualize cells of the RES by specific staining of the histologic sections (Marshall, 1956) failed to give a precise delineation. Attempts have been made to modify the variety of cell groups in the RES on the basis of cytogenesis and cytology without affecting the original concept of Aschoff (1924). Kiyono (1918) proposed the term "histiocytic system," on the basis of his belief that histiocytes originated from reticulum cells, and he included endothelial cells of the sinusoids within this system. In this sense, his concept was similar to Virchow's. Later, the similar term "reticulo-histiocytic system" was used by Rohr (1960) to include a group of nonendothelial cells. He justified this inclusion on the assumption that these cells originated from some immature reticulum cells and played an important role in the body-defense mechanism. In his concept, he included cells of heterogeneous morphology, such as fat cells, osteoclasts, mast cells, plasma cells, and fibroblasts. The "reticulo-histiocyte system" of Rohr differs markedly from the original concept of Aschoff. More recently, Langevoot *et al.* (1970) proposed the term "mononuclear phagocytic system," which includes mononuclear phagocytes and their possible precursors, monocytes. This system excludes both reticulum cells (or reticular cells) and sinus endothelial cells, which have been long regarded as contributing to the development of macrophages. They apparently assume that blood monocytes are precursors of most, if not all, macrophages. This seems an unwarranted assumption, and the term "mononuclear phagocytic system" suffers the vagueness of previous classification attempts.

In 1930, Roulet had distinguished reticulum cells from endothelial cells of specific sinuses and proposed a term "retothelium" to define the reticulum cells. He based his conclusions on observations made from a study of reticulum cell sarcoma, using the presence of reticulin fibers, regardless of their phagocytic activity. The term "retothelial system," later introduced by Rossle (1939), included only reticulum cells and was analogous to the original view of RES proposed by Aschoff. In this system, the association of reticulum cells to reticulum fibers is far more important than their phagocytic activity. The same term was used by Fresen (1960), who included the endothelial cells of the specific sinuses, on the basis of the assumption that they were actually reticulum cells. More recently, the term "retothelium" was used strictly for delineation of sinus endothelium of lymph nodes (Lennert, 1961; Mori and Lennert, 1969), in contrast to the original concept of Rossle.

Cells of the RES are frequently known as mother cells of blood-forming organs. Such an expression may be misleading, as it seems unlikely that cells with phagocytic activity have the capacity to regenerate hemopoietic cells. However, cells with phagocytic activity are believed to be capable of production of histiocytes (macrophages) by exfoliation from their original site. Fixed interstitial cells associated with reticulum fibers include both phagocytic and nonphagocytic types. Ultrastructurally, no clear distinction between immature mesenchymal elements and fibroblasts is possible. In bone marrow, interstitial cells with the classic characteristics of reticulum cells are incapable of regenerating new populations (Caffrey *et al.,* 1966; Tanaka, 1969). A large portion of macrophages in tissues and visceral cavities probably originate from blood-borne mononuclear cells, possibly monocytes or their precursors. These observations suggest that the classic view of hematopoietic activity imposed on cells of RES should be reconsidered.

MACROPHAGES AND PRECURSORS

Unattached cells with significant phagocytic activity can be recognized in interstitial tissue when stained with colloidal pigments. The term "histiocyte" was proposed for these cells by Kiyono (1918), who believed they originated from the fixed interstitial elements known as reticulum cells. The term "histiocyte" indicates the cytogenesis of the cells as well as their phagocytic function, so that the term "histiocyte" should not be used for vague descriptions of all types of cells that show significant phagocytosis. The nonspecific term "macrophage" (Metchnikoff, 1884) is more extensively used by morphologists to describe cells with significant phagocytosis. Extensive cytogenetic analyses made on free cells with active phagocytosis have generally concluded that macrophages in various organs originated from cells of the reticuloendothelial system. This was reviewed extensively by both Jaffe (1938) and Bloom (1938).

Recent kinetic studies have led to a revision of the classic concept of macrophage cytogenesis, and a greater number of these studies support the concept that many macrophages are cells of free circulating type which originate from the bone marrows—i.e., monocytes (van Furth, 1970). These cells apparently transform into macrophages in various tissues, such as subcutaneous connective tissues, serosal cavities, liver sinusoids, and alveolar spaces. Though the significance of blood monocytes is established, it is not clear that all mononuclear phagocytes in tissues were once blood monocytes. Daems and Brederoo (1971) have used the peroxidase stain to distinguish resident macrophages in peritoneal exudates of guinea pigs from the influx of mononuclear phagocytes from the blood following saline injection into the peritoneal cavity (Fig. 7-35). A contribution of phagocytes from lymphoid tissues has also been demonstrated (Howard *et al.,* 1967). These observations suggest that mononuclear phagocytes of bone marrow may not be an exclusive source of tissue macrophages.

There are many reports on electron microscopy of macrophages (Cohn, 1968; Fedorko and Hirsch, 1970). Tanaka (1958)

(text continues on page 388)

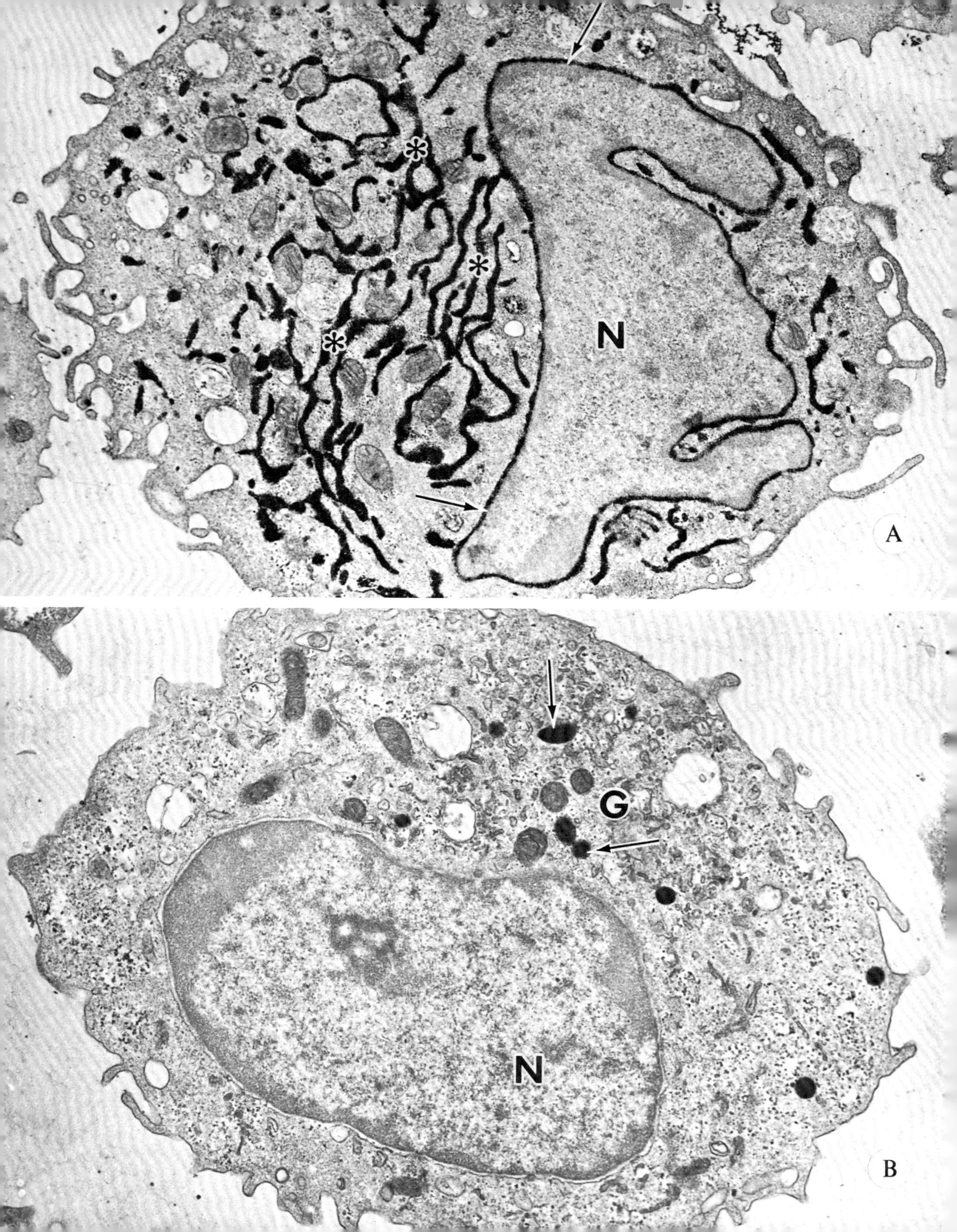
N
A
G
N
B

FIGURE 7-35. Peritoneal macrophages of guinea pig.

A. Normal resident macrophage from peritoneal exudates of guinea pig incubated for cytochemical localization of endogenous peroxidase activity. The cell is characterized by numerous cytoplasmic projections of the surface and an irregular nuclear (*N*) outline with a membrane containing many pores. The reaction product of peroxidase activity is the electron-dense material present in the nuclear envelope (*arrows*) and the cisternae of the endoplasmic reticulum (*asterisks*). × *20,000.*

B. The dominant macrophage, a mononuclear phagocyte from peripheral blood, in guinea pig exudates 16 hours after stimulation by sterile saline injection into the peritoneal cavity. This cell incubated for endogenous peroxidase activity has a smoother cytoplasmic surface and a rounded nucleus (*N*) with few nuclear pores. There are only a limited number of profiles of rough endoplasmic reticulum and Golgi vesicles (*G*), neither of which contain any peroxidase activity. However, there is intense activity in a few round or ovoid granules (*arrows*) limited by single membranes. This cell is considered to be a monocyte from the blood that has migrated into the peritoneal cavity and is distinguished from the resident macrophage (Fig. 7-35**A**) by the morphology and peroxidase activity. × *20,000.*

Supplied by Drs. W. Th. Daems and P. Brederoo, University of Leiden, Netherlands.

Figures 7-36 and 7-37 appear on the following pages

FIGURE 7-36. Serosal macrophage.
Free macrophage from pleural fluid has typical morphology. The crescent-shaped nucleus (*N*) partially encircles a large Golgi area (G). The cytoplasm has many vesicles, endoplasmic reticulum (*er*), numerous examples of ingested material (*asterisks*), and rounded mitochondria (*M*). × *19,000.*

FIGURE 7-37. Cytoplasm of serosal macrophage.
Macrophage cytoplasm has a pervasive vascular nature, mitochondria (*M*), larger vesicles containing amorphous material (*asterisks*), and saccules (*s*). The edge of the nucleus (*N*) is visible. The scattered electron-opaque particles are probably glycogen. × *38,000.*

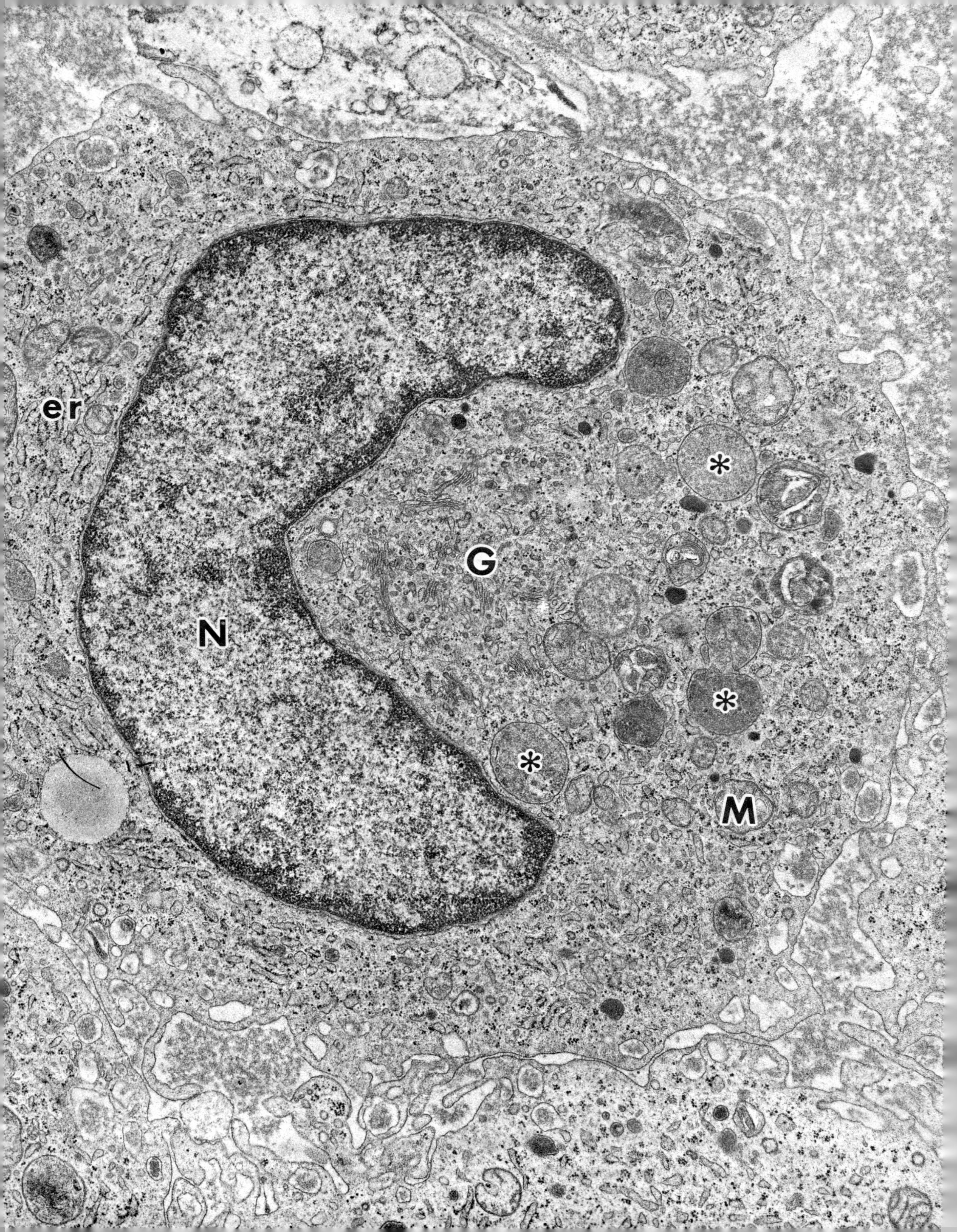
er
G
N
*
*
*
M

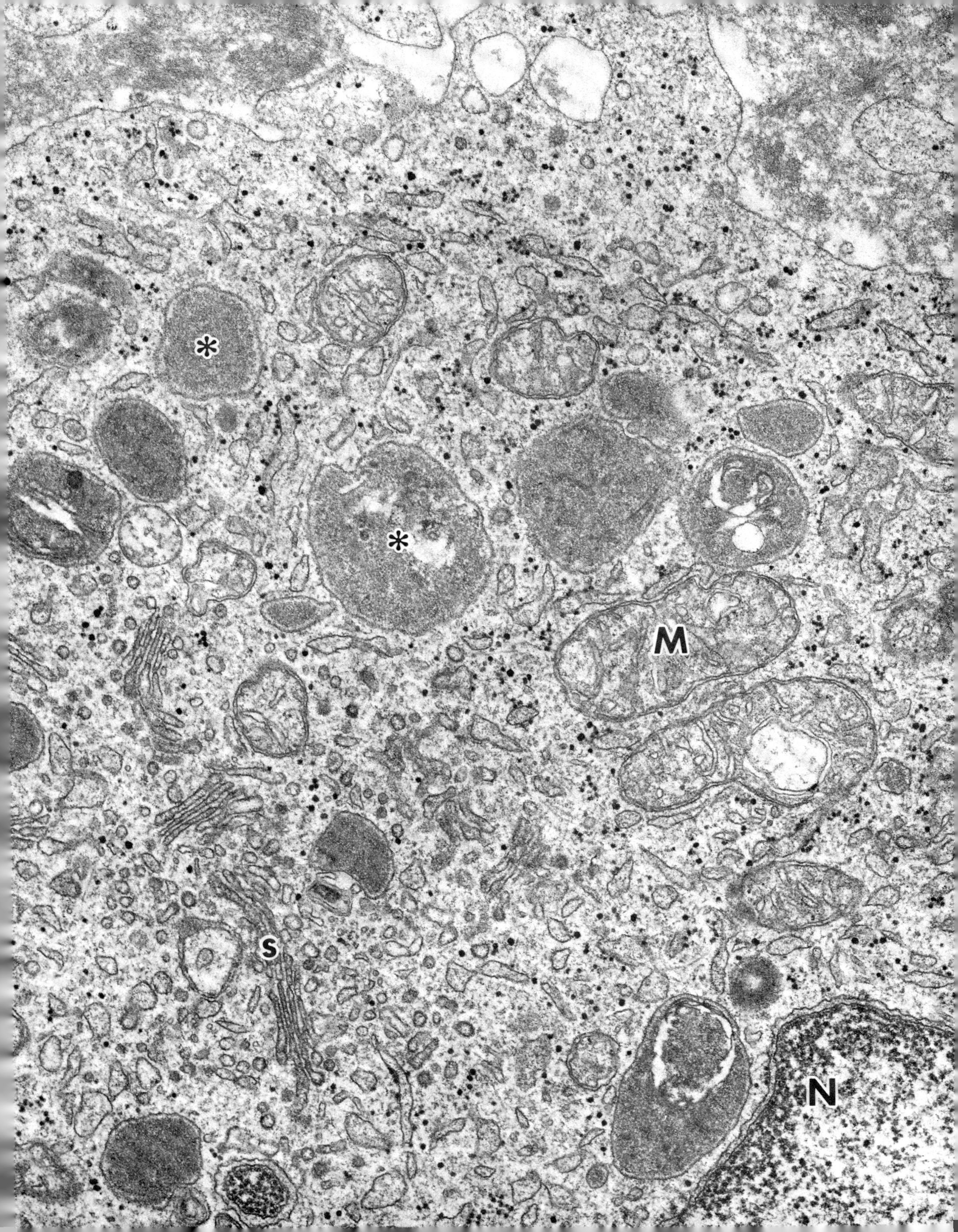

*
*
M
S
N

compared mononuclear phagocytes in various tissues and showed the presence of many characteristic vesicles. This observation has been confirmed by many (Dumont, 1969; Fedorko and Hirsch, 1970). Various morphological studies of these cells have related to their process of phagocytosis, lysosomal function, and transfer of antigenic information. Examples of serosal macrophages are shown in Figures 7-36 and 7-37.

FUNCTION

SUPPORTING STRUCTURE

The function of the vasculature in bone marrow is to provide oxygen and nutrients and remove newly formed blood elements. It also functions as a loose network, or frame, within which all other marrow elements proliferate and mature. Recovery of hematopoiesis after marrow destruction (Steinberg and Hufford, 1947; Mital and Cohen, 1966) has been observed during and following the repair of the marrow structure. This has also been noted in the reestablishment of hematopoiesis in bone marrow transplants (Tavassoli and Crosby, 1968, 1970; Crosby, 1970), and thus suggests that bone marrow structure may be essential for hematopoiesis.

CELL GENERATION

The chief function of bone marrow is blood cell generation, an activity which can be intermittent during the total life span of the body. Stimulation can provoke new hematopoiesis in some areas of marrow while other areas rest temporarily. Practically all types of blood cells can be produced in the bone marrow, although the production of plasma cells and lymphocytes is performed extensively in the lymphoreticular tissues.

The cells which generate and replicate various blood cells are called stem cells and, as a group, are called the stem cell compartment. Although the term appears to fit the previously described immature cells, the specific morphology of a stem cell compartment is not clearly established. Thus, the term remains merely functional though it is customarily adopted in kinetic studies to define a specific cell group. Visualization of the stem cell has been repeatedly attempted, and many hematologists claim to have identified it.

The immediate precursors of committed blastic forms in human bone marrow are large lymphoid cells with basophilic cytoplasm, called hemocytoblasts (Bessis, 1956; Caffrey *et al.,* 1966). Various non-self-generating blastic cells, proerythroblasts for erythrocytic cells, and myeloblasts for granulocytes, are believed to have originated from these elements. Hemocytoblasts can maintain their number and in emergency may be regenerated from the diffuse mesenchyma of the blood-forming organs. Studies on cell generation have used suspensions of myeloid and lymphoid tissues to produce hematopoietic colonies in the spleen of sublethally irradiated animals after 8 to 10 days of infusion (Till and McColloch, 1961). A similar phenomenon was also seen when peripheral blood was injected (Trobaugh and Lewis, 1964). Consequently, the diffuse mesenchyma of myeloid tissues is considered to be a possible, but less likely, immediate precursor (Loutit, 1968). Using the spleen colony method, many have shown that myelocytic and erythrocytic colonies can be produced when the marrow and splenic suspensions are injected (Becker *et al.,* 1963; Wu *et al.,* 1967), but hemopoietic activity was insignificant when only lymphocytes were used. The morphology of the colony-forming cells, both lymphocytic (Moffat *et al.,* 1967) and monocytic forms (Caffrey-Tyler and Everett, 1966), have been described. Though cells resembling the small lymphocyte have been observed repeatedly in animal marrows, they are rarely noted in human marrows even under reactive and malignant conditions. Their exact identity or genesis is not clearly established. (The origin of these cells is discussed under Morphology and under Cytogenesis in Chap. 5.)

STORAGE

Another function of the bone marrow is the storage of iron and fats in physiological conditions. Since the total amount of marrow tissue is comparable in size to the liver, the storage capacity for such metabolites is considerable. The function of bone marrow fat is not understood, although other fat cells have been shown to be metabolically very active and the stored fat is easily available. There are no data to indicate that marrow fat cells perform the same function as other fat cells. Harris (1960) suggested that fat cells in marrow, following sublethal irradiation, might be a source of energy and metabolites for the regeneration of other cell types in the regenerating marrow. The significance of bone marrow macrophages in iron metabolism and iron turnover have been discussed (Chap. 2).

PHAGOCYTOSIS

This phenomenon was discovered by Metchnikoff (1884), who correctly considered the mechanism to be important for body defense. The topics relating to phagocytosis have been reviewed by Berry and Spies (1949), Rowley (1962) and, more recently, by North (1970).

The recognition of the object to be phagocytized precedes the ingestion of the object. Macrophages can distinguish foreign cells from self cells and dead cells from living cells. It has been known for a long time that certain substances (opsonins) in serum are necessary to induce ingestion of bacteria by phagocytes (Wright and Douglas, 1904; Ecker *et al.,* 1942). These are now considered to be specific antibodies belonging to the IgG group (North, 1970). As yet, the mechanism for induction of phagocytosis by these globulins is not clearly understood. Recognition by macrophages could be based on differences in surface charges, as observed in phagocytosis of ejected erythroid nuclei (Skutelsky and Danon, 1969). The importance of surface activity was demonstrated by Vaughn and Boyden (1964), who showed that the attachment of aged and chemically modified erythrocytes on the macrophage surface was prevented by treatment with trypsin.

The process of phagocytosis has been studied electron microscopically in neutrophils (Goodman *et al.,* 1956a,b) and in macrophages of various species. Large objects, such as dead red cells, engulfed by macrophages are disintegrated within the cells. In studying erythrophagocytosis, one can see that the periphery of the phagocytized red cell is attacked by endocytosis, and myelin figures are rapidly formed in the macrophage cytoplasm (Policard *et al.,* 1956). Frequently, one may also see that erythroblasts are digested in the macrophages without further cellular fragmentation (Goodman *et al.,* 1968). During this process, large amounts of hydrolytic enzymes are supplied, possibly from the Golgi apparatus. During cell digestion, heterogeneous vacuoles and inclusions are formed in macrophages, and are frequently called lysosomes. Engulfed red cells are decomposed into iron complexes and other chemical constituents, some of which are reutilized in cell metabolism and cytogenesis. Cohn and Wiener (1963) observed that alveolar macrophages have a high content of hydrolases. They suggested functional heterogeneity of the macrophage population.

Macromolecules from the environment are imbibed by a process generally known as endocytosis or pinocytosis, which can create large cytoplasmic inclusions in macrophages. These develop by the fusion of small pinocytotic vesicles near the cell surface, forming large vesicles (Hirsch *et al.,* 1968). In human bone marrow, this phenomenon is best seen in patients with lipidosis. The speed of digestion of molecules in macrophages has been estimated by decomposition of labeled albumin by Ehrenreich and Cohn (1967), who found that the material was eliminated as peptide molecules—50 per cent activity loss in 5 hours, 90 per cent elimination in 10 to 12 hours.

TRANSFER OF ANTIGENIC INFORMATION

There are two main hypotheses for the mechanism of antibody formation: (1) the instructive or template, and (2) the selective or elective stimulation concepts. Both require an antigen to initiate the immunological process. Phagocytosis, endocytosis, or cell surface absorption may be important initial steps in this process, and the macrophages of the RES are the primary tissue cells involved in this action. Antigens that reach follicular macrophages are found on or adjacent to the macrophage surface (Nossal *et al.,* 1968a,b). Since nearly all circulating antibodies are produced by plasma cells and lymphocytes, and since macrophages probably do not transform into either of these cell types, there must be a transfer of antigenic information from macrophages to the immunologically competent cells. The observation that such a transfer can be achieved by a macrophage ribosomal fraction (Adler *et al.,* 1966) stimulated further investigation.

It is not clear how the transfer of antigenic information takes place. Askonas and Rhodes (1965) suggested that the addition of the antigen to a small RNA molecule makes it immunogenic. Others (Nossal *et al.,* 1968a,b) consider that the function of the macrophage is to hold the antigen on the cell surface, allowing efficient interaction of the different cell types involved in the immune response. Roelants and Goodman (1969) suggested that these RNA antigen complexes may be unrelated to the immunopotency of the antigen, that they are not an enzyme-dependent reaction, do not require the synthesis of RNA following the introduction of the antigen, do not seem to involve antigen-specific RNAs, and are not specific for macrophages. These observations raise doubts about the role of soluble RNA as a antigenic carrier. More data are necessary to clarify understanding of these mechanisms.

PATHOLOGY

NONMALIGNANT PROLIFERATION OF RETICULUM CELLS

Granuloma

Granulomatous lesions may be observed in bone marrow during the course of various infectious diseases. Granulomatous lesions consist of mononuclear cells, including small lymphocytes, large mononuclear cells, and, frequently, phagocytes and fibroblasts (Fig. 7-38). Investigation of granulomatous lesions in bone marrow is of interest, since blood monocytes are generated in this organ and macrophages may originate from monocytes and their precursors. Ultrastructural studies of these granulomatous foci reveal proliferation of various mononuclear cells with active phagocytosis in some (Figs. 7-39 through 7-41).

The most prominent cell types are large and small mononuclear cells with well developed vesicular elements (Fig. 7-39). The mononuclear cell has a round vesicular nucleus with an occasional indentation. The cytoplasm contains various organelles such as many mitochondria, developed Golgi apparatus, tubular endoplasmic reticulum, and vesicles and ribosomes, usually single. Ultrastructurally, none of these mononuclear cells resemble the typical blood monocytes. There is neither an accumulation of granulocytes around the granulomatous foci nor proliferation of elongated cells resembling fibroblasts. There are various intermediate forms between small mononuclear cells and giant epithelioid cells (Figs. 7-38*B*, 7-40, and 7-41), and also proliferating mononuclear cells resembling typical small lymphocytes (Fig. 7-39). Ultrastructurally, large epithelioid cells in bone marrow differ slightly from those of sarcoidosis. Many cytoplasmic inclusions are noted (Figs. 7-40 and 7-41). It is not known whether these mononuclear cells are produced locally or come from the circulation.

Lipidosis

Proliferation of large, lipid-containing cells can occur in bone marrow as well as in other lymphoreticular tissues in conditions of impaired lipid metabolism. The presence of lipid-containing macrophages in bone marrow is commonly considered to be diagnostic of lipidosis, a pathological condition generally considered to be a genetic defect. The lipid-containing macrophages may also be observed in other conditions in which hyperlipemia is induced secondarily to the primary disorders. Occasionally, macrophages resemble Gaucher's cells and can be observed in nonlipemic thrombocytopenic purpura (Dollberg *et al.,* 1965). Thus lipid-containing macrophages are not pathognomonic (Malinin, 1961) but suggestive of a dysfunction in lipid metabolism. Some of the most representative lipidoses are Gaucher's disease, Niemann-Pick disease, and Fabry's disease.

Gaucher's Disease. Unique macrophages containing cerebrosides are commonly noted in spleen as well as bone marrow in this disorder. The disease was described by Gaucher in 1882, and clearly distinguished from Niemann-Pick disease by Pick in 1927. The abnormal lipids in macrophages were identified by Epstein (1924) and Lieb (1924). The pathogenesis of this disorder was suggested by Brady *et al.* (1965) to be a defective enzyme needed for the breakdown of cerebrosides.

The unique morphology of these lipid-containing cells is well recognized in routine smears by phase microscopy as well as electron microscopy. Gaucher cells range from 20 to 80μ in diameter and have a large cytoplasm containing faintly eosinophilic, weblike substances. Fibrillar structures may be clearly recognized in the cytoplasm of these cells by phase microscopy. Histochemically, the cytoplasm appears PAS-positive; however, no strong reaction is demonstrated by Sudan black B staining. These cells show a diffuse blue color when the tissues are exposed to Perl's reagent, suggesting the presence of iron in the cytoplasm.

Electron microscopic studies (De Marsh and Kautz, 1957) show tubular

(text continues on page 398)

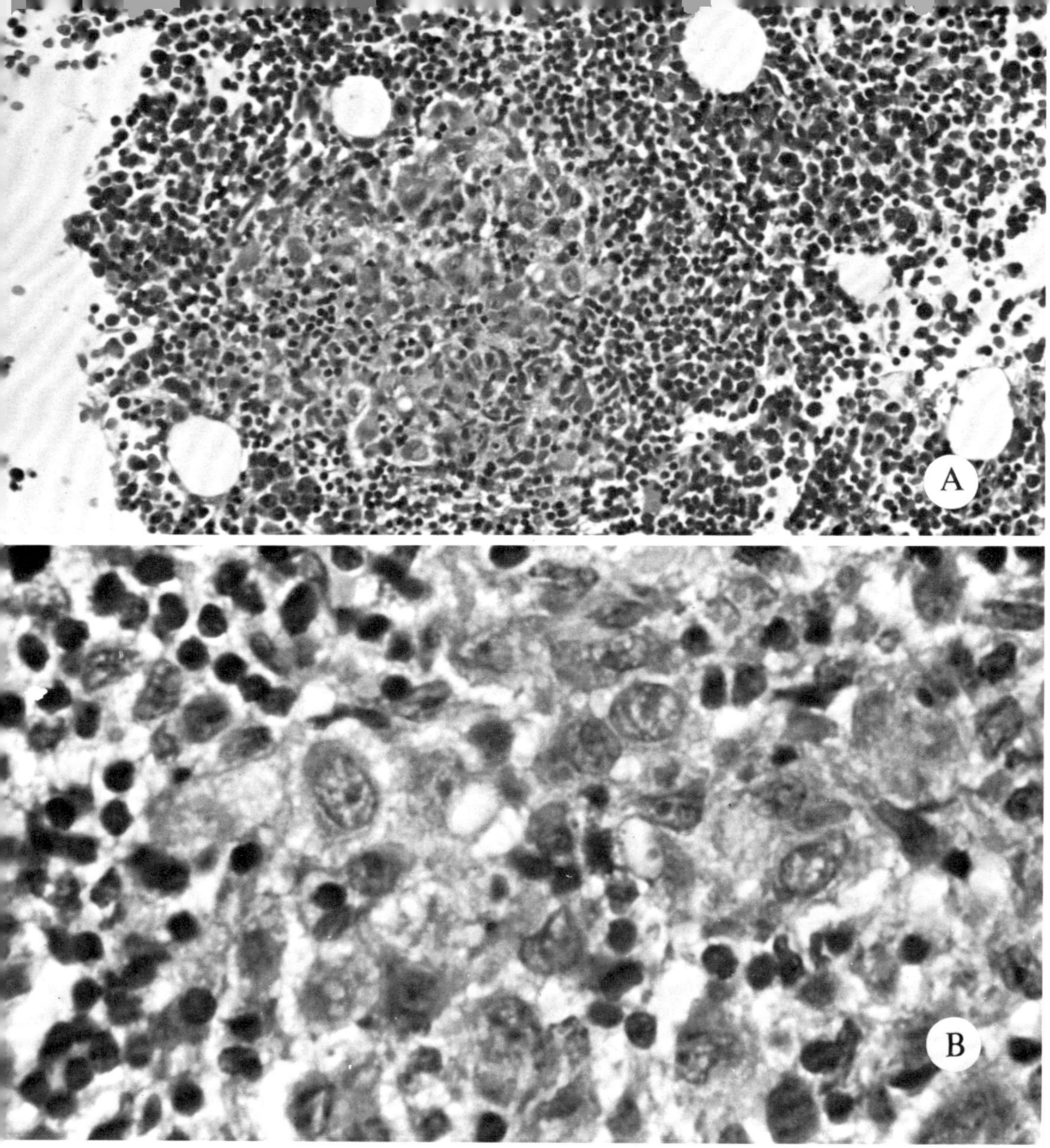

FIGURE 7-38. Granuloma in human marrow.
A. Light micrograph of marrow, fixed with formalin and stained with hematoxylin and eosin, shows an area of epithelioid cell hyperplasia surrounded by lymphoid cells. × *250.*
B. This light micrograph shows details of a portion of the epithelioid granuloma. × *1,000.*

FIGURE 7-39. Granuloma in human marrow.
Cells are from same lesion illustrated in Figure 7-38. Cytoplasm of several mononuclear cells—one with distinct nucleolus (*Nu*)—has many very small vesicles which suggests phagocytic activity. Some lymphocytes (*L*) and a macrophage (*Ma*) are intermixed with larger mononuclear cells. × *8,900.*

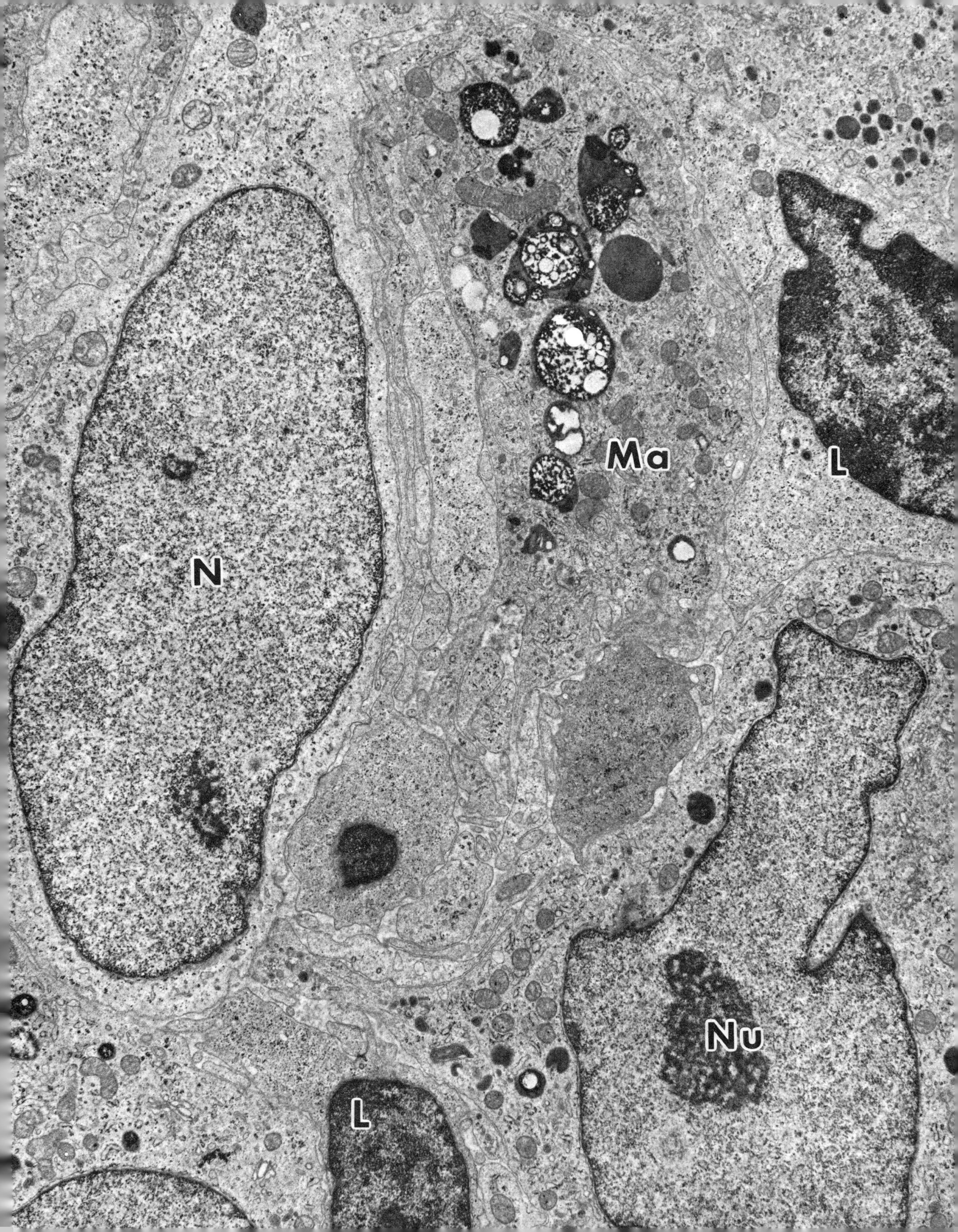
Ma
L
N
Nu
L

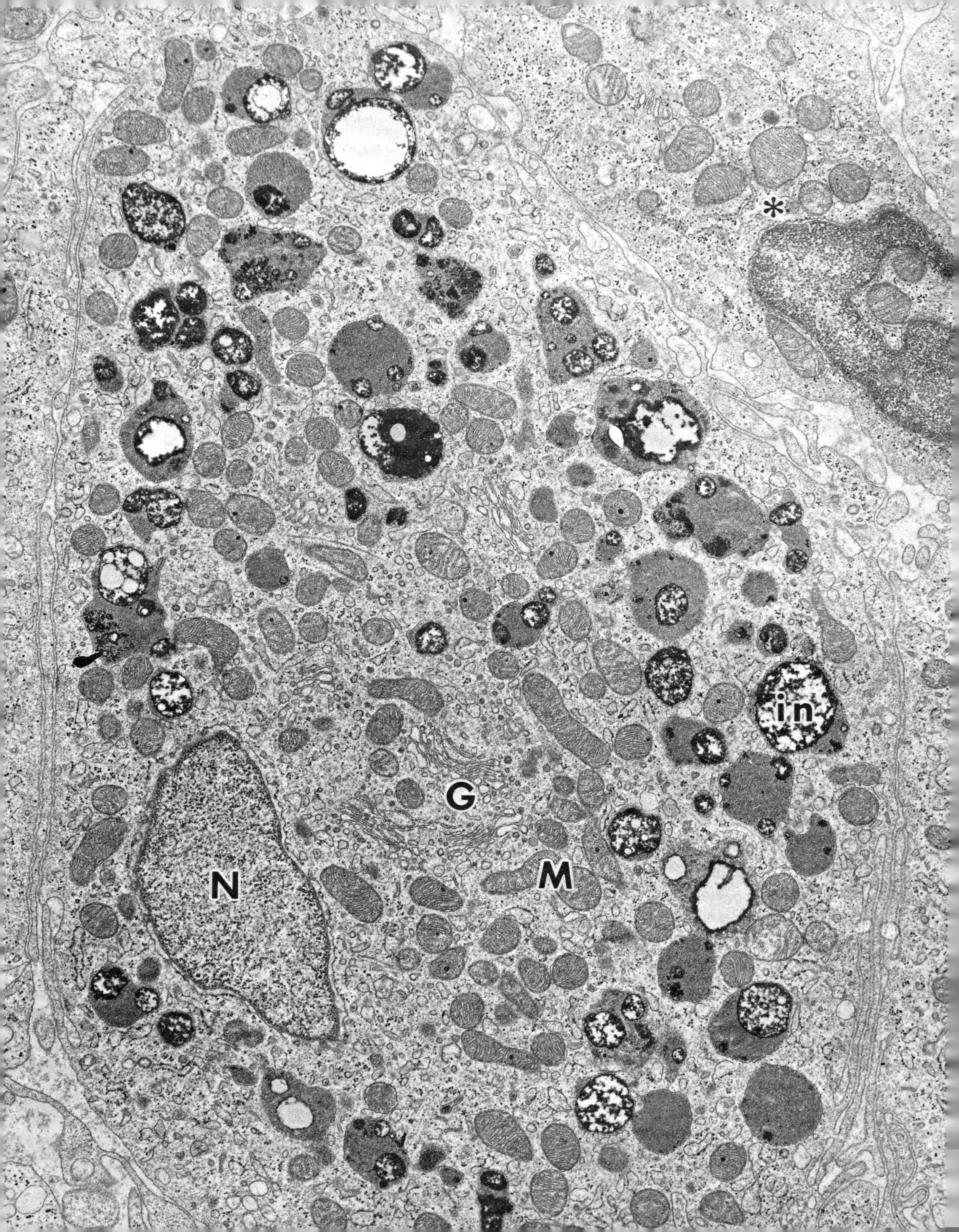

*
in
G
N
M

FIGURE 7-40. Granuloma in human marrow.
This macrophage and mononuclear cell (*asterisk*) are from same specimen shown in Figure 7-39. In addition to the nucleus (*N*), there are many inclusions (*in*), of nearly uniform size, containing ingested material. Small vesicles, numerous mitochondria (*M*), and a large Golgi apparatus (*G*) are present. This was interpreted as an epithelioid cell in smears and histologic sections. The mononuclear cell (*asterisk*) is more characteristic in this granuloma and does not appear to be either a typical monocyte or lymphocyte, nor was there any granulocytosis in the lesion. × *15,400.*

Figures 7-41 and 7-42 appear on the following pages ⇨

FIGURE 7-41. Granuloma in human marrow.
In this section from the same specimen shown in Figures 7-39 and 7-40, the cytoplasm has many mitochondria (*M*) and inclusions (*in*) containing unidentified amorphous and granular material. × *15,400.*

FIGURE 7-42. Macrophage in Niemann-Pick disease.
Large lipid-laden inclusions in macrophage from marrow of "adult" type Niemann-Pick disease are similar to lipid inclusions seen in the infantile form, although this size is uncommon. The nucleus (*N*) is eccentrically located. The Golgi complex (*G*) and mitochondria (*M*) are apparent. × *10,000.*

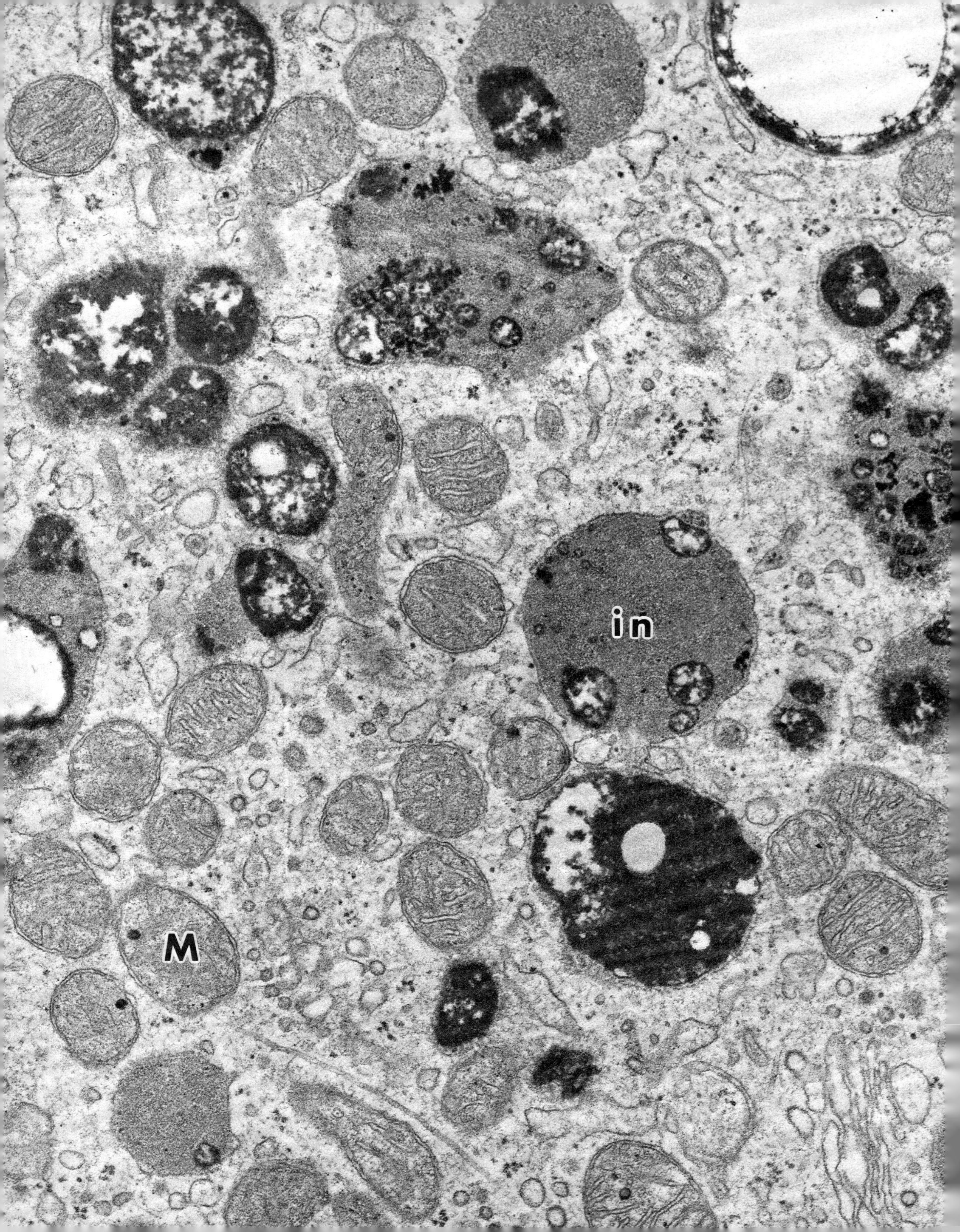
in
M

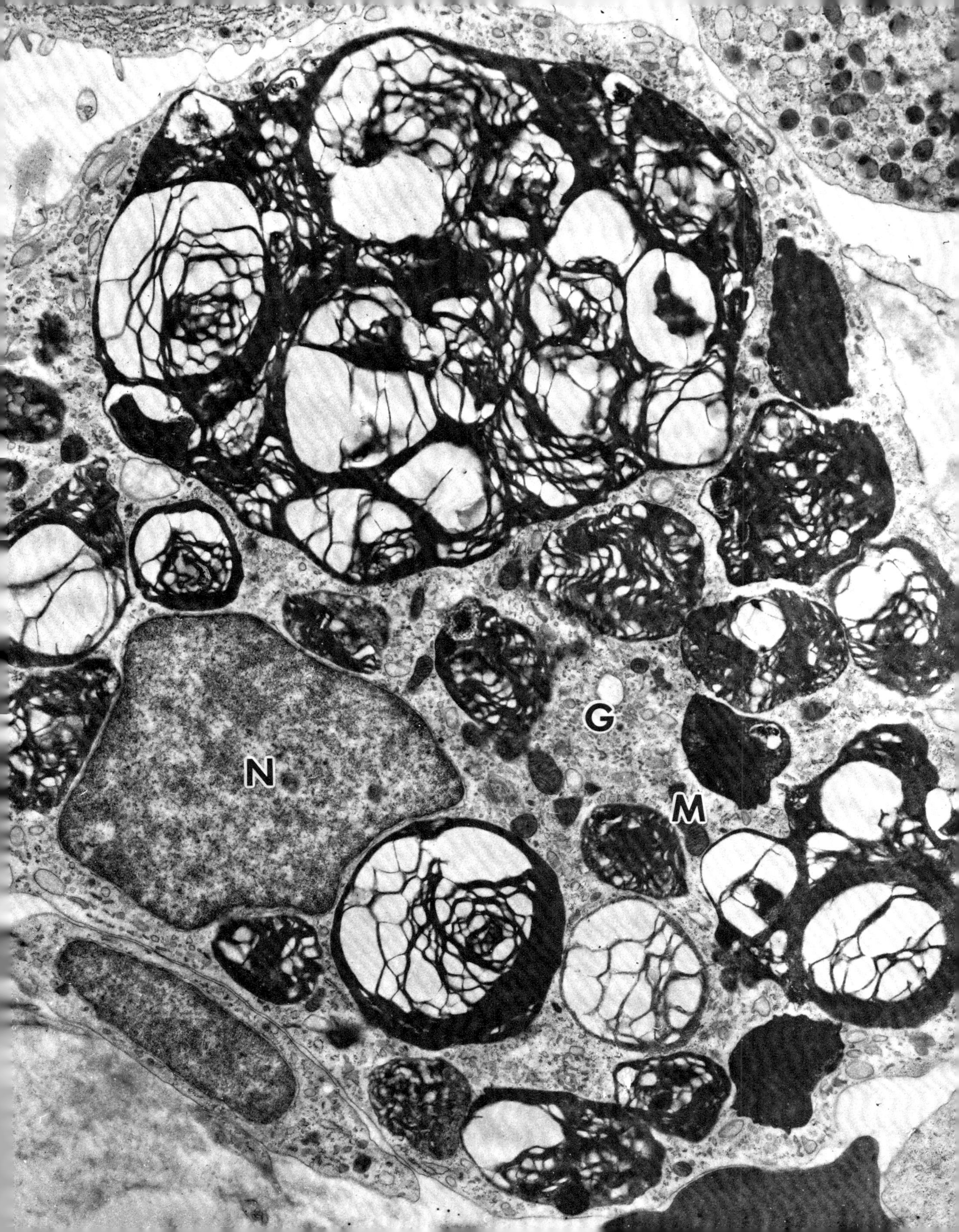
G
N
M

structures of about 130 to 400 Å in thickness. These ultrastructural characteristics of lipid granules have been confirmed by many (Fischer and Reidbord, 1962; Jordan, 1964; Pennelli *et al.,* 1969), with minor modifications. Similar tubules have been isolated from the abnormal lipid of Gaucher's disease (Lee *et al.,* 1967), but in contrast to the other lipidoses, no myelin figures have been identified in these lipid granules. This is possibly due to decreased water solubility of the monohexose sphingosine which is present in these lipid granules. The mechanism of formation of the tubular patterns is unknown, though it has been suggested that they may originate from mitochondria. This hypothesis is based on the study of forms intermediate between intact mitochondria and lipid granules (Fischer and Reidbord, 1962) whose origin is uncertain. However, monohexose sphingosine is a normal constituent of red blood cells, and the absence of a specific enzyme may result in the continuous accumulation of this cerebroside from degenerating red cells (Pennelli *et al.,* 1969) in the cytoplasm of macrophages.

Niemann-Pick Disease. Inherited abnormal lipid metabolism which causes the accumulation of sphingomyelin in tissues was first described by Niemann in 1914. The disease is separated from Gaucher's disease on the basis of the anatomical differences between the disorders (Pick, 1927). Thus the disease now bears the names of both investigators. The disease is rare, with strong predilection for Jewish families. The biochemical nature of the accumulated lipid was identified as sphingomyelin by Klenk in 1934. It manifests itself in early infancy, and patients generally die within several months after the onset of clinical symptoms. Those who survive to puberty are considered to have the adult type of Niemann-Pick disease. As in other lipidoses, the defect is apparently the lack of an enzyme, in this situation, required for the metabolic breakdown of sphingomyelin (Brady, 1966). No abnormal elevation of serum lipids has been demonstrated in these patients.

In this disease, proliferating macrophages are referred to as Niemann-Pick cells. They are more than 40μ in diameter and have a foamy or honeycomb appearance, in contrast to the wrinkled homogeneous appearance of Gaucher cells. The cells have one or two nuclei; rarely, a few are multinuclear. The lipid granules of these cells stain blue to colorless with the May-Grünwald-Giemsa stain. Histochemically, granules stain positively in Sudan black B and PAS. Double refractile bodies and Maltese crosses are recognized frequently in these granules. An electron microscopic study of Niemann-Pick cells by Tanaka *et al.* (1963) included one case of adult type and three of the infantile form. Considerable variation was noted in the morphology of lipid granules in the adult type, whereas lipid granules observed in three infants appeared more uniform. Lamellar arrangements of electron-opaque materials were seen in these

(*text continues on page 404*)

FIGURE 7-43. Inclusions in Niemann-Pick disease.
A. Spherical lipid inclusions with distinctive lamellar structures from Niemann-Pick disease (as in Figure 7-42) are uncommon in the infantile form. There are numerous clear areas in the cores of these inclusions. × *22,000.*
B. Inclusion has a large area of clear zones in honeycomb or crystal array. The clear spaces may represent substances lost in specimen preparation. × *48,000.*

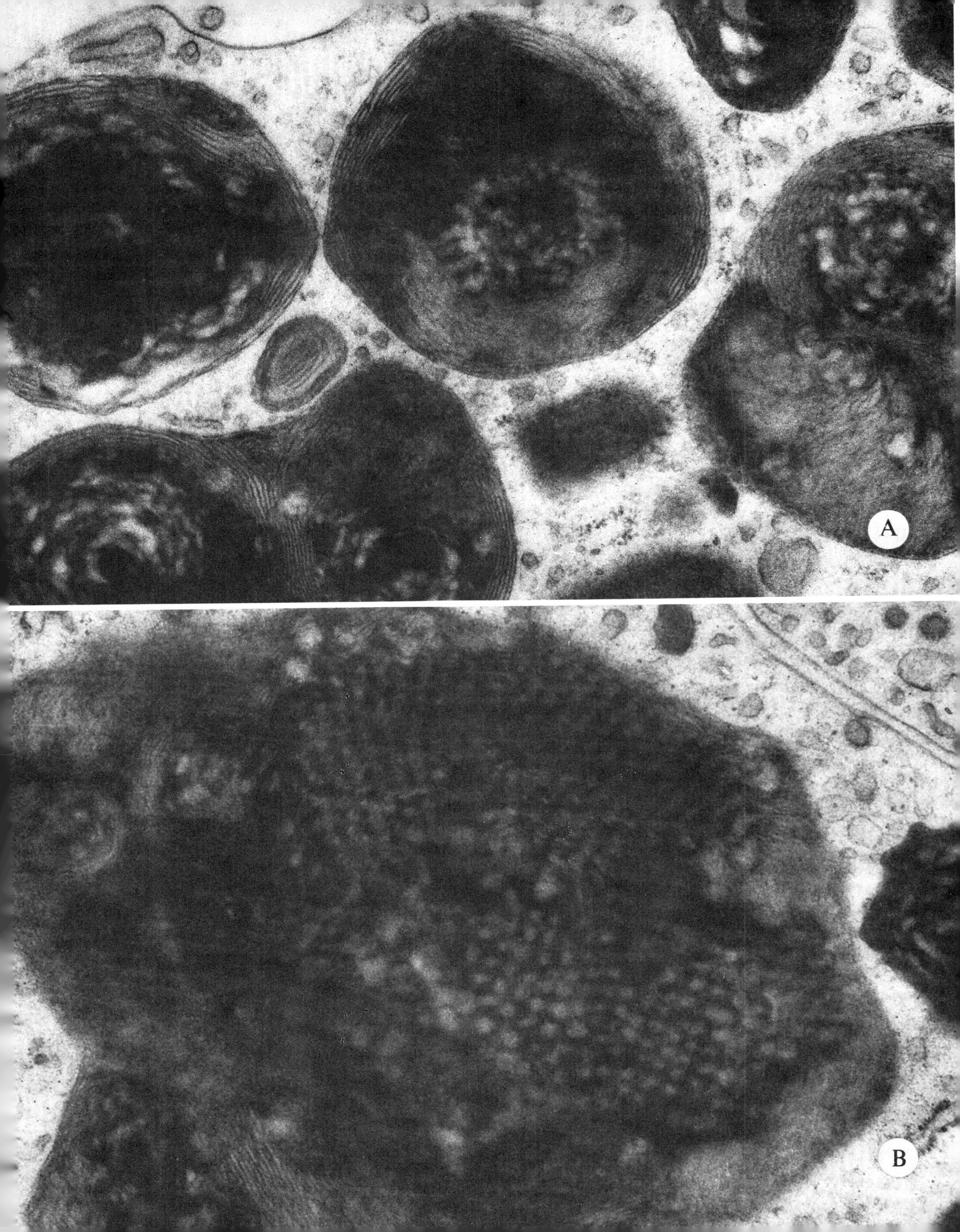
A
B

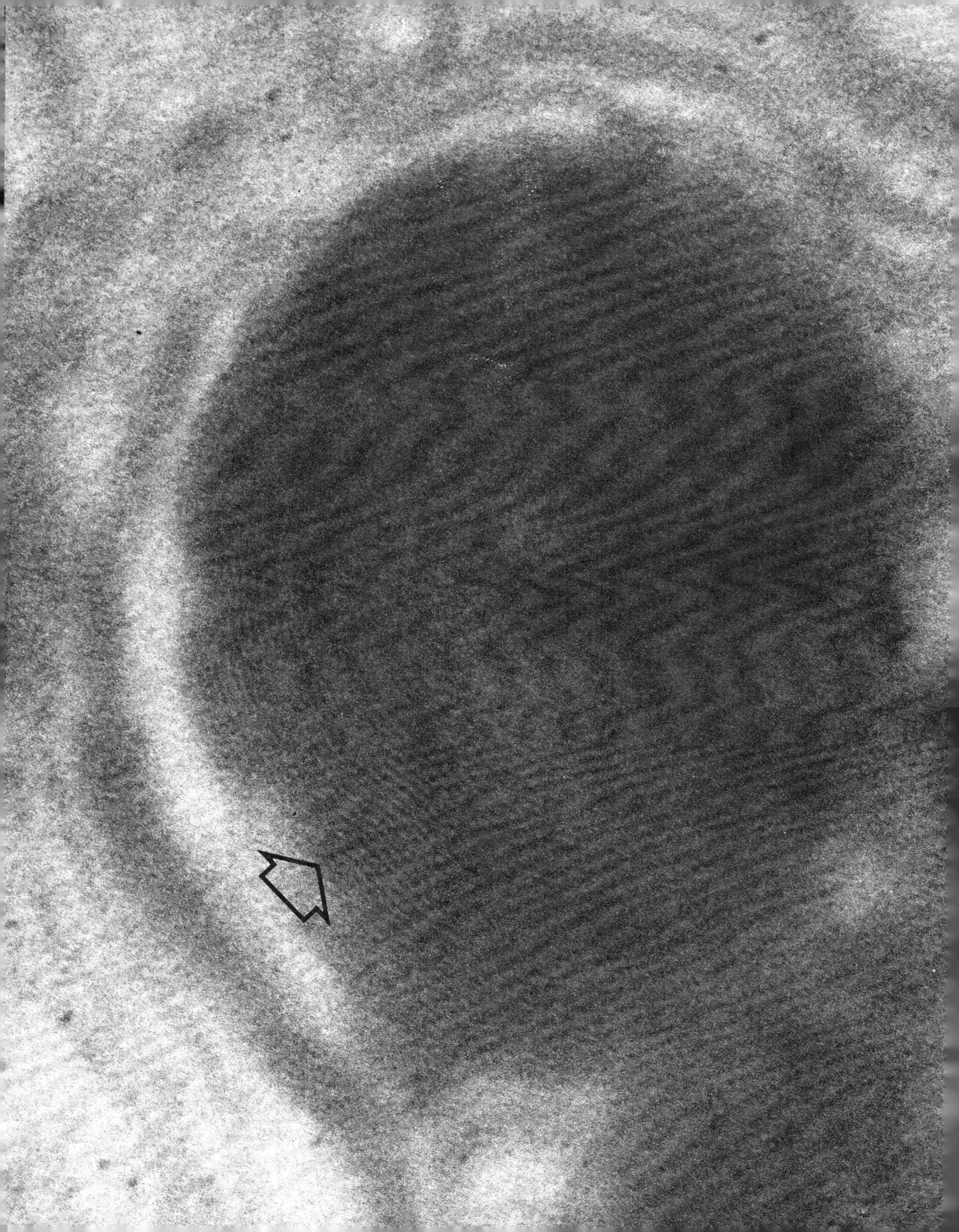

FIGURE 7-44. Inclusion in Niemann-Pick disease.
Electron-opaque spheroid has well-developed myelin-like structure (*arrow*) and 40 to 50 Å periodicity of layers. × *472,000.*

Figures 7-45 and 7-46 appear on the following pages

FIGURE 7-45. Inclusion in Fabry's disease.
These electron-dense lipid inclusions in macrophage from marrow in Fabry's disease have many small ring-like structures (*open arrow*) along with lamellar masses (*asterisks*). The fine dense granules are many ferritin particles free in the cytoplasm. A portion of a mitochondrion (*M*) is present. × *49,000.*

FIGURE 7-46. Lamellated structures in macrophages in Fabry's disease.
A. Small ring-like structures. × *472,000.*
B. Lamellar masses. × *472,000.*

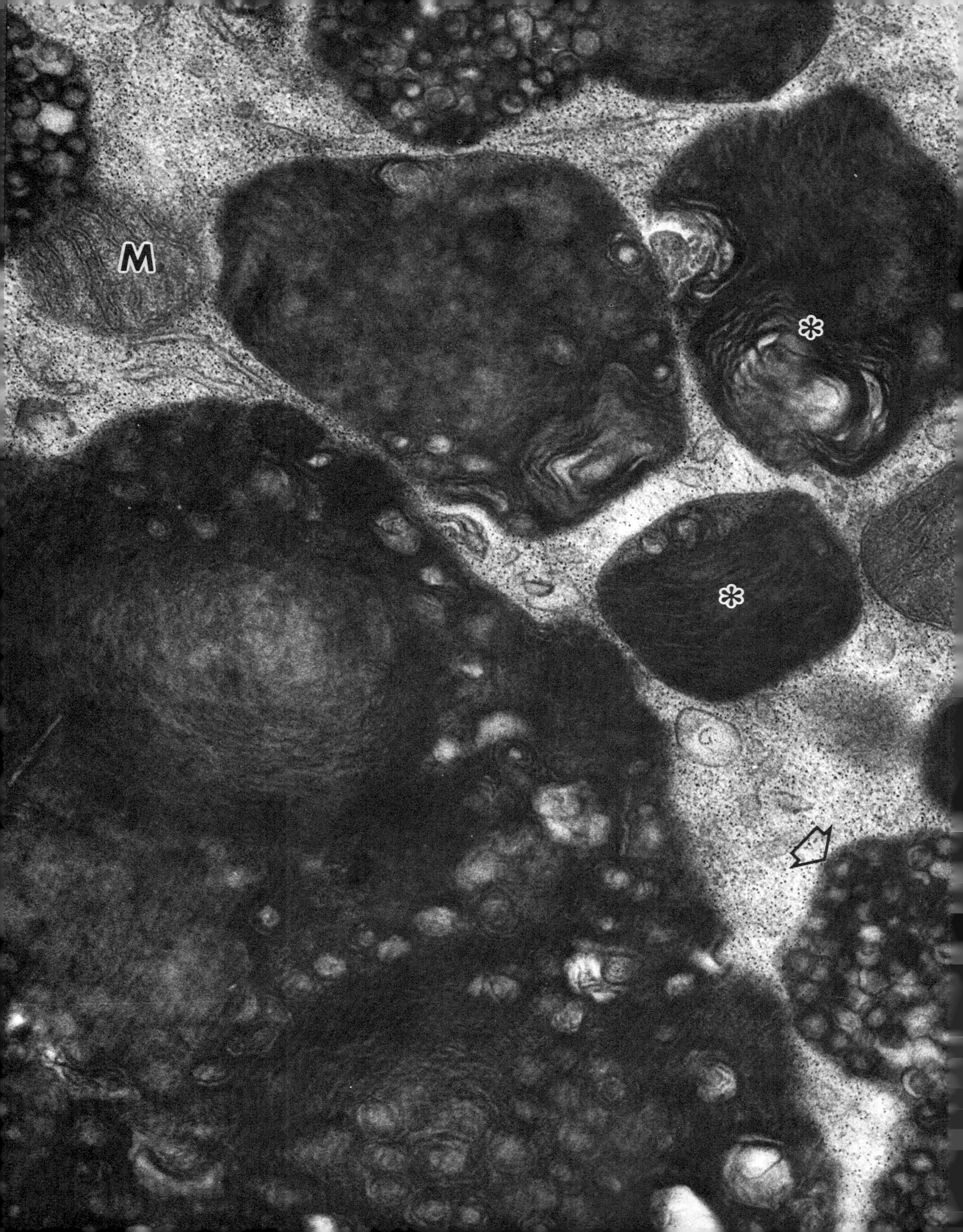
M

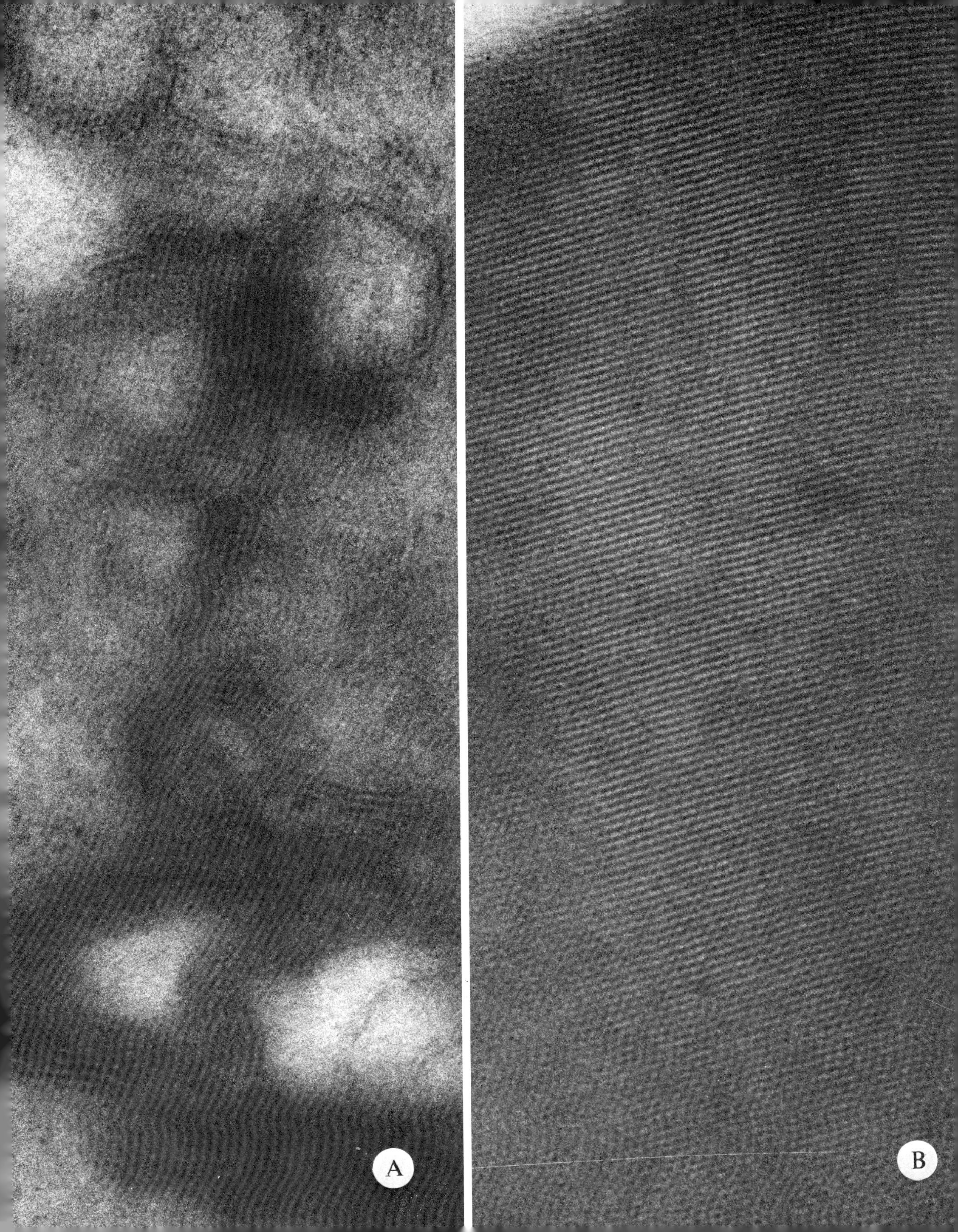
A
B

granules (Figs. 7-42 through 7-44). Some of the granules had myelin figures consisting of alternatively arranged, electron-opaque and translucent zones of about 40 to 50 Å (Lynn and Terry, 1964) (Fig. 7-44). Granules in the adult case showed clear spaces resembling crystals in the dense granule cores (Fig. 7-43). Deposition of lipid has also been observed in lymphocytes and neutrophils in the peripheral blood (Abt and Bloom, 1928; Lazarus *et al.*, 1967). The myelin figures are also found in the endothelial cells of the bone marrow (Tanaka *et al.*, 1963).

Fabry's Disease. Generalized deposition of abnormal lipid in Fabry's disease, also known as angiokeratoma corporis diffusum (Anderson, 1898), has been reported. It was first described by Fabry in 1898 under the term "purpura hemorrhagica nodularis," but is now categorized within the systemic disorders of lipid metabolism. Ceramide-trihexoside has been isolated from tissues of both biopsied and surgically removed specimens (Sweeley and Klionsky, 1963). Lipid deposits in various epithelial and interstitial cells have been reported (Frost *et al.*, 1966) which, histochemically, are positive to both Sudan black and PAS reaction. By these tests they cannot be distinguished from the lipid accumulations observed in Niemann-Pick disease. The unique feature of this disorder is the presence of lipid deposits in endothelial cells of systemic blood vessels (Frost *et al.*, 1966). These deposits lead to irreversible distention of small vessels and result in the abnormal skin eruptions known as angiokeratomas. Similar vascular involvement in the kidney results in dysfunction of the organ leading to uremic death.

Electron microscopy shows extensive intracellular deposition of electron-opaque material in various tissues. This material has an alternately arranged electron-opaque and pale periodicity of about 40 Å. Rarely, large macrophages containing these lipid granules are noted in bone marrow smears; they may be disrupted in preparation of the smear. Electron microscopic examination shows many interstitial cells with various forms of deposited lipids (Fig. 7-45). One of the most characteristic features of these granules is the presence of both honeycomb and lamellated structures consisting of many small myelin figures of about 40 to 50 Å in periodicity (Fig. 7-46) (Tanaka *et al.*, 1965). The honeycomb structures are rare in the other lipidoses which we have examined.

Sarcoidosis

Nonmalignant, non-necrotizing proliferation of large reticulum cells is observed in lymph nodes of various diseases. One of the most prominent examples of this condition is sarcoidosis, which is characterized histologically by numerous scattered miliary nodules consisting of both epithelioid and giant cells (Fig. 7-47). The morphology of the latter elements is similar to that of Langhans' cells in tuberculosis. No significant lymphocytic proliferation has been observed around the epithelioid cell nests. The condition was noticed by both Boeck and Hutchinson in 1869,* documented by Besnier in 1889, and described in detail by Boeck in 1905. The etiology of this disease is still unknown.

We have included illustrations of these cells because proliferating cells in sarcoidosis have a unique ultrastructural characteristic which may suggest another functional aspect of the reticulum cell. These cells have no significant phagocytotic activity. Production of an amyloid-like substance around the proliferating

* Cited by Siltzbach, L. E. Sarcoidosis. *Therap Notes* *15*:157, 1968.

(*text continues on page 414*)

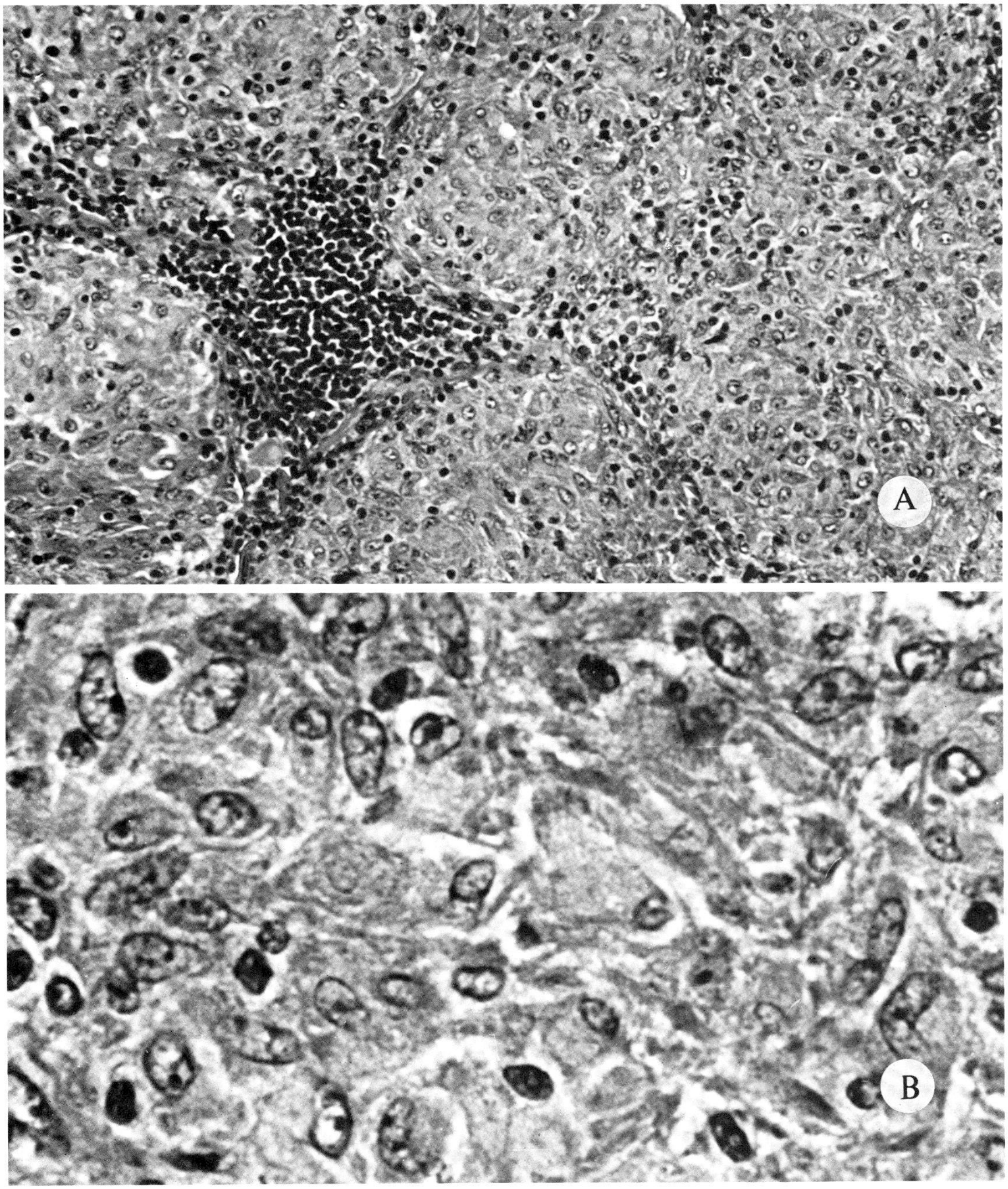

FIGURE 7-47. Typical sarcoidosis in human lymph node.
A. Nodular proliferation of epithelioid cell. × *250.*
B. Detail of epithelioid cell nodule. × *1,000.*

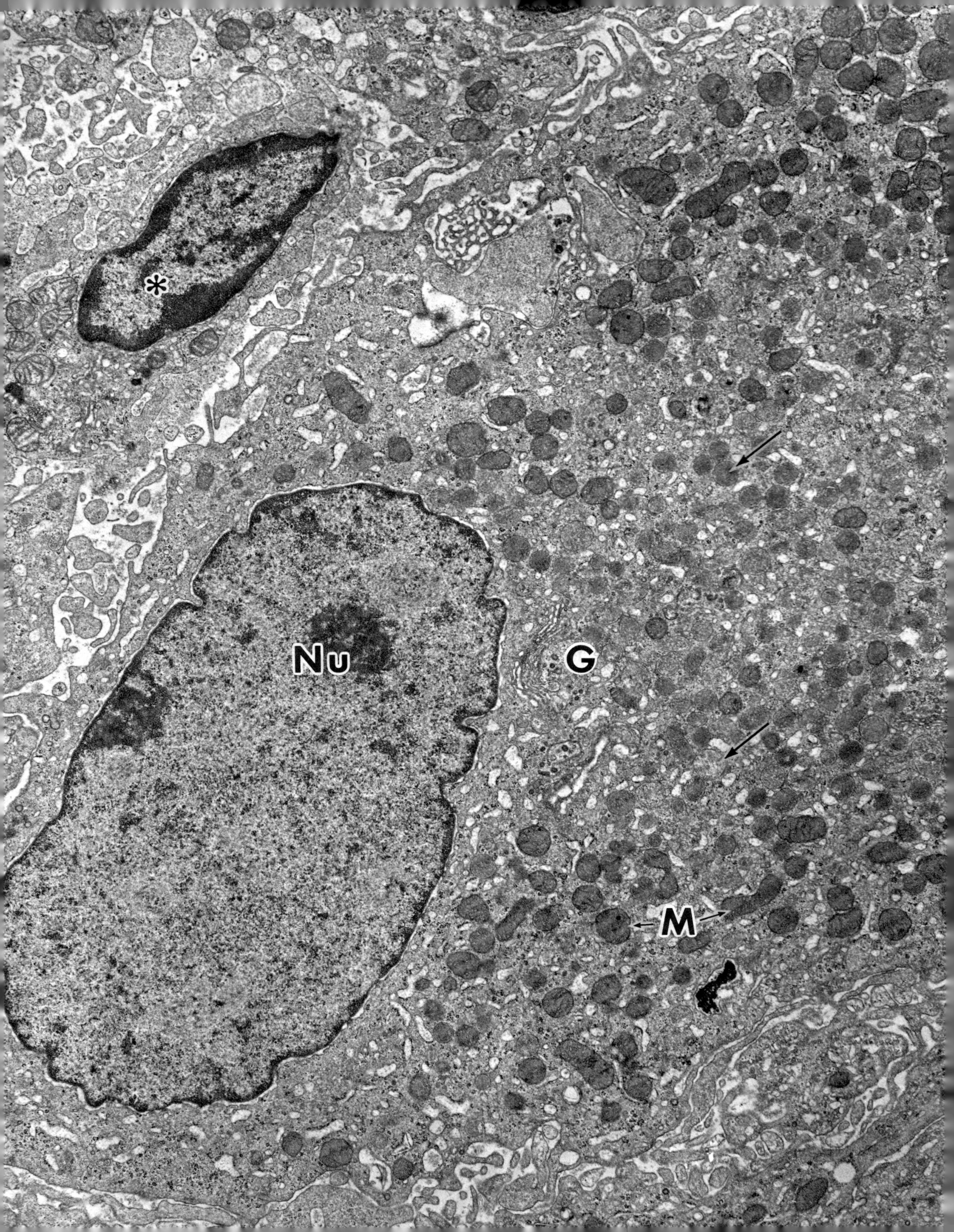
*
Nu
G
M

FIGURE 7-48. Sarcoidosis.
Large epithelioid cell is from lymph node shown in Figure 7-47. Cell surface is highly irregular, with many indentations and fine projections. The nuclear outline is slightly indented and two nuclei (*Nu*) are present. The cytoplasm has a vesicular appearance, with widespread smooth endoplasmic reticulum, many small rounded mitochondria (*M*), numerous spherical inclusions (*arrows*), several profiles of the Golgi apparatus (*G*), and a smaller unidentified mononuclear cell (*asterisk*). × *8,700.*

Figures 7-49 and 7-50 appear on the following pages ⇨

FIGURE 7-49. Sarcoidosis.
Cells are from same specimens shown in Figures 7-47 and 7-48.
A. Cytoplasmic detail reveals small mitochondria (*M*), many small single membrane inclusions (*in*) containing unidentified material, and smooth endoplasmic reticulum (*ser*) that is occasionally associated with ribosomes (*arrow*). × *46,000.*
B. In cytoplasm from a different cell, inclusions (*in*) contain more dense material in larger amounts, which may result from coalescence of smaller inclusions. × *29,000.*

FIGURE 7-50. Marrow in histiocytosis X.
The nucleus (*N*) of one of these malignant cells from bone marrow of a patient with histiocytosis X has two large prominent nucleoli (*Nu*) centrally located in reticular chromatin. The cytoplasm has many polyribosomes, a few round to ovoid mitochondria (*M*), and several distended cisternae in endoplasmic reticulum (*er*). × *21,000.*

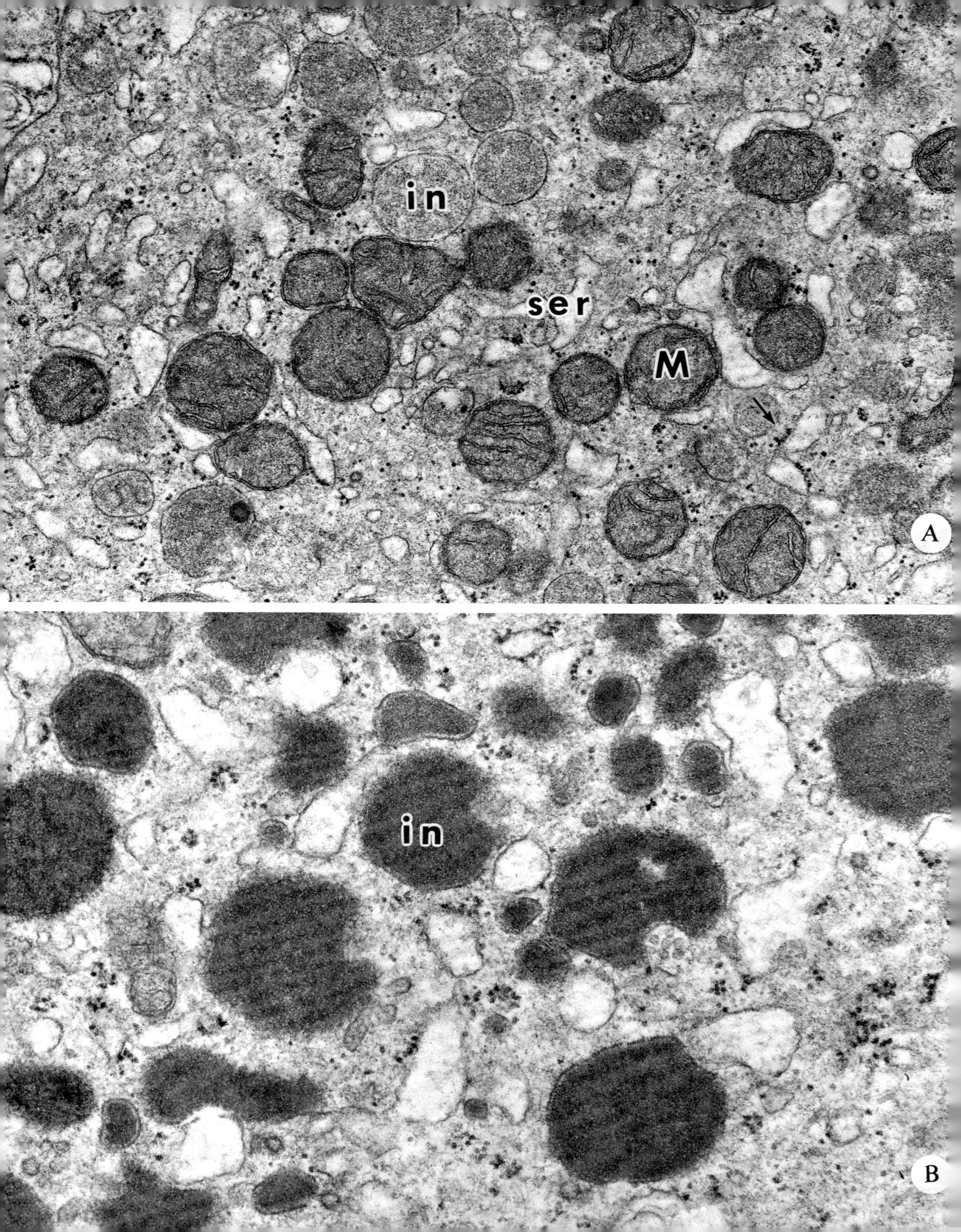

in
ser
M
A
in
B

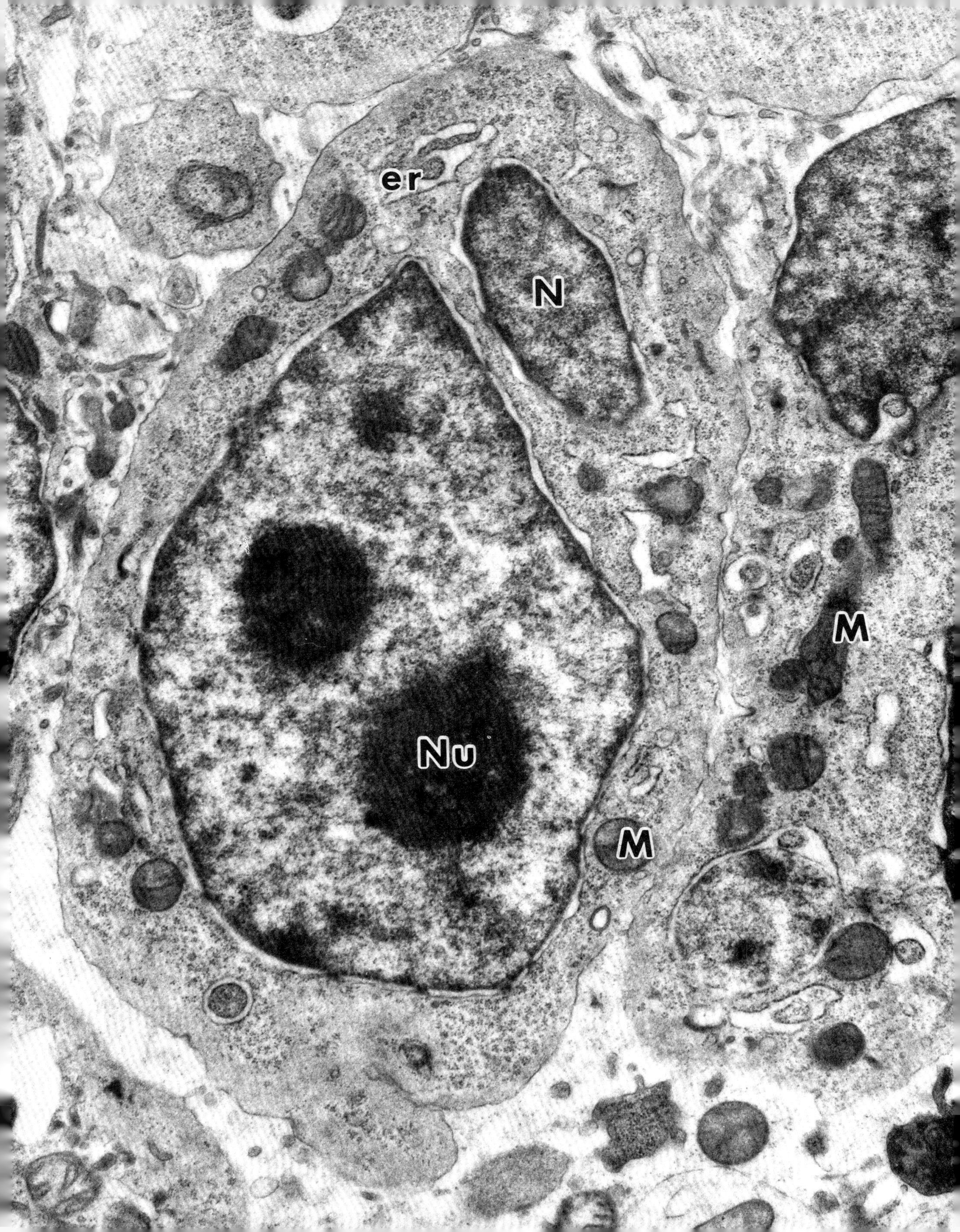
er
N
Nu
M
M

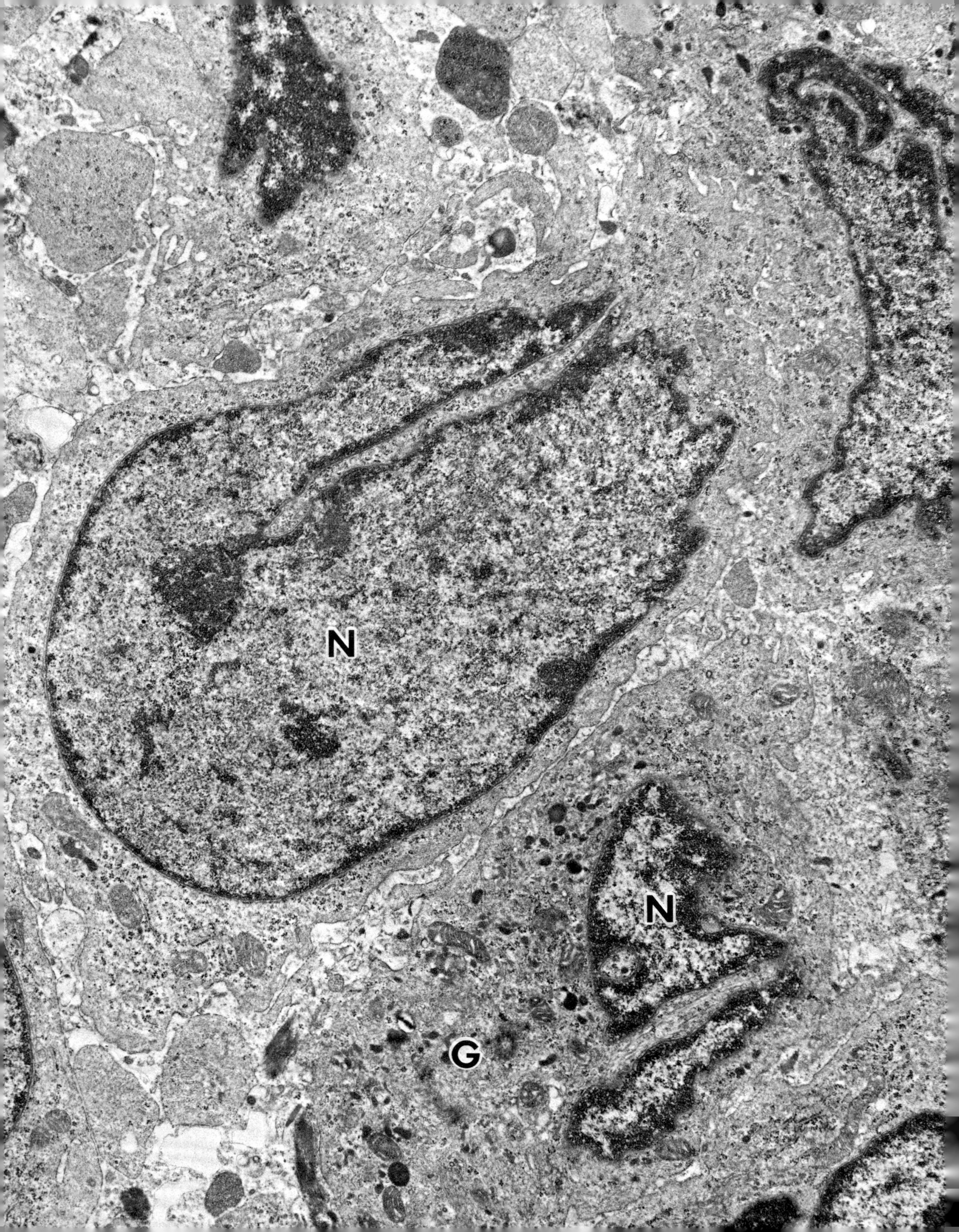
N
N
G

FIGURE 7-51. Oral mucosa in histiocytosis X.
In these characteristic cells from oral mucosa of another patient with histiocytosis X, the nuclei (*N*) are highly indented. The cytoplasm is extended in almost an ameboid manner, with numerous vesicles and fine fibrils (see Figs. 7-52 and 7-53), and dense mitochondria and Golgi areas (*G*). × *14,800.*

Figures 7-52 and 7-53 appear on the following pages

FIGURE 7-52. Oral mucosa in histiocytosis X.
This malignant cell is from the same specimen as that in Figure 7-51. Nucleus (*N*) and cell have irregular surfaces. There are numerous fine fibrils (*fb*), rough endoplasmic reticulum (*er*), and dense mitochondria (*M*). × *40,000.*

FIGURE 7-53. Histiocytosis X.
These cytoplasmic details are in cells from the same case illustrated in Figures 7-51 and 7-52.
A. Many small dense granules with lamellated internal structures (*open arrow*) and many fine tubular profiles (*arrow*) are scattered throughout. A mitochondrion (*M*), a tangential cut of centriole (*Ce*), and edge of the nucleus (*N*) are seen. × *48,000.*
B. Rough endoplasmic reticulum (*er*) is distended. There are irregular ribosome distribution, many small dense mitochondria (*M*), and portion of the nucleus (*N*). × *48,000.*

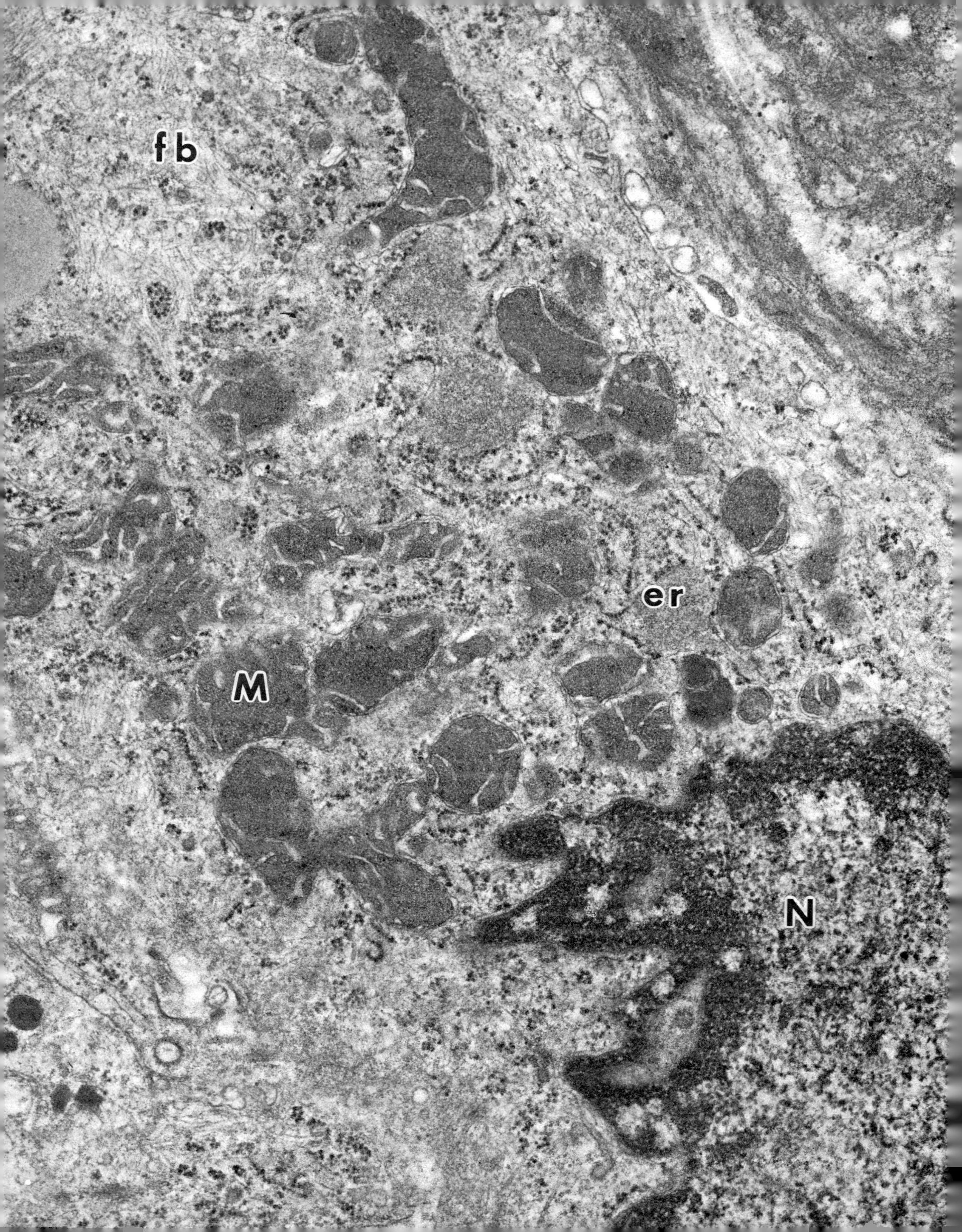

fb
er
M
N

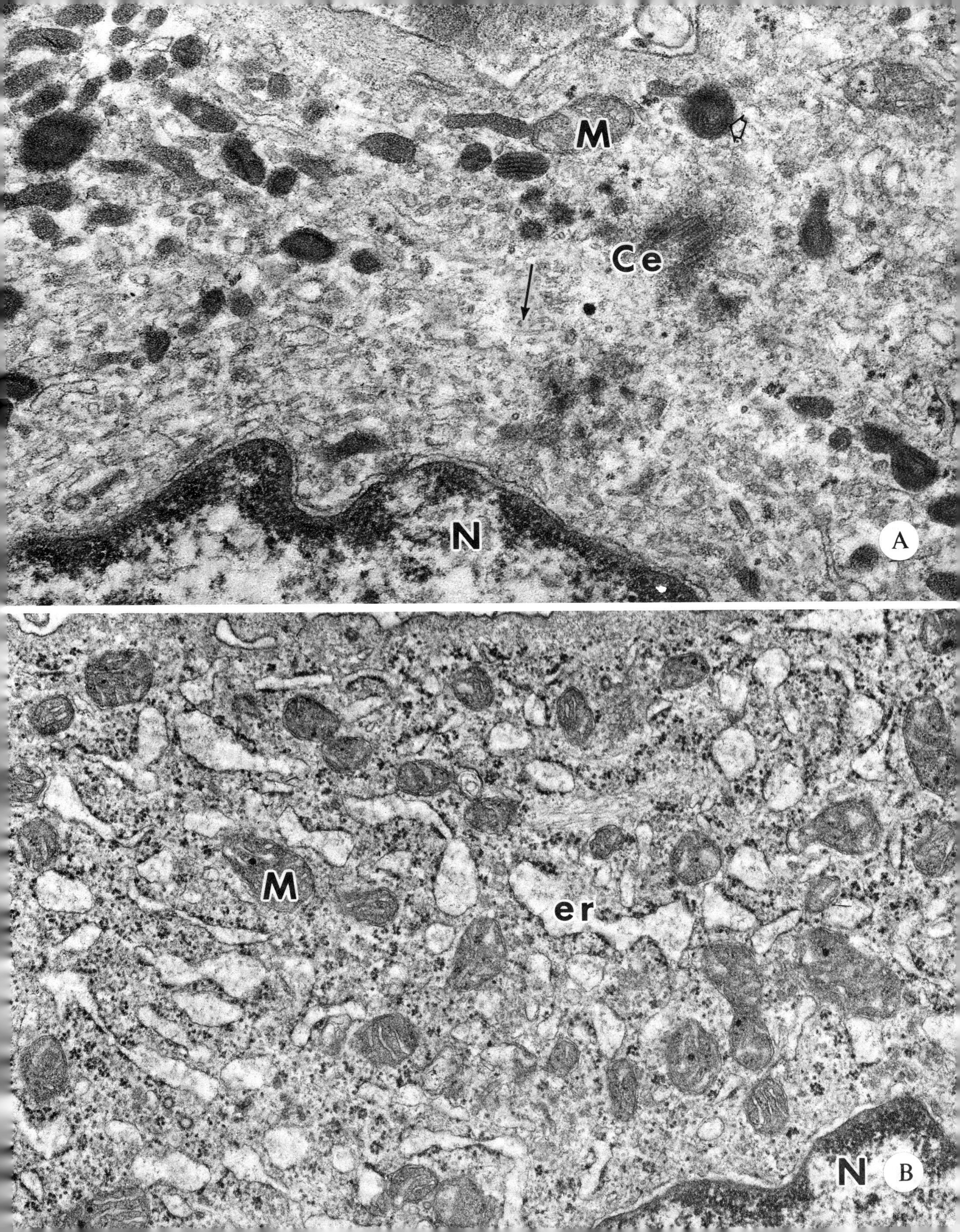
M
Ce
N
A
M
er
N
B

cell foci, the formation of crystalloid structures in the cells (astroid), and the association of hyperglobulinemia are common. These features suggest that the proliferating cells may produce a protein-like substance. The ultrastructural details of these proliferating cells have been described by Wanstrup and Christensen (1966) and Mori and Lennert (1969). These epithelioid cells are large and their endoplasmic reticulum (Fig. 7-48) has an accumulation of fine granular material in the cisternae (Fig. 7-49*A*). The cytoplasm also contains many mitochondria, cytoplasmic spheroids about 0.5 to 1μ in size (Fig. 7-49*B*), and fibrillar structures. These cells may represent a bizarre form of reticulum cell morphology. A collagen nature of the astroid bodies observed has also been suggested (Azar and Lunardelli, 1969). Though it has not been proved, it is possible that reticulum cells with similar morphology might participate in the production of IgM antibodies.

MALIGNANT PROLIFERATION OF RETICULUM CELLS

This type of malignancy, common in the lymph nodes, is seen rarely in bone marrow (less than 1 per cent of these malignancies are in marrow). The morphology of such malignant reticulum cells has been amply described (Bernhard and Leplus, 1964; Mori and Lennert, 1969). Malignant proliferation of reticulohistiocytic cells in bone marrow may appear as the local manifestation of the systemic disorder. Pathologically, two types of the disease can be distinguished. The first is a type involving blood-forming organs primarily, with occasional leukemic manifestations which are sometimes difficult to distinguish from monocytic leukemia. The second is a type involving the skin primarily, with proliferating histiocytic appearance. This type is more common in children than in adults, may be neoplastic, and is known by many related terms, including Letterer-Siwe and Hand-Schüller-Christian disease.

We examined a case diagnosed as histiocytosis X which involved the bone marrow, and found the cytological characteristics of the malignant cells in smears to be comparable to those of histiocytes described elsewhere. The ultrastructural detail of proliferating cells in bone marrow showed a lymphoid appearance with significant pleomorphism (Fig. 7-50). Frequent indentations of the nucleus and prominent nucleoli are common. Mitochondria appear as electron-opaque rods distributed at random throughout the cytoplasm. Polyribosomes in the cytoplasm and dilated endoplasmic reticulum are common. The ultrastructural appearance is comparable to that of immature cells observed in the interstitial space of lymphoreticular tissues. Proliferating cells in these lesions, which were histologically compatible with histiocytosis X, were studied in a specimen of submucosa from an infant. Mononuclear cells showed all the characteristics of histiocytes (Figs. 7-51 and 7-52) except for the absence of phagocytosis. The nucleus was highly indented and the cytoplasm contained many small vesicles, dense inclusions (Fig. 7-53*A*), polyribosomes, and fibrils (Figs. 7-51 and 7-52). The cell membrane was frequently distorted and irregular. Occasionally cells with a large amount of endoplasmic reticulum with distended cisternae were present (Fig. 7-53*B*). The frequent appearance of cells with distended endoplasmic reticulum in reticulum cell sarcoma suggests that they may produce some proteins. Cytoplasmic inclusions have also been described (Jarnowski and Hashimoto, 1967), called Langerhan's bodies, in cells of histiocytosis X. However, no similar structures were seen in cells studied in this case.

REFERENCES

Abt, A. F., and Bloom, W. Essential lipoid histiocytosis (type Niemann-Pick. *JAMA 90*:2076, 1928.

Adler, F. L., Fishman, M., and Dray, S. Antibody formation initiated *in vitro*. III. Antibody formation and allotypic specificity directed by ribonucleic acid from peritoneal exudate cells. *J Immun 97*:554, 1966.

Akazaki, K. Reticulo-endothelial system. *Acta Path Jap 2*:113, 1952.

Akazaki, K., and Watanuki, S. The concept of reticulo-endothelial system. (In Japanese.) *Handbook Hemat 1*:630, 1963.

Amano, S., and Tanaka, H. Further observation of plasma cell generation from the vascular adventitial cells through metamorphosis by ultrathin sections under electron microscope. *Acta Haemat Jap 19*:738, 1956.

Anderson, W. A case of "angio-keratoma." *Brit J Dermat 10*:113, 1898.

Aschoff, L. Das reticulo-endotheliale system. *Ergeb Inn Med Kinderheilk 26*:1, 1924.

Askonas, B. A., and Rhodes, J. M. Immunogenicity of antigen-containing ribonucleic acid preparations from macrophages. *Nature (London) 205*: 470, 1965.

Azar, H. A. and Lunardelli, C. Collagen nature of asteroid bodies of giant cells in sarcoidosis. *Amer J Path 57*:81, 1969.

Becker, A. J., McCulloch, E. A., and Till, J. E. Cytological demonstration of the clonal nature of spleen colonies derived from transplanted mouse marrow cells. *Nature (London) 197*:452, 1963.

Bergmann, W. Ueber den Feinbau der Knochenmarkskapillaren. *Z Zellforsch 11*:1, 1930.

Bernhard, W., and Leplus, R. *Fine Structure of the Normal and Malignant Human Lymph Node.* MacMillan, New York, 1964.

Berry, L. J., and Spies, T. D. Phagocytosis. *Medicine 28*:239, 1949.

Besnier, M. E. Lupus perino de la face. Synovites fongueuses (scrofulo tuberculosis) symétrique des extrémitiés supérieures. *Ann Derm Syph (Paris) 10* (Series 2):333, 1889.

Bessis, M. *Cytology of the Blood and Blood-Forming Organs* (Ponder, E., transl.). Grune & Stratton, New York, 1956.

Bloom, W. Fibroblasts and macrophages. *Handbook Hemat 2*:1337, 1938.

Boeck, C. Fortesetzte Untersuchungen über das multiple benigne Sarkoid. *Arch Derm Syph 73*: 71, 301, 1905.

Brady, R. O., Kanfer, J. N., and Shapiro, D. Metabolism of glucocerebrosides. II. Evidence of an enzymatic deficiency in Gaucher's disease. *Biochem Biophys Res Commun 18*:221, 1965.

Brady, R. O. The sphingolipidoses. *New Eng J Med 275*:312, 1966.

Brånemark, P. I. Bone marrow microvascular structure and function. *Advances Microcirc 1*:1, 1968.

Caffrey, R. W., Everett, N. B., and Rieke, W. O. Radioautographic studies of reticular and blast cells in the hemopoietic tissues of the rat. *Anat Rec 155*:41, 1966.

Caffrey Tyler, R. W., and Everett, N. B. Radioautographic study of hemopoietic repopulation using irradiated parabiotic rats. Relation to the stem cell problem. *Blood 28*:873, 1966.

Calvo, W. The innervation of the bone marrow in laboratory animals. *Amer J Anat 123*:315, 1968.

Cohn, Z. A. The structure and function of monocytes and macrophages. *Advances Immunol 9*: 163, 1968.

Cohn, Z. A., and Wiener, E. The particulate hydrolases of macrophages. I. Comparative enzymology, isolation and properties. *J Exp Med 118*: 991, 1963.

Crosby, W. H. Experience with Injured and Implanted Bone Marrow: Relation of Function to Structure. In *Hemopoietic Cellular Proliferation* (Stohlman, F. Jr., ed.) Grune & Stratton, New York, 1970, p. 87.

Daems, W. Th., and Brederoo, P. The fine structural and peroxidase activity of resident and exudate peritoneal macrophages in the guinea pig. In "The Reticuloendothelial System and Immune Phenomena" (Di Luzio, N. R. and Jacques, P. J., eds.). *Advances in Experimental Medicine and Biology.* Plenum Press, New York, 1971, vol. 15, pp. 19–31.

DeMarsh, Q. B., and Kautz, J. The submicroscopic morphology of Gaucher cell. *Blood 12*:324, 1957.

Doan, C. A. The capillaries of the bone marrow of the adult pigeon. *Bull Hopkins Hosp 33*:222, 1922.

Doan, C. A. The reticulo-endothelial system: Its physiology and pathology. *J Lab Clin Med 26*: 89, 1940.

Dollberg, L., Casper, J., Djaldetti, M., Klibansky, C. and de Vries, A. Lipid-laden histiocytes in the spleen in thrombocytopenic purpura. *Amer J Clin Path 43*:16, 1965.

Drinker, C. K., Drinker, K. R., and Lund, C. C. The circulation in the mammalian bone marrow. *Amer J Physiol 62*:1, 1922.

Dumont, A. Ultrastructural study of the maturation of peritoneal macrophages in the hamster. *J Ultrastruct Res 29*:191, 1969.

Ecker, E. E., Weisberger, A. S., and Pillemer, L. The opsonins of normal and immune sera. I. Methods. A comparison of the effects of normal and immune opsonins on staphylococcus aureus. *J Immun 43*:227, 1942.

Ehrenreich, B. A., and Cohn, Z. A. The uptake and digestion of iodinated human serum albumin by macrophages *in vitro*. *J Exp Med 126*:941, 1967.

Epstein, E. Beitrag zur Chemie der Gaucherschen Krankeit. *Biochem Z 145*:398, 1924.

Fabry, J. Ein Beitrag zur Kenntniss der purpura hemorrhagica nodulairs (purpura papulosa hemorrhagica Habrae). *Arch Derm Syph 43*:187, 1898.

Fedorko, M. E., and Hirsch, J. G. Structure of monocytes and macrophages. *Seminars Hemat 7*:109, 1970.

Ferrata, A. *Le Empatie*. Societa Editrice Libraria, Milano, 1918.

Ferrata, A. Sulla pathogenesi e sulla essenza della anemie a tipo pernicioso. *Haematologica 1*:48, 1920.

Ferrata, A. Studi sulle emopatie. I. Sulla istogenesi della leucemia granulocitica. *Haematologica 2*:242, 1921.

Fischer, E. R., and Reidbord, U. Gaucher's disease; pathogenetic considerations based on electron microscopic and histochemical observations. *Amer J Path 41*:679, 1962.

Fliedner, T., Sandkühler, S., and Stodtmeister, R. Unterschungen uber die Gefassarchitektonik des Knochenmarks der Ratte. *Z Zellforsch 45*: 328, 1956.

Franco, E. E., and Ferrata, A. Cellule istioidi (emoistioblasti) e loro derivati nel sangue circulante. *Arch Sci Med (Torino) 42*:109, 1919.

Fresen, O. The morphological determination of the retothelial system and its pathogenetic importance. *Tohoku J Exp Med 73*:1, 1960.

Fresen, O. The submicroscopical structure of the reticular cell tissue. *Acta Haemat 32*:193, 1964.

Frost, P., Tanaka, Y., and Spaeth, G. L. Fabry's disease—glycolipid lipidosis. Histochemical and electron microscopic studies of two cases. *Amer J Med 40*:618, 1966.

Gaucher, P. De l'Épithélioma Primitif de la Rate. Thèse de Paris, 1882.

Goodman, J. R., and Moore, R. E. Electron microscopic study of phagocytosis of staphylococcus by human leukocytes. *J Bact 71*:547, 1956a.

Goodman, J. R., Moore, R. E., and Baker, R. F. Electron microscopic study of phagocytosis of staphylococcus by human leukocytes. II. Virulent and non-virulent staphylococci. *J Bact 72*: 736, 1956b.

Goodman, J. R., Wallerstein, R. O., and Hall, S. G. The ultrastructure of bone marrow histiocytes in megaloblastic anemia and the anemia of infections. *Brit J Haemat 14*:471, 1968.

Harris, P. F. Quantitative studies of bone marrow cells in the early stages of final haemopoietic recovery in irradiated guinea pigs. *Brit J Haemat 6*:107, 1960.

Hirsch, J. G., Fedorko, M. E., and Cohn, Z. A. Vesicle fusion and formation at the surface of pinocytotic vacuoles in macrophages. *J Cell Biol 38*:629, 1968.

Howard, J. G., Boak, J. L., and Christie, G. H. Further studies on the transformation of thoracic duct cells into liver macrophages. *Ann NY Acad Sci 129*:327, 1967.

Hudson, G., and Yoffey, J. M. Reticulo-endothelial cells in the bone marrow of the guinea pig. *J Anat 97*:409, 1963.

Hudson, G., and Yoffey, J. M. Ultrastructure of reticuloendothelial elements in guinea pig bone marrow. *J Anat 103*:515, 1968.

Ito, U. Electron microscopic study on benzene intoxicated rat bone marrow, with special reference to its reticuloendothelial structure. *Bull Tokyo Med Dent Univ 12*:1, 1965.

Jaffe, R. H. The reticulo-endothelial system. Its role in pathologic conditions in man *Arch Path 4*:45, 1927.

Jaffe, R. H. The reticulo-endothelial system. *Handbook Hemat 2*:973, 1938.

Jarnowski, W. M., and Hasimoto, K. Langerhans' cell granules in histiocytosis X. The epidermal Langerhans' cell as a macrophage. *Arch Derm 96*:298, 1967.

Jordan, S. W. Electron microscopy of Gaucher's cells. *Exp Molec Path 3*:76, 1964.

Kiyono, K. Blood and tissue leukocyte with special

reference to the histiocytic cell. (In Japanese) *Trans Soc Path Jap 8*:1, 1918.

Klenk, E. Uber die Natur der Phosphatide der Milz bei der Niemann-Pickschen Krankheit. *Z Physiol Chem 229*:151, 1934.

Lambin, P. Recherches sur le rôle hématopoiétique du système réticulo-endothélial. I. Les cellules de Ferrata. *Haematologica 8*:349, 1927.

Langevoot, H. L., Cohn, Z. A., Hirsch, J. G., Humphrey, J. H., Spector, W. G., and van Furth, R. The Nomenclature of Mononuclear Phagocytic Cells. A Proposal for a New Classification. In *Mononuclear Phagocytes* (van Furth, R., ed.). Blackwell, Oxford, 1970, p. 1.

Lazarus, S. S., Vethamany, V. G., Schneck, L., and Volk, B. W. Fine structure and histochemistry of peripheral blood cells in Niemann-Pick disease. *Lab Invest 17*:155, 1967.

Lee, R. E., Balcerzak, S. P., and Westerman, M. P. Gaucher's disease. A morphologic study and measurements of iron metabolism. *Amer J Med 42*:891, 1967.

Lennert, K. Cytologie des ruhenden, aktivierten und entznudeten Lymphknotens. Lymphknoten, Diagnostik und Cytologie. *Handbuch der Speziellen Pathologischen Anatomie und Histologie.* Springer, Berlin, 1961.

Lieb, H. Cerebrosidspeicherung bei Splenomegalie, Typus Gaucher. *Z Physiol Chem 140*:305, 1924.

Loutit, J. F. Annotation: Versatile haemopoietic stem cells. *Brit J Haemat 15*:333, 1968.

Lynn, R., and Terry, R. D. Lipid histochemistry and electron microscopy in adult Niemann-Pick disease. *Amer J Med 37*:987, 1964.

Malinin, T. I. Unidentified reticuloendothelial cell storage disease. *Blood 17*:675, 1961.

Maloney, M. A., and Patt, H. M. Origin of repopulating cells after localized bone marrow depletion. *Science 165*:71, 1969.

Marshall, A. H. E. *An Outline of the Cytology and Pathology of the Reticular Tissue.* Thomas, Springfield, Ill., 1956.

Maximow, A. A. Bindegewebe und blutbildende gewebe. Die gewebe. *Handbuch Mikr Anat Mensch 2*:237, 1927.

Metchnikoff, E. Uber ein Sprobpilzkronkheiten der Daphnien. Beitrag zur Lehre über den Kampf der Phagocyten gegen Krankheitserreger. *Virchow Arch Path Anat 96*:177, 1884.

Mital, M., and Cohen, J. Repair of experimental boney intramedullary injuries varying in degree. *Surg Forum 17*:451, 1966.

Moffat, D. J., Rosse, C., and Yoffey, J. M. Identity of the hematopoietic stem cell. *Lancet 2*:547, 1967.

Mori, Y. and Lennert, K. *Electron Microscopic Atlas of Lymph Node Cytology and Pathology* (Kirchemann, K., transl.). Springer, Berlin, 1969.

Naegeli, O. Ueber rothes Knochenmark and Myeloblasten. *Deutsch Med Wschr 26*:287, 1900.

Neumann, E. Ueber die Bedeutung des Knochenmarkes für die Blutbildung. *Zbl Med Wiss 6*: 689, 1868.

Neumann, E. Das Gesetz der Verbreitung des gelben und roten Marks in den Extremitätenknochen *Zbl Med Wiss 20*:321, 1882.

Niemann, A. Ein unbekanntes Krankheitsbild. *Jahrb Kinderheilk 79*:1, 1914.

North, R. J. Endocytosis. *Seminars Hemat 7*:161, 1970.

Nossal, G. J. V., Abbot, A., and Mitchell, J. Antigens in immunity. XIV. Electron microscopic radioautographic studies of antigen capture in the lymph node medulla. *J Exp Med 127*:263, 1968a.

Nossal, G. J. V., Abbot, A. Mitchell, J. and Lummus, Z. Antigens in immunity. XV. Ultrastructural features of antigen capture in primary and secondary lymphoid follicles. *J Exp Med 127*:277, 1968b.

Penelli, N., Scaravilli, F., and Zachello, F. The morphogenesis of Gaucher cells investigated by electron microscopy. *Blood 34*:331, 1969.

Pick, L. Uber die lipoidzellige Splenohepatomegalie Typus Niemann-Pick als Stoffwechslerkrankung. *Med Klin 23*:1483, 1927.

Policard, A., Bessis, M., and Breton-Gorius, J. Structures myéliniques observées au microscope électronique sur des coupes de globules rouges en voie de lyse. *Exp Cell Res 13*:184, 1956.

Rindfleish, G. E. Ueber Knochenmark und Blutbildung. *Arch Mikr Anat 17*:1, 1880.

Ringeon, A. The hemohistioblasts of Ferrata. *Anat Rec 27*:216, 1924.

Ringeon, A. Further studies of Ferrata's hemohistioblasts. *Anat Rec 29*:372, 1925.

Roelants, G. E., and Goodman, J. W. The chemical nature of macrophage RNA-antigen complexes and their relevance to immune induction. *J Exp Med 130*:557, 1969.

Rohr, K. *Das menschlische Knochenmark* (3rd ed.). Thieme, Stuttgart, 1960.

Rössle, R. Das Retothelsarkom der Lymphdrüsen,

Seine Formen und Verwandtschaften. *Beitr Path Anat 103*:385, 1939.

Roulet, F. Das primäre Retothelsarkom der Lymphknoten. *Virchow Arch Path Anat 277*:15, 1930.

Rowley, D. Phagocytosis. *Advances Immun 2*:241, 1962.

Shimamine, T. Studies on the histogenesis of fat cells in bone marrow. *Acta Haemat Jap 15*:311, 1952.

Skutelsky, E., and Danon, D. Reduction in surface charge as an explanation of the recognition by macrophages of nuclei expelled from normoblasts. *J Cell Biol 43*:8, 1969.

Steinberg, B., and Hufford, V. Development of bone marrow in adult animals. *Arch Path 43*:117, 1947.

Sweeley, C. C., and Klionsky, B. Fabry's disease: classification as a sphingolipidosis and partial characterization of novel glycolipid. *J Biol Chem 238*:3148, 1963.

Tanaka, H. Comparative cytologic studies by means of an electron microscope on monocytes, subcutaneous histiocytes, reticulum cells in the lymph nodes and peritoneal macrophages. *Ann Rep Inst Virus Res Kyoto Univ* (Series A) *1*:87, 1958.

Tanaka, Y., Brecher, G., and Fredrickson, D. S. Cellules de la maladie de Niemann-Pick et de quelques autres lipoidoses. *Nouv Rev Franc Hemat 3*:5, 1963.

Tanaka, Y. Fibrillar structure in the cells of blood-forming organs. *J Nat Cancer Inst 33*:467, 1964.

Tanaka, Y., Frost, P., and Spaeth, G. L. Figures myéliniques dans les cellules spumeuses de la maladie de Fabry. *Nouv Rev Franc Hemat 5*:423, 1965.

Tanaka, Y., Brecher, G., and Bull, B. Ferritin localization on the erythroblast cell membrane and rhopheocytosis in hypersiderotic human bone marrows. *Blood 28*:758, 1966.

Tanaka, Y. Iron-laden mitochondria in reticulum cells of hypersiderotic human bone marrows. *Blood 29*:747, 1967.

Tanaka, Y. An electron microscopic study of non-phagocytic reticulum cells in human bone marrow. I. Cells with intracytoplasmic fibrils. *Acta Haemat Jap 32*:275, 1969.

Tavassoli, M., and Crosby, W. H. Transportation of marrow to extramedullary sites. *Science 161*: 54, 1968.

Tavassoli, M., and Crosby, W. H. Bone marrow histogenesis: A comparison of fatty and red marrow. *Science 169*:291, 1970.

Till, J. E., and McCulloch, E. A. A direct measurement of the radiation sensitivity of normal mouse bone marrow cells. *Radiat Res 14*:213, 1961.

Trobaugh, F. E., Jr., and Lewis, J. P. Repopulating potential blood and marrow. *J Clin Invest 43*: 1306, 1964.

Van der Stich, O. Nouvelles recherches sur la genese des globules rouges et das globules blancs du sang. *Arch Biol Band 12*:199, 1892.

van Furth, R. Origin and kinetics of monocytes and macrophages. *Seminars Hemat 7*:125, 1970.

Vaughan, R. B., and Boyden, S. V. Interactions of macrophages and erythrocytes. *Immunology 7*: 118, 1964.

Wanstrup, J., and Christensen, H. E. Sarcoidosis. I. Ultrastructural investigations on epitheloid cell granuloma. *Acta Path Micr Scand 66*:169, 1966.

Watanabe, Y. An electron microscopic study on the reticulo-endothelial system in the bone marrow. *Tohoku J Exp Med 89*:167, 1966.

Weiss, L. An electron microscopic study of the vascular sinuses of the bone marrow of the rabbit. *Bull Hopkins Hosp 108*:171, 1961.

Weiss, L. The structure of bone marrow. Functional interrelationships of vascular and hematopoietic compartments in experimental hemolytic anemia. An electron microscopic study. *J Morph 117*: 467, 1965.

Wells, H. G. Adipose tissue, a neglected subject. *JAMA 114*:2177, 1940.

Wetzel, N. C. Die Grosse des roten Markorgans. *Anat Anz 53*:82, 1920.

Wright, A. E., and Douglas, S. R. An experimental investigation of the role of blood fluids in connection with phagocytosis. *Proc Roy Soc [Biol] 72*:357, 1904.

Wu, A. W., Till, J. E., Siminovitch, L., and McCulloch, E. A. A cytological study of the capacity for differentiation of normal hemopoietic colony-forming cells. *J. Cell Physiol 69*:177, 1967.

Zamboni, L., and Pease, D. C. The vascular bed of red marrow. *J Ultrastruct Res 5*:65, 1961.

index

Subject Index*

* Numbers in italics indicate figures.

Text and cover designed by Maria S. Karkucinski

Composed in Helvetica by American Book–Stratford Press, Inc.
Printed by Pearl Pressman Liberty

HARPER & ROW, PUBLISHERS
72 73 74 75 76 77 78 10 9 8 7 6 5 4 3 2 1